Introduction to Medical Laboratory Technology

Sixth Edition

Introduction to Medical Laboratory Technology

F. J. Baker, OBE, FIMLS

R. E. Silverton, FIMLS, FBIM

With: **D. Kilshaw,** FIMLS, CBiol, MIBiol

In conjunction with:

R. Shannon, MPhil, FIMLS
Head MLSO, Public Health Laboratory Service,
Bristol

D. L. Guthrie, DMS, FIMLS
Senior Chief MLSO, Department of Haematology,
St. Thomas's Hospital, London

S. Egglestone, BSC, PhD
Principal SO, Public Health Laboratory Service,
Bristol

J. C. Mackenzie, FIMLS
Chief MLSO, Department of Blood Transfusion,
St. Thomas's Hospital, London

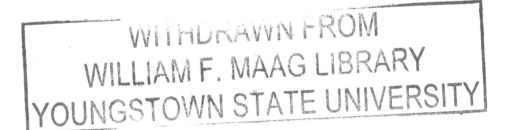
Butterworths
London   Boston   Durban   Singapore   Sydney   Toronto   Wellington

First published	August, 1954	Reprinted	September, 1970
Second Edition	August, 1957	Reprinted	August, 1971
Revised	January, 1960	Reprinted	August, 1972
Reprinted	March, 1961	Reprinted	February, 1974
Third Edition	August, 1962	Reprinted	January, 1975
Reprinted	March, 1964	Reprinted	August, 1975
Reprinted	April, 1965	Fifth Edition	August, 1976
Fourth Edition	May, 1966	Reprinted	1978
Reprinted	December, 1968	Reprinted	1980
Reprinted	December, 1969	Sixth Edition	1985

© Butterworth & Co (Publishers) Ltd 1985

British Library Cataloguing in Publication Data

Baker, F.J.
  Introduction to medical laboratory technology.—
  6th ed.
  1. Diagnosis, Laboratory
  I. Title   II. Silverton, R.E.
  616.07′5   RB37

  ISBN 0–407–73252–7

Library of Congress Cataloging in Publication Data

Baker, F. J. (Francis Joseph)
  Introduction to medical laboratory technology.

  Bibliography: p.
  Includes index.
  1. Medical technology. I. Silverton, R. E. II. Title.
III. Medical laboratory technology. [DNLM: 1. Diagnosis,
Laboratory. 2. Technology, Medical. QY 25 B167i]
RB37.B28 1985   616.07′5   84–27464
ISBN 0–407–73252–7

Typeset by Scribe Design, Gillingham, Kent
Printed and bound by Robert Hartnoll (1985) Ltd, Bodmin, Cornwall

Preface

When writing the Preface to the previous edition of this book we stated that 'during the twenty-two years which have elapsed since this work was first published, laboratory medicine has undergone many changes'. That was written nine years ago, but those words are probably even more applicable today than when first written. Not only have there been changes in medical laboratory sciences, but also in medicine itself: new diseases have been diagnosed, such as AIDS and Legionnaire's disease; new surgical transplant techniques have been developed; more safety legislation has been introduced. These and other changes have all contributed to an increase in the responsibility and scope of the medical laboratory scientist. The research into new techniques, the never ending introduction of automated procedures and the increased use of computers—all these advances have emphasized the need for highly skilled and highly trained laboratory personnel.

In the UK, many newcomers to the profession now enter with a degree in science. Others have either A- or O-levels. Whatever background the new entrant has, there is still a need for comprehensive training in the fundamentals of medical laboratory sciences to enable an appreciation of disciplines other than their own specialization.

Although it was originally written for students in the UK, this book is now also widely used by students overseas. In this respect we were privileged to have it recognized by the British Council and it is available to the developing countries in a paperback edition. For this reason, we have continued to include methods and techniques which to some may seem unnecessary but which we feel may be of assistance to those students in countries where fully automated procedures may not yet be available.

It is with these objectives in view that we offer this sixth edition, in the hope that it will prove to be as valuable to the many types of reader in the future as the earlier editions proved to be in the past. The contents have been expanded and updated, the layout changed to facilitate easier reading and handling, and some sections have been completely rewritten.

Despite the many advances in both the subject and the profession, the title under which this book was first published in 1954 remains the same. The possibility of changing the title to *An Introduction to Medical Laboratory Sciences* was discussed at length, but it was felt that the title by which it has become widely known should be retained.

In preparing this sixth edition we have again been very fortunate in the advice and encouragement so freely given by many of our friends and colleagues and wish to record our sincere thanks and appreciation to them all for their valuable contributions. In particular, our thanks are due to Mr J.M. Ashton, FIMLS, Senior Chief MLSO, Department of Histopathology and Clinical Cytology, Arrowe Park Hospital, Merseyside, and Mrs Heather D. Hawker, AIMLS, of Difco Laboratories, for their assistance in the preparation of the section on cellular pathology.

For administration and secretarial assistance we are deeply indebted to Mrs Audrey Garside, who has liaised with manufacturers on our behalf, and to whom we give our thanks. Mr D. Kitto, BA, AIMLS, provided valuable guidance on the first-aid section.

Once again, our publishers, with their customary patience and help, have been of great assistance in bringing this book to fruition. We especially wish to express our appreciation to Bob Pearson, the sub-editor responsible, with whom it has been a pleasure to work, and who has been particularly helpful and largely instrumental in keeping our noses to the grindstone during the long gestation period of this edition.

Authorship inevitably produces domestic disturbances and our final expression of gratitude is extended to our wives, who have shown patience, forbearance and understanding during the preparation of this and the previous five editions.

F.J.B.
R.E.S.

Contents

Introduction

Medical laboratory science is a complex subject embracing a number of different disciplines. The post-war years brought a dramatic increase in the use of the laboratory whose role is to assist in the diagnosis, treatment and control of disease. The increased demands on the laboratory have inevitably resulted in the introduction of more specialized and sophisticated procedures including mechanization, automation, data processing and computerization. To keep abreast with this modern development it has become necessary for students entering the profession in the United Kingdom to have a more academic background. Today, entrants generally possess either a relevant university degree or relevant A- or O-levels.

The professional body—the Institute of Medical Laboratory Sciences (IMLS)—is responsible for providing the opportunities to qualify by examinations. Until 1977, the National Certificate pathway was the main route to qualification. The IMLS, having members on the Joint Committees (who were responsible for the certificates in Medical Laboratory Subjects/Sciences) and the IMLS, also appointed Assessors for these various certificates. In 1977, the Joint Committee for Ordinary National Certificates and Diplomas in Sciences announced that 1980 would be the last year for entry to its examinations and that the new Technician Education Council's (TEC) courses and examinations would replace them. Subsequently, TEC became Business and Technician Education Council (B/TEC).

In Scotland, the Scottish Technical Education Council (SCOTEC) took over, and the first Ordinary Certificates in Medical Laboratory Sciences were awarded in 1982. Also in that year, courses for the Higher Certificate commenced and certificates were awarded in 1984. SCOTEC has now become the Scottish Vocational Educational Council (SCOVEC).

These examinations or qualifications, coupled with satisfactory experience in a recognized laboratory, lead to State Registration by the Council for Professions Supplementary to Medicine, without which a Medical Laboratory Scientific Officer is not allowed to practice in the National Health Service.

Newcomers to the profession are reminded that it is not a profession to be taken up lightly. Many leisure hours will have to be devoted to study, even when qualified, and the medical laboratory scientist will still have to keep abreast of modern developments and trends by the regular reading of the appropriate journals and by attending lectures and discussion groups. Considerable satisfaction, however, will be derived not only from the interesting nature of the work, but also from the knowledge that the duties undertaken during each working day are for the benefit of the community. The importance of this work and the obligations to the patient must therefore be remembered at all times and placed before any personal consideration.

In 1965, the Disciplinary Committee of the Medical Laboratory Technicians' Board of the Professions Supplementary to Medicine issued a statement to all registered practitioners of medical laboratory sciences, and in 1982 the IMLS issued a 'Code of Professional Conduct' which is given below with their permission.

Every member of the Institute shall always:

1. Exercise his professional judgement, skill and care to the best of his ability.
2. Fulfil his professional role with integrity, refraining from its misuse to the detriment of patients, employers or professional colleagues.

3. Seek to safeguard patients and others, particularly in relation to health and safety.
4. Treat with discretion all confidential and other information requiring protection, and avoid disclosing to any unauthorized person the result of any investigation or other information of a personal or confidential nature gained in the practice of his profession.
5. Act in good faith towards those with whom he stands in a professional relationship and conduct himself so as to uphold the reputation of his profession.
6. Strive to maintain, improve and update his professional knowledge and skill.
7. Promote the study and development of medical laboratory sciences and the education and training of medical laboratory scientists.

Section 1

General

1

General laboratory glassware, plastic ware and apparatus

Glassware and plastic ware

Glassware and plastic ware is widely used in medical laboratories, and it is essential to become thoroughly familiar with the common varieties. This chapter is concerned only with some of the more general types, and specialized equipment is not considered.

Composition of glass and types of plastic

Laboratory glassware is usually manufactured from borosilicate glass, a material developed to conform to certain well-defined characteristics. It is resistant to the action of chemicals, with the exception of hydrofluoric and phosphoric acid, and is made to withstand mechanical breakage and a sudden change of temperature. Resistance to thermal shock necessitates a low coefficient of thermal expansion. Glassware produced from the soda-lime type of glass does not meet this requirement and is easily broken by the mechanical stress produced by a sudden change of temperature.

Hardened glass, such as Pyrex, has a low soda content and is manufactured especially to resist thermal shock. The walls of the vessels are generally thicker than those made from soda-lime glass and the low soda content increases the chemical durability of the glass. With the less expensive soda-lime glassware, however, free soda is present on the walls, and must be neutralized before use.

Ingredients of borosilicate glass

	per cent
Silica (SiO$_2$)	80.6
Sodium oxide (Na$_2$O)	4.15
Boric oxide (B$_2$O$_2$)	12.6
Aluminium oxide (Al$_2$O$_3$)	2.2

Types of plastic

Polystyrene: rigid — non-autoclavable
Polypropylene: rigid — non-autoclavable
Polythene: rigid or flexible — non-autoclavable
Polyvinyl chloride (PVC): rigid or flexible — autoclavable
Polytetrafluoroethylene (PTFE): rigid or flexible— autoclavable

Care of glassware

All glassware must be handled carefully. Breakages can sometimes be dangerous, and they may result in the loss of valuable and irreplaceable material. Certain precautions must be observed.

1. Flasks and beakers should be placed on a gauze mat when they are heated over a bunsen flame.
2. Test-tubes exposed to a naked flame should be made of heat-resistant glass (such as Pyrex).
3. If liquids are to be heated in a bath of boiling water, the glass containers used should be heat-resistant. It is safer to immerse the containers in warm water, which is then brought to the boil, than to plunge them directly into boiling water. Similarly, sudden cooling of hot glass should be avoided, unless it is specifically required.
4. When diluting concentrated acids, thin-walled glassware should be used. The heat evolved by the procedure often cracks thick glass.
5. Heat expansion is liable to crack bottles if their caps are screwed on tightly. If heat is to be applied, flasks held in retort stands should not be tightly clamped.
6. Containers and their corresponding ground-glass stoppers should be numbered, to ensure correct matching when stoppers are replaced. When

3

these bottles or flasks are being used, the stoppers should be laid on clean filter paper, to avoid scratching them.

Cleaning of glassware

General glassware

The cleaning of all glassware is simplified by rinsing in tap water immediately after use. Contaminated material, however, must always be sterilized before cleaning is commenced.

New glassware may be cleaned by washing in a suitable laboratory detergent and then rinsed thoroughly in tap water. Soda-lime glassware should have the free alkali neutralized by standing the glass in a 5% solution of hydrochloric acid. This is followed by several rinses in tap water and in distilled water. If it is desired simply to neutralize free alkali given off by new glassware, it may be steeped in 1% hydrochloric acid for several hours. This is followed by thorough rinsing. The glass is then dried in a hot-air oven. To test that the free alkali has been neutralized, autoclave the glassware in neutral distilled water, and when cool, check the pH of the water. If excess alkali has been given off (the pH is high, see p. 47) re-steep the glassware in the hydrochloric acid. If free alkali still persists after several treatments the glassware should be discarded.

Automatic washing machines

These machines are widely used in laboratories. They are supplied with interchangeable heads, which allows many different types of glassware to be accommodated and to go through the washing and rinsing cycle. It is necessary with these machines to use low-foam detergents.

Biochemical glassware

Chemical cleaning is necessary for the following reasons:

1. Traces of reagents left in tubes and containers may interfere with later chemical investigations.
2. Air bubbles may be trapped between greasy surfaces and contained liquid, resulting in inaccurate volumetric readings.

The traditional method of cleaning laboratory glassware is by chromic acid solution. Although in many laboratories this has been superseded by cleaning with detergents, the method is given below.

Procedure for rendering glassware chemically clean

1. Preparation of cleaning fluid:

Potassium dichromate	10 g
Concentrated sulphuric acid	25 ml
Distilled water	75 ml

Grind the dichromate crystals in a pestle and mortar, and add the powder to the distilled water in a heat-resistant flask. Pour in the acid very slowly. The heat evolved hastens the dissolving of the potassium dichromate.

▰ Note

This fluid should be handled with caution, rubber gloves and apron being worn to protect the hands and clothes and an eyeshield to protect the eyes. If clothes or skin are splashed with the fluid, they should immediately be washed in water, and any residual acid neutralized with a weak alkali. This, in turn, is washed off with tap water.

After repeated use, the colour of the fluid may darken. When this occurs, fresh fluid should be prepared.

2. Steep the glassware in the cleaning mixture for several hours.
3. Remove the glassware, and wash it thoroughly in tap water, to remove all traces of acid and preferably leave in fresh water overnight.
4. Rinse twice in distilled water.
5. After allowing surplus water to drain off, dry the glassware in a hot-air oven.

Procedure for cleaning glassware with detergents

Detergents, which are available in either liquid or powder form, owe their cleansing action to the manner in which they reduce the interfacial tension of water with that of oily or greasy substances.

Detergents possess the following advantages over ordinary soaps: their cleansing action is unaffected by the temperature of the water; they are equally efficient in water which is either slightly alkaline or slightly acidic; they have no coagulative action on proteins.

One serious disadvantage of some detergents is their haemolytic action on red blood cells, the slightest trace of detergent being capable of producing haemolysis. This point must always be borne in mind, particularly with glassware destined to be used for haematology or blood transfusion work. The following procedure should be adopted when using detergents for cleaning glassware:

1. Rinse the glassware thoroughly in cold tap water.
2. Place in the detergent solution and brush thoroughly.
3. Wash thoroughly in running tap water.

4. Rinse three times in distilled water, using fresh distilled water for each rinse.
5. Drain off excess water and dry in the hot-air oven. Glassware dried in the hot-air oven should be packed, mouth downwards, in metal baskets, the bottoms of which are lined with thick blotting paper.

Recommended detergents are Decon 90 (Decon Laboratories Ltd) and RBS 25 (Chemical Concentrates Ltd)*. These are phosphate-free, surface-active agents suitable for cleaning all glassware and plastics including those contaminated with radioactive material.

It has been stated that accurately calibrated volumetric glassware should never be heated in the oven as the expansion and contraction of glass that occurs may render the graduations inaccurate. Some workers, however, have shown that this is not the case and that Grade A glassware may be sterilized in a hot-air oven.

Cleaning of pipettes

1. Steep the pipettes overnight in cleaning fluid.
2. The following morning, wash them thoroughly in tap water, preferably leave overnight in fresh water, and rinse in distilled water. To facilitate washing, connect the pipette to a water pump, using rubber tubing of suitable bore, and suck tap water through for several seconds. Follow this with two or three rinses of hot distilled water.
3. Dry the pipette with two or three brief rinses of acetone. Drying is best effected by sucking through small volumes of acetone and air successively. Repeat this procedure until the internal surface is quite dry. Alternatively, an electrically heated pipette dryer may be used.
4. Wipe the outside of the pipette.
5. To avoid breakage, store the pipettes in drawers lined with lint. It is convenient to fit the drawers with separate compartments for each size and type of pipette.

▓ Notes

Immediately after use, pipettes should be rinsed in tap water, especially when they have held proteinous fluid, for example blood. Should the pipette be heavily contaminated with such material, it may be cleaned by standing it in a strong solution of caustic soda. This treatment should not be prolonged, as the alkali dissolves glass and may cause an alteration in contained volume. A pipette which has been used for measuring stain can often be cleaned rapidly by rinsing it through with hydrochloric acid.

The cleaning procedures described above do not apply to Pasteur pipettes. After use with infected material, these are placed in a disinfectant solution.

*The addresses of manufacturers who are mentioned throughout the book are listed in Appendix I.

Standardized glassware

Apparatus used for the measurement of liquid volume, for example, pipettes, burettes, volumetric flasks and cylinders, is divided into three grades, depending on the accuracy of calibration.

The limits of these grades are defined by the British Standards Institution, and the manufacturers mark each piece of standardized glassware with the appropriate symbol. The maker's assurance, however, is the only guarantee that the product conforms with the BSI criteria. For example, tolerances laid down for bulb-type pipettes are given in *Table 1.1*.

Table 1.1 Tolerances for delivery pipettes (bulb type)

Capacity in ml	2	10	20	50
Time of outflow seconds, grade A	7–15	18–25	20–35	25–40
Tolerance ± ml, grade A	0.01	0.02	0.02	0.04
Time of outflow seconds, grade B	7–20	15–40	20–50	25–60
Tolerance ± ml, grade B	0.02	0.04	0.05	0.08

The most accurately calibrated glassware available in Britain carries certificates from the National Physical Laboratory. Each such piece of apparatus is etched with the letters NPL. This glassware is necessary only for the highest standards of accuracy.

Examples of the markings on an NPL Class A pipette are:

NPLA	NPL Class A
5 ml	5 ml volume
D20°C	Delivery pipette: volume correct at 20°C
10 + 15	10 s to deliver: 15 s to drain
32867	Certificate number

By international agreement, pipettes and vessels 'to deliver' are marked with the letters 'Ex', while those designed 'to contain' are marked with the letters 'In'. The delivery time is no longer given and indeed it is recommended that the tip of the jet be kept in contact with the inside of the receiving vessel for approximately 3 s after movement of the meniscus has appeared to cease.

General glassware

Beakers

These have capacities of 5–5000 ml. They are usually made of heat-resistant glass, and are available in different shapes. The type most commonly used is the *squat form*, which is cylindrical and has a spout. There is also a *tall form*, usually without a spout. Conical and flask-shaped types are available, but these are not widely used. Beakers are often supplied in sets or *nests* of assorted sizes. Some may be graduated, while others may be made of polystyrene.

Bottles

These are made in many shapes. Some of the more general types are described below.

Reagent bottles are supplied in 25–1000 ml capacities. They are cylindrical, have narrow necks and are fitted with ground-glass or polythene stoppers.

Screw-capped bottles are supplied in 5–1000 ml capacities, and may be round or flat (the 5 ml size is often called a 'bijou' bottle). The caps may be made of metal or plastic. These bottles are used for holding specimens, solutions and media. Metal caps should never be used on bottles containing mercuric chloride, as this substance will attack the metal.

Winchester quart bottles are of 2000 ml capacity, and are available in white or brown glass. They may be fitted with glass stoppers, corks or rubber bungs. They are useful for storing stock solutions and reagents, and for specimens, for example, samples of urine collected over 24 h.

Drop bottles are of about 50 ml capacity, and are made in white or brown glass, with a narrow neck and a grooved glass stopper. They are designed for delivery of drops of solutions, such as stains. After use the stoppers should be turned, so that the contents are not open to the air.

Polythene bottles are of various sizes and shapes, and some are fitted with a nozzle, for use as 'wash bottles'.

Burettes

These are used for measuring variable quantities of liquid, and are made in capacities of 1–100 ml. They are long graduated tubes of uniform bore and are closed at the lower end by means of a glass stopcock, which should be lightly greased for smooth rotation.

Technique of using burettes

1. Before use, half-fill the burette with distilled water, and allow it to be discharged through the tap. Droplets adhering to the glass indicate a greasy surface. If this is seen, chemical cleaning is necessary.
2. Rinse the burette two or three times with small volumes of the solution to be measured, discharging the washings through the tap.
3. With the tap closed, clamp the burette in a vertical position and pour in the liquid to be measured through a funnel, until the meniscus rises above the zero mark of the burette. Remove the funnel.
4. Open the stopcock tap until the meniscus of the liquid exactly coincides with the zero mark. Make sure that the tap is completely free of air bubbles, and that the tip has no droplets adhering to it. The burette is now ready for use.
5. When the work with the burette is complete, the fluid is drained out. The burette is rinsed through several times with tap water, and then with distilled water.
6. For storage, the burette is clamped in an inverted position.

Centrifuge tubes

These are made of hardened glass, nylon or plastic material that can withstand the centrifugal strain. The bottom of the tubes may be round or conical. The latter type is preferable, because the deposit is concentrated into a smaller volume. Some centrifuge tubes are calibrated up to 10 ml. These markings may be useful, provided the graduations have been checked for accuracy.

Desiccators

It may be necessary to dehydrate substances, or to keep them in an anhydrous state. This may be effected by storing them in a desiccator over a water-absorbent chemical, such as anhydrous calcium chloride or phosphorus pentoxide. Evacuation of air increases the rate of dehydration, and some desiccators are therefore made of glass strong enough to withstand a vacuum. Others are not designed for this purpose, and have no tap in the lid. The tap, when present, and the opposed surfaces of jar and lid are of ground glass.

Technique of using vacuum desiccators

1. Place the substance to be stored in an open container, and rest this on the zinc gauze sheet, which forms a platform above the desiccating chemical. Lubricate the tap and the opposing surfaces of jar and lid with Vaseline, petroleum jelly or stopcock grease, to ensure that all junctions are air-tight.
2. Slide the cover onto the jar, and rotate it into position.
3. Open the tap, and connect the outlet to a vacuum pump. If this is of the water type, always insert a trap-bottle between the pump and desiccator to prevent any backflow of water into the desiccator from a sudden fall in water pressure (see p. 10).
4. When the jar has been sufficiently evacuated, close the tap, turn off the pump, and disconnect the desiccator.
5. To open the vessel, release the vacuum. Turn the tap gradually, allowing air to be sucked in. Slide the lid off the jar. If the desiccator has been kept

in a refrigerator, allow the temperature of the glass to rise to that of the room, before opening the tap. This prevents condensation of moisture on the inside of the cold glass.

Evaporating basins

These are shallow vessels made of porcelain, silica or heat-resistant glass. They have a large surface area which facilitates evaporation.

Funnels

Filter funnels are used for pouring liquids into narrow-mouthed containers, and for supporting filter papers during filtration. Some funnels have a fluted inner surface.

Separating funnels are for separating immiscible liquids of different densities, for example, ether and water.

Technique of using separating funnels

1. Close the tap, and add the mixture of liquids until the bulb is about half full.
2. Insert the stopper, and holding both tap and stopper firmly in position shake to facilitate extraction.
3. Release the pressure from time to time by inverting the funnel and gently opening the tap.
4. Stand the funnel upright and allow the liquids to separate.
5. Remove the stopper and open the tap carefully, allowing the lower layer to run out slowly.
6. Close the tap just before the last drop of the lower layer has escaped.

Flasks

Flasks have capacities of 25–6000 ml.

Conical flasks (Erlenmeyer) are useful for titrations, and also for boiling solutions when it is necessary to keep evaporation to a minimum. Some have a side arm, suitable for attachment to a vacuum pump. Buchner or Seitz filters can be inserted into rubber bungs, and used in conjunction with these flasks.

Flat-bottomed round flasks are convenient containers in which to heat liquids. A gauze mat should be interposed between flask and flame. These flasks are widely used in the preparation of bacteriological culture media.

Round-bottomed flasks can withstand higher temperatures than the flat-bottomed type. They may be heated in a naked flame, or in an electrothermal mantle.

Volumetric flasks are flat-bottomed, pear-shaped vessels with long narrow necks, and are fitted with ground-glass or plastic stoppers. Most flasks are graduated to *contain* a certain volume, and these are marked with the letters 'C' or 'In'. Those designed to *deliver* a given volume are marked with the letters 'D' or 'Ex'. A horizontal line etched round the neck denotes the stated volume of water at a given temperature, for example, 20°C. The neck is narrow, so that slight errors in reading the meniscus result in relatively small volumetric differences.

Technique of using volumetric flasks

To prepare an accurate solution of known concentration, proceed as follows:

1. Using a watchglass, accurately weigh the substance and transfer to the flask by means of a funnel.
2. Using a little of the solvent, wash any residual traces of the weighed substance from the watchglass and funnel into the flask. Half-fill the flask with further solvent.
3. Stopper the flask, and shake it until the weighed substance is completely dissolved.
4. Add solvent until the lower margin of the meniscus reaches the etched line on the flask neck. Invert to mix.

Variations of temperature cause changes in volume. If the solution is warm, it should be allowed to cool to room temperature, or ideally the temperature at which the glass was calibrated, before the volume is made up to the line.

Measuring cylinders

These are supplied in 10–2000 ml capacities. Some are made of heat-resistant glass, and some are fitted with ground-glass or plastic stoppers. Measurement of liquids can be made quickly with these vessels, but a high degree of accuracy is impossible because of their wide bore.

Pestle and mortar

These are used for grinding solids, for example calculi and large crystals of chemicals. Those of unglazed porcelain have a porous surface, and those of heavy glass are made with roughened surfaces. Some are of agate, and these are uniformly smooth. After use, always clean the pestle and mortar thoroughly, for chemicals may be driven into the unglazed surfaces during grinding, resulting in contamination when the apparatus is next used.

Petri dishes

Petri dishes are flat glass or plastic containers which have a number of uses in the medical laboratory. They are used predominantly for the cultivation of organisms on solid media. They are made with diameters of 5–14 cm. For further details reference should be made to Chapter 23.

Pipettes

These are used to measure liquid volumes of up to 50 ml. There are several types, each having its own advantages and limitations. Some of them are now made of plastic and are disposable, but whichever type is used, pipetting *must never* be performed by mouth.

Automatic pipettes and dispensers

These are designed to measure and deliver variable volumes of fluids. There are many types on the market (*Figures 1.1–1.3*) which will deliver micro and macro volumes. With many of them, disposable tips are available.

Another type of automatic pipette is that shown in *Figure 1.4*. These pipettes are compact, versatile units, designed for rapid repetitive work. Their working principle is that pressure from the reservoir moves the piston contained within the graduated barrel. The position at which the piston is set can be adjusted by means of a micro-adjustor, thereby allowing the volume of the reagent delivered to be changed. Turning the stopcock key to the left, drives the piston along from the right end of the barrel until it reaches the stop, forcing the volume of liquid

before it out of the delivery jet. Turning the stopcock key in the opposite direction reverses the procedure, thereby producing a rapid and continuous delivery of the reagent.

Delivery pipettes

Delivery pipettes are made in 1–50 ml capacities. They are calibrated to *deliver* a constant volume of liquid under certain specified conditions. These pipettes are marked with the letter 'D', the temperature at which the pipette was calibrated, that is, 20 °C unless otherwise stated, and a letter denoting the grade. Pipettes are calibrated using water, and consequently their use for fluids of different viscosity results in inaccurate measurements. Such liquids, for example glycerol and ether, are most accurately measured with pipettes designed to be rinsed out.

There are two types of delivery pipette: the volumetric and the graduated types.

The *volumetric (bulb) type* is the most accurate type of pipette in everyday use. The outflow and drainage times are usually marked on the bulb.

Technique of using volumetric pipettes

1. Rinse out the pipette with the fluid to be measured.
2. Fill it by suction, until the liquid rises above the graduation mark. Retain the liquid at this level

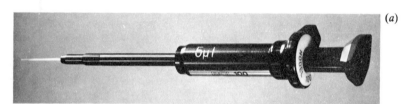

(a)

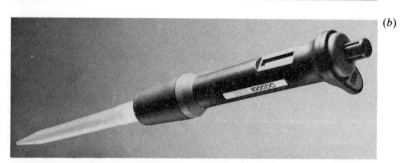

(b)

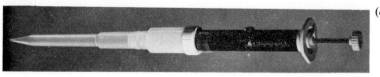

(c)

Figure 1.1. (a) BCL 100 ultra-micro-pipette; (b) BCL 1000DG adjustable pipette; (c) BCL 3000 macropipette (reproduced by courtesy of Boehringer Corp. (London) Ltd)

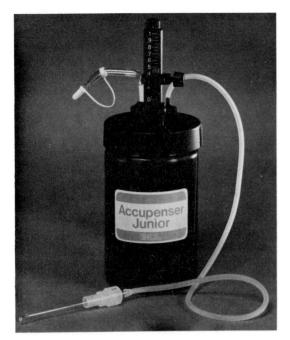

Figure 1.2. Accupenser Junior dispenser (reproduced by courtesy of Boehringer Corp. (London) Ltd)

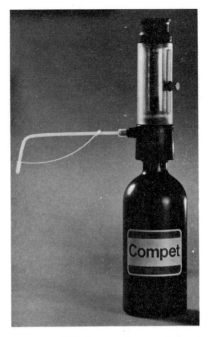

Figure 1.3. BCL Compet dispenser (reproduced by courtesy of Boehringer Corp. (London) Ltd)

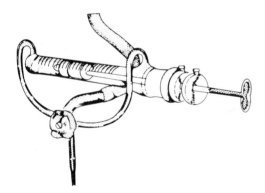

Figure 1.4. Exelo all-glass double-action automatic pipette

by placing the dry forefinger over the mouthpiece of the pipette.

3. Reduce the pressure of the finger, allowing the liquid to run slowly down to the mark.
4. Read the meniscus at eye-level, to avoid any error due to parallax.
5. Wipe the outside of the stem with a clean cloth, and remove any drops on the tip by touching it against a glass vessel.
6. Remove the finger, and the pipette will deliver its contents. Hold the tip of the pipette against the inside of the receiving vessel, until the liquid has run out.
7. When the free flow has ceased, hold the pipette against the side of the receiver for a further 15 s,

allowing it to drain. The entire volume will now have been delivered.
8. The residual drop in the tip is discarded.

The graduated type

These pipettes are satisfactory for most routine purposes, if a high degree of accuracy is not essential. They are used in the same way as the volumetric pipette, but the graduations along the stem enable variable amounts of liquid to be delivered.

The least accurate sector of the graduated stem is the tapering point. Some pipettes are made with graduations that do not extend down to the tip.

Pipettes 'to contain'

Some pipettes are not designed for delivery of a given volume of liquid, but are made to *contain* it. A pipette of this type holds a stated volume, and in order to transfer its contents completely, one must rinse out the pipette after it has drained. There are two types of pipette made *to contain*: the bulb type and the graduated type.

Bulb-type pipettes are made to contain a specified volume. They are available in 0.2–10 ml volumes.

Many micro-methods of blood analysis, for example blood sugar and urea methods, require accurate measurement of 0.2 ml of blood and a 'wash-out' pipette should be used for this purpose.

Technique of using bulb-type wash-out pipette

1. Fill the pipette with liquid and allow the meniscus to fall to the mark 'O' and wipe the outside with a cloth.
2. Run the liquid slowly into the receiving vessel, until the pipette is empty but for a residual drop at the tip.
3. Remove the last traces of solution in the pipette by rinsing it out two or three times, and add the rinsings to the delivered volume in the receiving vessel.

Graduated pipettes

Graduated pipettes are made for measuring volumes of 0.2–25 ml. They are used in the same way as the bulb-type (Ostwald) pipette.

Haemacytometer pipettes are of the wash-out type.

Water-vacuum pump (water Venturi pump)

This indispensable piece of laboratory equipment may be made of metal or glass. The principle of its action is illustrated in *Figure 1.5*.

If the vacuum pump fails during use, negative pressure in the system will cause water to be sucked back. To safeguard this, a 'trap-bottle' is interposed, which will receive the water, and prevent it from flowing back into the vessel being evacuated. A glass Venturi pump is available incorporating an all-glass non-return valve, making a trap-bottle unnecessary.

Apparatus

Autoclaves

The autoclave is used for sterilization by steam under pressure (see Chapter 22).

Centrifuges

Centrifuges are used to hasten the deposition of substances suspended in liquids. The suspended matter is deposited in order of weight, the heaviest element being the first to settle.

There are many types of centrifuge, but the basic principle is the same, that is, the use of centrifugal force. Centrifugal force speeds up the settling process that would normally occur slowly under natural gravity.

For the purpose of comparison, centrifugal force is referred to as RCF (relative centrifugal force). The RCF is taken as a guide to the separating capacity of a centrifuge and the RCF value for any centrifuge may be calculated from the following equation:

$$RCF \text{ (in g)} = 1.118 \times R \times N^2 \times 10^5$$

where R is the radius in cm from the centre of the centrifuge shaft to external tip of the centrifuge tube, and N is the number of revolutions per minute (rpm) of the centrifuge head.

Small models are designed to centrifuge a series of 15 ml amounts in conical tubes or 30 ml amounts in thick-walled round-bottom tubes at speeds of 3000–5000 rpm. Larger free-standing models will centrifuge total volumes of up to 2000 ml at 3000–5000 rpm. Laboratory centrifuges with speeds up to 20 000 rpm are not uncommon and much higher speeds still can be reached in ultracentrifuges, as with the refrigerated type used in virus studies.

Most modern centrifuges have inbuilt safety features to satisfy changing needs and to meet national and international standards. It is now quite common to find even the simplest of bench centrifuges fitted with such devices as electrical interlocked lid catches, out-of-balance protection, built-in speed indicators and electric brakes. These features make the units much safer and easier to use. Of particular importance is the availability of 'sealed' cups or buckets to provide for safe handling of potentially hazardous samples.

Centrifuges are used with two types of head— 'swing-out' and 'angle'—based on the principles of horizontal or angle sedimentation.

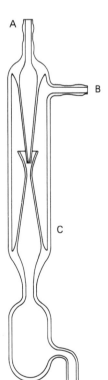

A

B

C

Figure 1.5. The principle of the Venturi pump. Inlet A is connected to the water-tap. When the tap is turned on fully, water flows rapidly into tube C which has a constriction near its upper end. Air is sucked into the rapidly flowing jet of water, and the negative pressure created inside the jacket of the pump causes air to be sucked in through inlet B

In angle sedimentation, particles only move a short distance through the liquid before reaching the outer wall of the container where they join the stream of particles travelling towards the bottom of the tube. In horizontal sedimentation, particles have to travel a longer path through the liquid but the deposit is evenly compacted at the bottom of the tube, whereas in angle sedimentation the wedge-shaped sediment spreading up the side of the container may easily be disturbed when centrifuging stops and the tube is removed.

The angle-head centrifuge is capable of higher speeds than the swing-out models, owing to less air resistance, but the speed of the swing-out head can be increased in certain machines by the attachment of a wind shield.

Technique for centrifugation

1. Remove all the metal cups or buckets from the centrifuge head.
2. Ensure rubber cushions are present in all metal cups.
3. Insert the tubes or bottles to be centrifuged into buckets, and place one on each pan of a crude balance.
4. With a pipette, add disinfectant to the lighter *bucket*, not to the tube or bottle, until the weight of the two buckets and contents are balanced.
5. Place the buckets containing the tubes in diametrically opposite positions in the centrifuge head, and close the lid. If using the swing-out head, position the trunnions (or bucket carriers) carefully before inserting the buckets.
6. Start the motor, and *gradually* increase the speed until the required number of revolutions per minute is reached.
7. When the tubes have been centrifuged sufficiently, switch off the motor, and allow the centrifuge to stop.

Points on care and maintenance

The siting of the centrifuge is important, bench models being positioned on a firm base.

■ Notes

Despite out-of-balance protection, a feature of most modern centrifuges, it is still desirable to balance the buckets.

Do not increase the speed of revolution too rapidly, and never slow the revolving head manually. Wait until it has stopped before attempting to remove the buckets or tubes.

The interior bowl of the centrifuge should be frequently wiped with a disinfectant.

The carbon brushes need replacing periodically and a supply of these should always be available.

Lubrication on the modern centrifuge is seldom necessary, the manufacturers having fitted sealed grease units.

In certain procedures it is necessary to prevent aerosols from being blown out into the laboratory. It is now possible to use capped centrifuge tubes and buckets. Alternatively, the centrifuge should be housed in an exhaust inoculating cabinet. Buckets should be examined frequently for any flaws.

The production of chemically pure water

As tap water contains many dissolved salts and gases, it is unsuitable for most laboratory work. The water must therefore be purified, generally by one of the following methods—distillation or the use of ion exchange resins.

Distillation

Using a still, the water is boiled and the resultant steam condensed onto a cold surface. The condensed steam is then collected as 'distilled water'. The condenser of a still should preferably be made of pure tin or fused quartz, as pure water readily absorbs ions from glass. A knife point of potassium permanganate and a few pellets of sodium hydroxide added to the tap water before commencing distillation will oxidize steam-volatile organic compounds which might otherwise be carried over into the distilled water receiver. It is also a good plan to discard the first and last portions of the distillate. If really pure water is desired, it may be distilled three times (triple distilled). If 'pyrogen-free' distilled water is required (see p. 368), the still must be equipped with a suitable anti-splash device which allows only pure steam to pass through and prevents any droplets from passing into the condensate. In the simplest form of 'still', tap water is heated in a flask and the steam given off is conveyed by glass tubing to a Liebig condenser. This consists of a central tube into which the steam is passed. An outer glass jacket provides for circulation of cold tap water around the inner tube. The fall in temperature causes condensation of the steam into distilled water which is collected into the receiving flask.

The rate of distillation with this apparatus may not be adequate to supply the routine needs of a large laboratory. There are several commercial stills available which deliver distilled water at rates ranging from 2 to 200 l/h. These may be heated by gas or electricity, and incorporate an automatic water feed which maintains the volume of boiling water.

For some purposes, water must be glass-distilled, that is, at no stage must the steam or distillate come into contact with any surface other than glass.

De-ionization by ion exchange resins

Although this technique, which is used routinely in many laboratories, produces water free from ions,

not all non-electrolyte contaminants may be removed, that is, the water is not pyrogen-free. There
may also be some extraction of organic impurities
from the resins, but under normal circumstances the
water obtained by this method is purer than that
obtained by distillation. Water purified by ion
exchange resins is sometimes called 'conductivity
water' as it has such a low electrical conductivity that
it is suitable for use in such measurements.
Although the theoretical pH of pure water is 7.0, in
practice, pure water rapidly becomes acidic when
exposed to air, due to the absorption of carbon
dioxide and the formation of carbonic acid.

Ion exchange resins are of two types: (a) cation
exchange resins $(R—SO_3)^-H^+$ which are insoluble
acids, and (b) anion exchange resins $(R—
NH_3)^+OH^-$ which are insoluble bases. R represents
a polystyrene resin.

The mode of action of ion exchange resins may be
illustrated by the following. If, for instance, water
containing sodium chloride is passed through a
column of cation exchange resin, the Na^+ cations
replace the H^+ cations of the resin

$$(R—SO_3)^-H^+ + Na^+ \rightarrow (R—SO_3)^-Na^+ + H^+$$

The emerging water now contains H^+ ions (obtained
from the resin) together with the original Cl^-
anions. If this water is now passed through the anion
exchange resin, the Cl^- replaces the OH^- anion of
the resin

$$(R—NH_3)^+OH^- + Cl^- \rightarrow (R—NH_3)^+Cl^- + OH^-$$

The water now contains H^+ and OH^- ions which
combine to form H_2O. In this way the water is made
ion-free.

In practice, the two resins are usually mixed
together in one column, as a 'mixed-bed' de-ionizer.
To obtain pure water, simply pour the water to be
purified onto the mixed polystyrene resins, and the
water emerging after passing through this column is
pure.

Ion exchange resins may be regenerated by
passing HCl through the cation resin, followed by
washing well with water, and by passing NaOH
through the anion resin, and washing with water. If
the resins are of the mixed-bed type, it is necessary
to separate the two resins first by passing an upward
flow of water through the mixture. The two resins,
being of unequal density, will separate out.

Reverse osmosis

Reverse osmosis (RO) is rapidly becoming the
method of choice in a number of water-treatment
applications. It will be remembered that if two equal
volumes of fluids are separated by a semi-permeable
membrane, the purer fluid will flow through the
membrane to balance the concentrations of the two
fluids. The pressure required to equalize the two
volumes again, after equilibrium has been reached,
is called the 'osmotic pressure' (*Figure 1.6a*). If
physical pressure is applied in excess of osmotic

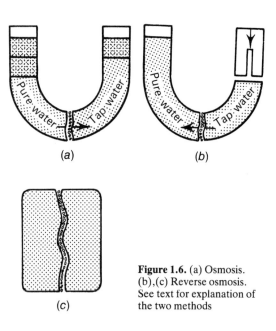

(a)   (b)

(c)

Figure 1.6. (a) Osmosis.
(b),(c) Reverse osmosis.
See text for explanation of
the two methods

pressure, reverse osmosis occurs as water is forced
through the membrane, leaving contaminants concentrated upstream. The concentrate is diverted to
drain—rejecting contaminants from the system
altogether (*Figure 1.6b,c*).

Apart from laboratory and pharmacy use, water
prepared by this method is used in dialysis
machines, where not only is the removal of dissolved
inorganics and heavy metals required, but also the
removal of bacteria and pyrogens.

2

Elementary microscopy

Principles of the microscope

The modern compound microscope is an indispensable piece of apparatus in all medical laboratories, and a theoretical knowledge of its working principles is essential. It is a precision instrument, and its efficient use requires some measure of skill and training. The magnification and clarity of the image depend upon the quality of its lenses, but definition is readily lost if the instrument is improperly used.

Time spent in the systematic setting up of the microscope and light source is amply repaid by the results obtained. Microscopes are made in two forms, monocular and binocular. Although binocular microscopes are generally available, monocular models are still used in many parts of the world, and for this reason they are described in this chapter. In essence, a microscope consists of an objective lens and eyepiece, with the mechanism necessary for focusing them. A bright light is passed through the object under examination and into the objective lens, which is the main magnifying agent. The rays of light emitted at the upper end of the objective form an image which is viewed through the eyepiece.

Many advances have been made in the design of microscopes in recent years. The limb or tube of the modern monocular microscope is now usually fixed rigidly to the base, which is constructed to contain a built-in illuminant. The eyepiece is held in an inclined tube which is attached to a tube head into which the objectives are screwed. Focusing is accomplished by raising or lowering the stage, the coarse and fine adjustment being situated in the stage support together with the mechanism for supporting and focusing the substage condenser (*Figure 2.1*).

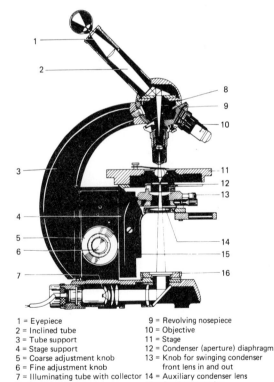

1 = Eyepiece	9 = Revolving nosepiece
2 = Inclined tube	10 = Objective
3 = Tube support	11 = Stage
4 = Stage support	12 = Condenser (aperture) diaphragm
5 = Coarse adjustment knob	13 = Knob for swinging condenser
6 = Fine adjustment knob	front lens in and out
7 = Illuminating tube with collector	14 = Auxiliary condenser lens
8 = Tube head	15 = Condenser carrier
	16 = Diaphragm insert

Figure 2.1. Diagram of a modern monocular microscope

In the older type of monocular microscope, many of which are still in use, the construction is different. The base or foot is sufficiently solid to hold the instrument stable, even when tilted in use. The limb is pivoted to the foot and its lower end carries the stage, substage condenser and reversible mirror with

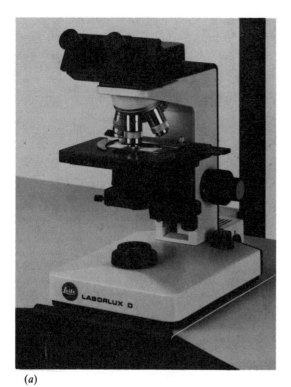

(a)

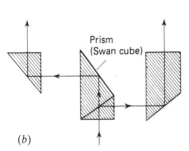

Prism
(Swan cube)

(b)

Figure 2.2. (a) The Laborlux D modern binocular microscope (reproduced by courtesy of E. Leitz (Instruments) Ltd). (b) Principle of the binocular microscope

A sliding adjustment is provided enabling the operator to set the eyepieces at a comfortable interpupillary distance.

With modern instruments, both oculars can be focused. This allows the interpupillary distance to be read from a scale between the eyepieces and adjustments made for variations in tube length by setting the eyepiece tube scale at the same reading. Should the observer's vision be at fault the image is first focused with the normal (emmetropic) eye and the necessary adjustment made for the abnormal (ametropic) eye. If the instrument has only one focusing collar, it is set up as for the monocular microscope using the fixed eyepiece. The adjustment on the other is used to correct any discrepancy between the observer's eyes.

Before dealing with the components of a microscope, it is necessary to explain certain terms.

Refraction

Refraction is the change in direction of light passing obliquely from one medium to another of different optical density. *Figure 2.3a* shows the path of a ray of light passing from air into a glass plate and out

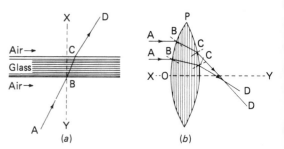

Figure 2.3. Refraction of light rays passing through (a) a glass plate, and (b) a biconvex lens

plane and concave surfaces. The body is attached to the upper end of the limb and contains coarse and fine adjustments by which the body-tube is raised or lowered.

The body-tube houses the draw-tube, in which the eyepiece rests. An objective mount or nosepiece is attached to the lower end of the body-tube and objectives of varying focal length may be screwed into this mount.

In the modern binocular microscope (*Figure 2.2a*), the rays reflected from the object are equally divided between the two eyepieces. This is achieved by the use of a prism, known as a Swan cube. All models are based on the principle illustrated in *Figure 2.2b*.

into the air again. At B, the point of entry of the ray into the glass, a line XY, called the 'normal', is perpendicular to the surface of separation of the media. The ray AB is refracted towards the normal along BC in the glass, and away from the normal along CD in the air.

In general, a ray of light passing from a rarer to a denser medium is refracted *towards* the normal, but when passing from a denser to a rarer medium is refracted *away* from the normal.

Refractive index

In *Figure 2.3a*, the ray AB is termed the incident ray, and the ray BC is the refracted ray. The angle ABY is therefore termed the angle of incidence (*I*), and CBX the angle of refraction (*R*). The sine of the angle of incidence divided by the sine of the angle of refraction is a constant quantity for any two given media and is called the refractive index (RI):

$$RI = \frac{\sin I}{\sin R}$$

In *Figure 2.3a*, the sine of the angle ABY divided by the sine of the angle CBX determines the refractive index of the glass. The refractive index of air is 1.00, of water 1.30 and of glass 1.50.

Spherical aberration

Spherical aberration is the indistinct or fuzzy appearance of the outer part of the field of view of a lens, which is caused by the non-convergence of rays to a common focus.

Figure 2.3b shows rays of light ABCD entering and leaving a biconvex lens. Because of the curvature of the lens, 'normals' at points along the surface are not parallel to one another. The direction which rays of light will take when refracted by the lens will therefore vary according to their place of entry. It will be seen that rays entering the

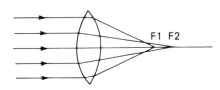

Figure 2.4. Spherical aberration by a biconvex lens. The marginal rays intercept the axis at a point closer to the lens (F1) than the more central rays (F2)

lens near the centre O are refracted less than those entering the lens at the more peripheral part, towards P. Rays from an object therefore tend not to be brought to a common focus, and the result is a distorted image (*Figure 2.4*).

Chromatic aberration

When white light is passed through a prism it is split into a spectrum of colours ranging from red (wavelength 700 nm) through orange, yellow, green, blue, indigo, and violet (wavelength 350 nm). These colours when combined reproduce white light. A biconvex lens also splits white light into its component colours, the blue light being refracted more than the red so that it comes to a focus nearer to the lens (*Figure 2.5*). This non-convergence of the coloured components of white light to a common focus is termed chromatic aberration. This term is used to describe the coloured fringes sometimes seen around the edge of an object viewed through a lens.

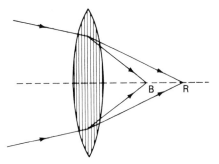

Figure 2.5. Chromatic aberration in a biconvex lens. R = Red component of light coming to a common focus. B = Blue component of light coming to a common focus

Principal focus of a converging lens

A biconvex lens has two spherical surfaces which curve outwards (*Figure 2.6*). It is called a *converging lens* as rays of light passing through the lens converge to a focal point. The centre of the lens surfaces are called the *centres of curvature*. A straight line between these two centres is the *principal axis*. A line, at right angles to this axis, which passes through the centre of the lens is termed the *principal plane*. The diameter or width of the lens is called its *aperture*.

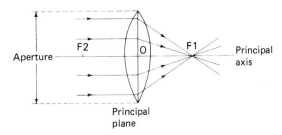

Figure 2.6. The principal axis and plane of a biconvex lens. F1 and F2 are the principal foci. O is the optical centre and the distance O–F1 the focal length

Rays of light entering a converging lens parallel to the principal axis are refracted towards and across this axis. The point at which they cross is called the *principal focus*. A biconvex lens has two principal foci, one on either side.

Optical centre

A ray of light that enters one side of a lens or lens system and emerges parallel to the entering ray, will pass through the *optical centre*. A ray acting similarly when entering the opposite side of the lens, will also pass through the optical centre. The point at which these two rays cross will therefore be the optical centre (*Figure 2.7*).

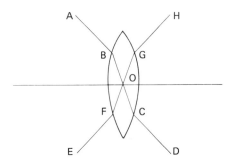

Figure 2.7. Optical centre of a converging lens. AB is parallel to CD; EF is parallel to GH; O = optical centre

Focal length

The distance between the optical centre and the principal focus (the focal point) is the *focal length* of that lens. This must not be confused with *working distance* which is the distance between the surface of the lens and the focal point.

Principal focus of a diverging lens

A biconcave lens has two surfaces which curve inwards (*Figure 2.8*) and is called a diverging lens. Rays passing parallel to the principal axis of a diverging lens are refracted away from the principal axis as though originating from the principal focus.

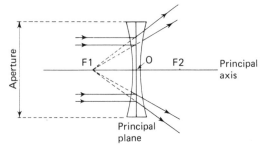

Figure 2.8. Manner in which rays are refracted away from the principal axis by a diverging lens. The principal focus of the lens is shown by the use of broken construction lines

Image formation

Real image

A converging lens can produce either a *real image* or a *virtual image*. A real image is an inverted image, which can be projected onto a screen, and is formed when the object is placed outside the focal length of the lens or lens system (*Figure 2.9*). The size of the image produced depends on the distance between the lens and the object. For example,

if u = distance between object and lens
2f = twice the focal length of the lens.

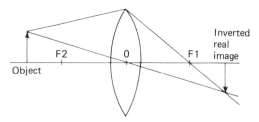

Figure 2.9. Diagram showing the formation of a real image

Then when

u is greater than 2f a diminished image is produced
u is equal to 2f an image of the same size is produced
u is less than 2f (but more than f) a magnified image is produced.

Virtual image

If the object is placed within the focal length of the converging lens, then a *virtual image* is formed which has no physical existence, and cannot be projected onto a screen (*Figure 2.10a*).

A diverging lens will always produce a virtual image which is erect (not inverted) but which is diminished (*Figure 2.10b*).

In the compound microscope two sets of lens systems produce the magnified image, namely the

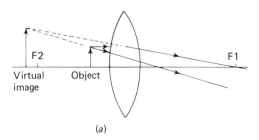

(a)

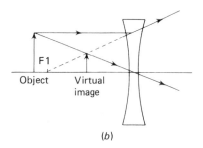

(b)

Figure 2.10. (a) Diagram illustrating (by the use of broken construction lines) formation of a magnified virtual image by a converging lens when the object is within the focal length of the lens. (b) Diagram illustrating (by the use of broken construction lines) diminished virtual image by a diverging lens

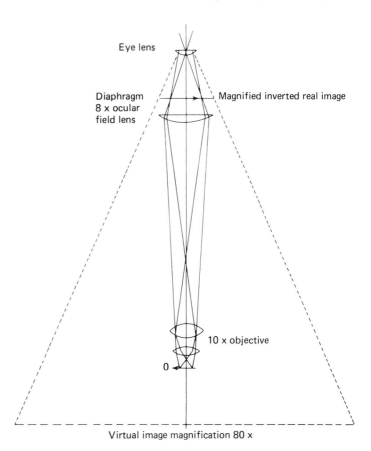

Eye lens

Diaphragm
8 x ocular
field lens

Magnified inverted real image

10 x objective

0

Virtual image magnification 80 x

Figure 2.11. Rays from the object O are brought to a focus by the field lens in the plane of the eyepiece diaphragm as an inverted, magnified real image. The image is within the focal length of the eye lens, resulting in the production of an inverted, magnified virtual image

objective and the ocular. The objective produces the primary image, which is brought to focus in the plane of the eyepiece diaphragm by the field lens, and is then viewed with the eye lens. The primary image is a real, magnified image of the object, which must therefore be at a greater distance from the objective than the focal length ($u < 2f$ produces a magnified image, see above). The primary image when viewed by the eye lens is within the focal length of the lens and a magnified virtual image is produced (*Figure 2.11*).

Components of the microscope

Optical components

The optics of the compound microscope can be most easily understood by considering the components in stages. The optical system consists essentially of a condenser, an objective and an eyepiece (*Figure 2.12*).

Rays from a light source are directed into the substage condenser, which brings them to a common focus on the object, for example, blood film. Having illuminated the object, light rays pass through the

objective, and produce the primary image in the plane of the eyepiece diaphragm. The eye lens magnifies the image and brings it into focus on the retina of the eye as a virtual image.

The retina forms the inner coat of the eyeball and acts as a screen. It is composed of small, highly specialized cells of which two types, the rods and cones, are sensitive to light. Under normal conditions and when the eye is at rest, distant objects are registered as being in focus. Magnification is achieved by the simple process of reducing the distance between the eye and the object, thereby increasing the visual angle and spreading the image over a larger area of the retina (*Figure 2.13*).

The eye has a minimum focusing distance of 25 cm, however, and objects brought closer than this appear indistinct. Further magnification can only be achieved by placing a lens, or system of lenses such as a microscope, between the object under examination and the eye (*Figure 2.14*).

Objectives

The aberrations mentioned previously are corrected to greater or lesser degree, in the modern microscope, by using combinations of lenses of different

18

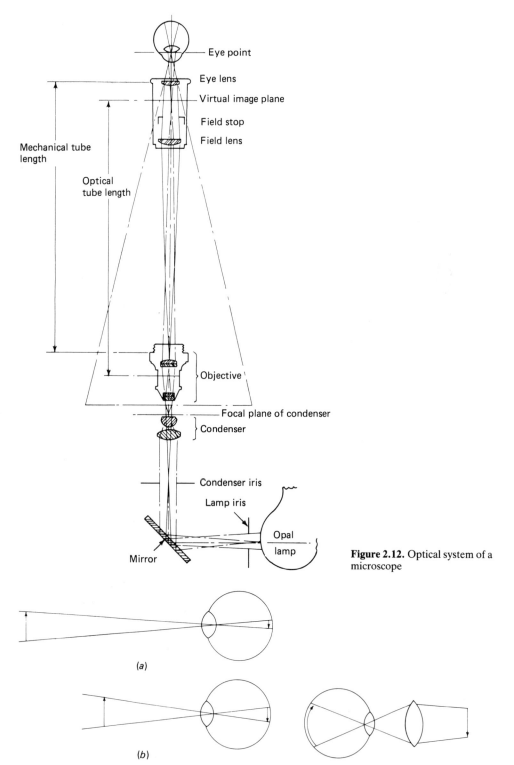

Eye point

Eye lens

Virtual image plane

Field stop

Field lens

Mechanical tube
length

Optical
tube length

Objective

Focal plane of condenser

Condenser

Condenser iris

Lamp iris

Opal
lamp

Mirror

Figure 2.12. Optical system of a
microscope

(a)

(b)

Figure 2.13. Diagram illustrating the manner in which the
retinal image is increased as the object is brought closer to
the eye, thereby increasing the visual angle

Figure 2.14. Diagram illustrating the manner in which a
convex lens interposed between the object and the eye
increases the visual angle and size of the retinal image

shape and types of glass. The average objective (achromatic) brings to a common focus the rays of red and blue light, that is, it is corrected for two spectral colours. In addition, spherical aberration is corrected for light of one colour. Flat-field achromatic objectives are now in common use.

For highly critical work, apochromatic objectives are necessary. The lenses employed in these objectives bring rays of three different colours to a common focus, and are said to be corrected for three spectral colours. In addition, they correct the spherical aberration for two spectral colours, that is, spherical aberration is minimized provided the light used consists only of these two colours. They necessitate the use of a compensating eyepiece. Apochromatic lenses are usually reserved for oil immersion or high-powered objectives, preferably in conjunction with a compensating eyepiece. Of recent development are planochromatic objectives which are designed to provide the flattest possible field. *Figure 2.15* illustrates the lens arrangement in the common objectives.

The focal length of a lens is the distance between its centre, or in the case of a system of lenses their optical centre, and the point where a parallel beam of light is brought to focus. The focal length of a high-power objective is shorter than that of a low-power one (*Figure 2.15*). The focal length should not be confused with the working distance,

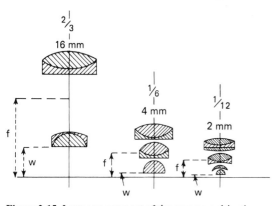

Figure 2.15. Lens arrangement of the common objectives showing the relative focal lengths and working distances. f = Focal length; w = working distance

which is the distance between the front lens of an objective and the object on which it is sharply focused (*Figure 2.15*). The working distance is relative to the numerical aperture; the higher the numerical aperture of the objective, the shorter the working distance.

Objectives of focal length over 3 mm have air between the front lens of the objective and the object under examination (dry objective).

Objectives with focal length under 3 mm use fluid between the front lens and the object under examination. This fluid should have the same refractive index as glass. Special cedarwood oil is generally used, unless otherwise stated on the objective, for example, water immersion. The chromatic aberration produced by this procedure is corrected in the lens system.

Resolving power

The power of a lens to reveal detail is referred to as the resolving power or resolution of the lens. It may be defined as the ability to reveal closely adjacent structural details as being actually separate and distinct.

The resolving power of a microscope is largely dependent upon the angle of light entering the objective. It will be seen from *Figure 2.16* that the presence of oil between objective and slide conserves many of the light rays, which would otherwise be lost by refraction. In *Figure 2.16a*, ABCD is the path of a ray of light through a glass slide. It is refracted towards the normal on entering the glass, BC, and away from the normal, CD, on entering the rarer medium, air; this ray of light would not enter the objective. In *Figure 2.16b* a similar ray of light, ABCD, behaves exactly the same on entering the glass, BC. It is not refracted when leaving the slide, however, as oil has the same refractive index as the glass. The ray CD will, therefore, pass into the objective.

Numerical aperture

The resolution, or resolving power, of an objective is partly dependent upon the cone of light collected by the front lens. The numerical aperture (NA), an

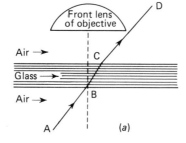
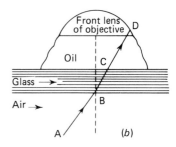

Figure 2.16. Diagram to illustrate angle of light entering objective

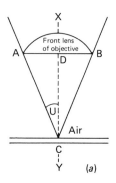
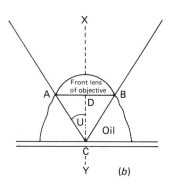

Figure 2.17. Refractive index of objectives (a) without oil, (b) with oil

optical constant, is defined as the product of the refractive index of the medium outside the lens (n), and the sine of half the angle of the cone of light absorbed by the front lens of the objective (U), that is, NA = $n \times \sin U$ (*Figure 2.17*).

The wider the cone of light, the greater the NA. Thus, if two objectives of the same focal length have lenses of different diameters, one will admit a greater angle of light, and therefore have a higher NA. In *Figure 2.17a*, ACB is the angle of the cone of light entering the front lens of the objective, AB is the diameter of the front lens of the objective and C is the object being viewed. The NA of that objective is, therefore, $n \times \sin U$. As the external medium is air, the value of n is unity. Therefore

$$\text{NA} = \sin U \equiv \frac{AD}{AC}$$

In *Figure 2.17b*, as the external medium is oil with a refractive index of 1.5, the NA of that objective is

$$1.5 \times \frac{AD}{AC}$$

The NA for dry lenses may be calculated by measuring the angle U with an apertometer. As the external medium is air, the value for n is unity. The NA is normally marked on the objective.

With oil-immersion objectives, somewhat higher values are obtained for NA, owing to the higher figure for n. Most oils used have a refractive index of about 1.5.

Eyepieces

The eyepiece most commonly used is of the Huygenian pattern. This is composed of two planoconvex lenses which are arranged with their convex surfaces facing the objective. The two lenses are of different sizes, the front (or field) lens having a focal length twice or three times that of the eye lens. A diaphragm is situated within the eyepiece at the focal plane of the eye lens (*Figure 2.18a*).

Compensating eyepiece

This is primarily designed for use with apochromatic objectives. The apochromatic objectives are under-corrected for the magnification of light of various colours, and compensating (overcorrected) eyepieces are designed to rectify this (*Figure 2.18b*). The overcorrection can be seen by looking through the eyepiece at a distant light source. A red fringe will usually be seen at the edge of the diaphragm, in contrast to the blue fringe produced with an ordinary Huygenian ocular.

Mechanical tube length

This is the distance which separates the top lens of the eyepiece from the point where the objective screws into the revolving nosepiece (see *Figure 2.12*). Most objectives are made to be used with a mechanical tube length of 160 mm.

Optical tube length

This is the distance between the upper focal plane of the objective and the lower focal plane of the eyepiece (see *Figure 2.12*) and is of a similar distance to that of the mechanical tube length. The magnifying power of the microscope is dependent in part on the optical tube length. In practice, however, the mechanical tube length is used for calculating the total magnifying power of the

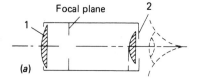
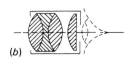

Figure 2.18. Eyepieces: (a) Huygenian type (1, field lens; 2, eye lens); (b) compensating eyepiece

microscope, or the individual power of the eyepiece and objectives.

The use of the draw-tube

Extension of the draw-tube in older types of monocular microscopes increases magnification of the final image, but its primary function is the elimination of spherical aberration when using coverglasses of incorrect thickness. Objectives are usually corrected for coverglasses of 0.17 mm thickness, and shortening of the tube length is desirable if very thick coverglasses are used.

Condensers

The substage condenser is the most neglected part of the optical system in a microscope. The important role which it plays is frequently overlooked, and as a general rule, while a great deal of attention is given to the optical qualities of the objectives, very little care is taken to ensure that the condenser is of a sufficiently high quality to allow maximum resolution to be achieved by the other optical components.

Only two working errors are possible with components situated above the stage: (1) the tube length may be set incorrectly, and on modern instruments this is no longer adjustable, and (2) the front lens of the objective may be racked down too far, resulting in damage to the objective and the specimen; this is also allowed for in many modern objectives which have the front component spring loaded.

In the case of the substage condenser, many major errors may be committed when working with the microscope. Incorrect centring, failure to adjust it correctly for Köhler illumination, indiscriminate use of the auxiliary lens, top lens or the iris diaphragm—each of these factors can separately or collectively reduce the resolution of which the objective may be capable.

Condensers fall into two categories, bright-field and dark-field.

Bright-field condensers

These are used with transmitted light for routine work. The most common type is the Abbé condenser, designed by Professor E. Abbé in 1872. It consists of two lenses and an iris diaphragm. As no correction is made for chromatic or spherical aberration, a considerable amount of scattering occurs. This can be reduced by partly closing the iris diaphragm or by placing immersion oil on the top lens of the condenser, under the object slide. For critical work, an achromatic condenser which consists of a series of lenses is essential.

The NA quoted for Abbé condensers is frequently as high as 1.20 but, due to the lack of correction, the iris diaphragm must be partly closed in order to produce an aplanatic cone of light. This reduces the working NA of the condenser markedly and with it the effective working NA of the objective.

For critical work, a three-lens type of Abbé achromatic condenser may be used, but for the best results an aplanatic condenser should be selected. The maximum working NA of the objective/condenser system is then obtained.

The working NA of the objective/condenser system is the arithmetic mean of the two. Thus an objective with NA 1.2 and a condenser with working NA of 0.4 is equal to

$$\frac{1.2 + 0.4}{2} = 0.8$$

This means that only two-thirds of the possible NA of the objective is being utilized.

Low-power objectives necessitate the use of low-power condensers if the whole field is to be illuminated. This may be achieved by removing the top lens of the condenser. Some manufacturers produce condensers with top lenses which may be flipped in or out of the optical train as required.

Dark-field condensers

These are designed so that the object under examination is illuminated very obliquely. The light rays passing through the condenser are lost unless they are deflected or refracted into the objective by the object. The field as seen under the microscope is therefore black, but any solid material present is clearly illuminated (*Figure 2.19*).

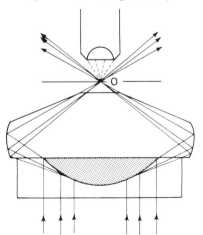

Figure 2.19. Diagram illustrating the way in which light rays are reflected from the central spherical surface and outer cardioid reflecting surface in the cardioid dark-field condenser. The rays of light strike the object O at an oblique angle

Most dark-field condensers have a fixed focus and must be used with thin slides and coverglasses, being usually corrected for slides 1.2 mm in thickness and a coverglass of 0.17 mm. A more expensive type of focusing condenser is available, however, which will allow slides and coverglasses of varying thickness to be used. All types should be used as immersion condensers, cedarwood oil being the usual immersion fluid. The type of dark-field condenser usually available in medical laboratories cannot give a perfectly black background when used in conjunction with an objective which has a numerical aperture higher than 0.90. Such objectives should have their aperture decreased by the insertion of a funnel stop—a small metal tube. Some high-power objectives incorporate an iris diaphragm for this purpose (Davis diaphragm).

An intense source of light is necessary for dark-field illumination. Objects examined by dark-field illumination appear larger than they actually are: this is due to their light-scattering properties.

Filters

A variety of light filters is available for use with the microscope. Light filters may be used to (a) increase resolution and contrast; (b) decrease light intensity and glare; and (c) absorb excess heat.

Neutral filters

These are used to decrease the brilliance of the illuminant without reducing the operating voltage of the bulb. They are manufactured in a number of densities, two or more of which may be used together to obtain the effect of their combined strength.

Coloured filters

These have a number of different functions. 'Daylight blue' is the most commonly used filter in medical laboratories. By absorbing those light rays of longer wavelengths and only transmitting the shorter, resolution is increased. Green filters similarly increase resolution but also decrease glare. Increased contrast can be obtained with coloured filters by selecting one that is complementary to the colour of the object under examination.

Colour correction filters

These cover a very wide range. They are used mainly in colour photomicrography in order to correct the colour temperature of the light source to agree with that of the film.

Heat-absorbing filters

These are used in conjunction with medium and high-intensity lamps. Their purpose is to absorb the heat rays.

Exciter filters

These are used in fluorescence microscopy for transmitting light of a selected wavelength.

Barrier filters (secondary filters)

These are used to protect the retina from injury by preventing the passage of ultraviolet light. They must, therefore, only transmit light of a longer wavelength than the exciter filter. In addition, they serve to increase the brilliance of the fluorescent image by producing a dark background.

Source of illumination

The resolution achieved by the optical components of the microscope is dependent in part upon the intensity and adjustment of the light source. Correct alignment is therefore essential when the microscope is set up.

Daylight is a poor illuminant for microscopy as it imposes strict limitations on the use of the instrument and makes standardization impossible. It should only be used when no alternative light source is available and then only with low-power objectives. Most microscope lamps use electricity as the source of energy and good lamps possess the following features.

The base is of sufficient size and weight to ensure perfect stability. The lamphouse has good ventilation to prevent overheating, but is light-tight, except for the working orifice, and is supported on a stand which permits smooth adjustment of the height. Facilities are provided which permit adjustment in both a vertical and horizontal direction, and provision is made for coloured filters to be interposed in the light path. The better lamps are fitted with a condenser and an iris diaphragm and have a focusing mechanism for providing Köhler illumination. A rheostat, or variable voltmeter, is also incorporated to give control over the intensity.

Electric light bulbs of 10–100 W are used in the simplest form of student lamps; the bulb should be of an opal type rather than a frosted glass one, as the latter do not give even illumination and the filament, which can be seen, is in focus when the microscope is adjusted for critical illumination. Most microscopes in medical laboratories have a coil filament bulb as the illuminant. This is of low voltage, usually 6–12 V, and must be used in conjunction with a transformer and variable voltmeter. Lamps of this nature have a small but intense light source which is

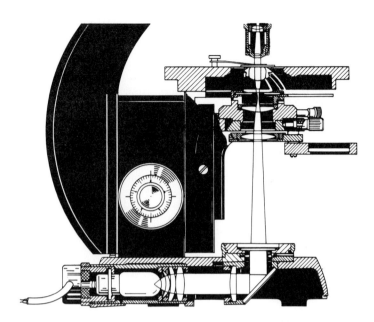

Figure 2.20. Built-in illumination

very often of uneven brilliance. It is therefore essential to use Köhler illumination with this form of illuminant (see p. 25). Microscopes manufactured with built-in illumination are invariably provided with this type of light source, which is pre-centred. To comply with the conditions necessary for Köhler illumination, a condenser is provided and an iris diaphragm is built into the foot of the instrument. If the condenser is not adjustable, provision is made for varying the position of the bulb in relation to the condenser (*Figure 2.20*).

A widely used type of illuminant in microscopy is the quartz–iodine vapour lamp. This may be a 6 V 10 W, 6 V 20 W or 12 V 100 W illuminant which is used in conjunction with a variable voltmeter. The tungsten–iodine filament is enclosed within a quartz envelope. The lamp is rich in light at the 400 nm level of the spectrum and is therefore useful for blue light fluorescence.

The most efficient source of intense illumination is undoubtedly the high-intensity mercury vapour lamp (50 W super-pressure mercury vapour bulb). The main application of this lamp in medical laboratory work is in ultraviolet microscopy, particularly for studying immunofluorescence reactions.

Mechanical components

To complete the microscope, certain mechanical details must be considered.

The coarse adjustment is a rack and pinion utilized in older models for connecting the body-tube to the body. A similar device is used for attaching the substage condenser to the base of the limb. The fine adjustment, allowing precision in

focusing, may be of several different designs. Modern microscopes are different in construction. The body-tube is permanently fixed to the limb, and focusing is performed by racking the stage up or down.

The fixed stage is a basic component of the microscope, but only allows manual movement of the object slide. This disadvantage can be overcome by the mechanical stage.

Mechanical stages are fitted with two scales and Vernier plates running at right angles to each other, for the purpose of recording a particular field in the specimen under examination. For this reason, the habit should be adopted of always placing the slide on the stage with the label at the same end. Some workers also use these scales for making approximate measurements of relatively large objects, for which purpose the eyepiece should be fitted with cross-wires or a marker.

The Vernier system consists of a main scale, which is divided into millimetres, and a Vernier plate which has a scale 9 mm in length but divided into ten equal divisions. The zero mark on the Vernier plate is used as the reference point for recording. When this falls between two divisions on the main scale, the lower one should be recorded, and the Vernier plate scale examined to see which of

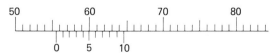

Figure 2.21. The Vernier system. The main scale shows a reading of 55 and the Vernier scale a reading of 5. The reading is recorded as 55.5

its divisional lines coincides with a reading on the main scale. The reading from the Vernier plate is then recorded as a decimal reading. Thus, if the zero on the Vernier scale falls between 55 and 56 on the main scale and the Vernier plate reading is 5, the reading recorded is 55.5. Readings from both Vernier scales should be taken in order to re-locate a particular field in a slide (*Figure 2.21*).

Micrometry

Vernier scales are not suitable for making accurate measurements with the microscope and, when this is necessary, specialized equipment is required. The most widely used type in medical laboratories is the stage micrometer and micrometer eyepiece. The actual measuring is done with the micrometer eyepiece, but it must be emphasized that the scale used is a transfer scale to be compared against a known standard with which it must first be calibrated.

Micrometer eyepiece

This may be one of several types of eyepieces (Ramsden, Huygenian, compensating) containing an engraved micrometer scale at the level of the diaphragm. The eye lens is provided with a means of adjustment in order to bring the scale into sharp focus (*Figure 2.22*).

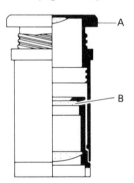

Figure 2.22. Eyepiece micrometer. A = Eye lens which can be focused. B = Graticule with scale

Stage micrometer

This consists of a 3 × 1 in (76 × 25 mm) slide, in the centre of which is an engraved scale with finely divided divisions mounted beneath a coverglass. The scale is usually 2 mm in length and the divisions are 0.1 mm and 0.01 mm in width (100 μm and 10 μm, respectively).

Method of use

1. Focus the eye lens sharply on the engraved scale by pointing the eyepiece towards an illuminated surface and adjusting the eye lens.
2. Place the eyepiece in the draw-tube and ensure

that the tube is set to the correct working distance.
3. Place the stage micrometer in position and focus on the scale.
4. Turn the eyepiece until both scales are parallel.
5. Study the two scales carefully and record the number of larger divisions on the eyepiece scale that corresponds to a whole number on the stage micrometer. When necessary the draw-tube can be adjusted to ensure that an accurate reading is obtained (*Figure 2.23*).

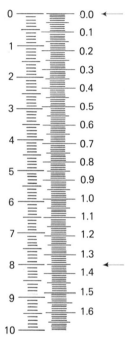

Figure 2.23. Diagram illustrating the manner in which the eyepiece micrometer is calibrated with the stage micrometer. In this example, 80 divisions correspond to 1350 μm, each division therefore being 16.9 μm in length

6. From the readings obtained, calculate the ratio of the two scales.
7. Having calculated the size of the division on the eyepiece micrometer, place the specimen to be examined on the stage and make the necessary reading. The eyepiece micrometer should be calibrated for each objective used.

For example, from *Figure 2.23* it will be seen that 80 small eyepiece divisions are equal to 135 small stage-divisions; as each small stage division is 10 μm in width,

$$80 \text{ eyepiece divisions} = 1350 \text{ μm}$$
$$\therefore 1 \text{ eyepiece division}$$
$$= \frac{1350}{80} \text{ μm}$$
$$= 16.9 \text{ μm}$$

Magnification

At the normal optical tube length of 160 mm, the total magnifying power of the compound microscope is the product of the magnification of the objective and eyepiece; for example, with objective ×40 and eyepiece ×10, the magnification would be 40 × 10 = 400. If the tube length is varied, the final magnification is

$$\left(\begin{matrix}\text{Magnification of}\\\text{objective}\end{matrix}\right) \times \left(\begin{matrix}\text{Magnification of}\\\text{eyepiece}\end{matrix}\right)$$
$$\times \left(\frac{\text{Working tube length}}{\text{Normal optical tube length}}\right)$$

For example, with objective ×40, eyepiece ×10 and working tube length 180 mm, total magnification is

$$40 \times 10 \times \frac{180}{160} = 450$$

If objectives are marked with focal length only, total magnification is

$$\left(\begin{matrix}\text{Magnification of}\\\text{eyepiece}\end{matrix}\right) \times \left(\frac{\text{Working tube length}}{\text{Focal length of objective}}\right)$$

For example, with eyepiece ×10, objective of focal length 4 mm and working tube length of 160 mm, total magnification is

$$\frac{10 \times 160}{4} = 400$$

Empty magnification

This is the term used to describe magnification which produces an increase in the apparent size of an object without revealing any new detail. In other words, empty magnification is magnification without resolution.

Setting up the microscope

If the best results are to be obtained it is of the utmost importance that the microscope is set up correctly. The most widely used method of adjusting the illumination is that of Köhler. Köhler illumination is named after the German scientist August Köhler, who was famous for his photomicrography and who introduced the method in 1892. With Köhler illumination the whole field is illuminated evenly, a condition which is essential for photomicrography. In order to obtain Köhler illumination it is necessary for the lamp to be fitted with a condenser and an iris diaphragm. The lamp condenser is used to project an enlarged image of the lamp filament, which is brought to focus on the iris diaphragm of the substage condenser. When so focused, the

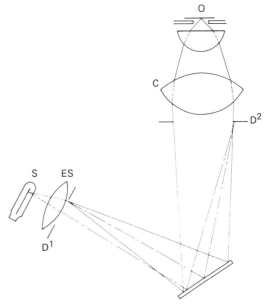

Figure 2.24. Köhler illumination. An image of the actual light source S is formed in the plane of the substage iris diaphragm. D^1 serves as a field diaphragm, the substage iris diaphragm D^2 being the aperture diaphragm

effective source is imaged in the object plane, the whole field being flooded with parallel light. The lamp diaphragm, which should have a large aperture and be mounted as near as possible to the lamp condenser, serves as a field diaphragm; the substage iris diaphragm is used as an aperture diaphragm (*Figure 2.24*).

A *field diaphragm* controls the area illuminated but does not change the brilliance of the illumination or affect the working numerical aperture of the system.

An *aperture diaphragm* controls the brilliance of the illumination and the working numerical aperture of the system, but does not affect the size of the area illuminated.

Köhler illumination

■ **Note**

If the microscope is equipped with built-in lighting designed to work on the Köhler principle, steps 2 and 7 of the following procedure are omitted.

1. The microscope bench should be firm, of suitable height and free from vibration.
2. Place the microscope about 25 cm in front of the lamp diaphragm and direct the beam onto the centre of the plane surface of the mirror.
3. Place a 16 mm objective and a low-power eyepiece in the optical train, insert a neutral filter in the light path and adjust to obtain maximum illumination.

4. Place a stained slide on the stage and focus on the specimen. Close the substage iris diaphragm, remove the eyepiece and by means of the centring screws ensure that the substage condenser is correctly aligned.
5. Rack up the substage condenser, replace the eyepiece and adjust the lamp condenser until an enlarged image of the light source is focused on the substage diaphragm. This can be observed by using a small hand-mirror.
6. Open the substage diaphragm, close the lamp diaphragm and focus the substage condenser to obtain a sharp image of the lamp diaphragm in the object plane.
7. Adjust the mirror to bring the centre of the lamp diaphragm image into the centre of the field.
8. Open the lamp diaphragm until the field is just filled with light, remove the eyepiece and adjust the substage diaphragm until the back lens of the objective is just filled with light.

Setting up the microscope for dark-field illumination

1. Switch on the electric current, place a piece of lens paper over the eyepiece and adjust the illuminant until the maximum illumination is obtained. Remove the bright-field condenser.
2. Fix the dark-field condenser into position and swing the 10× objective into the optical train.
3. Place a drop of oil on the top lens of the condenser and lower surface of the slide to be examined and carefully place the slide in

position, taking care to avoid the formation of air bubbles between the oiled surfaces.
4. Examine the specimen and adjust the condenser until a small but intense area of illumination is obtained, centring the condenser if necessary.
5. Swing the 40× objective into the optical train and focus. Correct for maximum illumination by closing the lamp diaphragm and refocusing the light spot with the condenser. Recentre the condenser if necessary.
6. Open the lamp diaphragm until the minimum working field is illuminated and examine the specimen.
7. Rack up the body-tube slightly, apply a drop of oil to the area of the slide to be examined and swing the immersion objective into the optical train. Carefully lower the body-tube until the front lens of the objective is just less than the working distance from the slide. Complete the focusing with the fine adjustment by *raising* the body-tube. When the specimen is in focus, make any final adjustment necessary to the condenser.

Fluorescence microscopy

The term 'fluorescence' was first introduced by George Gabriel Stokes in 1852 to describe the reaction of fluorspar when illuminated with ultra-violet light. Basically, fluorescence is the absorption and re-emission properties possessed by certain substances, whereby short-wave radiation is absorbed and re-emitted as light of a longer visible wavelength, resulting in the object acquiring a luminous appearance.

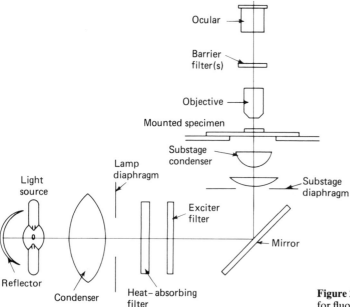

Figure 2.25. Essential requirements for fluorescence microscopy

The development in recent years of intense light sources rich in short-wave radiation, has given a tremendous impetus to the development of the fluorescence microscope as a diagnostic and research instrument. As a result, many companies now market microscopes especially designed for this purpose. The essential requirements for fluorescence microscopy (*Figure 2.25*) are the following: (a) a suitable light source; (b) a heat-absorbing filter; (c) exciter filters; (d) condenser; (e) objective; (f) barrier filter; (g) eyepiece.

The light source

A variety of light sources is available, the final selection being dependent upon the work to be undertaken. At the present time the two most widely used lamps are the mercury vapour lamp and the quartz–iodine lamp. Of these the latter, which is relatively cheap, is quite adequate for a great deal of work in the medical laboratory, such as screening for mycobacteria. For detailed research work, however, particularly in the field of immunology where ultraviolet light of a shorter wavelength is desirable, the mercury vapour lamp is preferable.

Heat-absorbing filter

This must be interposed between the lamp and the exciter filters. When using the mercury vapour lamp, the exciter filter should be at least 4 mm in thickness to provide adequate protection. Examples of glass filters are Chance–Pilkington OX 2 and Schott KG 2.

Exciter filters

The correct selection of the exciter filters is perhaps the most important single factor in fluorescence microscopy. The filter, or combination of exciter filters used, depends upon a number of factors, including the light source, the specimen under examination, the fluorochrome used as the staining reagent and the barrier filter. Instructions for the use of exciter filter combination are supplied by the manufacturers and the student should follow their directions. In addition, the original papers in which the staining procedure in use was first described should be consulted, in order to establish the filter combination originally recommended.

Condenser

Special quartz condensers are manufactured for use in fluorescence microscopy, but are only necessary for specific purposes. In general, condensers made from crown glass are adequate, but it is important that the condenser does not contain too many components which are cemented together. In many

instances, a cardioid dark-field condenser is to be preferred, as this provides greater contrast.

Objective

This should be of simple construction. When available, planochromatic objectives should be used to provide a flatter field. If immersion objectives are used, the immersion oil must be 'fluorescence-free'. Special immersion oil is manufactured for this purpose, but oxidation can cause it to fluoresce after the bottle has been opened a few months.

Barrier filter (secondary filter)

A barrier filter is an essential item for fluorescence microscopy and specimens should not be examined by ultraviolet light without a barrier filter being positioned in the optical train. Microscopes manufactured especially for fluorescence microscopy usually have a turret or slide in the body, in which the filters are housed. Instruments adapted for fluorescence normally have the barrier filter located in the eyepiece either as a clip-on attachment or resting on the diaphragm. The latter is in direct focus of the eye lens and must therefore be free from specks of dust and fingerprints.

The barrier filter is complementary to the exciter filter and selection should therefore be made with care. The facilities provided in research microscopes for having a series of barrier filters is one of the many advantages of purchasing specially designed equipment.

Eyepiece

For fluorescence microscopy low-power oculars are to be preferred. The construction should be as simple as possible, the most widely used being the Huygenian pattern.

Fluorochromes

Mention was made earlier of the use of fluorochromes as staining reagents in fluorescence microscopy. These are organic dyes which fluoresce when subjected to short-wave radiation, and which have an affinity for certain substances. Fluorescence produced by the use of fluorochromes is termed 'secondary fluorescence'. A knowledge of the wavelength at which fluorochromes absorb the exciting radiation and re-emit the absorbed energy is of great importance when selecting the exciter and barrier filter combination. Ideally, the transmission of the exciter filter should match the emission peak of the fluorochrome being used.

Using the fluorescence microscope

There is no special technique for using the fluorescence microscope other than applying the general rules for good microscopy, adjusting it for Köhler illumination and ensuring that the correct filters are in position prior to switching on the lamp. The art in obtaining high-quality results lies more in a thorough knowledge of the fluorochromes and filters in use. When using a mercury vapour lamp, a record should be kept of the number of hours for which the lamp is used.

Incident light fluorescence

The use of incident light or epifluorescence is a simple yet highly efficient fluorescent technique becoming more widely applied in medical laboratories. By the use of this method the specimen is illuminated from above by using an interference beam splitter or dichroic mirror (*Figure 2.26*).

Short wave light from the light source is directed onto the mirror and reflected onto the specimen. Visible light from the reflected specimen is then passed back to the mirror and through the ocular.

The light source is normally either a 100 W halogen lamp for blue light excitation or a 50 W mercury vapour burner for ultraviolet blue–green excitation.

The optical system is corrected so that incident light fluorescence may be used without affecting either the magnification or the size of the field.

The relative properties of transmitted light fluorescence and incident light fluorescence (*Figure 2.26*) are given below.

Transmitted light fluorescence

1. Good intensity at all magnifications.
2. Ease of interchangeability to white-light and dark-ground illumination.
3. Interchangeable bright-field and dark-field condensers.

Incident light fluorescence

1. Good intensity at all magnifications, but particularly with high-power lenses.
2. Ease of use.
3. More efficient for thicker specimens.
4. No substage condenser required.
5. The objective acts as a condenser.

The interference microscope

The optical principle of the interference microscope is as follows (*Figure 2.27*): light from a light source (LS) is divided by means of a beam splitter (BS)

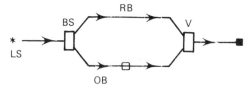

Figure 2.27. Optical principle of the interference microscope

forming a reference beam (RB) and an object beam (OB); RB travels direct to a point (V), where it is recombined with OB which has been caused to traverse the object and has hence become retarded relative to RB. As the beams are coherent, interference can take place and the object becomes invisible.

The system is similar to phase contrast microscopy, but with the fundamental difference that the interference microscope does not rely on diffraction by the object but produces the contrast by generating mutually interfering beams.

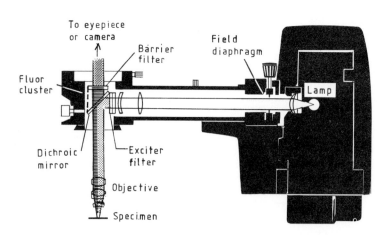

Figure 2.26. Epifluorescence— illumination by means of dichroic mirror

Phase contrast microscopy

Phase contrast microscopy is used to examine living cells and organisms in detail without previous treatment—such as staining—and reveals minute structures not seen by 'ordinary' microscopy. To understand how phase contrast microscopy works, it is necessary to explain certain properties of light rays.

Amplitude governs brightness and wavelength governs colour. This can be represented diagrammatically, as shown in *Figure 2.28*. The brightness of light rays can be altered by passing them through a block of glass (*Figure 2.29*).

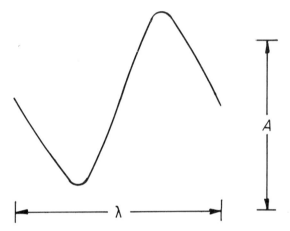

Figure 2.28. Sine curve representing a ray of light (A, amplitude or brightness; λ, wavelength or colour)

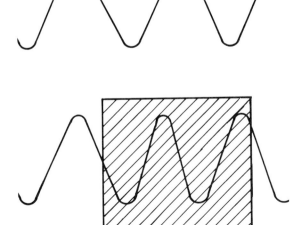

Figure 2.29. Retardation of lower light by a block of glass—the lower ray, having passed through the glass, is retarded by half a wavelength

The principles of interference microscopy were explained above and this property of interference—which may result in complete extinction of the light or in a reduction of it, depending on the relative amplitudes of the light rays—is used in phase contrast microscopy.

Standard phase contrast outfits consist basically of the following items of equipment: (a) phase contrast objectives; (b) condenser; (c) auxiliary microscope.

Phase contrast objectives

These objectives are fitted with a phase plate, which consists of an optically plane glass disc which has a channel cut to a thickness that will retard the rays of light going through the thicker part of the plate one-quarter of a wavelength, relative to these rays passing through the channel. Although this annulus will give interference, the brightness (amplitude) between the two sets of rays will be different, and therefore the channel has a light-absorbing deposit which reduces the brightness without affecting the diffracted light, thus giving the maximum contrast.

Condenser

The condenser is usually fitted with a rotating changer carrying separate annular diaphragms matching each of the phase objectives to be used. The rotating changer is provided with a means of centring, so that each condenser annulus may be brought into accurate register with the annulus of each phase plate.

Auxiliary microscope

A simple auxiliary microscope is used in place of the eyepiece to enable the light from the condenser annulus to coincide with the ring of the phase plate in the objective.

Figure 2.30 demonstrates the application of the component parts of the phase contrast by showing the passage of light rays through the optical components of the phase contrast microscope. An intense source of light is necessary and a green filter with a peak of about 550 mm should be inserted in front of this light source. The green filter will ensure optimal image contrast, as the phase components have been computed for use in green light.

Setting up the microscope

1. With the specimen in position, make the necessary adjustments to achieve Köhler illumination (see p. 25).
2. Substitute the auxiliary microscope for the eyepiece and adjust so that the phase plate annulus is in sharp focus.

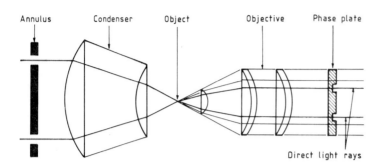

Annulus   Condenser   Object   Objective   Phase plate

Direct light rays

Figure 2.30. Passage of light rays through the optical components of the phase contrast microscope

3. Rotate the changer to bring the appropriate matching condenser annulus in position and using the centring device register the bright ring of the condenser annulus exactly coincident with the annulus of the phase plate.
4. Replace the eyepiece and check that the illuminating cone of light is appropriate to the size of field by adjusting the lamp when necessary.

Some do's and don'ts of microscopy

Do cover the microscope when not in use.

Do remove all immersion oil from the objective immediately after use. This may easily be done by wiping with lens paper or a soft cloth. Xylene may be used sparingly.

Do clean the optical parts with lens paper before use.

Do support the microscope carefully, when moving it.

Don't rack the objective downwards to bring the object into focus while looking down the microscope.

Don't attempt to dismantle objectives.

Don't use a high-power objective when a low-power one is sufficient.

Don't lubricate the microscope with any oil other than that provided for the purpose.

Don't place wet preparations on the stage without wiping the undersurface of the slide.

3

Health and safety in the laboratory

In the UK, the Health and Safety at Work Act 1974 requires employers to provide adequate safety precautions and regulations. Workers in medical laboratories are exposed to many dangers, not only from infected material, dangerous compounds and apparatus which they use routinely, but also from the common dangers that apply to any home, office or factory.

These precautions must be observed by all members of the staff, not only for themselves as individuals but for the safety of all concerned. While the application of safety precautions is mainly a matter of common sense, it is necessary to lay down general rules for guidance which must be maintained at all times. Although safety is the responsibility of every member of the laboratory, the Head of Department or, through him, a Safety Officer is responsible for the safety measures adopted by the laboratory. The duty of the Safety Officer is to instigate a Code of Practice in the conduct of safety for the laboratory, and to ensure that all members of staff are familiar with the code and adhere to it at all times.

All laboratory staff should be familiar with the publication *The Code of Practice for the Prevention of Infection in Clinical Laboratories and Post-Mortem Rooms* (1978), more popularly known as the Howie Report, issued by the Department of Health and Social Security (DHSS), the Scottish Home and Health Department, the Department of Health and Social Services N. Ireland and the Welsh Office.

Some of the contents of the booklet have been modified and these modifications have been notified in bulletins issued by the DHSS.

In May 1981, an Advisory Committee on dangerous pathogens was set up to advise Health and Agriculture Ministers, the Health and Safety Commission and the Health and Safety Executive on all classes of pathogens dangerous to humans. Its first report, entitled 'Categorisation of Pathogens According to Risk and Categories of Containment' outlines a fourfold classification of organisms according to risk. It also contains lists of pathogens assigned to risk groups and a model Code of Practice, setting out physical containment levels in laboratories and animal rooms which are appropriate for work with pathogens in each of the four risk groups.

It is essential that all personnel working in medical laboratories are familiar with the contents of these codes and reports, as it is not possible to give more than a cursory appraisal in this book.

Health of staff

Before commencing employment, a prospective employee must have a medical examination or provide a statement from his own doctor that he is medically fit for the type of employment he is undertaking.

A chest X-ray must be taken, or evidence produced of having had one taken in the previous 12 months. It is essential that X-rays are kept to a minimum.

Staff handling tuberculous material must have an annual X-ray and must have a skin test for tuberculosis or produce evidence of having a positive reaction.

If the work necessitates it, staff must be offered protective immunization.

Rubella antibody tests must be offered to all female staff of child-bearing age and immunization offered if results are negative.

Sickness records, and records of immunization, chest X-rays and job-associated injuries must be kept by a designated person or persons.

Protective clothing

When working in the laboratory, all staff must wear protective clothing.

Protective clothing worn in the laboratory must be taken off before visiting rest rooms, recreation rooms, canteen, libraries and other parts of the premises including wards.

When handling dangerous organisms, the traditional front-buttoned laboratory coat must not be worn—a gown or wrapover coat fastened by press studs must be used. It must not be worn for more than 2 days and should be discarded into a receptable prior to autoclaving.

Washing facilities

Hand basins with wrist lever taps or foot pedals must be fitted in each laboratory or office where specimens are handled.

Paper towels must be provided and single or roller towels must not be used.

Safety precautions

Smoking, eating and drinking must not be allowed in the laboratory.

Mouth pipetting must never be performed. Glassware with damaged edges should not be used. All broken glassware should be discarded into a clearly identifiable impermeable container.

Hypodermic needles must be placed in commercially available containers with imperforate, not readily penetrable, walls. When full, they must be incinerated.

Bottles should be wiped before returning them to the shelf. Never leave bottles of acids or alkalis where they may be overturned.

Label all bottles clearly to show their contents when working.

Certain dyes, stains and chemicals must be considered as possible harmful substances, for example *corrosive, carcinogenic, highly flammable*, etc. International hazard symbols covered by the EEC are given in *Figure 3.1* and should be clearly labelled on all bottles and containers having these products.

Always use a fume cupboard when working with chemicals which evolve a toxic or irritant vapour.

Keep the working space on the bench clear, so that if an accident occurs the minimum number of articles will be involved.

Spillage from specimens should be covered with a cloth soaked in a suitable disinfectant and left for at least 10 min.

All vessels that have contained specimens must be sterilized by autoclaving at 121°C for 15 min.

Corrosive   Harmful   Oxidising   Irritant

Highly
Flammable   Toxic   Explosive

Figure 3.1. International hazard symbols; these symbols should be in black on an orange-yellow background

Preferably use disposable loops which can be discarded after use, rather than those that require flaming.

Discard cultures into an appropriate receptacle for sterilizing. Cultures must never be removed, once discarded, until they have been sterilized.

The exhaust protective cabinet

All work involved in the handling of infective specimens suspected of harbouring ACDP Group III organisms (see p. 31) should be performed under cover of an exhaust protective cabinet. A warning note 'Danger of infection' within the international 'Biohazard' symbol (*Figure 3.2*) must be permanently displayed on the outside of all doors giving access to rooms dealing with such infective organisms.

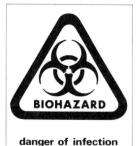

Figure 3.2. 'Danger of infection' warning. The 'Biohazard' symbol has the word 'Biohazard' in black against a black-edged yellow-filled triangle, with the message wording, e.g. 'danger of infection', in black on a general white background

Precautions against fire

When working with highly flammable chemicals in the laboratory the danger of fire should always be kept in mind and adequate precautions taken. Flammable chemicals include benzene, xylene, toluene, acetone, ether and alcohol. It should be remembered that the greater fire hazard is from the vapour given off from the chemical. To guard against this, all flammable chemicals must be securely stoppered when not in use. When working with flammable chemicals all naked flames in the near vicinity should be extinguished. A waste bottle should be kept in all laboratories for the purpose of discarding flammable chemicals. When full, the contents of the waste bottle may be disposed of in a safe place. On no account smoke when handling flammable chemicals.

Fire emergency measures

In the event of fire the following steps should be taken:

1. Sound the alarm.
2. Evacuate from the immediate vicinity of the fire.
3. Close all the doors and windows, turn off all gas and electrical appliances. Attack the fire if possible with the appliances available, but without taking personal risk.

The following equipment for dealing with all minor fires and controlling larger ones should be available in all laboratories. All members of the staff should also be familiar with the location of the fire apparatus adjacent to their own laboratory in cases of emergency.

Hoses

These must be checked regularly to ensure that they are in good working order.

Water and sand buckets

These must be kept filled and covered, checked and refilled periodically.

Fire blankets

These must be fixed in easily accessible positions. They are effective in smothering and preventing the spreading of fires. They are particularly useful for extinguishing fires involving clothing or cotton wool.

Fire extinguishers

Foam type

Used on fires started by solvents immiscible with water, for example xylene. They should *not* be used where live electrical circuits are exposed.

Soda–acid type

Used on fires involving solid material such as paper and wood. They may also be used on water-miscible solvents, but *not* where live electrical circuits are exposed.

Carbon dioxide type

Used on small fires and where live electrical circuits are exposed. They should *not* be used on liquid fires.

Storage of chemicals

Acids must be kept in glass-stoppered bottles preferably in a drip tray. Winchester quart bottles should be stored at floor level.

Alcohol. Duty-free alcohol must be kept locked, and all details of its use recorded. Customs and Excise officials periodically inspect the stock.

Ammonia must be kept tightly stoppered and away from heat and other chemicals.

Bromine ampoules must be stored in absorbent material.

Cyanide and all other poisonous chemicals must be clearly marked 'poison' in red letters, and kept locked in a poisons cupboard; details of all poisons issued should be entered in a poison record book.

Deliquescent and hygroscopic chemicals must be stored in air-tight containers. Such chemicals include potassium and sodium hydroxide, sodium carbonate, phenol and phosphorus pentoxide.

Ether must be kept in a glass bottle, stoppered with a tinfoil-covered cork or a wax-lined bakelite screw top. Never use a rubber bung, as ether attacks rubber, and never store in a refrigerator.

Flammable liquids must be kept well stoppered in a metal container clearly marked 'flammable'. Stocks of such fluids should be kept in a store used solely for this purpose. The store room should have a sunken floor so that in the event of breakages no liquid will flow from the room. Keep the bottles as cool as possible; never use the liquids near a naked flame.

Hydrogen fluoride attacks glass and must be stored in a gutta-percha or polythene bottle.

Hydrogen peroxide must be kept in a brown glass bottle in a refrigerator. Exposure to warmth and light causes oxygen to be evolved, and a pressure sufficient to cause the bottle to explode may be built up.

Iodine must be kept in a brown glass bottle with a glass stopper. Never use a rubber bung, as iodine attacks rubber.

Potassium hydroxide solution should be stored in bottles waxed on the inside, as it attacks glass, forming sodium silicate. Glass stoppers must never be used, as the CO_2 in the air combines with the NaOH, forming Na_2CO_3 which acts as a cement, firmly fixing the stopper into position. The solution in daily use should be stored in an aspirator. A soda-lime guard tube will absorb and prevent any CO_2 from entering the aspirator.

Potassium permanganate must be stored in a dark, glass-stoppered bottle, as it decomposes when exposed to light.

Silver nitrate solution must be kept in a dark, glass-stoppered bottle. Exposure to light decomposes the silver nitrate to silver oxide.

Sodium must *never* be allowed to come into contact with water, as spontaneous combustion will result. Keep completely covered with ligroin, naphtha or xylene.

Sodium hydroxide solution (see Potassium hydroxide, above).

Sodium nitroprusside must be stored in a dark, glass-stoppered bottle, as it decomposes upon exposure to light.

First aid in the laboratory

In the UK, the Health and Safety (First Aid) Regulations 1981 came into effect on 1 July 1982. This means that in the UK an employer is responsible for providing both equipment and trained personnel to satisfy the requirements of the regulations. The minimum requirements must be (a) the provision of first-aid boxes; (b) the appointment of a person to look after the boxes and take charge in cases of serious injury or major illness; (c) to inform employees of the arrangements (local Code of Practice); (d) to keep adequate records of all first-aid treatment.

The definition of 'first aid' is the treatment by people not necessarily qualified to (a) preserve life; (b) minimize the consequences of injury and sudden illness until a qualified person is available; (c) deal with minor injuries that do not need professional attention.

First-aid treatment

All accidents which occur in the laboratory *must* be reported and entered in the accident book according to the local Code of Practice. It is emphasized that the procedures described below are only emergency measures and must be followed immediately by adequate treatment given by a qualified person.

General treatment of superficial wounds

If a limb is involved, raise it to reduce the bleeding. To arrest the flow of blood apply digital pressure with a clean dressing to the wound. Fragments of glass should be left unless they can be easily removed with a sterile dressing. Blood clots which form should not be disturbed. Place a dry sterile dressing over the wound and, if the bleeding is profuse, back the dressing with cotton wool. Bandage firmly into position and obtain further treatment in the casualty or out-patients department.

Nose bleeds

Sit the person upright with the head slightly forward, and get him to pinch the soft part of the nose firmly and to breathe through the mouth.

General treatment of burns and scalds

Dry burns and scalds

Pain produced by burns may be reduced by immersing in cold water as soon as possible or applying a cold compress. Burn dressings, such as tannic acid, should only be applied under a doctor's supervision and blisters must not be punctured.

Chemical burns

Dab away as much of the chemical as possible and bathe with water. If the corrosive chemical is an acid, sprinkle powdered sodium bicarbonate over the site of injury. Phenolic burns should be washed with surgical spirit. If the corrosive chemical is an alkali, sprinkle powdered boracic acid over the affected area. In the event of an alkali entering the eye, immediately wash the eye with water or 1% acetic acid. If acid splashes into the eye, wash with water from a wash bottle and bathe with 5% sodium bicarbonate in an eyebath.

All cases of burns must be referred to a doctor as quickly as possible.

Corrosive poisoning

This is caused by swallowing strong acid or alkali. Treatment consists of rinsing the mouth immediately, followed by copious draughts of water. If acid has been swallowed, milk of magnesia should be given. For alkali poisoning, very dilute acetic acid should be administered. Vomiting should *not* be encouraged. Obtain medical help quickly.

Contamination by infected material

In the event of an accident involving infected material occurring, for example cutting a hand, medical treatment must be obtained immediately.

Electric shock

Switch off the power at source. If the patient is unconscious send for medical assistance immediately and if necessary apply artificial respiration.

Artificial respiration

Mouth-to-mouth resuscitation

If a person has stopped breathing for any reason it is important that resuscitation (*Figure 3.3*) is commenced as quickly as possible—*remember, seconds count*:

1. Pull the victim clear of any immediate danger of further injury.
2. Lay the victim on his back and remove any obstructions from the mouth and throat, for example, loose dentures.
3. Tilt the head back, with the heel of one hand on the forehead and the thumb and forefinger of the same hand pinching the nostrils together to close the air passage. With the other hand push the jaw upwards so that the chin juts out (*Figure 3.3a*).
4. Take a deep breath. Seal your lips around the victim's mouth and blow steadily, watching for chest movements (*Figure 3.3b*).
5. Remove your mouth and watch the chest of the victim fall, at the same time taking another deep breath. Repeat this process a further three times as quickly as possible to saturate the lungs with oxygen (*Figure 3.3c*).
6. This process should be repeated steadily at the normal breathing rate of about 10–15 times per minute.
7. If for any reason, for example injury, you cannot seal your mouth over the victim's mouth, close the victim's mouth and blow in through his nose using the same technique as for mouth-to-mouth resuscitation. Resuscitation should be carried out until (a) the victim starts to breathe for himself again, (b) the arrival of a qualified person, (c) for as long as is possible. If after the first four inflations there is no response, the pulse running along either side of the windpipe in the neck should be checked. If this is absent, the pupils dilated and the victim remains or becomes blue/grey, then the circulation has arrested. External compression of the heart should then be started, while *continuing to ventilate the lungs*.

External cardiac compression

Take up a position to the side of the victim. Place the heel of one hand over the lower half of the breastbone. Cover this hand with the other hand, and with straight arms rock forward and press the lower half of the breastbone down towards the spine (*Figure 3.4*).

Repeat the pressure once a second. If only one person is present, a ratio of two inhalations to fifteen compressions should be aimed for; if two people are present, a ratio of one inhalation to five compressions should be achieved. When a casualty has been successfully resuscitated he should be placed in the recovery position to ensure maintenance of a clear airway (*Figure 3.5*).

If it is suspected that a victim has taken cyanide or other poison by mouth, mouth-to-mouth resuscitation *should not be attempted*, due to the obvious danger to the operator. Alternative methods of resuscitation should be employed, for example, the Holger–Nielsen method (*Figure 3.6*) which is as follows:

1. Place the victim face downwards on a flat surface.
2. Cross his hands level with his forehead, his head being turned to one side so that his cheek rests on the uppermost hand (*Figure 3.6a*).
3. Kneel on one knee at the victim's head, putting your other foot near his elbow (*Figure 3.6b*).
4. Place your hands parallel with his spine, just below the shoulder blades. Keeping your elbows straight, rock forwards until the arms are approximately vertical, exerting steady pressure on the victim's back for 2 seconds (*Figure 3.6c*).
5. Slide your hands along the victim's arm to just

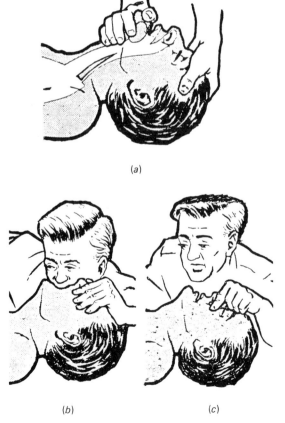

(a)

(b)   (c)

Figure 3.3. Mouth-to-mouth resuscitation (reproduced by courtesy of St John Ambulance)

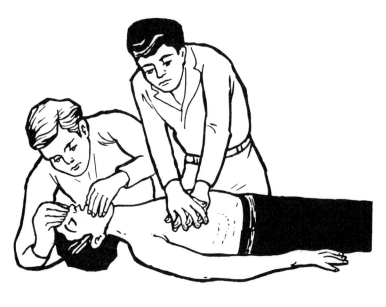

Figure 3.4. External cardiac compression: technique (reproduced by courtesy of St John Ambulance)

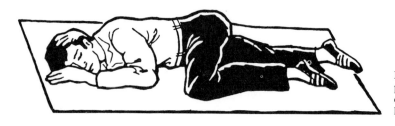

Figure 3.5. External cardiac compression: recovery position (reproduced by courtesy of St John Ambulance)

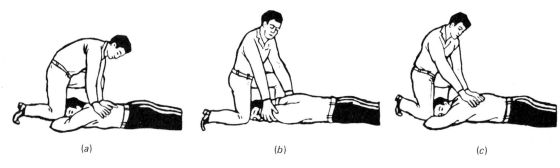

(a)   (b)   (c)

Figure 3.6. Holger-Nielsen resuscitation method (reproduced by courtesy of St John Ambulance)

above the elbow and rock backwards, raising his arms until resistance and tension are felt at his shoulders.

6. The arms are then dropped and the operator's hands returned to the victim's spine.

The phases of expansion and compression should each last 2½ seconds and the complete cycle repeated 12 times per minute. Again, when the victim recovers he should be placed in the recovery position (see *Figure 3.5*) and transported to hospital.

4

Collection and reporting of specimens

Many different types of specimen are received daily in a routine pathology department, and it is necessary to observe certain details to ensure an accurate report with the minimum of delay:

1. The specimen should be clearly labelled with the patient's name, hospital number, ward, date and time of collection.
2. A fully completed 'request form' should accompany each specimen with the details mentioned above, together with the nature and origin of the specimen, the provisional diagnosis, the investigation required, and any other relevant information that can aid the laboratory in setting up the correct test.

In all routine laboratories the quality of the specimen has an effect on the tests that are performed and their results. For example, a sputum for bacteriological examination would be of little value if the specimen was mainly saliva; a urine for culture whose delivery to the laboratory had been delayed for a considerable time would again be of little value as any organisms present would be multiplying within that urine, giving a false picture of possible infection; a clotted blood sample would be of little value for a white cell count, etc.; therefore, for a laboratory to give an adequate service, there must be two-way communication. It is essential that physicians know what specimens to send for a particular investigation, what container should be used and how quickly it should be delivered to the laboratory.

On the other hand, it is equally important that the laboratory help the physician in these matters. One way of achieving this is to issue to the medical staff lists similar to those in *Tables 4.1* and *4.2*, which cover the majority of tests performed in laboratories. Not all of these tests, however, are included in this book.

Receipt of specimens

Hospitals vary with the way in which specimens are collected from the wards, but the following requirements must be fulfilled:

1. The specimen containers must be robust and leak-proof.
2. Special collecting trays or boxes must be used and they must be leak-proof and able to withstand repeated autoclaving or disinfection.
3. All specimens must be carried upright, and therefore the tray or box must have bottle or tube racks fitted.
4. The trays or boxes must be sterilized weekly or after any visible leak or spillage.
5. Requisition forms should be kept separate from the specimens—to prevent them from becoming contaminated. Plastic envelopes for specimens, with a separate sleeve for the request form, are ideal for this purpose.

Specimens that are suspected or contain dangerous pathogens must have a 'Danger of Infection' label affixed and be inserted into a plastic envelope (see above). The reception staff must not handle such labelled specimens. On receipt of the specimen, many hospital laboratories have a central area where it is given a laboratory number, the information on the request form accompanying the specimen is checked, and the specimen and form despatched to the appropriate laboratory. It is essential that the staff working in the reception area are trained to wear protective clothing and must not be permitted to handle leaking or broken specimens.

In most routine histopathology departments, specimens are received in a container of fixative. This should be of a suitable size to contain a volume of fixative approximately 10 times that of the specimen.

Table 4.1 Examination, type and blood volume required

Examination required (1)	Type of blood	Volume required (ml)
Microbiology		
Culture	Into special blood culture bottles see p. 288	10
Virus agglutination		
VD and other serology	C	10
Widal		
Clinical chemistry		
Acid phosphatase, total	C (2)	5
Alcohol	H (3)	10
Aldolase	C	2.5
Alkaline phosphatase	C	2.5
Aminotransferases	C	2.5
Amylase	C	2.5
Ascorbic acid	Consult laboratory	
Barbiturates	H	5
Bicarbonates	see Electrolytes	
Bilirubin	C	2.5
Blood gases	Consult laboratory	
Bromide	C	2.5
Calcium	C (4)	2.5
Chloride	see Electrolytes	
Cholesterol	C	2.5
Cholinesterase	C or H (5)	2.5
Copper	C	2.5
Cortisol	C	5
Creatine	C	2.5
Creatine kinase	C	2.5
Creatinine	C	2.5
Digoxin	C (6)	5
Electrolytes	C	10
Glucose	Oxalated (7)	2.5
γ-Glutamyl transpeptidase	C	2.5
Glycosylated haemoglobin	H	5
Hydroxy butyrate dehydrogenase	C	2.5
Immunoglobins	C	5
Iron		
Iron-binding capacity	C	5
Isoenzymes	C	2.5
Lactate	Consult laboratory	
Lactate dehydrogenase	C	2.5
Lead	H	5
Lipase	C	5
Lithium	C	2.5
Liver function tests	C	10
Magnesium	C	2.5
Methaemalbumin	see Schumm's test	
Methaemoglobin	see Haemoglobin spectroscopy	
Paracetamol	H	5
Phosphatase	H or C	2.5
Proteins/albumin/globulin	C	2.5
Pyruvate	Consult laboratory	
Salicylate	C	2.5
Sodium	see Electrolytes	
Sulphaemoglobin	see Haemoglobin spectroscopy	
Thyroid stimulating hormone		
Thyroxine	C	10
Tri-iodothyronine		
Triglycerides/neutral fat	C	5
Urea	see Electrolytes	
Uric acid	C	2.5
Vitamin A	C	10
Zinc	C	2.5

Table 4.i continued

Examination required (1)	Type of blood	Volume required (ml)
Haematology		
Full blood count (FBC), including		
Haemoglobin		
Red cell count		
White cell count		Volume to line indicated
Platelet count	E	on EDTA bottle (may be
Mean cell volume		2.5, 4 or 5 ml)
Absolute values		
Differential and/or film (8)		
Reticulocyte count		
Erythrocyte sedimentation rate	S (9)	Volume to line
Plasma viscosity	E (10)	Volume to line
Coagulation studies	S (9)	Volume to line. Two bottles required for coagulation screen or factor assays
Fibrin(ogen) degradation products		Special bottle from laboratory. Volume to line
Blood grouping		
Compatibility testing (cross-matching)	C	10
Coombs test (direct or indirect)		
Cold agglutinins	C (11)	10
IM screen (modified Paul Bunnell)	C	5
Serum B_{12}		
Serum folate	C	10
Intrinsic factor antibodies		
Haemoglobinopathy screening	E	Volume to line. Supply details of patient's ethnic origin
Haemoglobin A_2 and F levels		
Platelet function tests	S (10)	Volumes to line. Special bottle may be available from the laboratory for the larger volume of blood (10 ml) required
Osmotic fragility	H	5–10
LE screening test	C	5–10
LE cells	H (or may be special bottle from lab.)	10
Haptoglobins	C	5–10
G-6-PD		
Pyruvate kinase	E	Volume to line
Glutathione reductase	Screening tests	
2,3-DPG	E	Volume to line
Glutathione assay and stability		
Haemoglobin spectroscopy	E	Volume to line
Schumm's test for methaemalbumin	C	10
Ham's test for PNH	E and C	EDTA to line and 5–10 ml clotted

C = clotted; E = EDTA (sequestrene); H = heparinized; S = sodium citrate.

(1) Specimens should be sent to laboratory as quickly as possible to minimize deterioration.
(2) Enzyme degrades very quickly—send promptly to laboratory.
(3) Use an enzyme inhibitor.
(4) Do not use a tourniquet.
(5) Red cell cholinesterase must be kept cold and sent to the laboratory straight away.
(6) Sample must not be taken within 6 h of last dose. Digoxin levels with potassium concentration.
(7) Sodium fluoride is added to prevent glycolysis.
(8) Some recent blood counting instruments perform differential counts automatically as part of their operating cycle.
(9) ESR and coagulation study bottles contain different volumes of sodium citrate and must not be confused.
(10) Specimens must not be refrigerated.
(11) Specimens must be kept at 37°C and sent to the laboratory immediately.

Notes:
(a) Profile tests are carried out for certain groups of estimations and therefore less blood is required.
(b) Micro methods are used in a large number of laboratories, so the above volumes are only to be used as a guideline.
(c) Some laboratories may use a different sample depending upon the methodology used.

Table 4.2 Other specimens; examination and containers required

Specimen and examination required	Specimen container
FAECES	
Microbiology	
Organisms	Sterile wide-mouth screw-capped container
Amoeba	Fresh specimen sent immediately
Clinical chemistry	
Faecal fat	In a plastic carton and consult laboratory
Occult blood	See p. 117
GASTRIC CONTENTS	
Microbiology	
Tuberculosis	Universal container
For other investigations the laboratory should be consulted	
HAIR	
Microbiology	
Fungi	Fold the hairs into clean white paper
PLEURAL, PERITONEAL AND OTHER EFFUSIONS	
Microbiology	
Organisms	20 ml into sterile bottle containing anticoagulant
Histology	Container large enough to accommodate the whole specimen; no sodium citrate
PUS	
Microbiology	
Organisms	Sterile universal container or swab
SALIVA	Sterile universal or disposable container
SPUTUM	
Microbiology	
Organisms	Sterile universal or disposable container
Tuberculosis	Sterile disposable wide-mouth screw-capped container
Histology	
Tumour cells	Sterile universal container
URINE	
Microbiology	
Organisms	Sterile universal container
Tuberculosis	Early morning specimen
Clinical chemistry	
Routine examination	Sterile universal container
Electrolytes	24 h specimen, no preservative
Pregnancy test	Early morning specimen, at least 12 days after last expected menses

The most common incidence of unfixed specimens coming to the laboratory is when specimens for frozen section are sent: here, the theatre should make arrangements with the laboratory so that the staff and equipment are at hand to deal with the specimen. Some specimens are not placed in fixative before sending to the laboratory, such as specimens for histochemistry (muscle biopsies) or specimens in which cytological imprints may be made, e.g. lymph nodes may be bisected, smears made and then a slice(s) of the tissue is put into fixative.

In all cases where specimens are not fixed it is essential that the laboratory staff and theatre staff have an abundantly clear understanding that these specimens must be delivered to the laboratory immediately.

Once the specimens have arrived at the laboratory, they should be correctly identified along with their request forms which have been suitably completed. In many laboratories it is usual to sign the theatre book to acknowledge receipt of correctly identified specimens and forms. Multiple specimens from a patient should be collated, in order that they will ultimately be reported together. They should then be identified with self-adhesive numbered labels on the specimen container (not the lid) and request form.

In general terms, specimens received for cytology are designated gynaecological or non-gynaecological. Almost all gynaecological specimens are received in the laboratory as fixed smears labelled with a pencil. The smears should be transported to the laboratory in a suitable container together with the request form.

Reporting

After the specimen has been processed in the laboratory, it is essential that the information obtained be conveyed to the physician. The 3 Rs of reporting are reliability, rapidity and relevance. Reliability of course speaks for itself. The results must be reliable and they must be transmitted as rapidly as possible. Relevance is of vital importance. Although many tests may be performed on a specimen, it is advisable that only those relevant to the request should be sent. For example, if several antibiotic susceptibility tests are performed on an organism, it is not always advisable to give every result. Only those relevant and consistent with the antibiotic policy of the hospital should be mentioned. The need for information to be given as rapidly as possible often means telephoning results to the ward. This can be a highly dangerous procedure. There are many examples of misinterpretation of results due to either the speaker not being precise, or the recipient misunderstanding. A classic example of this was when the specimen was received from the theatre for a rapid result. The result was phoned through as an adenocarcinoma which was interpreted as 'had no carcinoma'. If results are telephoned, it is essential for the person to read back what has been said so that no mistakes can occur. A written report should be sent as soon as possible.

Reporting systems vary from hospital to hospital and no universal reporting system would necessarily be accepted by everyone. Cumulative reporting, if carried out correctly, is probably the most helpful way both to laboratory and physician. This necessitates each patient having a master card for each discipline and the results are entered onto this card and photocopied, the photocopy being delivered to the ward. By this method the physician can see at a glance any changing pattern of results and this also gives the laboratory a check on their results when compared with the previous ones. Today, more and more laboratories are reporting by computer. This has many advantages, particularly with the storage of reports. If wards have a visual display unit (VDU), reports can be obtained even more rapidly. Whichever system is used, an adequate check must be made that (a) the correct details of the patient's name, ward, hospital number, etc., have been filled in, and (b) the correct result has been entered and the report delivered to the right place.

Postal specimens

The sending of specimens by post is governed by regulations laid down by the Postmaster General. These rules must be strictly adhered to at all times:

1. The specimen must be sent by first class letter post only and must be labelled clearly 'Fragile with Care' and 'Pathological Specimen'.
2. The specimen must be in a sealed container which is robust and leak-proof.
3. The sealed container must be placed in a plastic bag, packed in a fibreboard, wood or metal box which contains sufficient absorbent material such as cotton wool to prevent any possible leakage should the container be damaged en route.

The full regulations may be obtained from the Post Office and if any doubt about a type of box or container in general use exists, the person in charge should submit it to the Secretary of the General Post Office for confirmation of its suitability. Failure to do so may lead to the loss of the specimen and prosecution of the person sending it.

Preparation of specimen containers

It is invariably the duty of the pathology department to issue the many varied containers used for the collection of specimens. Most laboratories in the UK use commercially prepared anticoagulant bottles (disposable), which saves valuable preparation time. For those who have to prepare their own bottles the method of preparation is listed below.

Sterile universal bottles

These are 1 oz glass or plastic bottles, with screw caps. After suitable cleaning and drying the glass bottles are capped and autoclaved at 121°C for 20 min. The plastic bottles are purchased sterilized.

Sequestrene (EDTA) bottles

Dry salt

Sequestrene (disodium salt of ethylenediamine):

Ethylenediamine tetra-acetic acid	10 g
Distilled water	100 ml

Dissolve the salt in the distilled water. Deliver 0.05 ml of solution into small bottles or tubes marked at the 2.5 ml level. Allow the water content of the solution to evaporate at room temperature. Fix screw caps or corks to tubes and label as containers for 2.5 ml of blood.

Heparin bottles

Disposable bottles obtainable commercially. Heparin is a physiological anticoagulant and is used in a concentration of 0.1–0.2 mg per ml of blood. Lithium heparin is to be preferred for electrolyte studies.

Sodium fluoride–potassium oxalate

Sodium fluoride	1.2 g
Potassium oxalate, neutral	6.0 g

Grind the two salts to a fine powder and dissolve in 100 ml of distilled water. Distribute in screw-capped bottles in volumes of 0.05 ml for each ml of blood. Evaporate to dryness in an oven which does not exceed 60°C.

■ Notes

1. Ammonium oxalate should not be used as an anticoagulant for blood which is to be examined biochemically, as it prevents the determination of nitrogen and ruins any analysis which requires the use of Nessler's reagent.
2. Sodium fluoride prevents glycolysis. It should not be used as a preservative, however, when the blood is to be examined for urea by a urease method.

Sodium citrate

Sodium citrate	3.8 g
Distilled water	100 ml

Dissolve the salt in the distilled water. Distribute in small screw-capped bottles in 5 ml or 10 ml amounts and sterilize by autoclaving. Label according to the volume.

Swabs*

Throat, eye, vaginal swabs

A swab for one of these areas consists of a plastic applicator around which a small wisp of absorbent wool is wound to give a small pledget approximately 12 mm in length and 2–3 mm in width.

Ready made and sterilized disposable swabs are available commercially.

Laryngeal swabs

Laryngeal swabs are made from approximately 22.5 cm of brass wire which is slightly bent 5 cm from one end. Absorbent cotton wool is wrapped round this end which is then inserted into a large test-tube, plugged with non-absorbent cotton wool and sterilized by dry heat. Alternatively, calcium alginate wool can be used in place of absorbent cotton wool. This wool will dissolve in a sodium salt solution, and has proved very effective for laryngeal swabs for mycobacteria. The whole swab is investigated, and there is no loss of material by immersion into acid and alkali. Sterilize by autoclaving.

Pernasal swabs

These consist of a small piece of absorbent cotton wool mounted on a fine wire. The wire used should be polished nicrome SWG 22 roughened at one end to prevent the wool from slipping. The wire must be thin and flexible to ensure easy passage into the nares. Place in a 150 × 15 mm tube, plug with non-absorbent wool and sterilize in the hot-air oven.

Pharyngeal (post-nasal) swabs

These consist of a piece of absorbent cotton wool attached to a 20 cm length of flexible wire. The wire

*All the swabs described in this section are available commercially and very rarely made and sterilized in the laboratory.

used should be copper SWG 18 prepared as for pernasal swabs. The cotton wool end should be bent like a hockey stick for easy passage into the pharynx. The whole swab is then enclosed in a piece of curved glass tubing and plugged at both ends with non-absorbent wool. Sterilize in the hot-air oven.

Transport swabs

These may be purchased commercially in pack form, sterilized and ready for use. Each pack contains a tube of solidified transport medium and swab. Various combinations of media and swabs are available, e.g. Stuart's transport medium and Amies medium and plain, charcoal-coated or serum-coated swabs.

Collection of autopsy specimens

Histology

Small pieces of tissue: in bottle containing a suitable fixative.

Whole organs: preserved in Wentworth's solution or 10% formol saline (see p. 184).

Bacteriology

Small pieces of tissue: in sterile universal container.

Collection of biopsy specimens

Histology

In bottle containing a suitable fixative.

Bacteriology

In sterile universal container.

Section 2

Clinical chemistry

5

Some fundamentals of chemistry

The student should have previous knowledge of the following—elements, atoms, isotopes and formulae; chemical units such as atomic weight, molecular weight, gram-atom and gram-molecule*.

Fundamental laws of chemistry

Familiarity with the fundamental laws of chemistry is assumed, but only two have been included because of their particular importance.

1. Law of conservation of mass

Mass can neither be created nor destroyed. This means that in a chemical reaction, there are the same number of atoms of each element in the products as there were in the reactants.

2. Law of constant composition

A given chemical compound, however it is prepared, always contains by weight the same elements in the same proportions.

Note

Many compounds do not obey this law, e.g. ferrous sulphide has variable composition and rarely has the precise formula FeS. Such compounds are called non-stoichiometric or Berthollide compounds.

*In SI units the mole (mol), unit of amount of substance, has replaced gram-atom, gram-molecule, gram-equivalent, etc.

The gas laws

Although an ideal gas is purely hypothetical, the usefulness of the laws is that they are obeyed very closely by gases under normal conditions.

1. Boyle's law

The volume of a given mass of gas at constant temperature is inversely proportional to its pressure, i.e.

$$pv = k$$

where p is the pressure and v is the volume of a fixed quantity of gas at constant temperature; k is the constant.

2. Charles' law

At constant pressure the volume of a given mass of any gas is proportional to its temperature on the absolute scale.

If t is the temperature on the Celsius (centigrade) scale, then the absolute temperature T (K) is equal to $t + 273$. Therefore Charles' law can be expressed as

$$v = k(t + 273)$$
$$v = kT$$

Boyle's and Charles' laws can now be combined to give the following relationship:

$$pv = kT \quad \text{or} \quad \frac{pv}{T} = k$$

The absolute temperature (Kelvin) scale is, as mentioned above, obtained by adding 273 to the temperature in degrees Celsius. For example

$$20°C = (20 + 273) = 293 \text{ K}$$
$$-10°C = (-10 + 273) = 263 \text{ K}$$

Boyle's and Charles' laws can be further elucidated by the following calculation: a gas occupies 250 ml at 30°C and at a pressure of 730 mmHg; calculate the volume of gas at 760 mm and 0°C:

$$\frac{p_1 v_1}{T_1} = \frac{p_2 v_2}{T_2}$$

$p_1 = 730 \text{ mm}$ $v_1 = 250 \text{ ml}$ $T_1 = (273 + 30) = 303 \text{ K}$ $p_2 = 760 \text{ mm}$ $T_2 = 273$

$$v_2 = \frac{730 \times 250 \times 273}{303 \times 760} = 216 \text{ ml}$$

3. Avogadro's law

Equal volumes of all gases at the same temperature and pressure contain equal numbers of molecules. One gram-mole of any gas at a given temperature and pressure will therefore occupy a definite volume, which will be the same for all gases. Therefore, the value k in the equation $pv = kT$ will also be the same for all gases. This standard value k is usually indicated by a special symbol R, the gas constant.

General gas equation

The three gas laws combine to give

$$pv = nRT$$

where p = pressure of gas, v = volume of the gas, n = moles of gas molecules, R = gas constant, and T = absolute temperature. The value of R depends upon the units of p and v:

$$R = \frac{pv}{nT}$$

Numerical value of the gas constant

Experimentally, the volume of 1 mole of a perfect or ideal gas occupies 22.4 litres at 0°C and at 1 atmosphere (standard temperature and pressure, STP).

The value R is then

$$R = \frac{pv}{nT} = \frac{1 \times 22.4}{1 \times 273} = 0.082 \text{ litres/atm/degree/mole}$$

Find the volume of 3.2 g of oxygen at 0°C and 100 atm:

$$pv = nRT$$

One mole of oxygen weighs 32 g,

Therefore, moles of oxygen $= \dfrac{3.2}{32} = 0.10$

$$v = \frac{nRT}{p} \quad \text{or} \quad v = \frac{0.10 \times 0.082 \times 273}{100}$$

$$v = 0.0224 \text{ litres or } 22.4 \text{ ml}$$

Acids and bases

There are several definitions of acids and bases, but the one which is particularly helpful is that of Brønstead-Lowry, who defined acids and bases in terms of proton exchange.

An acid is a substance existing as molecules or ions which can donate a proton, i.e. a proton donor; a base is a molecule or ion which can accept a proton, i.e. a proton acceptor, i.e.

$$\text{acid} \rightleftharpoons \text{base} + \text{proton}$$

where $\rightleftharpoons$ is the reversible reaction sign. This can be considered further by the interaction of acetic acid and water:

$$\underset{\text{acid}}{CH_3COOH} + \underset{\text{base}}{H_2O} \rightleftharpoons \underset{\text{base}}{CH_3COO^-} + \underset{\text{acid}}{H_3O^+}$$

Acetic acid is the proton donor and water the proton acceptor; therefore, water is a base. However, the hydroxonium ion (H_3O^+) is also a proton donor and the proton acceptor is the acetate ion.

Other examples are:

$$\left.
\begin{array}{llll}
\underset{\text{acid}}{HCl} + \underset{\text{base}}{H_2O} \rightleftharpoons \underset{\text{base}}{Cl^-} + \underset{\text{acid}}{H_3O^+} \\
\underset{\text{acid}}{HNO_3} + \underset{\text{base}}{H_2O} \rightleftharpoons \underset{\text{base}}{NO_3^-} + \underset{\text{acid}}{H_3O^+} \\
\underset{\text{acid}}{H_2SO_4} + \underset{\text{base}}{H_2O} \rightleftharpoons \underset{\text{base}}{HSO_4^-} + \underset{\text{acid}}{H_3O^+}
\end{array}
\right\} \quad (1)$$

The essential constituent of acidic solution in water is the hydroxonium ion (H_3O^+). It is responsible for the typical acidic properties namely: (a) sharp taste; (b) ability to change the colour of blue litmus to red; (c) ability to evolve carbon dioxide when added to carbonates.

HCl, HNO_3, H_2SO_4 are termed *strong acids* because they are ionized almost completely in dilute solutions so that there are virtually no molecules of the acid present. Examples of weak acids are lactic and acetic because they do not completely dissociate even in dilute solutions. In the presence of bases stronger than itself, water can function as an acid. This is illustrated by the donation of protons to such bases as ammonia and the carbonate ion (CO_3^{2-}):

$$H_2O + NH_3 \rightleftharpoons NH_4^+ + OH^-$$
$$H_2O + CO_3^{2-} \rightleftharpoons HCO_3^- + OH^-$$

The essential constituent of bases (alkaline solutions) is the hydroxyl ion (OH^-). It is responsible for the typical properties of alkaline solutions, namely: (a) soapy feeling; (b) ability to change the

Table 5.1 Acid–base chart

	Acid	Formula	Base	Formula	
Increasing acid strength ↓	Water	H_2O	Hydroxide ion	OH^-	Increasing basic strength ↑
	Bicarbonate ion	HCO_3	Carbonate ion	CO_3^{2-}	
	Ammonium ion	NH_4^+	Ammonia	NH_3	
	Acetic acid	CH_3COOH	Acetate ion	CH_3COO^-	
	Phosphoric acid	H_3PO_4	Dihydrogen phosphate ion	$H_2PO_4^-$	
	Hydroxonium ion	H_3O^+	Water	H_2O	
	Nitric acid	HNO_3	Nitrate ion	NO_3^-	
	Hydrochloric acid	HCl	Chloride ion	Cl^-	
	Sulphuric acid	H_2SO_4	Bisulphate ion	HSO_4^-	

colour of red litmus to blue; (c) ability to neutralize acids.

NaOH, KOH are termed *strong bases* because they completely dissociate in water liberating the hydroxyl ion.

In the equations (1) the bases Cl^-, NO_3^- and HSO_4^- are termed weak bases because their power of accepting a proton is low.

The trends in acid strength and basic strength are shown in *Table 5.1* which illustrates the important principle: the stronger the acid the weaker the base.

The dissociation of water

Pure water is a bad conductor of electricity. The presence of small amounts of dissolved substances, however, increases the conductance considerably. Distilled water rapidly acquires impurities from the air and from the walls of the containing vessels. Water used as a solvent has to be specially prepared so that its own conductance will be as small as possible. For example, water obtained by deminer-alizing ordinary water by ion exchange resins is described as *conductivity water*.

Pure water is very slightly ionized due to the slight dissociation into H_3O^+ and OH^- ions. For simplic-ity it is usually written

$$H_2O \rightleftharpoons H^+ + OH^- \tag{2}$$

Applying the law of mass action

$$K = \frac{[H^+][OH^-]}{[H_2O]} \tag{3}$$

Since the degree of dissociation is very small $[H_2O]$ can be considered to be constant, so therefore we have a constant K_w which is the ionic product of water, expressed as

$$K_w = [H^+][OH^-] \tag{4}$$

It can be calculated from conductivity experiments that at 25°C, 1 litre of water contains approximately 1×10^{-7} moles of both hydrogen and hydroxyl ions. Hence from (4)

$$K_w = 10^{-7} \times 10^{-7} = 10^{-14}$$

K_w increases with rise in temperature, but as 25°C is commonly used for carrying out experiments, the value at this temperature is the one most frequently used. As the K_w for all aqueous solutions at 25°C will always equal 10^{-14}, if an acid is added to water the H_3O^+ ion concentration will rise but there will be a proportionate decrease in OH^-. Likewise, if alkali is added, there is a rise in OH^- concentration but a proportionate decrease in H_3O^+.

Hydrogen ion concentration and pH

As hydrogen ion concentrations of solutions are a matter of great practical importance, expressing values in terms of 10^{-7} moles per litre is not very convenient.

Sørensen devised the convenient units of pH (puissance d'hydrogen), strength of hydrogen, or pOH (puissance d'hydroxyl) to overcome this difficulty. pH is therefore defined as the logarithm to the base 10 of the reciprocal of the hydrogen ion concentration or the negative value of the logarithm to the base 10 of the hydrogen ion concentration:

$$pH = \log \frac{1}{[H^+]} = -\log[H^+]$$

$$pOH = \log \frac{1}{[OH^-]} = \log[OH^-]$$

But we have said that $[H^+][OH^-] = K_w$

Therefore, $[pH][pOH] = -\log K_w$

Now if $[H^+] = 10^{-7}$
$pH = \log 10^{-7} = pH\ 7.0$

or $[H^+] = 10^{-2}$
        $pH = log 10^{-2} = pH 2.0$

It follows therefore that

A neutral solution has a pH of 7.0
An acid solution has a pH less than 7.0
An alkaline solution has a pH greater than 7.0

Now if we consider 0.1M HCl:
This acid completely dissociates and the $[H^+]$ concentration is 10^{-1} moles per litre. Therefore, pH = 1.0.

Likewise, 0.1M NaOH completely dissociates and the $[OH^-]$ concentration is 10^{-1} moles per litre. Since

$[H^+][OH^-] = 10^{-14}$
$[H^+] = 10^{-13}$

Therefore, pH = 13.0.

In the case of 0.15M HCl, its $[H^+]$ concentration is 1.5×10^{-1} moles per litre:

$log [H^+] 0.15 = \bar{1}.1761$
$- 1 + 0.1761 = - 0.8239$
$pH = 0.8239$

As weak acids and bases are not completely dissociated, the concentration of ions and hence 'acidity' and 'alkalinity' are less. For example:

the pH of 0.1M acetic acid = pH 2.9
pH of 0.1M ammonia   = pH 11.1

Find the pH of 0.1M acetic acid, when the degree of dissociation is 2.0%:

$[H^+] = 0.020 \times 10^{-1} = 0.0020$ g moles per litre

Now if the acid was completely dissociated, the ionic concentration would be 10^{-1} g moles per litre:

$[H^+] = 0.002 = 2.0 \times 10^{-3}$

$pH = log \dfrac{1}{2.0 \times 10^{-3}}$

$= log \dfrac{1}{0.301 \times 10^{-3}} (- 3 + 0.301)$

$pH = 2.699 (2.70)$

Measurement of pH

For the measurement of pH see Chapter 6.

Buffer solutions

It is possible to prepare solutions of known pH by making up solutions of strong acid or alkali of known concentration. For example, 0.0001M HCl has a pH of 4.0, while 0.0001M NaOH has a pH of 10.0. However, these solutions do not retain a constant hydrogen ion concentration for long, as they accept impurities from the air and the walls of the containers. This can best be illustrated by the following examples.

When small amounts of a strong acid or base are added to water, there is a considerable increase in H^+ ion and OH^- ion concentration resulting in a lower and higher pH, respectively. On the other hand, when an equal amount of *acid* is added to a solution of a salt of a weak acid such as sodium hydrogen carbonate ($NaHCO_3$), the pH is lowered only slightly. This is because the salt of the weak acid is freely dissociated in solution and the anion HCO_3^- is a strong base which readily takes up H^+ ions.

$$NaHCO_3 \rightleftharpoons Na^+ + HCO_3$$
$$HCl \rightleftharpoons H^+ + Cl^-$$
$$H^+ + HCO_3^- \rightleftharpoons H_2CO_3$$
carbonic
acid

The result is the replacement of a strong acid freely dissociated by a weak acid only slightly dissociated.

The solution of the salt of a weak acid which absorbs hydrogen ions in this way is a *buffer*. A buffer solution can therefore be described as a mixture of substances in solution which controls the H^+ ion concentration of that solution and maintains it on the addition of reasonable amounts of acid or alkali. It usually contains a mixture of a weak acid and a salt of a strong base, or a weak base and its salt with a strong acid, for example, a mixture of acetic acid and sodium acetate.

Mode of action of acetic acid and sodium acetate

The above-mentioned buffer contains both acetate ions and acetic acid molecules. On the addition of acid to the buffer, the acetate ions combine with the H^+ ions to form undissociated acetic acid:

$$H^+ + CH_3COO^- \rightleftharpoons CH_3COOH$$

while upon the addition of base, the OH^- ions combine with the H^+ ions from acetic acid to form water and an acetate ion:

$$OH^- + H^+ \rightleftharpoons H_2O$$

In this way the additional H^+ ions and OH^- ions are removed from the solution. Other examples of buffers are (a) hydrochloric acid and potassium hydrogen phthalate; (b) hydrochloric acid and potassium chloride; (c) sodium dihydrogen phosphate and disodium hydrogen phosphate.

Buffering capacity and range of buffer action

Different buffers have a different 'buffering capacity'; that is, they vary in their resistance to the addition of H^+ and OH^- ions. By varying the proportions of the constituents in a buffer system, solutions of different pH may be prepared. For example, in Appendix II it can be seen that if 50 ml 0.2M potassium hydrogen phthalate is added to 46.60 ml 0.2M hydrochloric acid and diluted to 200 ml with distilled water, a pH of 2.2 is obtained. On the other hand, pH 8.3 is obtained when the same amount of phthalate is added to 2.65 ml of hydrochloric acid and diluted to 200 ml. However, the range of buffer action of a particular system is limited because the buffering capacity reaches a maximum at a certain pH and falls off on either side of its maximum point.

Solutions

Solute and solvent

In a solution of one substance in another, the dissolved substance is called the solute and the substance in which the solute is dissolved is called the solvent.

Saturated solutions

If a few grams of sodium chloride are added to 100 ml of water the salt will dissolve, but if further quantities are added a stage is reached when solid sodium chloride remains and no more dissolves. Such a solution is said to be saturated. A saturated solution, therefore, is one which contains as much solute (dissolved substance) as it can dissolve, in the presence of the solid solute. This last proviso is very important, because it is possible to prepare, sometimes quite easily, supersaturated solutions containing more solute than the saturation value. However, supersaturated solutions are metastable, and the addition of solute to them causes precipitation of excess dissolved solute until the concentration falls to the saturation value; that is, a supersaturated solution cannot exist in the presence of solid solute. Therefore, when making a saturated solution always make sure that some solute remains undissolved.

Solubility

The concentration of a saturated solution at a particular temperature is called the solubility of the solute in the particular solvent.

Solubilities are usually expressed as the number of grams of solute dissolved in 100 ml of distilled water (see Appendix II).

Temperature effects

Usually solubility rises with temperature. For example, the solubility of sodium hydroxide at 100°C is eight times higher than it is at 0°C. The temperature effect is very variable; however, the solubility of sodium chloride increases hardly at all between 0°C and 100°C, and for a few compounds, such as lithium carbonate, the solubility decreases with rise in temperature.

Concentrations of solutions

The concentration of a solution is the amount of solute in a given amount of solution. There are several ways of expressing concentrations:

1. Percentage solutions (w/v) contain x g of solute in 100 ml of solution, for example, 20% Na_2CO_3 is made by dissolving 20 g of solid sodium carbonate in distilled water and making the final volume up to 100 ml with distilled water.
2. Weight per cent solutions (w/w) contain x g of solute in 100 g of solution.
3. Molar solutions (mol/l; M) contain 1 mole of the solute dissolved in and made up to 1000 ml with solvent. For example:

   M Na_2CO_3 contains 105.988 g/l
   M NaCl   contains 58.44 g/l

4. Millimoles per litre (mmol/l) expresses the strength in terms of the molecular weight in milligrams per litre of solution. For example:

   A solution containing 1 mmol/l of NaCl contains 58.44 mg/l
   A solution containing 1 mmol/l of Na_2CO_3 contains 105.988 mg/l

5. A mole (mol) is the molecular weight of a substance expressed in grams.

   When studying chemical changes it is often desirable to consider the *numbers* of reacting atoms, ions and molecules rather than their masses. Numbers are measured in *moles* and 1 mole is the number of carbon atoms in 12 g of neutral atoms of carbon 12. This number $= 6.023 \times 10^{23}$; that is, a mole of O_2 means 6.023×10^{23} oxygen molecules; of Na: 6.023×10^{23} sodium atoms; of NO_3^-: 6.023×10^{23} nitrate ions.

   The mass of a mole of a substance is obtained from the fact that a mole of atoms of carbon 12 (the basis of the atomic weight scale) has a mass of 12 g. Hence, there is 1 mole of atoms in 1.008 g H; 16 g O; 32.06 g S; 23 g Na; 35.45 g Cl. Similarly, there is 1 mole of molecules in 32 g O_2; 98.08 g H_2SO_4; 18.015 g H_2O, and 1 mole of sodium ions and 1 mole of chlorine ions in 58.443 g NaCl.

■ Note

'Normal saline' usually refers to a physiological saline (0.85%), which is isotonic with body fluids.

Simple qualitative analysis

Simple tests to identify certain cations and anions.

Cations

Flame test—moisten the substance with concentrated hydrochloric acid, dip a platinum wire or porcelain rod into the mixture and apply it to the base of a non-luminous bunsen flame (*Table 5.2*).

Table 5.2 Results of flame test

Flame coloration	Colour seen through blue glass	Inference
Persistent yellow	Invisible	Sodium
Violet	Crimson	Potassium
Brick-red	Light green	Calcium
Green flashes	Bluish green	Barium
Green (blue zone)	Bluish green	Copper

Ammonium NH_4^+—boil with 5M sodium hydroxide solution. Ammonia gas, which turns moistened red litmus paper from red to blue and has a characteristic smell, is evolved:

$$NH_4^+ + OH^- \rightarrow NH_3 + H_2O$$

Calcium Ca^{2+}—to a concentrated solution of the substance made alkaline with ammonium hydroxide add a 3% solution of ammonium oxalate. A white precipitate of calcium oxalate, $CaC_2O_4.H_2O$, is formed.

Iron—when freshly prepared, all ferrous solutions are pale green in colour; on standing in air they are oxidized to the yellowish-red ferric state.

Fe^{2+}—a solution of a ferrous salt gives a dirty-green gelatinous precipitate of ferrous hydroxide when made alkaline with sodium hydroxide solution.

Fe^{3+}—a ferric salt solution gives a reddish-brown gelatinous precipitate of ferric hydroxide with sodium hydroxide.

Fe^{3+}—intense blue precipitate (Prussian blue)

$$KFe[Fe(CN)_6].H_2O$$

formed with a 5% solution of potassium ferrocyanide $K_4[Fe(CN)_6].3H_2O$:

$$Fe^{3+} + Fe(CN)_6^{4-} \rightarrow Fe[Fe(CN)_6]^-$$

Anions

Halides—to a solution in distilled water, add dilute nitric acid, followed by silver nitrate solution.

Chloride—white curdy precipitate of silver chloride, which is readily soluble in M ammonia solution:

$$AgCl + 2NH_3 \rightarrow Ag[(NH_3)]_2^+ + Cl^-$$

Bromide—whitish-yellow precipitate of silver bromide, not readily soluble in M ammonia solution, but will dissolve easily in concentrated (0.880) ammonia solution.

Iodide—yellow precipitate of silver iodide, insoluble in ammonia solution of any concentration.

Sulphate—to a solution in water, add dilute hydrochloric acid, followed by a 6% solution of barium chloride. White precipitate of barium sulphate:

$$Ba^{2+} + SO_4^{2-} \rightarrow BaSO_4 \downarrow$$

Nitrate—brown ring test: to a cold solution add an equal volume of a freshly prepared saturated solution of ferrous sulphate. Pour a few ml of concentrated sulphuric acid into a boiling tube, and then very carefully, so as to avoid mixing, pour the prepared solution down the side of the tube to form a layer on top of the sulphuric acid. A brown ring forms at the junction of the two liquids, due to the formation of the unstable compound $Fe(NO)SO_4$. On shaking and warming, nitric oxide, NO, is evolved, and the brown colour disappears.

Carbonate—to the solid add dilute nitric acid. Effervescence occurs, and carbon dioxide, which is liberated, can be detected by passing the gas into 'limewater' (saturated solution of calcium hydroxide), when a white precipitate of calcium carbonate is formed:

$$CO_3^{2-} + 2H^+ \rightarrow H_2O + CO_2$$
$$CO_2 + Ca(OH)_2 \rightarrow CaCO_3 \downarrow + H_2O$$

Quantitative analysis

Volumetric (titrimetric) analysis

In volumetric analysis, the volume of a solution of accurately known concentration is allowed to react

Table 5.3 Reagents for titration of primary standards

Primary standards	For titration with	Indicator
Anhydrous sodium carbonate (Na_2CO_3)	Hydrochloric acid (HCl)	Methyl orange
Sodium chloride (NaCl)	Silver nitrate ($AgNO_3$)	Potassium chromate
Sodium oxalate ($Na_2C_2O_4$)	Potassium permanganate ($KMnO_4$)	None needed
Silver nitrate ($AgNO_3$)	Potassium thiocyanate (KCNS)	Ferric alum
Potassium hydrogen phthalate ($KHC_8H_4O_4$)	Bases	Phenolphthalein
Disodium tetraborate (borax) ($Na_2B_4O_7.10H_2O$)	Hydrochloric acid (HCl)	Methyl red

quantitatively with a solution of the substance being titrated. The solution of known concentration is the standard solution containing a definite number of moles per litre. The unknown substance is titrated by adding standard solutions until the reaction is just complete (*Table 5.3*). This 'end-point' is shown by a colour change, due either to the standard solution or a colour change given by an indicator, or the end-point may be revealed by the deposition of a precipitate. The complete process is called a *titration*. There are three main categories of titration: (a) neutralization reactions; (b) oxidation–reduction reactions; and (c) precipitation reactions.

In volumetric analysis there are always two types of standard solutions, primary and secondary.

Primary standards

To obtain a reference for volumetric analysis, certain primary standards are used, each of which should satisfy the following requirements:

1. It must be stable, easy to obtain, to dry and to preserve in a pure state.
2. It should have a large molecular weight, to lessen the effect of errors in weighing.
3. It must not be altered in air during weighing (i.e. absorb moisture during weighing).
4. It must be readily soluble in the solvent.
5. The titration reaction with the standard solution should be stoichiometric (theoretical end-point) and practically instantaneous.
6. It should not give rise to any product likely to interfere with the titration.

Ideal primary standards are difficult to obtain and hence a substance meeting as closely as possible the ideal requirements is usually made.

Secondary standards

Unlike primary standards, which can be accurately weighed, some substances cannot be made directly into solutions of known concentrations. They must first be prepared to an approximate concentration and then titrated against a primary standard to obtain the precise concentrations. Such substances are known as 'secondary standards'. Various acid solutions, for example hydrochloric (not the constant boiling point mixture), nitric, sulphuric and acetic acid, can be distilled to a given approximate concentration, and by suitable titration against the base, a secondary standard of precise concentration can be prepared. On the other hand, sodium and potassium hydroxide for example, although in solid form, cannot be weighed accurately, as the material deliquesces and combines with the carbon dioxide in the air. Solutions of greater concentration than those finally required are prepared, titrated against a suitable standard solution and then diluted to give the required standard solution. The concentration is again checked by repeating the titration procedure. This is rather a cumbersome way of standardization and it may be more convenient to work out a factor for the secondary standard (see p. 52). Sodium and potassium hydroxide solutions are not stable unless kept in a suitable container (polythene) and if required for daily use, the vessel must be fitted with a soda-lime guard tube to prevent carbon dioxide from entering the solution.

Neutralization indicators

Neutralization indicators are substances which dissociate in solution into two (or more) different coloured forms, the nature of the form present being governed by the pH of the solution. An indicator may be used for determining the pH of a solution or for determining the end-point of an acid–base titration.

Theory of indicators

Indicators are either very weak acids or very weak bases. Let HIn represent the weak acid indicator. In water this will be ionized as follows:

$$HIn + H_2O \rightleftharpoons H_3O^+ + In^-$$

where HIn and In^- have different colours. The equilibrium constant is

$$\frac{[H_3O^+][In^-]}{[H_2O][HIn]} = K$$

If an acid is added to the indicator solution, the effect of the added H_3O^+ ions will be to decrease the concentration of In^+ and increase the concentration of HIn. That is, the indicator will be almost completely in the HIn coloured form.

On the other hand, if an alkali is added the H_3O^+ itself is neutralized and further ionization promoted, i.e. more In^- is produced and its colour predominates.

Let In represent the weak base indicator. In water this will be ionized as follows:

$$H_2O + In \rightleftharpoons HIn^+ + OH^-$$

where In and HIn^+ have different colours.
The equilibrium constant is

$$\frac{[HIn^+][OH^-]}{[H_2O][In]} = K$$

If an alkali is added, the OH^- ions will force the point of equilibrium to the left, and the In-coloured form will predominate. If acid is added, the base OH^- is neutralized and the dissociation left to right is favoured, with the HIn^+ colour predominating.

Each indicator has a pH range over which a visible colour change occurs called the 'colour change interval'. Some of the properties of the more common indicators are given in *Table 5.4*.

Table 5.4 Quantitative analysis

Indicator	Colour in 'acid' solution	Colour in 'alkaline' solution	Colour change interval
Methyl orange	Red	Orange-yellow	3.1–4.6
Methyl red	Red	Yellow	4.2–6.3
Bromothymol blue	Yellow	Blue	6.0–7.6
Phenol red	Yellow	Red	6.8–8.4
Phenolphthalein	Colourless	Red	8.0–9.8

Acid–base titrations

At the equivalence point, the ions in solution are the same as if the pure salt of the base and acid had been dissolved, and the resultant pH depends on the extent to which the salt is hydrolysed.

Strong acid: strong base (for example, sodium hydroxide and hydrochloric acid)

The pH at the equivalent point is 7 because the salt, for example sodium chloride, is not hydrolysed. Also, a very small amount of titrant at the equivalence point causes a large change in pH from about 3 to 10, so it is not necessary to employ an indicator having a colour change interval covering pH = 7. In practice, any indicator between methyl orange and phenolphthalein is satisfactory. This assumes that carbon dioxide from the air is not dissolved in the alkali because dissolved carbon dioxide acts as an acid to phenolphthalein. If the alkali is not carbon dioxide-free, then methyl orange is a suitable indicator. In the titration of sodium carbonate with hydrochloric acid the solution is saturated with carbon dioxide at the equivalence point causing a pH of about 3.5, and again methyl orange is the indicator that should be used.

Weak acid: strong base (for example, acetic acid and sodium hydroxide)

The pH at the equivalence point is >7, that is, alkaline because the anion of the weak acid, for example acetate ion, combines with water to form un-ionized acid and hydroxyl ions:

$$AcO^- + H_2O \rightleftharpoons AcOH + OH^-$$
Acetate ion   Acetic acid

Because the relationship $[H_3O^+][OH^-] = 10^{-14}$ always holds, the formation of OH^- ions by the hydrolysis is accompanied by a decrease in H_3O^+ concentration, and hence a pH > 7.

Apart from the fact that the equivalence point occurs on the alkaline side, the change in pH for a small addition of titrant at the equivalence point varies from about 6 to 11. Methyl orange is quite valueless for this titration, since it completes its colour change before the equivalence point is reached. Phenolphthalein should be used for this class of titration.

Strong acid: weak base (for example, hydrochloric acid and ammonium hydroxide)

The pH at the equivalence point is <7, that is, acidic, because the cation of the weak base, for example ammonium, combines with water to form un-ionized base and hydroxonium ions:

$$NH_4^+ + H_2O \rightleftharpoons NH_3 + H_3O^+$$
Ammonium   Ammonia

The addition of a small quantity of titrant at the equivalence point causes a pH change from about 4 to 8. Phenolphthalein is not satisfactory and methyl red or methyl orange should be used.

Weak acid: weak base (for example, acetic acid and ammonium hydroxide)

The pH at the equivalence point is 7, but the change in pH is so gradual that no indicator gives a sharp colour change. For this reason such titrations are not practicable.

Preparation of volumetric solutions

Volumetric analysis, like many other types of analysis, has changed over the past few years, the change being mainly in the introduction of molar instead of normal solutions.

A molar solution contains 1 g mole of the solute dissolved in and made up to 1000 ml with solvent, e.g.

1M HCl contains 36.5 g
1M H_2SO_4 contains 98.0 g
1M NaOH contains 40.0 g
1M $Ba(OH)_2$ contains 171.36 g

The use of factors in volumetric analysis

Factors are very important in volumetric analysis because they save all the problems of preparing exactly standardized volumetric solutions, i.e. diluting down a solution of sodium hydroxide after the initial titration until it is exactly 0.1 M, a step which is very difficult to carry out satisfactorily.

Rules in volumetric analysis

Finding a factor (F): method 1

If we have in our laboratory 0.02M NaOH with a factor value of 1.032 and we require to standardize a solution of approximately 0.02M sulphuric acid, we then have to find the factor for the sulphuric acid:

$$H_2SO_4 + 2NaOH \rightarrow Na_2SO_4 + 2H_2O$$

In the above equation

$$1M\ H_2SO_4 = 2M\ NaOH$$

Therefore, 1000 ml M H_2SO_4 = 2000 ml M NaOH.
If 20 ml aliquot of approximately 0.02M H_2SO_4 required 38.4 ml 0.02M NaOH of factor 1.032, then from the equation we know that

$$1\ ml\ 0.02M\ H_2SO_4 = 2\ ml\ 0.02M\ NaOH$$

Therefore, 20 ml approximately 0.02M H_2SO_4 = 38.4 × 0.02M NaOH (factor 1.032). Then

$$1\ ml\ 0.02M\ NaOH = \frac{38.4 \times 1.032}{2^* \times 20}$$

$$= 0.9907\ ml\ of\ exactly\ 0.02M\ H_2SO_4$$

or F for 0.02M H_2SO_4 is 0.9907.

Finding a factor (F): method 2

By standardization of a substance, e.g. NaOH, using a pure solid primary standard. First of all calculate the weight of primary standard to be weighed out:

$$1\ mole\ of\ primary\ standard = 1000\ ml\ M\ NaOH$$

Then

$$\frac{MW}{1000} = 1\ ml\ M\ NaOH$$

As the titres are usually around 20 ml we then need to weigh out (MW/1000) × 20 of primary standard to give a reasonable titration figure.
Example using potassium hydrogen phthalate (PHT) ($C_6H_4COOHCOOK$):

$$1000\ ml\ M\ PHT\ contains\ 204.22\ g$$

Therefore, 1000 ml 0.1M PHT contains 20.422 g. Then 20 ml 0.1M PHT will contain

$$\frac{20.422}{1000} \times 20 = 0.40844\ g$$

If 0.405 g of PHT were weighed out accurately, transferred to a conical flask, dissolved in distilled water and titrated with approximately 0.1M NaOH and a titre of 19.5 ml was obtained, then

$$F\ for\ NaOH = \frac{0.4050}{0.4084 \times (19.5/20)} = 1.017$$

*2 is included in the calculation because of the difference in equivalence.

Therefore, to find the F for a substance using a solid primary standard, the following calculation can be used:

$$F = \frac{\text{Weight of primary standard actually used}}{\text{Calculated weight should have used} \times (\text{Titre/Calculated titre})}$$

Primary standards can easily be weighed out because they conform to the criteria laid down on p. 51, but in the case of secondary standards such as strong acids, a known volume of acid is usually diluted to a given volume to give an approximate solution. The volume of acid required can be readily calculated from the specific gravity and the percentage composition.
The specific gravity of concentrated hydrochloric acid is 1.18; the percentage composition is 35.4% (w/w), and the molecular weight is 36.5; therefore, the volume of acid required to make a litre of molar solution is as follows:

Sp. gr. of concentrated HCl = 1.18   i.e. 1 ml HCl weighs 1.18 g
percentage composition = 35.4

Then, number of ml concentrated HCl equivalent to 36.5 g is

$$36.5 \times \frac{100}{1.18} \times \frac{100}{35.4} = 87.2\ ml$$

Thus, if 87.2 ml of concentrated HCl are diluted to 1 litre, an approximately molar solution is obtained.
The specific gravity of concentrated sulphuric acid is 1.83; the percentage composition is 96.0% (w/w) and the molecular weight is 98. Therefore, the volume of acid required to be diluted to a litre to prepare an approximately molar solution is as follows:

$$98 \times \frac{1.0}{1.83} \times \frac{100}{98} = 54.6\ ml$$

Preparation of approximately 0.1M hydrochloric acid

Measure out from a burette 9 ml pure concentrated hydrochloric acid into a litre volumetric flask containing about 500 ml of distilled water and dilute to 1 litre. Mix well and this will give an approximately 0.1M hydrochloric acid solution.

Standardization against pure anhydrous sodium carbonate

$$Na_2CO_3 + 2HCl \rightarrow 2NaCl + H_2O + CO_2$$

From the above equation, 1 mole of Na_2CO_3 is equivalent to 2 moles of HCl; therefore,

1000 ml 0.05M Na_2CO_3 = 1000 ml 0.1M HCl
20 ml 0.05M Na_2CO_3 =   20 ml 0.1M HCl

Then

$$\frac{0.05\ MW}{1000} \times 20\ g\ of\ Na_2CO_3 = 20\ ml\ 0.1M\ HCl$$

or

$$\frac{0.05 \times 106}{1000} \times 20 = 0.106\ g\ Na_2CO_3$$
$$= 20\ ml\ 0.1M\ HCl$$

Therefore, if 0.106 g Na_2CO_3 was weighed out, dissolved in water and then titrated with the HCl solution, a reasonable titre should be obtained. This is a far better technique than making up an accurate 0.05M solution of Na_2CO_3, because one does not need to weigh out exactly 0.106 g of solid; any weight around this figure can be used, provided it is accurately weighed (see below).

Procedure

1. AR grade of anhydrous sodium carbonate is 99.9% pure, but it does contain a little moisture and must be dehydrated by heating at 260–270°C for 1 h and then allowed to cool in a desiccator before use.
2. Dry 5–6 g of anhydrous sodium carbonate as above.
3. Prepare three 250 ml conical flasks (A,B,C) with a funnel in the neck of each.
4. Weigh out accurately from a weighing bottle about 0.110 g of the pure sodium carbonate and transfer quantitatively, with washing, to the conical flask. Rinse the funnel thoroughly with distilled water, allowing washings to run into the flask. Add a total of about 50 ml of distilled water to dissolve completely.
5. Repeat the same procedure for flasks B and C.
6. Add a few drops of methyl orange indicator to each flask, or preferably methyl orange indigo carmine indicator.*
7. Rinse out a 25 ml burette with the approximately 0.1M acid solution several times; fill the burette to a point 2–3 cm above the zero mark and open stopcock until the jet is completely filled with liquid. Refill if necessary to bring the liquid above the zero mark; then slowly run out the excess acid until the liquid meniscus is at the zero mark. Read the position of the meniscus to 0.01 ml.

*Preparation of indicators:
1. Methyl orange—0.1 g methyl orange per 100 ml water.
2. Methyl orange–indigo carmine—0.1 g methyl orange and 0.25 g indigo carmine per 100 ml water. The colour change on passing from alkaline to acid solution is from green to magenta with a neutral grey colour at pH of about 4.0.

8. Place a white tile beneath the flask in order to see the colour changes more readily. Run the acid slowly into flask A from the burette. During the addition of the acid, the flask must be constantly rotated with one hand while the other hand controls the stopcock. When the orange colour lightens to a yellow tint or the green colour of the mixed indicator becomes paler the end-point is near. Rinse the walls of the flask with a little distilled water, and continue the titration drop by drop, until the colour becomes orange or a faint pink or in the case of the mixed indicator grey. This marks the end-point of the titration and the burette reading is noted.
9. Repeat the titration, using flasks B and C, and note the titration readings. Calculate the molarity from each titre. Average the values.
10. *Calculation of molarity of HCl solution:*

$$Molarity = \frac{w \times t \times M}{W \times V}$$

where w is the weight of primary standard used, t the theoretical titre, W the calculated weight, V the actual volume used, and M the assumed molarity.
Example: 0.125 g of Na_2CO_3 required 19.5 ml HCl solution. Therefore,

$$Molarity = \frac{0.125 \times 20}{0.106 \times 19.5} \times 0.1 = 0.121M$$

11. The bulk of the hydrochloric acid solution can then be diluted with distilled water to obtain a theoretically exact 0.1M solution by using the following calculation.
12. As the acid is 0.121M, it must be diluted with distilled water to obtain a concentration closer to 0.1M. The acid is 1.21 times too concentrated; therefore, dilute the acid to the proportion of 1.00/1.21 = 0.826.
13. Place 826 ml of the 0.121M HCl into a litre volumetric flask and carefully dilute to 1000 ml with distilled water and thoroughly mix.
14. If this diluted solution of acid is then titrated against Na_2CO_3 and it is found to be 0.105M, further dilutions are unnecessary as the bottle is labelled 0.1M HCl:

F = 1.05

Preparation of 0.1M sodium hydroxide

A standard solution of sodium hyroxide cannot be made from direct weighing because it is hygroscopic and contains sodium carbonate formed from atmospheric carbon dioxide. Also a solution for titration should be carbonate-free, otherwise it is not possible to obtain an exact end-point with phenolphthalein. For most purposes the AR sodium hydroxide (which contains 1.2% of sodium carbonate) is sufficiently pure.

Procedure

1. The molecular weight of NaOH is 40 and therefore 0.1M NaOH contains 4.0 g per litre.
2. Weigh out about 5 g of dry sodium hydroxide pellets on a watch glass and transfer quantitatively to a 500 ml Pyrex beaker and dissolve in about 300 ml carbon dioxide-free distilled water. Warm if necessary. Cool and transfer quantitatively to a 1 litre volumetric flask. Wash out the beaker with more carbon dioxide-free water and transfer the washings to the volumetric flask; dilute to the mark and mix well. Transfer to a reagent bottle fitted with a rubber stopper.

Standardization of sodium hydroxide solution

Using 0.1M HCl

1. Pipette 20 ml 0.1M HCl into each of four 250 ml conical flasks, add a few drops of phenolphthalein indicator. The solution should be colourless.
2. Fill a 25 ml burette in the same way as described on p. 6 and titrate until a permanent light pink coloured end-point is obtained. Note the titre.
3. Repeat the titration until duplicate determinations agree to within 0.05 ml of each other.
4. *Calculation of molarity of sodium hydroxide solution:*
Suppose 19.0 ml of sodium hydroxide were required to neutralize 20.0 ml 0.1M HCl of factor 1.05:

20.0 ml 0.1M HCl of factor 1.05 = 21.0 ml 0.1M HCl

Therefore, as 21.0 ml 0.1M HCl = 19.0 ml of approx. 0.1M NaOH,

$$\text{Molarity of NaOH} = \frac{21.0 \times 0.1}{19.0} = 0.1105M$$

0.1105M NaOH is the same as 0.1M NaOH of factor 1.105 and the reagent bottle should be labelled as such.

Using potassium hydrogen phthalate (PHT)

$$NaOH + C_6H_4COOHCOOK \rightarrow$$
$$C_6H_4COONaCOOK + H_2O$$

From the above equation 1M NaOH is equivalent to 1M PHT; therefore, 20 ml 0.1M NaOH = 20 ml 0.1M PHT):

20 ml 0.1M NaOH

$$= \frac{0.1MW\ PHT}{1000} \times 20\ g\ of\ PHT$$

$$= \frac{0.1 \times 204.22}{1000} \times 20\ g\ of\ PHT$$

20 ml 0.1M NaOH = 0.4083 g of PHT.

Procedure

1. AR PHT has a purity of at least 99.9%; it is almost non-hygroscopic, but it should be dried at 120°C for 2 h and allowed to cool in a desiccator.
2. Weigh out three 0.4–0.5 g accurately and transfer to 250 ml flasks in the same way as described on p. 54.
3. Add 75 ml boiled distilled water and shake gently to dissolve.
4. Titrate with the sodium hydroxide solution using phenolphthalein* as indicator. Note the titre.
5. Repeat the titration with the other two weighings.
6. Calculation of molarity as for hydrochloric acid (see p. 54).
Example: 0.45 g of PHT required 20.0 ml of approximately 0.1M NaOH; therefore,

$$\text{Molarity} = \frac{0.45 \times 20.0}{0.4083 \times 20.0} \times 0.1$$
$$= 0.1103M\ (0.110M)$$

7. Calculate the molarity from each weighing and average the values. Label the reagent bottle accordingly.

Preparation of 0.1M silver nitrate solution

AR silver nitrate has a purity of at least 99%. Although it is an excellent primary standard, it is still advisable to dry some finely powdered $AgNO_3$ at 250°C for 1–2 h, allowing to cool in a desiccator.

Procedure

1. The molecular weight of $AgNO_3$ is 169.876 and therefore 0.1M $AgNO_3$ contains 16.9876 g per litre (in theory this weight should be multiplied by the purity factor for AR silver nitrate, e.g. 1/0.999).
2. Weigh out accurately 8.4938 g dissolved in distilled water and transfer quantitatively to a 500 ml volumetric flask. Dilute to the mark and mix well.

---

*Preparation of indicator: phenolphthalein—0.5 g in 50% alcohol.

Titration of silver nitrate solution

Mohr's method

Principle

In this method potassium chromate (5% w/v) is used as an indicator and silver chromate, although only sparingly soluble, is more soluble than silver chloride. Consequently, when chloride is titrated with silver nitrate no silver chromate is precipitated until all the chloride has been precipitated. The next drop of silver nitrate after the end-point then produces a deep red precipitate of silver chromate. The solution then darkens due to the masking effect of the white chloride precipitate.

Potassium chromate should only be used in neutral solution. In acidic solution the chromate is converted into dichromate and the end-point is poor. In alkaline solution, the hydroxide ion precipitates silver oxide:

$$AgNO_3 + NaCl \rightarrow AgCl + NaNO_3$$

From the above equation 1M $AgNO_3$ is equivalent to 1M sodium chloride; therefore, 20 ml 0.1M $AgNO_3$ = 20 ml 0.1M sodium chloride:

$$20 \text{ ml } 0.1\text{M } AgNO_3 = \frac{0.1 \text{ MW}}{1000} \times 20 \text{ g of NaCl}$$

$$= \frac{0.1 \times 58.46}{1000} \text{ 20 g of NaCl}$$

$$20 \text{ ml } 0.1\text{M } AgNO_3 = 0.1168 \text{ g of NaCl}$$

Procedure

1. AR sodium chloride has a purity of 99.9–100%. Although an excellent primary standard, it is slightly hygroscopic and should be dried at 250°C for 1–2 h, then allowed to cool in a desiccator.
2. Weigh out three 0.125 g accurately and transfer to 250 ml flasks in the same way as described on p. 54.
3. Dissolve in about 50 ml of distilled water and shake gently to dissolve.
4. Add 1 ml of 5% potassium chromate solution.
5. Slowly add the silver nitrate solution from a burette with constant shaking until the red colour formed by the addition of each drop begins to disappear more slowly: this is an indicator that most of the chloride has been precipitated.
6. Continue the addition of the silver nitrate until a faint but distinct change in colour occurs. The faint reddish-brown colour should persist after brisk shaking. Note the titre.
7. Repeat the titration with the other two weighings.
8. Calculation of molarity as for hydrochloric acid (see p. 54).

Example: 0.125 g of sodium chloride required 20.5 ml of 0.1M $AgNO_3$. Therefore,

$$\text{Molarity} = \frac{0.125}{0.1168} \times \frac{20.0}{20.5} \times 0.1$$

$$= 0.1\text{M NaCl}$$

9. Calculate the molarity from each weighing and average the values. Label the amber reagent bottle accordingly.

Alternative procedure

Weigh out accurately about 2.923 g pure dry sodium chloride from a weighing bottle, dissolve in water and dilute to 500 ml. Pipette 20 ml portions into 250 ml conical flasks, add 1 ml of 5% potassium chromate and titrate as above. Note the titre. Repeat the titration until duplicate determinations agree to within 0.05 ml of each other.

Calculation

2.923 g NaCl dissolved in 500 ml water is an exact 0.1M solution. If 2.900 g is the exact amount weighed out, then the molarity of the resulting solution is

$$\frac{2.900 \times 0.100}{2.923} = 0.0993\text{M}$$

Suppose 19.7 ml of the silver nitrate solution were required to precipitate 20 ml of 0.0993M NaCl, then the molarity of the silver nitrate is:

$$\frac{20.0 \times 0.0993}{19.7} = 0.1008\text{M (0.1M)}$$

Volhard's method

Chloride is precipitated from acidic (nitric acid) solution by excess standard silver nitrate solution, and the excess nitrate back-titrated with a standard solution of ammonium or potassium thiocyanate. The indicator is ferric ammonium alum (ferric alum). At the end-point, when all the silver ion has been precipitated, the thiocyanate ion reacts with the ferric ion to produce a reddish-brown colorization, due to the formation of a complex ferri-thiocyanate ion:

$$Fe^{3+} + SCN^- \rightleftharpoons (FeSCN)^{2+}$$

When the chloride ions have precipitated the silver ions, the excess silver ions during titration form silver thiocyanate, after which the thiocyanate may then react with the silver chloride, since silver thiocyanate is the less soluble salt:

$$Ag^+ + Cl^- \rightleftharpoons AgCl$$
$$Ag^+ + SCN^- \rightleftharpoons AgSCN$$

and so

$$AgCl + SCN^- \rightleftharpoons AgSCN + Cl^-$$

This will take place before the reaction occurs with the ferric ions and therefore there will be a considerable titration error. To prevent this, an immiscible liquid nitrobenzene is added to the reaction mixture to 'coat' the silver chloride particles and thereby protect them from the interaction with the thiocyanate.

Thiocyanates are slightly deliquescent and are unsuitable as primary standards.

Preparation of 0.1M ammonium thiocyanate

$$AgNO_3 + NaCl \rightarrow AgCl + NaNO_3 \qquad (1)$$
$$AgNO_3 + NH_4SCN \rightarrow AgSCN + NH_4NO_3 \qquad (2)$$

From equations (1) and (2) 1 mole of $AgNO_3$ is equivalent to 1 mole of NaCl and 1 mole of $AgNO_3$ is equivalent to 1 mole of NH_4SCN. Therefore, 1 mole of $AgNO_3$ is equivalent to 76.12 g of NH_4SCN. Then 0.1 mole of $AgNO_3$ is equivalent to 7.612 g of NH_4SCN.

As ammonium thiocyanate is deliquescent, weigh out about 8.5 g of AR ammonium thiocyanate (or 10.5 g of AR potassium thiocyanate), dissolve it in water and dilute to 1 litre in a volumetric flask. Shake well.

Standardization against 0.1M AgNO₃

Procedure

1. Pipette 20 ml of standard 0.1M $AgNO_3$ into a 250 ml conical flask, add 5 ml of 6M HNO_3 and 1 ml ferric alum indicator*.
2. Slowly add the ammonium thiocyanate from a burette with constant shaking. At first a white precipitate is produced and as each drop of thiocyanate is added, it produces a reddish-brown colour. As the end-point approaches, the precipitate coagulates and settles; eventually, one drop of thiocyanate solution produces a faint reddish-brown colour which no longer disappears on shaking. This is the end-point.
3. Note the titre and repeat the titration with two other 20 ml portions or until duplicates agree to within 0.1 ml of each other.
4. Calculation of molarity of ammonium thiocyanate. Suppose 20 ml of 0.1M $AgNO_3$ required 19.5 ml of ammonium thiocyanate. Then

$$\text{Molarity of } NH_4SCN = \frac{20 \times 0.1}{19.5}$$
$$= 0.1026M \ (0.103)$$

*Preparation of indicator: Ferric alum indicator—40 g of ferric ammonium sulphate AR per 100 ml of distilled water to which a few drops of 6M HNO_3 has been added.

5. Transfer the solution to an amber reagent bottle and label accordingly, i.e. 0.1M NH_4SCN:

   F (factor) = 1.03

Titration of chlorides (Volhard's method)

Principle

See above.

Procedure

1. Pipette 20 ml of approximately 0.1M NaCl solution into a 250 ml conical flask.
2. Add 5 ml 6M HNO_3.
3. Run into the flask from a burette 25 ml standard 0.1M $AgNO_3$ (sufficient to give about 5 ml excess).
4. Add 3 ml nitrobenzene AR and 1 ml ferric alum indicator and shake the flask vigorously to coagulate the precipitate.
5. Titrate the excess silver nitrate with the 0.103M ammonium thiocyanate until a permanent faint reddish-brown colour appears.
6. Note the titre and repeat the titration with two other 20 ml portions of sodium chloride solution or until duplicate titres agree to within 0.1 ml of each other.
7. *Calculation of molarity of sodium chloride solution:*
   25 ml of standard 0.1M $AgNO_3$ were used in the titration. If 4.8 ml of 0.1M NH_4SCN of factor 1.03 were required to titrate the residual silver nitrate (i.e. $4.8 \times 1.03 = 4.94$ ml of 0.1M NH_4SCN), then volume of silver nitrate equivalent to chloride

   $$= (25 - 4.94) \text{ ml of 0.1M } AgNO_3$$
   $$= 20.06 \text{ ml of 0.1M } AgNO_3$$

   Therefore,

   $$\text{Molarity of NaCl} = \frac{20.06 \times 0.1}{20.0} = 0.1003M$$

Titration of chlorides (adsorption indicator method)

Indicator 0.1% dichlorofluorescein in 70% alcohol.

Procedure

1. Pipette 20 ml of chloride solution into a 250 ml conical flask.
2. Add 5–10 drops of indicator.
3. Titrate with the silver nitrate solution in diffuse light with constant swirling. As the end-point is near, the silver chloride coagulates appreciably and the development of the pink colour upon the

addition of each drop of silver nitrate solution becomes more and more pronounced.

4. Continue the titration, dropwise, until the precipitate suddenly becomes a pronounced pink or red colour. Note the titre.
5. Repeat the titration with two other 20 ml portions of chloride solution or until the individual titrations agree to within 0.1 ml of each other.

Preparation of 0.02M potassium permanganate solution

Potassium permanganate ($KMnO_4$) is a very powerful oxidizing agent and, in acid solution, the reduction can be represented by the following equation:

$$MnO_4^- + 8H^+ + 5e^- \rightarrow Mn^{2+} + 4H_2O$$

Procedure

1. The molecular weight of $KMnO_4$ is 158.03 and therefore 0.02M $KMnO_4$ contains 3.1606 g per litre.
2. Weigh out 3.2–3.25 g of AR $KMnO_4$ and transfer to a litre beaker, add about 500 ml of distilled water and boil.
3. Allow to cool, filter the solution through a plug of purified glass wool into a clean litre volumetric flask.
4. Add further distilled water to the beaker and transfer quantitatively to the filtrate and finally dilute to 1000 ml.
5. Mix well and keep in the dark or in diffuse light until standardized.
6. Alternatively, the solution can be kept in an amber reagent bottle.

Standardization against sodium oxalate

Sodium oxalate* is a primary standard, whereas oxalic acid is not. An acidified solution of an oxalate is for purposes of titration with $KMnO_4$ solution equivalent to a solution of oxalic acid itself:

$$Na_2C_2O_4 \rightleftharpoons 2Na^+ + C_2O_4^{2-} \quad (1)$$
$$\text{sodium}$$
$$\text{oxalate}$$

$$C_2O_4^{2-} + 2H^+ \rightleftharpoons H_2C_2O_4 \quad (2)$$
$$\text{acid}$$

The oxidation of oxalic acid is represented as follows:

$$H_2C_2O_4 + [O] \rightarrow 2CO_2 + H_2O \quad (3)$$
$$\text{from}$$
$$KMnO_4$$

Caution! Oxalic acid and oxalates are toxic.

$$2KMnO_4 + 3H_2SO_4 + 5H_2C_2O_4 \rightleftharpoons K_2SO_4$$
$$+ 2MnSO_4 + 8H_2O + 10CO_2 \quad (4)$$

Thus

$$2KMnO_4 = 5H_2C_2O_4 \quad (5)$$

or

$$2KMnO_4 = 5Na_2C_2O_4 \quad (6)$$

From the molecular equations (4)–(6) it can be seen that 2 moles of potassium permanganate ($KMnO_4$) are equivalent to 5 moles of sodium oxalate ($Na_2C_2O_4$). But 20 ml 0.02M $KMnO_4$ is equivalent to 20 ml 0.05M $Na_2C_2O_2$; therefore,

$$\frac{0.05 \times MW}{1000} \times 20 \text{ ml of } Na_2C_2O_4$$
$$= 20 \text{ ml } 0.02M \ KMnO_4$$

or

$$\frac{0.05 \times 134}{1000} \times 20 = 0.134 \text{ g } Na_2C_2O_4$$
$$= 20 \text{ ml } 0.02M \ KMnO_4$$

Procedure

1. Dry about 2 g AR sodium oxalate at 105–110°C for 2 h and allow to cool in a desiccator.
2. Weigh out accurately three 0.135–0.140 g of sodium oxalate and transfer to 250 ml conical flasks in the same way as described on p. 54.
3. Add about 50 ml recently prepared distilled water, shake well to dissolve then add about 50 ml molar (M) sulphuric acid and heat the mixture to about 60–70°C.
4. Potassium permanganate does not oxidize oxalate readily in cold solution; a temperature of 60–70°C is necessary in order to perform the titration. This temperature can be best judged by testing with the palm of the hand. When the bottom of the flask is just too hot to hold, the temperature of the liquid is approximately correct.
5. Titrate with the $KMnO_4$, heating again as the liquid cools, until a permanent pink coloration is obtained.
6. For the most exact work, determine the excess $KMnO_4$ required to reach the end-point by adding permanganate solution to the same volume of water and dilute acid at 60–70°C—this is usually about 0.05 ml.
7. Note titre and repeat the titration with the other two weighed samples.
8. *Calculation of molarity of KMnO₄:*

$$\text{Actual molarity} = \frac{w \times t \times m}{W \times V}$$

where w is the weight of substance used, W the

weight of substance calculated, t the theoretical titre, V the volume used, and m the assumed molarity. If $0.140\,g$ of $Na_2C_2O_4$ requires $19.5\,ml$ of approximately $0.02M$ $KMnO_4$ and $0.134\,g$ of $Na_2C_2O_4$ is equivalent to $20\,ml$ $0.02M$ $KMnO_4$, then

$$\text{Molarity} = \frac{0.140 \times 20 \times 0.02}{0.134 \times 19.5}$$
$$= 0.0214M\ KMnO_4$$

$$\text{F for } KMnO_4 = \frac{0.140 \times 20}{0.134 \times 19.5} = 1.07$$

SI units

The International System of Units (Système International, SI) was adopted in 1960 by a General Conference of Weights and Measures as being a logical, coherent system and is basically divided into the following seven units: metre, kilogram, second, ampere, kelvin, candela and mole (*Table 5.5*). All other units are derived from these. Some derived SI units have special names and symbols; the ones we are concerned with are given in *Tables 5.5* and *5.6*.

Table 5.5 Basic SI units

Physical quantity	Name of SI unit	Symbol for SI
Length	metre	m
Mass	kilogram	kg
Time	second	s
Electric current	ampere	A
Thermodynamic temperature	kelvin	K
Luminous intensity	candela	cd
Amount of substance	mole	mol

Table 5.6 Some derived SI units

Quantity	Name of SI unit	Symbol
Work, energy, quantity of heat	joule	J
Power	watt	W
Electric charge	coulomb	C
Electric potential, potential difference	volt	V
Electric resistance	ohm	Ω
Pressure	pascal	Pa

The system has now been adopted by most international scientific bodies, including the International Federation of Clinical Chemistry (IFCC) and the International Union of Pure and Applied Chemistry (IUPAC). Multiples or fractions of the basic units or sub-units have also been defined. These are shown in *Table 5.7* and *5.8*, respectively.

Table 5.7 Prefixes for multiples of SI units

Multiple	Symbol	Prefix
10^1	da	deca
10^2	h	hecto
10^3	k	kilo
10^6	M	mega
10^9	G	giga
10^{12}	T	tera
10^{15}	P	peta
10^{18}	E	exa

Table 5.8 Prefixes for fractions of basic SI units

Fraction	Symbol	Prefix
10^{-1}	d	deci
10^{-2}	c	centi
10^{-3}	m	milli
10^{-6}	μ	micro
10^{-9}	n	nano
10^{-12}	p	pico
10^{-15}	f	femto
10^{-18}	a	atto

Although the SI unit of volume was given as the cubic metre (m^3), the litre (l) is still more generally recognized as the unit of volume and is exactly equal to 1 cubic decimetre (dm^3), i.e. $1000\ \text{litre} = 1\ m^3$. Because of its convenience the litre is used as the unit of volume in the laboratory. Multiples and submultiples of the litre should be used for all measurements of volume (*Table 5.9*).

Table 5.9 Units of volume

SI unit	Old unit
dl	100 ml
ml or cm^3	cc
μl	lambda, λ
nl	—
pl	$\mu\mu l$

The SI unit for mass is the kilogram (kg); the working unit is the gram (g). Multiples and submultiples of the gram should be used and not the kilogram (*Table 5.10*).

Table 5.10 Multiples and submultiples of the gram

SI unit	Old unit
kg	k, kg, kilogramme
g	gr, gm, gms, gramme
mg	mgm, mgms
μg	gamma
ng	mug
pg	$\mu\mu g$

Mass should not be confused with weight, which is measured in newtons. The SI unit for amount of substance is the mole (mol); this unit replaces the gram-molecule, gram-ion, gram-equivalent and so on. It is recommended that the use of the equivalent and its submultiples commonly used for reporting the monovalent electrolyte measurements (sodium, potassium, chloride, bicarbonate) should be replaced by molar concentrations (mmol/l). For these four measurements, the numerical value will not change (*Table 5.11*).

Table 5.11 Units of molar concentrations and their former equivalents

SI unit	Old unit
mol	M, g-mol, eq
mmol	mM, mEq
μmol	μM
nmol	nM

The SI unit for length is the metre (m). The ångström unit (Å) should not be used and the measurements should be converted to nanometres (nm): $1 \text{ Å} = 10^{-1} \text{ nm}$.

SI unit	Old unit
nm	mμ
μm	μ (micron)

The SI symbol for day (i.e. 24 hours) is 'd', but urine and faecal excretion of substances should be expressed as 'per 24 hours' (e.g. g/24 h). The basic unit for thermodynamic temperature is the kelvin (K), not degree Kelvin (°K). The customary working unit in medical laboratories is the degree Celsius (formerly centigrade) (°C).

In medical laboratory sciences SI units have caused changes in reporting results, the biggest and most important occurring in clinical chemistry, whereby analyses previously reported in conventional units such as mg/100 ml or μg/100 ml are now expressed in mmol/l or μmol/l, respectively. Determinations reported in mg/100 ml are converted into SI units by the following formula:

$$\frac{\text{mg/100 ml} \times 10}{\text{Molecular weight of substance}} = \text{mmol/l} \quad (1)$$

e.g. 210 mg/100 ml of urea:

Molecular weight of urea = 60

$$\frac{210 \times 10}{60} = 35 \text{ mmol/l}$$

To reconvert mmol/l back into mg/100 ml, the following formula is used:

$$\frac{\text{Conc. in mmol/l} \times \text{Molecular weight of substance}}{10} = \text{mg/100 ml} \quad (2)$$

e.g. 35 mmol/l of urea:

$$\frac{35 \times 60}{10} = 210 \text{ mg/ml}$$

In certain instances the molecular weight of a substance cannot be accurately determined (as in mixtures), in which case values are reported as the weight of the substance per litre, e.g. albumin will be reported as g/l. For example, 5 g/100 ml of albumin will become 50 g/l of albumin.

Another change is in reporting pressures, mmHg being replaced by the pascal unit or, because this is too small, the kilopascal (kPa) is used.

The molecular weight of enzymes is also difficult to determine, hence in 1966 the Commission on Clinical Chemistry of the IUPAC recommended that all activities should be expressed in terms of an international unit (U) which is defined as follows:

An international unit (U) is the amount of enzyme activity which brings about the consumption of 1 micromole of substrate or formation of 1 micromole of product per minute under defined conditions. Enzyme concentration is therefore expressed as units per ml (U/ml) or milli-international units (mU) can be used if this is a more convenient figure, in which case these are femtomoles consumed or formed per minute. One mU/ml is therefore equivalent to one U/l. This unit has been changed to an SI unit, the katal, but as yet the katal unit has not generally been adopted. One katal of activity causes a change in concentration of substrate or product of 1 mole per second. Because this is a large unit, measurements are made in nkat/l:

$$1 \text{ U/l} = 16.67 \text{ nkat/l}$$

6

Analytical procedures

Elementary colorimetry, absorptiometry and spectro-photometry

Many biochemical methods produce solutions of coloured compounds; others are involved in a chemical reaction to yield coloured substances. The measurement of a coloured solution forms the basis of a quantitative method of analysis and is used in the practice of colorimetry. There are various methods available for measuring the concentrations of coloured solutions, the first two of which are now only of historical interest, but are included so that the basic principles can be understood.

Visual comparison

This is a procedure where solutions are matched against a set of standards using test-tubes of similar diameter. Values intermediate between a set of standards can then be approximated. This principle is used in the Lovibond comparator, but in place of liquid standards coloured glass standards are utilized.

Lovibond comparator

This apparatus (*Figure 6.1*) consists of a box with compartments for tubes of the test and blank solutions, and it has a rotatable disc mounted in front of the two tubes. The central window of the box is in front of the test solution; the other window lies in front of the 'blank' solution and rotation of the disc permits the superimposition of the coloured glass standards.

Various discs are manufactured, but a standard solution of known strength should always be carried through in parallel with the test. This standard solution enables one to check the permanent

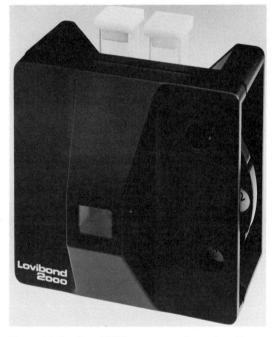

Figure 6.1. Lovibond 2000 comparator (reproduced by courtesy of Tintometer Ltd)

standard and also ensures that no error in technique has been made.

Visual colorimeter

The visual colorimeter (*Figure 6.2*) was widely used for many years, but has now been totally superseded by photoelectric absorptiometers of one kind or another.

One type of visual colorimeter is the Dubosq, which consists essentially of two glass containers each of which contains a solid glass plunger, capable

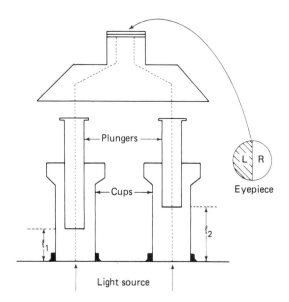

Figure 6.2. Visual colorimeter

of being raised or lowered. Light from an even source of illumination concealed at the base of the instrument passes through the two solutions to be tested and through the plungers. Some of the light is absorbed in passing through the solutions, the amount of absorption being dependent upon the concentration and the depth of the solution. The two beams of light are brought to a common axis by a prism system, which is focused onto an eyepiece. On looking through the eyepiece, a wide circular field is visible, light from one cup illuminating one half and light from the second cup illuminating the other half of the field. The depth of solution may be varied by raising or lowering the plungers (or cups) until the two sides of the field are evenly illuminated or matched, i.e. until the dividing line practically disappears. The depth of the solution through which the light passes to the plunger is then read on the vernier scale attached to the plungers or cups. It is usual to set either the test or standard at one particular vernier reading and then raise or lower the other plunger or cup until identical illumination is reached. When this condition is achieved, one of the laws of colorimetry is obeyed, namely Beer's law (see below).

To determine the concentration of the unknown (test) the following calculation can be used:

$$c_1 d_1 = c_2 d_2$$

or

$$c_2 = c_1 \times \frac{d_1}{d_2}$$

i.e.

Concentration of unknown

$$= \text{Conc. of standard} \times \frac{\text{Depth of standard}}{\text{Depth of test}}$$

where c is the concentration of substance and d is the depth of the plunger in the solution. Further on, one can see how the calculation is reversed in photoelectric measurements.

Photoelectric absorptiometers

These instruments are called absorptiometers since it is the amount of light absorbed which is measured and not colour. In this way many errors are eliminated due to the personal characteristics of each individual. Photoelectric absorptiometers use photoelectric cells either of the barrier layer or the emissive type. Light falling on these cells generates an electric current, which can be made to deflect a galvanometer needle, the deflector being proportional to the light density. Light on passing through a coloured solution is absorbed, the amount of absorption depending upon the concentration of the solution. The more light absorbed, the less light is transmitted to the photoelectric cell and the smaller the current generated. From this the second law of colorimetry is derived, namely Lambert's law (see below).

Theory of absorptiometry

When white light is passed through a coloured solution, some of the frequencies (wavelengths) of the white light will be absorbed, while others will be transmitted through the solution. If one passes monochromatic light of a frequency which is preferentially absorbed by the molecules in a solution, some of the light will be absorbed, while the excess light is transmitted.

Thus, if I_0 is the incident light, I_a the absorbed light and I_t the light transmitted, then

$$I_0 = I_a + I_t$$

The above relationship obeys two laws—Beer's law and Lambert's law.

The Beer–Lambert laws

Beer's law

The intensity of a solution when viewed through monochromatic light is directly proportional to the concentration of the substance.

Or

The proportion of the incident light absorbed by the molecules in a solution is directly proportional to the number of absorbing molecules in the light path.

In this law, the light path remains constant and the concentration varies.

Lambert's law

When monochromatic light passes through a transparent medium, the rate of decrease in intensity with the thickness of the medium is proportional to the intensity of light.

Or

Each successive layer, of equal thickness, of the same homogeneous solution, will absorb the same proportion of the light incident upon it.

In this law, the proportion of light absorbed is independent of the intensity of the incident light, but the amount of light absorbed is dependent on the intensity of the incident light.

In combining Lambert's law with Beer's law the basic laws of colorimetry, absorptiometry and spectrophotometry are obtained.

Beer–Lambert law

When monochromatic light passes through a coloured solution the amount of light transmitted decreases exponentially with the increase in the concentration of the solution and with the increase in the thickness of the layer of solution through which the light passes. (The first statement follows from Beer's law and the second from Lambert's law.)

Mathematically, this law can be expressed as

$$T = e^{-kct} \tag{1}$$

in which T is the transmission, k a constant, the absorption coefficient, c the concentration of solution, t the thickness of the solution or light path, and e the base of natural or Napierian logarithms.

Transmission (T) is defined as the ratio of the intensity of the transmitted (emergent) light to that of the incident light, thus equation (1) can be expressed in another way, namely:

$$\frac{I_e}{I_i} = e^{-kct} \tag{2}$$

where I_e is the intensity of the emergent light and I_i is the intensity of the incident light.

Rearrange equation (1)

$$T = e^{-kct}$$
$$\log_e T = -kct$$
$$-\log_e T = kct$$
$$-\log_{10} T = kct \tag{3}$$

Now $-\log_{10} T$ is the term used for absorbance (A) or the older terms of extinction (E) and optical density (OD). Although transmission is linear (0–100%) and absorbance is logarithmic (0–∞), there is a relationship between the two, namely:

$$A = \log \frac{(1)}{(T)} \quad \text{or} \quad \log \frac{100}{\%T}$$

or

$$A = 2 - \log \%T \tag{4}$$

Since $A = -\log T$, then, by substituting this into equation (3),

$$A = kct \tag{5}$$

In medical laboratory sciences k is usually constant, since the same conditions apply for both the test and standard solutions. As the standard and test solutions are always compared in identical cuvettes or tubes the same light path or thickness of solution is used and therefore t is also a constant value. Equation (5) can thus be rewritten:

$$A = c \tag{6}$$

Now

$$A_{test} = c_{test} \text{ and } A_{std} = c_{std}$$

Then

$$\frac{A_{test} = c_{test}}{A_{std} = c_{std}} = A_{test} \times c_{std} = c_{test} \times A_{std}$$

Therefore

$$c_{test} = \frac{A_{test} \times c_{std}}{A_{std}}$$

Expressed another way,

Concentration of unknown
$$= \frac{\text{Absorbance of unknown}}{\text{Absorbance of standard}} \times \text{Conc. of standard}$$

This is the standard formula used in photoelectric absorptiometry and spectrophotometry, provided Beer's law is obeyed. Since sets of measurements are made at a constant light path, it is the concentration which varies and therefore it is usual to say that Beer's law is obeyed or is not obeyed. The absorbance scale is always used, but some absorptiometers and spectrophotometers are provided with two scales, one from 0 to 100 showing percentage transmission, and the other 0 to ∞, showing absorption (*Figure 6.3*). The 100% transmission always corresponds to zero absorbance, and on the absorbance scale corresponds to zero transmission. When Beer's law is obeyed and the

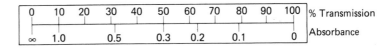

Figure 6.3. Photoelectric absorptiometer scale

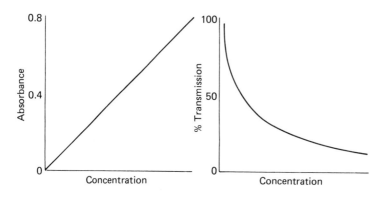

Figure 6.4. Graphs showing the relationships between absorbance and concentration and percentage transmission

concentrations are plotted against absorbance, a straight-line relationship is obtained. On the other hand, if percentage transmission is plotted against concentration a curve is obtained (*Figure 6.4*).

Absorptiometers

These have five essential parts.

A. Light source

This can vary in intensity, depending upon the type of instrument used. The source of radiant energy can be either a tungsten filament lamp, hydrogen or deuterium discharge lamp or a mercury–xenon arc lamp.

B. Wavelength selection

In most instruments filters are used for this purpose, but in the more expensive type of equipment a diffraction grating or prism is used to obtain approximately monochromatic light.

1. Light filters

The filter chosen is usually complementary to the colour of the solution to be measured (see *Table 6.1*).

Table 6.1 Complementary colours

Colour of solution	Usual filter
Blue	Yellow
Bluish-green	Red
Purple	Green
Red	Bluish-green
Yellow	Blue
Yellowish-green	Violet

Table 6.2 Maximum transmission of Ilford spectrum filters

Number	Type	Peak of maximum transmission (nm)
600	Spectrum deep violet	420
601	Spectrum violet	430
602	Spectrum blue	470
603	Spectrum blue-green	490
604	Spectrum green	520
605	Spectrum yellowish-green	550
606	Spectrum yellow	580
607	Spectrum orange	600
608	Spectrum red	680

Filters are made of glass, or dyed gelatin between glass plates, and have a limited transmission band, at which they transmit maximally (see *Table 6.2*). To understand the use of light filters, consider a bluish-green solution which absorbs light in the red part of the spectrum. Such a solution when

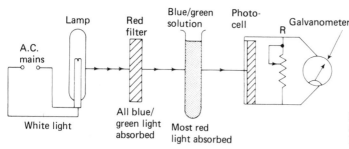

Figure 6.5. Single cell photoelectric absorptiometer: diagram showing light path and the use of a colour filter

illuminated by white light absorbs red colour wavelengths and emits bluish-green light, together with a small amount of red. The greater the concentration of the solution, the smaller the amount of red light transmitted.

The most sensitive readings of the galvanometer will therefore be obtained by allowing only the transmitted red light to activate the photoelectric cell. The red filter achieves this by stopping the transmission of bluish-green light and allowing only the red light to pass through the solution (see *Figure 6.5*). Before the correct filter is chosen for any investigation, further studies are required with respect to sensitivity and linear relationship (see p. 67).

2. Interference filters

These filters have narrower transmitted light bands than coloured filters. They are essentially composed of two highly reflecting but partially transmitting films of metal, usually of silver separated by a spacer. The amount of separation between the films determines the wavelength position of the band of light and therefore the colour of light the filter will transmit. This optical arrangement is called interference, resulting in a high transmission of light when the optical separation of the metal films is effectively a half-wavelength. Light which is not transmitted is for the most part reflected. While the light filters cover the range 400–680 nm, wavelength of the interference filters is from 330 to 1200 nm.

3. Diffraction grating or prism

See the text on spectrophotometers (p. 66).

C. Cells and cuvettes

These are used to hold the coloured solutions and must be scrupulously clean. They have two parallel flat clear sides made of optical glass; the other two parallel sides are opaque and must not be placed in the light path. The set of cells used should be optically matched before placing the cuvettes into the light path; the outside of the cells must be wiped clean with a lens tissue and held up to the light to ensure there are no dirty finger marks or spillage of fluid on the outside of the optical side. Spillage of fluid or dirty finger marks will absorb light and interfere in the measurement of the colour.

The cells must be carefully cleaned and scratches on the optical glass must be avoided. A badly scratched cuvette must be discarded. Never clean cuvettes with chromic acid—always use a good detergent.

Test-tubes are used in some of the simpler instruments, but they must be interchangeable. Although test-tubes are more convenient to use than cells they are not as satisfactory.

D. Photoelectric cell

There are three types of photoelectric element—the barrier layer cell, the photoemissive tube and the photomultiplier tube. Light falling on these elements generates an electric current which deflects a galvanometer needle, the deflection being proportional to the light intensity.

1. Barrier layer cell (selenium cell)

The commonest form of barrier cell consists essentially of a metal disc upon which is deposited a thin layer of selenium. This is covered by a thin transparent layer of metal, which is lacquered except for a thicker portion near the periphery. At this thick portion of the disc one of the terminals to the galvanometer is connected, the other connection being made to the underside of the disc which is covered by a non-oxidizing metal. When light passes through the thin metal layer to the selenium layer beneath, electrons are liberated which pass across the 'barrier' between the selenium and transparent metal layer to become negatively charged, while the thicker metal disc becomes positively charged. If the cell is connected to a galvanometer, a current will pass, the strength of which is proportional to the intensity of light falling on the selenium. The 'EEL' selenium photocell is an example of the barrier layer cell, sensitive to the visible part of the spectrum.

Absorptiometers using this type of cell may either be direct reading, single photocell instruments or of the double cell type. The double cell or null point instruments have two closely matched selenium cells balanced against each other. Light from a single source reaches both photocells; some light will be absorbed by the coloured solution inserted in front of one of the cells and this will be reflected by the galvanometer needle. By varying a resistance in the circuit, or by closing a diaphragm, the two currents may be balanced, the galvanometer acting as a null point indicator. Unlike the photoemissive tube they do not require the use of a battery.

2. Photoemissive tubes

These are similar to radio valves and are composed of an evacuated glass tube or a tube containing an inert gas at low pressure. The tubes are coated internally with a thin sensitive layer of either caesium or potassium oxide and silver oxide to act as the cathode. A metal ring inserted near the centre of the valve forms the anode and is maintained at a high voltage by a battery. When light penetrates the valve it falls on the sensitive layer, electrons are emitted, thereby causing a current to flow through

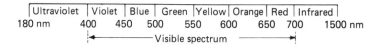

Figure 6.6. The spectrum of a spectrophotometer

an outside circuit; this is then amplified by electronic means and is a measure of the amount of light falling on the photosensitive surface.

The current from the phototube is smaller than that from the selenium cell and hence the amplification. They are sensitive to light outside the visible part of the spectrum and are more reliable than the selenium cell.

3. Photomultiplier tube

This is a further development of the photoemissive tube in which the sensitivity is greatly increased by connecting the elements within the tube in series. When the electrons hit the first element, secondary electrons are emitted in greater numbers than initially, with the net result that there is an increased current output from the cell. The output from the tube is limited to several milliamperes, therefore it will measure intensities of light about 200 times weaker than that measured by the photoemissive tube.

E. Galvanometers

The galvanometer measures the output of the photosensitive element, and in most instruments a very sensitive one is used.

As well as the single cell absorptiometer, as shown in *Figure 6.5*, there are also twin cell instruments which are used to eliminate fluctuations in cell fatigue, temperature changes and most importantly current variation in the light source.

Spectrophotometers

Spectrophotometers are instruments which measure absorbance at various wavelengths. The major difference between this type of equipment and the absorptiometers is the method of producing monochromatic light.

The colour filters are dispensed with and either a diffraction grating or glass prism produces the monochromatic light. A diffraction grating disperses the white light into a continuous spectrum, by turning a wavelength adjustment. The grating is rotated and different parts of the spectrum are allowed to fall onto the photocell.

In the glass prism spectrophotometers, light is focused onto the prism which then passes through and forms an extended spectrum. On adjusting the exit slit (wavelength adjustment) light can pass through the cuvette and illuminate the photocell.

This is the cheapest form of selecting monochromatic light and is only usually fitted to a spectrophotometer reading in the visible part of the spectrum (*Figure 6.6*).

These precision instruments are of two types: (a) visible spectrophotometers covering the range 360–1000 nm, having one light source and two photocells; and (b) ultraviolet spectrophotometers covering the range 185–1000 nm, having two light sources and two photocells.

Infrared spectrophotometers

These are very specialized pieces of equipment which are used for measuring groups of substances in the infrared region of the spectrum. They are of special construction and are used mainly in research establishments.

Flow-through colorimeters

In order to speed up analytical procedures, flow-through cells have been introduced into absorptiometry. These cells enable readings to be taken more speedily, since the cells or cuvettes can be drained without being removed from the instruments. Examples of this type of cell can be found in the Technicon Auto-Analyser system, the Hilger Chemispek J 200 multichannel analyser and in simpler instruments such as the SP6 spectrophotometers and the Gallenkamp linear scale colorimeters.

Maximum absorption

The selection of the correct wavelength of filter is one of the most important steps in colorimetric analysis. This is determined by measuring the absorbance of the coloured reaction throughout the visible spectrum and then deciding the wavelength or filter which gives the highest absorbance, an example of which can be seen in *Figure 6.7*. The absorbances of a solution of methyl red as used as secondary standards in bilirubin estimations have been plotted on a piece of graph paper against the wavelength settings. From the graph it can be seen that maximum absorption is at 525 nm.

Selectivity

Once the correct filter or wavelength has been chosen to give maximum absorption, its selectivity is determined by taking further readings at various

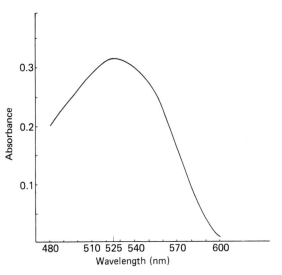

Figure 6.7. Graph showing maximum absorption at 525 nm

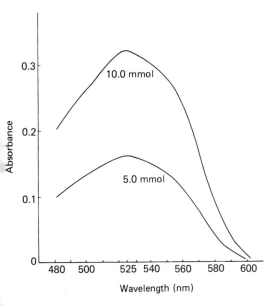

Figure 6.8. Graph showing maximum selectivity

wavelengths with two different concentrations of the same solution. These are then plotted on a piece of graph paper and the results can be seen in *Figure 6.8*. Here one can see that the filter or wavelength chosen for maximum absorption also gives maximum selectivity as the 5 mmol and 10 mmol readings are equidistant from each other, i.e. the 5 mmol absorbance is 0.160 and the 10 mmol absorbance is 0.320.

Linear relationship

With every colorimetric or spectrophotometric analysis carried out in the laboratory it is essential that calibration curves are prepared to confirm that Beer's law is obeyed.

If a straight-line relationship is obtained between absorbances and concentrations Beer's law is obeyed and therefore a linear relationship has been confirmed.

Calibration curves

The preparation of calibration curves is a procedure which causes students some concern, so an outdated method for the estimation of glucose in the UK has been retained, as it contains a protein precipitation stage and still uses the old units. This is a good example of learning from first principles and the method as quoted on p. 68 is still used in certain parts of the world, like the SP600 spectrophotometers which are still giving good service but are now replaced by the SP6 type of instrument.

The greatest care must be taken in the preparation of a calibration curve. Always use freshly prepared reagents and standards and scrupulously clean glassware.

One of the biggest problems in most colorimetric analyses is the presence of protein in biological fluid, since protein will in the majority of cases interfere with the final colour reaction.

Standard preparations are usually prepared in an aqueous medium so there is no problem with protein, but as the standards, tests and blanks must be treated in the same way with the colour reagent, the protein must be removed from either blood, serum or plasma. This step is called protein precipitation and used in the estimation of blood glucose (see p. 125).

In this method 2.0 ml of protein-free supernatant are required for colour development. To obtain this protein-free supernatant 0.05 ml blood or plasma is pipetted into 3.9 ml of isotonic sodium sulphate–copper sulphate solution; 0.05 ml of sodium tungstate is then added to the diluted sample and thoroughly mixed. Copper tungstate is formed which acts as a protein precipitant, leaving the glucose and other diffusable components in solution when the protein precipitate has settled out. This is hastened by centrifuging.

In the above-mentioned procedure 0.05 ml of blood or plasma has been diluted to 4.0 ml and therefore 2.0 ml of protein-free supernatant will only contain the equivalent of 0.025 ml of whole blood or plasma.

The unknown solution of glucose is compared against a standard solution of glucose which has been similarly treated (except for protein precipitation). From the absorbances of the standard and unknown, the concentration of glucose can be determined.

Let x = the concentration of glucose in the test sample.

Then 2.0 ml of supernatant (= 0.025 ml of blood or plasma) will contain x mg glucose.

If 2.0 ml of glucose standard solution (containing 0.025 mg glucose per ml) were used for colour

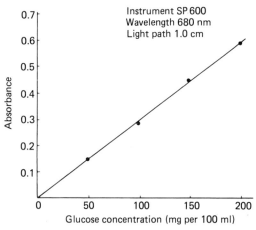

Figure 6.9. A correctly labelled graph showing a linear relationship between absorbance and concentration

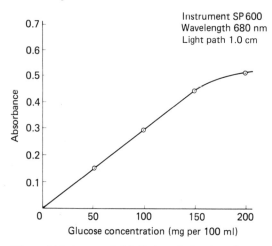

Figure 6.10. A correctly labelled graph showing a linear relationship up to 150 mg per 100 ml

comparison, then the standard is equivalent to 0.05 mg of glucose.

Using the standard formula:

$$\frac{\text{Absorbance (A) of unknown}}{\text{Absorbance (A) of standard}}$$

$$\times \; \frac{\text{Strength of standard used}}{\text{in the colour development}}$$

$$\times \; \frac{100}{\text{Amount of blood in reaction mixture}}$$

or

$$\frac{\text{A of unknown}}{\text{A of standard}} \times 0.05 \times \frac{100}{0.025} = \begin{array}{l}\text{mg glucose} \\ \text{per 100 ml} \\ \text{of blood}\end{array}$$

Then

$$\frac{\text{A of unknown}}{\text{A of standard}} \times 200 = \begin{array}{l}\text{mg glucose per 100 ml} \\ \text{of blood}\end{array}$$

This then means that when 2 ml of the standard glucose (0.025 mg/ml) solution is treated with the colour reagent in the same way as 2 ml of protein-free supernatant, it will be equivalent to not 0.025 mg/ml but 200 mg/100 ml of blood glucose.

Likewise 0.5 ml, 1.0 ml and 1.5 ml of the same standard glucose solution will be equivalent to 50, 100 and 150 mg of glucose per 100 ml under the conditions of the test.

Preparation of calibration curve

From the above it can be seen that in the estimation of blood glucose (p. 125) a calibration curve can easily be constructed by using the following volumes:

mg glucose per 100 ml	0	50	100	150	200
ml of glucose standard (0.025 mg/ml)	0.0	0.5	1.0	1.5	2.0
ml of distilled water	2.0	1.5	1.0	0.5	0.0

The solutions are thoroughly mixed and the colour development carried out as per test sample.

The absorbances for each standard preparation are recorded and, after subtracting the blank (zero value) from each reading, the results are plotted on a piece of graph paper as can be seen in *Figure 6.9*. It is important to label the graph correctly as shown, as this is good clinical chemistry practice.

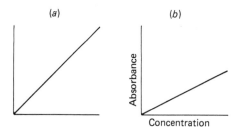

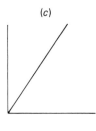

Figure 6.11. Calibration curves used to determine the degree of sensitivity of a method

Figure 6.9 shows a linear relationship between absorbance and concentration and therefore Beer's law is obeyed, while in *Figure 6.10* there is only a linear relationship up to a concentration of 150 mg per 100 ml and above this concentration Beer's law is not obeyed. Only when Beer's law is obeyed must you use the formula shown on p. 68.

When absorbances fall on a nonlinear part of a curve, the sample should be analysed again after dilution.

From the calibration curve, the sensitivity of the method can usually be determined. The line through the 0 should be ideally at 45° (see *Figure 6.11a*) and at this angle the method is said to be of ideal chemistry, because for each alteration in absorbance reading, a satisfactory increase in concentration is found. The same cannot be said for *Figure 6.11b* and *Figure 6.11c*. If good linearity is not obtained, the filter or wavelength next to maximum absorption may have to be used.

Excluding personal errors, the accuracy of any result in an analytical procedure using colorimetry depends upon the accurate preparation of a calibration curve. Always use volumetric glassware whenever possible and avoid pipetting small volumes of standard; for example, if the following dilutions have to be made:

| ml of dilute standard | 0.1 | 0.2 | 0.4 |
| ml of distilled water | 4.9 | 4.8 | 4.6 |

This is bad procedure and is not recommended; it is far more accurate to dilute the standard 1 in 10 so that the following dilutions can be made:

| ml of dilute standard | 1.0 | 2.0 | 4.0 |
| ml of distilled water | 4.0 | 3.0 | 1.0 |

Conversion of mg glucose to mmol/l glucose can be performed by using the formula on p. 126.

Requirements of colorimetric analysis

When colorimetric determinations are made, it is essential to ensure that the colour being measured is only due to the substance under investigation and is not due to any of the reagents used. It is therefore essential to include the following solutions.

1. *Test solution.* This contains the unknown concentration of the substance, together with the reagents used in the test.
2. *Standard solution.* This is usually identical to the test solution, except that it contains a known amount of the substance being determined and is approximately equal in concentration to that expected in the test solution.
3. *Blank solution.* This solution is identical to both the test and standard solution in that it is carried through the complete test procedure and contains all the reagents used, but without any test or standard substance. Any colour given by the reagents used in the analysis can be detected and eliminated.

It is essential to avoid any errors due to dirty glassware, turbidity of solution or air bubbles, as all these factors will seriously interfere with light absorption. It is especially important to remember not to handle the cuvette by its absorptive surfaces, which must be clean and dry.

In order to be sure that the absorbance is due solely to the substance under test, the reading given by the 'blank' solution must be considered with the reading obtained from the 'test' and 'standard' solutions. The photoelectric absorptiometer is set to read zero absorbance with distilled water. The blank, test and standard absorbance readings are recorded, rechecking the zero absorbance between each reading. The blank reading is then subtracted from the test and standard reading as follows:

$$\frac{\text{Test} - \text{Blank}}{\text{Standard} - \text{Blank}} \times \text{Concentration of standard}$$

This procedure will usually ensure that only the substance under investigation is being measured; however, in certain instances, e.g. in the estimation of protein, the instrument is set at zero absorbance with the blank solution, and not distilled water. Satisfactory results are only obtained with absorbances ranging from 0.2 to 0.8, so that if possible the determination should be modified in order that the lower and upper limits of detection fall within this range. The actual details of using a spectrophotometer or absorptiometer will vary with each instrument, so that the manufacturer's instructions must be followed.

Spectroscopy

When white light is passed through certain coloured solutions, part of the light is absorbed in relatively narrow areas of the spectrum, giving dark regions known as absorption bands. The position of these bands can be used to identify the coloured material in solution.

The absorption bands are conveniently observed through a direct vision spectroscope (*Figure 6.12*) which has some means of determining the position of the bands in terms of the corresponding wavelength of light.

Use of the direct vision spectroscope

1. Place the eye to the eyepiece, and view the sky through the instrument but do not point towards direct sunlight.
2. Close the slit 'S' by turning the milled ring, then reopen the slit slightly until the spectrum is visible.

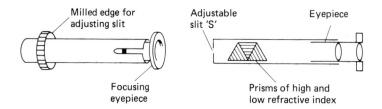

Figure 6.12. The direct vision spectroscope

3. Adjust the eyepiece until the colours are focused and the Fraunhofer lines can be clearly seen.

■ **Note**

Fraunhofer lines, which are due to absorption of light by different elements in the sun's atmosphere, are seen as fine vertical black lines across the spectrum. They will be invisible unless a very narrow slit is used.

4. Check that the D line of the sun's spectrum, which occurs at 589 nm in the orange-yellow, corresponds with the position of the 589 reading on the scale.
5. Place the solution in a test-tube or glass cup. (When examining blood, a dilution greater than 1 in 50 is usual.)
6. Position the tube in front of the slit, and observe through the eyepiece. Record the position of any absorption bands seen in relation to the spectral colours and Fraunhofer lines. If possible check against a solution of known composition.

■ **Note**

A graduated centrifuge tube makes a suitable fluid container as varying depths of solution may be viewed through the spectroscope.

Spectral colour	*Wavelength* (nm)
Red	760–620
Orange	620–595
Yellow	595–560
Yellow-green	560–540
Green	540–500
Blue-green	500–470
Blue	470–430
Violet	430–380

Flame emission spectroscopy (flame photometry)

Sodium and potassium solutions when placed in a bunsen burner impart characteristic colours and the brightness of the flame varies according to the concentration of the element in solution. Flame photometry is concerned with the measurement of individual elements as the emission intensity correlates to the concentration of the element. In the clinical chemistry laboratory of today the estimations of these two elements are probably two of the most commonly requested investigations and their determination must be simple, accurate and precise and these criteria are achieved by using the technique of flame emission spectroscopy.

Principle

When an element, in its atomic state, is placed in a flame the atoms increase in energy, become 'excited' and emit energy in the form of light in order to attain their original energy state. The light energy emitted is specific in wavelengths for each element, e.g. sodium emits light of wavelength 589 nm and potassium emits light of wavelengths 404 and 767 nm. The light emitted is proportional to the number of excited atoms present.

Basis of the technique

A dilution of the sample, usually in de-ionized water, is converted to an aerosol. This aerosol is mixed with gas used as a fuel, usually propane. The mixture is then ignited in a burner chamber; the heat from the flame releases free atoms from the molecular vapour and increases their energy state. As the atoms return to their ground state they emit energy in the form of light; the emitted light is then quantitated in the same way as a photoelectric absorptiometer.

Instrumentation

There are two types of instrument for measuring emission, the photometer and the spectrophotometer.

1. Flame photometer

Although design varies from manufacturer to manufacturer, all the instruments have a similar layout, which can be seen in *Figure 6.13*. The design includes a *nebulizer–burner system* which consists of a nebulizer (atomizer), cloud chamber with condensation vanes, and a burner suitable for the fuel to be employed; and a *detector system* which consists of a monochromator in the form of a filter, orange for sodium and deep red for potassium, and a photodetector which can vary from a simple photoelectric cell to photomultiplier tubes depending on design. The output from the photodetectors is fed to either a galvanometer or digital display electronic tubes.

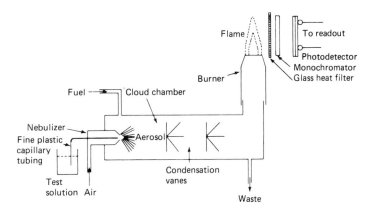

Figure 6.13. Diagram of a flame emission photometer

(a) *Internal standard.* In the majority of cases the precision of the method is improved by the use of an internal lithium standard, two filters and two photocells (one for the internal standard and one for the unknown) which are incorporated into the electronic circuit to give a direct reading for the unknown. Lithiums are now becoming another common estimation so the internal standard can be changed to caesium, thereby allowing the simultaneous estimation of sodium, potassium and lithium to be made by equipment such as the flame photometer from Instrumentation Laboratory (IL 943).

(b) *Temperature of the flame.* The temperature of the flame can vary between 1000°C and 3000°C. Mixtures of coal gas and air do not give very hot flames because of the nitrogen present; hence the use of propane. Maximum flame temperatures for various gas mixtures are as follows:

Fuel	Temperature (°C)	
	In oxygen	In air
Gas	2800	1800
Methane	2700	2000
Propane	2800	1925
Acetylene	3050	2200

Elements which are not easily excited therefore require higher temperatures.

2. Flame spectrophotometer

In this type of instrumentation, which has a variable slit and wavelength control, light from the burner passes into a monochromator of high light-gathering power incorporating a spherical mirror and a 60° prism; this, in conjunction with a photomultiplier tube and a red sensitive photocell, makes it suitable for measurements between 250 and 1020 nm.

Method of estimation. This varies from instrument to instrument; some manufacturers include an automatic diluter in the system, which simply requires the

sample to be presented to the instrument for suitable dilution. Sample volumes range from 20 µl to 100 µl and dilution ratios vary from between 1:500 to 1:100. The original basic flame photometer required dilution of 1:500 for sodium estimation and 1:25 for potassium levels.

Another newer type of instrumentation for estimating elements such as sodium and potassium will be discussed under ion-selective electrodes on p. 76.

Atomic absorption spectrophotometry

Principle

This procedure is based on flame absorption rather than flame emission. Metal atoms absorb strongly at discrete characteristic wavelengths which coincide with the emission spectra of the metal in question. A solution of the sample is converted into an aerosol which is injected into a flame which then converts the sample into an atomic and molecular vapour. The atomic vapour absorbs radiation from a hollow cathode lamp at specific wavelengths. This beam then traverses the flame and is focused on the entrance slit of a monochromator, which is set to read the intensity of the chosen spectral line. Light with this wavelength is absorbed by the metal in the flame and the degree of absorption is a function of the concentration of the metal in the sample.

Instrumentation

Figure 6.14 shows the layout of a simple atomic absorption instrument, the principal components of which are as follows:

(a) Light source

In the majority of procedures, hollow cathode lamps are used. These consist of an anode of tungsten and a hollow cylindrical cathode consisting of, or lined

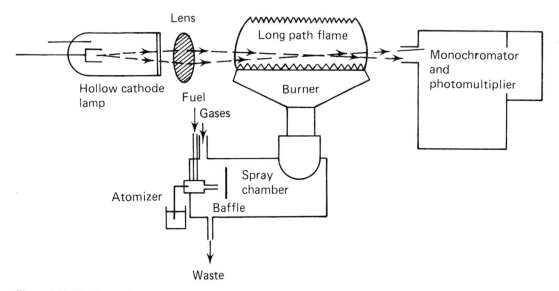

Figure 6.14. Simple atomic absorption flame photometer

with, the metal whose emission spectrum is required. The anode and cathode are sealed in a glass tube filled with argon or neon at a pressure of 1–3 mmHg. When an electric current is passed across the electrodes, the gases ionize and positively charged ions bombard the cathode. Free atoms of the metal are sputtered off the cathode, collide with the atoms of the inert gas, become excited, and emit light characteristic of the metal atom on returning to the ground state or lower level.

(b) Burner aspirator

This aspirates the test sample into the flame which should be sufficiently hot to vaporize the solute and dissociate the molecules to yield free neutral atoms in the ground state. Ground state occurs when the solution evaporates; the substance is then converted into an atomic state where the outermost ring of the electrons is in the position nearest to the nucleus. If the temperature is increased the thermal energy is increased and those outer electrons absorb more energy and then move to a higher energy orbit, further away from the nucleus. These electrons are therefore in a non-stable state and return to a lower level or ground state and release the previously absorbed energy.

With the burner it is important that the flame temperature is not too high as to excite the atoms in the flame, causing flame emission, or to produce ions, which will not absorb light.

There are several types of burner, including the fish-tank type which gives a long horizontal flame, providing a deep light path for the absorption of light, and the total consumption burner in which a narrow vertical flame is produced. To increase the

light path a multipass optical system is employed so that the light beam traverses the flame several times.

(c) Monochromator

This is usually a silica or quartz grating to select the most intense emission line from the hollow cathode lamp, e.g. 422.7 nm for calcium and 285.2 nm for magnesium.

(d) Detector

This is a photomultiplier tube.

(e) Readout system

The output of the detector may be measured either potentiometrically or directly on a meter, either as transmittance or absorbance on the meter, as a trace on a recorder or in digital form.

Double beam instruments

Double beam instruments, as in *Figure 6.15*, are more sophisticated than the simple types in that the double beam arrangement is designed to eliminate the effects of variation in the intensity of the light emitted by the hollow cathode lamp.

Precautions

Interference by other atoms in the flame may occur in this form of instrumentation and this can be divided into three types:

1. *Ionization*—due to excessive heat of the flame,

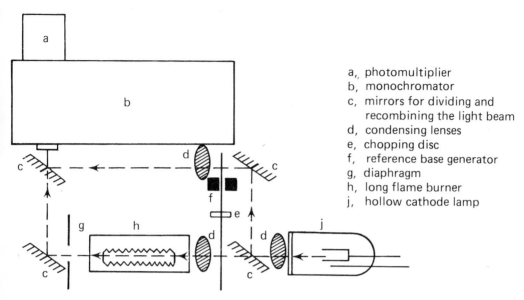

a,, photomultiplier
b, monochromator
c, mirrors for dividing and
   recombining the light beam
d, condensing lenses
e, chopping disc
f, reference base generator
g, diaphragm
h, long flame burner
j, hollow cathode lamp

Figure 6.15. Double beam atomic absorption flame spectrophotometer

some of the atoms may ionize and become non-absorbing. This can be overcome by carefully controlling the temperature of the flame or by adding to the solution under investigation a solute which is more readily ionizable, such as lanthanum or strontium salts.

2. *Chemical*—due to the presence of sulphate or phosphate radicals in the flame which combine with the test atoms, the absorbing characteristic of the flame is reduced. This can partly be overcome by adding a large excess of a competing metal which will combine with the interfering groups forming non-dissociating molecules, for example, lanthanum salts, or alternatively by adding a chelating agent, such as EDTA, when the metal chelate is sprayed into the flame and vaporizes to yield ground-state absorbing atoms.

3. *Physical*—due to the presence of proteins in biological solutions, the increase in velocity due to the protein causes changes in the rate of aspiration and the amount of aerosol entering the flame. This is overcome by precipitating the proteins with trichloracetic acid, centrifuging and then spraying the protein-free supernatant.

In all these cases the additive to the test solution must also be added to the standard and reference solutions.

Methods

These vary depending on the ion or metal to be estimated. If specimens for the estimation of calcium are mixed with lanthanum chloride at a dilution of about 1 in 50, interference from both protein and phosphate is eliminated. The solution is then sprayed into an air–acetylene flame and compared against suitably treated standards.

Turbidimetry and nephelometry

These are methods of analysis which depend upon the phenomenon whereby light passing through a turbid solution is attenuated (diminished) in intensity due to scattering.

Turbidimetric analysis refers to the measurement of unscattered light, i.e. the light which is transmitted through a solution. It can be quantitated by measuring the light transmitted, using an ordinary absorptiometer as described above, provided certain precautions are observed such as strictly adhering to the method of production of turbidity in order to obtain uniform particle size. If the average size of the particles is reproducible, then quantitative assays can be carried out.

When scattered light is measured, a special instrument is required called a nephelometer. The degree of light scattering is dependent on the size of the particle, the shape of the particle and on the concentration of the particles in suspension. It is also dependent on the wavelength of the incident light, in that short wavelengths (blue light) are scattered more easily than long wavelengths (red light).

Turbidimetric measurements may be used in the determination of trace proteins (CSFs and urines) in lipid assessments (chylomicrons) and in assessing the end-point of prothrombin assays, to name just a few.

Fluorimetry

Fluorescence is a phenomenon caused by the scattering and re-emission of light in random directions. A suitable quantum of light energy is absorbed by the molecule and an electron is raised to a higher energy level. Some of the absorbed energy is dissipated due to rotational changes within the molecule. When the electron falls back to the ground state, the excess energy is emitted as light, namely, fluorescence. The return to the ground state may be influenced by mechanisms other than fluorescence, in which case the quantum efficiency of fluorescence exhibited is less than unity. If, however, all the excited molecules fluoresce, then the process efficiency is unity.

There are two types of fluorescence—primary and secondary. Primary fluorescence, which may be pH dependent, refers to the capacity of some compounds to fluoresce intrinsically, e.g. vitamin A, riboflavin, porphyrin and quinine sulphate. Secondary fluorescence results from the interaction of compounds not normally fluorescent with other compounds; for example, cortisol with ethanolic sulphuric acid reagent, and catecholamines with alkaline ethylenediamine solution.

Measurement of fluorescence

Primary fluorescence

In this type of measurement, taking urinary riboflavin as an example, the urine is extracted with a solvent mixture containing acetic acid, pyridine and butanol. The upper alcohol layer is removed and the fluorescence from riboflavin is read against suitably treated standards at a fluorescent wavelength of 535 nm.

Secondary fluorescence

Cortisol is removed from serum or plasma by extracting with dichloromethane. The extract is then treated with an ethanolic sulphuric acid reagent and the resultant fluorescence is measured at 470 nm against suitably treated standards.

When estimating compounds by fluorescence, one important phenomenon to be aware of is quenching, which is a reduction in the amount of emitted light reaching the detector. This can happen in a number of ways; for example, other substances in the solvent may absorb some of the fluorescence or the presence of ions in the reaction mixture may reduce or abolish the fluorescence.

The measurement of pH

The pH meter is designed to measure the concentration of hydrogen ions in a solution. Basically, three parameters are involved in the effective measurement of pH, the actual molar concentration of hydrogen ions, the dissociation constant of the acid (pK_a) and temperature.

pH is defined as the negative value of the logarithm to the base 10 of the hydrogen ion concentration:

$$pH = -\log_{10}(H^+)$$

Water at 25°C has 0.0000001 mol of hydrogen ions per litre (10^{-7}), i.e. the log of the hydrogen ion concentration is -7; therefore, the pH is 7.0 at 25°C. A strong alkaline solution such as sodium hydroxide would have a higher concentration of hydroxyl ions and a lower concentration of hydrogen ions. Such a solution might have

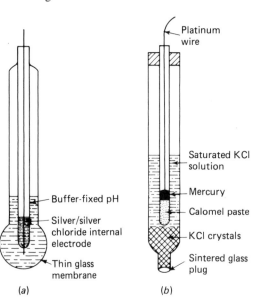

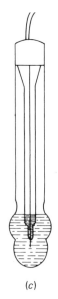

Figure 6.16. (a) Simple glass electrode. (b) Calomel reference electrode. (c) Modern glass electrode

0.000 000 000 000 6 mol of hydrogen ions per litre and this would therefore have a pH of 13. The stronger the acid the lower the pH.

The measurement of pH is called potentiometric analysis. Since the early twentieth century various workers have reported that a difference in electrical potential could be measured between two solutions of different pH separated by a thin glass membrane. The potential thus produced varies with the hydrogen ion concentration of the two solutions, i.e. the glass membrane is H^+ ion-sensitive. It is on this principle that the glass electrode is constructed. The type of glass is important—it must be a soft, hygroscopic glass, with a relatively low electrical resistance. Modern glass electrodes are constructed from glass containing lithium oxide. The inner surface of the glass membrane is in electrical contact with a buffer solution of fixed pH. Into this buffer dips a silver/silver chloride electrode, the internal reference electrode (*Figure 6.16a*). It has been suggested that the glass electrode functions like a semipermeable membrane, permeable only to hydrogen ions (possibly hydrated) which enter the lattice of the glass (i.e. selective for H^+ ions only). A calomel (mercurous chloride) reference electrode (*Figure 6.16b*) consists of mercury in contact with a solution of potassium chloride saturated with calomel. It is surrounded by an outer vessel containing saturated potassium chloride which acts as a salt bridge between the reference and test solution (this electrode is not dependent upon pH).

Only when the glass electrode is coupled with a calomel electrode is the potentiometric measurement of pH possible. We then have the arrangement as shown in *Figure 6.17*.

The potential difference (or electrical voltage) between the two electrodes depends upon the hydrogen ion concentration of the test solution or standard. Because of the small differences produced, an amplifier is included in the circuit to detect the point of balance between the two electrodes. It is a logarithmic response, measured in millivolts, which on the pH meter is calibrated both in mV and pH.

Figure 6.16c shows a simple glass electrode, but the better types of glass electrode are now constructed of two glasses; the working part of the electrode is made of special pH-responsive glass and this is sealed to a stem of harder high-resistance glass. This will exhibit a much greater resistance to ion transfer and therefore eliminate errors due to various depths of immersion. By this arrangement the working part of the electrode is always immersed in the solution. A good glass electrode will measure up to pH 14.

There is also available for use with most pH meters a combined glass and calomel reference electrode, i.e. two electrodes in one.

pH measurements vary with temperature and all measurements should be made at a temperature of 25°C. With increasing temperature there will be a fall in pH. Variations of pH with temperature can be seen as follows:

Temperature (0°C)	pH value
0	7.47
10	7.27
25	7.00
30	6.92
50	6.61

It is therefore important to record the temperature of the liquid before measuring the pH, adjusting the dial on the pH meter, and then record the pH. Some pH meters have facilities whereby a temperature thermometer can be incorporated into the circuit and variations above or below 25°C are automatically corrected by the meter itself.

Precautions with glass electrodes

The sensitivity of the glass electrode will be affected by the following:

1. Continuous use, when the electrode may need regenerating.
2. Protein solution: protein solution will poison the glass membrane and therefore must be removed.
3. Dehydrating agents or concentrated acids which dehydrate the membranes. The presence of water in the glass is essential; pH function is impaired when the glass is dehydrated, but can be restored by subsequent immersion in distilled water for several hours or overnight.
4. Temperature—see above.
5. Scratching or fracturing of the glass membrane. Under these circumstances a new glass electrode is required. When not in use the electrode should

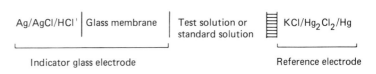

Ag/AgCl/HCl | Glass membrane | Test solution or standard solution | $KCl/Hg_2Cl_2/Hg$

Indicator glass electrode   Reference electrode

Figure 6.17. The arrangement of electrodes in the potentiometric measurement of pH

is the boundary between the two miscible phases (liquid junction)

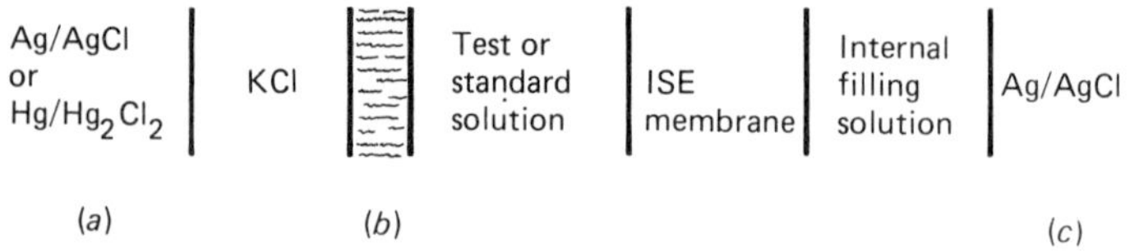

Ag/AgCl or Hg/Hg$_2$Cl$_2$	KCl		Test or standard solution	ISE membrane	Internal filling solution	Ag/AgCl
(a)		(b)				(c)

Figure 6.18. Layout of an ion-selective electrode system: (a) reference electrode; (b) liquid function; (c) internal reference solution

be left with the membrane immersed in distilled water. New electrodes will need generating by placing them in 0.1M hydrochloric acid overnight.

Standardization of the pH meter

Standardization should be carried out at least once a day and preferably before a series of measurements are to be made.

Always use two buffer solutions; for example, one at pH 4.0 and the other at pH 7.0. If higher or lower pHs are being measured, use buffer solutions in the appropriate pH ranges.

Ion-selective electrodes

The potentiometric measurement of pH involves use of an electrode which is a hydrogen ion-selective electrode. Selective electrodes have been developed for many ions such as, for example, sodium, potassium, calcium and fluoride. Ion-selective electrodes like other electrodes have one thing in common—the formation of a potential that obeys the Nernst equation* which measures ionic activity not ionic concentration.

They are electrochemical sensors, the potentials of which have a linear relationship with the logarithm of the activity of the particular ion in solution, despite the presence of other ions. An important requirement for ion-selective electrodes is that the membrane must be able to separate the solution containing the unknown ion from other ions in the detecting system. These membrane junctions (membrane electrodes) are electrochemical sensors which measure the activity and isolate the electrode space from the solution being measured. Their function is to allow selective attraction only of those ions whose activity is to be measured.

*The Nernst equation is expressed as follows:

$$E = E_0 + \frac{2.303RT}{nF} \log a_b$$

where E is the electrode potential measured, E_0 the constant for electrode system (including reference electrode), R the molar gas constant, 8.31 J/K, T the temperature (K), F the farad (96 487 coulombs), n the number of charges on the ion (positive or negative), and a_b the activity of the ion b to which the electrode responds.

The membrane electrodes are classified according to the nature of the material in the membrane, and can be of the following composition:

1. Glass membranes, which are usually composed of silicate or aluminosilicate glass, as in the hydrogen and sodium electrodes.
2. Liquid organic ion-exchanges; these utilize an organic water immiscible liquid phase which incorporates ionic or ionogenic compounds, as in some calcium electrodes.
3. Solid-state membranes, which consist of crystalline materials, either in the form of a single crystal or a fused pellet or the active material may be incorporated into an inert matrix, e.g. PVC, as can be found in the fluoride electrode.
4. Neutral-carrier liquid membranes, which consist of an organic solution of electrically neutral, ion-specific complexing agents incorporated into an inert polymer, as found in the potassium electrode.
5. Special membranes, which incorporate the features described in items 1–4. They are used in conjunction with gas permeable membranes and enzymes, similar to the pCO$_2$ electrode and glucose probe in the glucose analyser.

Each form of ion-selective electrode usually works in the same way as the glass electrode, the selectivity of an ion-selective electrode being dependent upon the electroactive substance used. This material must have some basic affinity for the sensed ion. It may be glass, an insoluble salt, a complexing agent that is highly selective for the ion, such as the antibiotic ionophore valinomycin, used in potassium electrodes, or a synthesized neutral carrier used in calcium electrodes. The ion-selective electrodes, therefore, work as shown in *Figure 6.18*.

In potentiometric analysis, instead of constructing a calibration curve, a two-point calibration is usually carried out, in which the two points chosen are those on each side of the unknown. This is a very similar procedure to that used in pH measurements.

Ion-selective methods are now well established in clinical medicine for the analysis of sodium, potassium and calcium ions in body fluids, using either whole blood, plasma, serum or urine. In this area, flame photometric methods of analysis have been dominant for many years, but sophisticated instrumentation using microprocessors is now gradually taking its place alongside the pH and blood gas analysers. Since the reference range for blood cations is so small, high precision is necessary, even for sodium when only about 2.4 mV charge is involved at 37°C. The advantage over the flame photometer is the speed, sample size and the possible use in *in vivo* measurements.

These are very brief comments and further information should be obtained from suppliers of ion-selective electrodes.

Blood glucose analysers

These analysers are instruments which use an oxygen-sensing electrode, as described on p. 75, and quantitatively measure the amount of glucose in biological fluids. There are three different suppliers of this form of instrumentation: Beckman Instruments, Yellow Spring Instruments (YSI) and Alpha Laboratories. The latter supplies the only British model, the Analox GM 7 oxidase analyser*. As they basically work on the same principle, only one will be described in this chapter, the YSI Model 23 AM glucose analyser.

YSI Model 23 AM glucose analyser†

Principle of operation

Glucose in the presence of oxygen is converted to gluconic acid and hydrogen peroxide, as shown in reaction 1:

$$\beta\text{-D-glucose} + \text{oxygen} \xrightarrow[\text{oxidase}]{\text{glucose}} \text{gluconic acid}$$
$$+ H_2O_2 \tag{1}$$

The dissolved oxygen in the diluted sample is then monitored electrochemically and the glucose level is computed from the rate of disappearance of oxygen. This is done by the probe oxidizing a constant proportion of hydrogen peroxide at the platinum anode, as shown in reaction 2:

$$H_2O_2 \rightarrow 2H^+ + O_2 + 2e^- \tag{2}$$

The circuit is completed by a silver cathode at which oxygen is reduced to water in reaction 3:

$$4H^+ + O_2 \rightarrow 2H_2O + 4e^- \tag{3}$$

While oxygen is present in great excess in those reactions involving oxygen, the 23 AM glucose analyser does not measure oxygen.

A YSI Model 23 AM is supplied complete with instructions for use. The 23 AM gives readings in SI units (mmol/l), while the 23 A model gives readings in mg/dl. A new model, YSI 24, is also available

*Distributor: Alpha Laboratories, 40 Parham Drive, Eastleigh, Hants. SO5 4NU
†Distributor: Clandon Scientific Ltd, Lysons Avenue, Ash Vale, Aldershot, Hants. GU12 5QR.

which is a fully automated system for the measurement of glucose in up to 40 samples of blood plasma or serum.

Conductivity analysis

The electrical conductance of a solution is the power of that solution to conduct an electric current, which will depend upon the number of ions in solution and the mobility of these ions. Strong acids and bases or the salts of strong acids and bases are completely dissociated in solution. Weak acids and bases and their salts are slightly dissociated and neutral organic substances other than salts do not ionize. Beckman Instruments have made use of this principle for determining urea in biological solutions. This method is based upon the difference in electrical conductivity of urea and ammonium carbonate produced from urea by the enzyme urease.

Beckman BUN (blood urea nitrogen) analyser

Principle of operation

Estimating urea with this instrument (Beckman–RIIC Ltd) eliminates many of the problems associated with other methods, some of which are described in Chapter 10. The BUN chemistry analyser uses the Beckman developed enzymatic-conductivity rate method, employing a Beckman conductivity electrode to measure the rate of increase of conductivity when a known sample of biological fluid is introduced into a precise quantity of urease reagent. When a sample is injected into the reaction cup containing the urease reagent, the urea in the sample reacts according to the following equation:

$$\underset{\substack{H_2N \quad NH_2}}{\overset{\overset{\displaystyle O}{\displaystyle \|}}{C}} + H_2O \xrightarrow{\text{urease}} (NH_4)_2CO_3$$
$$\rightarrow NH_4^+ + HCO_3^-$$

This results in the conversion of urea (non-ionic) to ammonium carbonate (ionic). During the reaction, the timed rate of increase of solution conductivity is directly proportional to the concentration of urea present in the reaction cup. The instrument measures the rate of time t, and this is converted into corresponding urea concentration either in mg urea nitrogen (BUN) per 100 ml or mmol urea per litre. A typical instrument is shown in *Figure 6.19* which Beckman supply with a full instruction manual.

This chemistry module is also incorporated into the Beckman Astra TM4 and TM8 automated

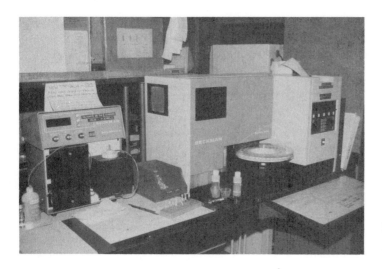

Figure 6.19. Beckman BUN analyser (reproduced by courtesy of Beckman-RIIC Ltd)

clinical analysers. These two instruments can also contain the Beckman oxygen rate analyser for estimating blood glucose.

Radioactive isotopes and their detection

Radioactive isotopes have been used in biochemical analysis for a number of years and are now of increasing importance in most clinical chemistry departments.

Lord Rutherford and his colleagues first discovered radioactivity in approximately 1920. The Curies in France continued with this work and, following the invention of the cyclotron by Lawrence in 1932, it became possible to apply the use of radioactive isotopes to biochemical analysis.

Isotopes are of two kinds, stable and unstable (radioactive)—see *Table 6.3*.

Table 6.3 Some stable and radioactive isotopes

Stable isotopes		Radioactive isotopes		Particles
Iodine	^{127}I	^{125}I		gamma
Carbon	^{12}C	^{14}C		beta
Calcium	^{40}Ca	^{15}Ca		gamma
Cobalt	^{59}Co	^{57}Co		gamma
Tritium	H	^{3}H		beta

Stable isotopes

Isotopes are atoms of the same element, having identical atomic numbers but different atomic weights. Stable isotopes are permanent substances, which do not disintegrate with time and are not radioactive.

Unstable isotopes

These isotopes can be prepared from stable elements in a cyclotron, when they become unstable because of their radioactivity. Radioactive isotopes disintegrate spontaneously, the rate of decay being proportional to the number of radioactive atoms present.

Radioactive isotopes can occur naturally as, for example, uranium.

The radiation emitted during disintegration can be of three types, alpha (α), beta (β) or gamma (γ).

Alpha particles are helium atoms (He^{2+}) with very low penetrating power. Preparations using these emitting particles are not commonly used. Beta particles are either positive or negative electrons; they have more penetrating power than alpha particles but are stopped by a very light shielding. Gamma particles are electromagnetic radiations similar to X-rays and have a high penetrating power.

The types of radioactive isotopes used in medicine are those which emit β- and γ-type radiations. The naturally occurring isotopes are the source of α-radiation.

Units of activity

The activity of a radioactive isotope preparation is measured by the number of nuclear disintegrations per second. The curie (Ci) is the unit of activity commonly used.

One curie is 3.7×10^{10} disintegrations per second. This is a great deal of activity and smaller units such as a millicurie (mCi) or microcurie (μCi) are much more commonly used.

SI unit of activity

Traditionally, radioactivity has been measured in curies and although the curie is still commonly used the SI unit of radioactivity is the becquerel (Bq) which corresponds to one disintegration per second. Therefore

1 mCi is equivalent to 37 MBq
1 MBq is equivalent to 27 µCi

Radioactive half-life

The half-life of a radioactive substance refers to the length of time required for the isotope to decay to half its activity. This can vary from a few seconds to one of 1000 years. Isotopes used in medicine usually have a half-life of about six weeks, e.g. ^{125}I.

Biological half-life

The biological half-life of a compound is the measure of the disintegration of the compound itself and has no relation to its radioactive properties.

Methods of measurement

The simplest way of detecting radiation is the use of photographic films or plates. The familiar radiation protection badges worn by all staff in isotope departments are the commonest application.

This method of detection, however, cannot be used for quantitative estimation of radioactive disintegrations; in that type of assay, a gamma or beta counter is required.

The essential part of a counter is the Geiger–Muller tube, a tube consisting of a fine wire anode surrounded by a coaxial cylindrical metal cathode. These are completely encased into a glass casing filled with gas at low pressure. Radiations entering the counter strike the Geiger–Muller tube, ionizing molecules of gas contained in it, and the negative ions move towards the positively charged anode. This causes a drop in potential which, when connected to a measuring device, is recorded as a pulse. By counting the number of pulses produced in a specific time, the radioactivity of a compound can be calculated. This is usually expressed in terms of counts per min.

^{125}I, for example, emits high-energy radiations which are therefore measured in a conventional gamma counter, as shown in *Figure 6.20*. In the case of low-energy radiations, for example from ^{14}C and ^{3}H, a scintillation (beta) counter is required. In the method, the compound to be estimated is dissolved in a suitable solvent (toluene), along with another compound (organic phosphor) which then undergoes a scintillation reaction. In this reaction the phosphor fluoresces or scintillates, i.e. emits light photons which are collected by the photomultipliers and converted into a pulse and recorded in the usual way.

Radioactive reagents are made use of in the determination of minute quantities of substances in biological fluids, such as ^{125}I-labelled hormone in radioimmunoassay methods, and for *in vitro* use in measurements and administration to patients.

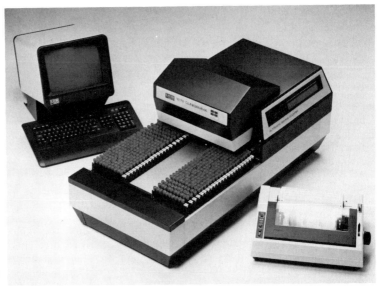

Figure 6.20. LKB 12720 CliniGamma (reproduced by courtesy of LKB)

Isotope laboratory design and safety

There are four booklets available for consultation, which will adequately cover the problems and precautions:

1. 'Safety in pathology laboratories', DHSS, May 1972.
2. 'The design of laboratories for radioactive and other toxic substances', Hughes, D. and Cullingworth, R., Koch–Light Laboratories Ltd, 1970.
3. 'Code of practice for the protection of persons against ionising radiations arising from medical and dental use', HMSO, 1972.
4. 'Health and Safety at Work etc. Act 1974', Chapter 37, HMSO, 1980.

Immunoassay

Over the past few years laboratories have seen the gradual introduction of new techniques, one of which is the highly specific and sensitive immunological procedure. The immunological response of the body to the introduction of foreign substances or *antigens*, either in the pure or mixed form, leads to the development of specific antagonists to the antigen which are referred to as *antibodies*. These humoral antibodies therefore combine with the antigens to reduce their biological activity, either directly by inactivation or by phagocytic action. This antigen–antibody reaction can therefore be utilized in radioimmunoassay procedures.

All methods using antibody binders are collectively called immunoassays; therefore when a radioactive isotope is used it is called radioimmunoassay. An enzyme label product is called enzyme immunoassay. If the label takes the form of a free radical it is called free radical immunoassay technique (FRIAT) or spin immunoassay. The use of fluorescent labels gives us fluoroimmunoassay and a bacteriophage label when used in virus assays is called viroimmunoassay.

Radioimmunoassay (RIA)

Before 1960, most assays in the laboratory for the estimation of hormones in biological fluid were carried out by bioassay which was crude and inaccurate. In 1960, methods were reported for the estimation of insulin and thyroxine which were based on a new principle which was described as 'saturation analysis'. Several varieties of this procedure have been developed in the past decade and they may be applied to the measurement of the amount of antigen (Ag) or antibody (Ab) in a specimen and involve the addition of a radioactive-labelled reagent in the form of the antigen or antibody. The final step is the measurement of the radioactive-labelled product following a separative

step and, in order to be applicable to the measurement of small quantities of antigen or antibody, the labelled product must be such that it can be detected in very low concentrations.

Basically, RIA can be illustrated as described in the following paragraphs. If the antigen is Ag, the labelled antigen is Ag' and the antibody is Ab, then, in this type of assay, the reactants are the Ag to be determined, the Ag' in a radioactive form, for example, ^{125}I, and the antiserum containing Ab to the antigen. Therefore,

$$Ag + Ag' + Ab \underset{K_2}{\overset{K_1}{\rightleftharpoons}} AgAb + Ag'Ab$$

This reaction results in the formation of a labelled antigen–antibody complex. If the amounts of Ag' and Ab added are kept constant, provided that optimal conditions are chosen, the binding sites on the Ab will be limited and the Ag and Ag' will complete for them. Once equilibrium has been reached, Ag and Ag' will either be in the free form (F), as shown on the left-hand side of the reaction above, or combined with the Ab in the bound form (B), as in the right-hand side of the reaction. Thus, the ratio of the labelled antigen bound to the antibody (B) to the free antigen (F) will progressively fall in proportion to the increase in concentration of the unlabelled antigen.

After separating the B and F forms by one of the standard methods of separation, the radioactivity of one or the other can then be measured and quantitated in an appropriate radioactive counter, after adding known amounts of Ag, to produce a calibration curve. In this assay, the B and F forms are determined and the ratio of B:F plotted against the antigen content of the standard or unknown preparation or, alternatively, %B is plotted against the antigen concentration.

By using this technique, levels down to picogram quantities can be detected and estimated.

Similar methods are also available for the measurement of specific antibodies rather than the antigen. Radioimmunoassay methods can also be used for the determination of specific enzyme proteins, but, as the preparation of purified enzymes for antibody production is costly, this technique is limited.

Enzyme immunoassay

There are two basic assays in this group—EMIT and ELISA. EMIT, or enzyme multiplied immunoassay technique, is a homogeneous enzyme immunoassay when the molecule is labelled with an enzyme. ELISA, or enzyme linked immunosorbent assay, is a heterogeneous enzyme immunoassay which uses labelled antibodies. The basic immunochemical reaction is as follows:

$$Ag + Ab \underset{K_2}{\overset{K_1}{\rightleftharpoons}} Ag{:}Ab$$

where Ag is the antigen or drug, Ab the antibody and Ag:Ab the immune complex.

The difference between a homogeneous and heterogeneous system can be summarized as follows: Ag + Ab:Ag-L (homogeneous) and Ab:Ag + Ag-L (heterogeneous). Here, Ag is the drug or antigen, Ab the antibody, L the label (enzyme) and Ag-L the labelled antigen.

Then, if the label L is active in both the bound product (Ab:Ag-L) and free form (Ag-L), then a physical separation technique is required and the assay is called heterogeneous. ELISA utilizes labelled antibodies and an antigen which has been made insoluble by attaching it to a solid support (e.g. tubes, insoluble polymers) and therefore necessitating the physical separation of the free from the bound antigen. If, however, the activity of the label L is reduced or eliminated in either the free or bound form, then no separation is required and the assay is called homogeneous.

EMIT

All immunochemical techniques require the preparation of specific antibodies (first component), as shown in *Figure 6.21*. In the antibody production, haptens of low molecular weight (e.g. drugs, steroids) do not generally elicit an immune response in an animal and therefore must be attached to a protein carrier, e.g. bovine serum albumin, to produce a larger antigen.

The second component in the system is the labelled antigen and to avoid the use of radioactive isotopes, enzymes make suitable labels because their catalytic properties allow them to act as amplifiers. *Figure 6.22* shows the chemical coupling of the hapten or antigen to an enzyme to produce the enzyme-labelled antigen.

A variety of enzymes have been used, such as lysozyme, malate dehydrogenase and glucose-6-phosphate dehydrogenase.

The EMIT assay procedure is simple; the reaction times are quite short due to the high specific activity of the enzyme label and the specific antibodies available. This type of assay has been developed for a wide variety of substances such as phenytoin, phenobarbital, digoxin, amphetamines, barbiturates, cortisol, thyroxine, thyroxine binding globulin and gentamicin.

Coulometric analyses

This form of analysis carried out in the clinical laboratory is in the estimation of chloride in biological fluid. Potentiometric titrations (coulometric titrations) are used every day in the form of chloride meters, automatic instruments based on the application of Faraday's law of electrolysis. The chloride meter is an easily operated instrument, containing a digital readout, various operating controls and a measuring head. Into the measuring head are fitted four silver electrodes, two silver generating electrodes (one an anode, the other a cathode) and two end-point detection electrodes. A linear current flows between two silver

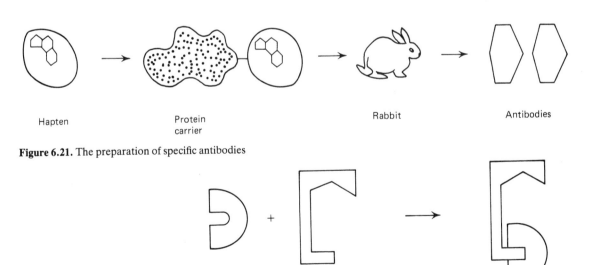

Hapten   Protein carrier   Rabbit   Antibodies

Figure 6.21. The preparation of specific antibodies

Figure 6.22. The chemical coupling of antigen/hapten to an enzyme   Antigen   Enzyme   Enzyme labelled antigen

generating electrodes. Silver ions are released from the anode and combine with the chloride ions in the sample during titration. The digital display starts registering as the silver and chloride ions combine ion to ion until all the chloride has been precipitated as silver chloride. The free silver ions in the solution cause a change in conductivity which is sensed by the two end-point detecting electrodes. This abrupt change in conductivity stops the digital readout, displaying the result directly in mmol chloride per litre.

The Corning 925 chloride meter (Corning Medical and Scientific) is the most popular instrument in use, and this differs from the earlier models in that magnetic followers are now replaced on the 925, with a built-in stirrer. For use with the estimation of chloride in biological fluids consult the manufacturer's instruction manual.

Osmometer

An osmometer is an instrument for measuring the concentration of solutes in a solution. When solutes are dissolved in a solvent the resulting solution changes because the freezing point is lowered and the osmotic pressure is increased. These are called colligative properties and they have a specific value since they are closely related to the osmolality of a body fluid.

Measurement of osmolality

The instruments available measure osmolality of body fluids by indirect means, by measuring the depression of freezing point, since the freezing point of a liquid is dependent upon its solute concentration. Water is first cooled without stirring to below freezing point. At a definite degree of supercooling, a vibration is activated to induce freezing and the temperature of the water then rises to the freezing point of 0°C, which is recorded on a galvanometer. In biological fluids the freezing point is below 0°C; this depression of freezing point is therefore a measure of the osmolality of the solution. The galvanometer is usually calibrated to read directly in milliosmoles (mosmol), 1 mosmol being equivalent to a depression of freezing point of 0.00186°C.

Automated analysis

Most medical laboratory scientists are thankful that many of the boring repetitive tests in the clinical laboratory have now been automated in one form or another. If the routine tests are not completely automated some form of semi-automation is used, such as the use of diluters, automatic pipettes and burettes, dispensers, mixers, shakers, etc. This approach is often called work simplification, involving not only a change in equipment, but also a reorganization of work practices to eliminate inefficient procedures and reduce technical errors.

Since the introduction of a complete form of automated analysis after Skeggs (1957), many more tests are now carried out per patient than was even thought of several years ago.

Automation has many advantages, two of which are (a) rapid throughput of investigations, and (b) increased accuracy and precision of the estimation compared with conventional manual methods. However, with the introduction of automation, 'bottlenecks' in processing clinical chemistry samples occurred, both with handling the patient samples before analysis and with the data generated by the analysers. One way of alleviating these bottlenecks was the introduction of data handling equipment or computerization.

As automatic equipment has grown in size, it must never be forgotten that in many laboratories manual methods of some form or other may need to be available for emergency cases. Some laboratories, however, may be in a position where they can purchase automated stat/routine analyser equipment similar to the Astra TM4 (Beckman) for their emergency procedures. This is a bench-top discrete microprocessor-controlled analyser which estimates electrolytes, enzymes or other chemistries depending on modules selected.

Automation can be of two different forms, namely, continuous flow or discrete (discontinuous) systems.

Continuous flow systems

Historically, the first real continuous flow system in clinical chemistry was manufactured by the Technicon Instruments Corporation of New York and this system was given the trade name AutoAnalyser. The AutoAnalyser uses a combination of modules where a sequence of standards and test samples are 'picked up' in a stream of fluid moved along a tube by a peristaltic pump, mixed at appropriate stages with a series of reagents, then passed through the various modules and finally analysed colorimetrically. To separate the samples in the moving stream and to assure that cross-contamination does not ocur between samples, a non-wettable plastic tube is used into which air bubbles are introduced at regular intervals. The air segments are large enough to completely fill the lumen of the tube.

With manual procedures every reaction must generally be brought to completion, but with the AutoAnalyser system it is never necessary, since it continuously measures and compares on a moving graph the level of concentration of a given component in the test solution against a known

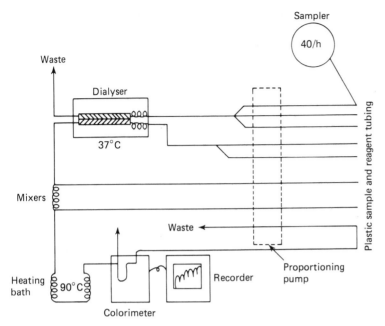

Figure 6.23. Flow diagram for an AA I system

concentration of that component in a standard control solution.

The function of the original AutoAnalyser has not changed in more than 25 years, in that the module used to determine a single substance in an AutoAnalyser I system (AA I) is as follows: (a) sampler, (b) proportioning (peristaltic) pump, (c) dialyser (to remove protein), (d) constant temperature heating bath, (e) colorimeter and (f) recorder. This arrangement is shown in *Figure 6.23* which is a flow diagram. This system existed essentially from about 1957 to 1970 when more than 10000 were installed throughout Europe alone.

Sequential Multiple Analysis system

The increasing demands on the clinical laboratory for faster rates of analysis and flexibility of procedures, along with increased accuracy of results, led to a newer generation of AutoAnalysers, the Sequential Multiple Analysis system (SMA). This system, the SMA 12/60, is capable of performing 12 simultaneous colorimetric tests on one sample and can introduce samples at the rate of 60 per h. Although the AA I system could be so constructed as to estimate four different parameters at the same time (e.g. Na, K, CO_2, urea), the SMA system gives steady-state conditions in which the concentration of the sample in the colorimeter flow cell remains constant for a period of time, and the result can therefore be reported directly into concentration on the recorder chart paper (see *Figure 6.24*). The introduction of the first SMA system was in 1966 and the next generation of multi-channel analysers came onto the market in 1974. This was the SMAC, a

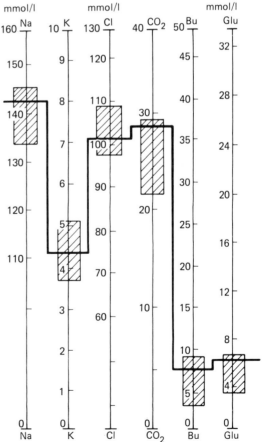

Figure 6.24. Recorder chart paper of the SMA system of analysis. Shaded areas are the 'normal' ranges

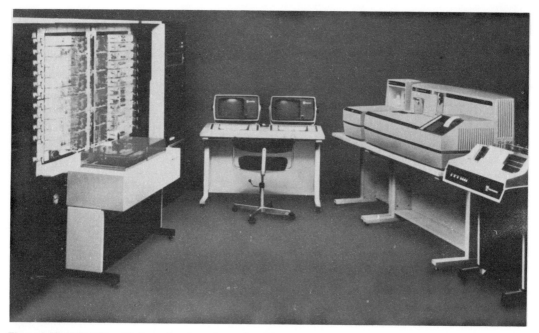

Figure 6.25. SMAC II multi-channel analyser (reproduced by courtesy of Technicon Instruments Co. Ltd)

computer-controlled SMA system achieving a high speed of analysis of 150 samples per hour with a total of 20 test profiles from the same sample. Later generations of these two systems, the SMA II and SMAC II (*Figure 6.25*), launched in 1978 and 1981, respectively, were developed to fully alleviate the problems associated with data generated by an increased throughput of samples.

Another multi-channel continuous flow system of UK design is the Chemispek J 200 multi-channel analyser (Hilger Analytical) which makes use of different continuous flow kinetics.

AutoAnalyser II system (AA II)

After the experience of the SMA system, the second generation of the AA I system was introduced in 1970. This analyser combines many of the virtues of the SMA system—improved pumping system, reduced reagent consumption and an improved flow cell arrangement. The AA II system brings to the single channel analysis the benefits of steady-state measurement with improved accuracy and reduced carryover. Samples are placed on a sample tray and sequentially aspirated into the continuous flow analytical stream. A wash solution is introduced between each sample to separate the specimens, along with air bubbles, at two-second intervals to separate each sample into segments and to clean the hydraulic tubing. The samples are then passed through a manifold system, a measurement module

(colorimeter, flame photometer and fluoronephelometer), after which the individual test outputs are recorded as traces on chart paper (*Figure 6.26*) or/and with a modular digital printer as digital values of the concentration units. A flow diagram is shown in *Figure 6.27*, while the layout of a typical AutoAnalyser II system is shown in *Figure 6.28*.

Discrete (discontinuous) systems

A further advancement from the work simplification equipment is the incorporation of dispensers, etc., into an automatic system whereby each sample is processed separately and the reactions carried out in individual tubes, reaction chambers or specially constructed cells. The chemistries involve protein precipitation or else the amount of protein in the sample reaction mixture is so minute that it does not interfere with the test.

The AutoAnalysers have had one significant advantage over other systems, in that protein is removed by dialysis whereas other instrument makers have difficulty in breaking the patent on the Technicon dialyser and therefore have to use other means of deproteinization. Basically, the main units in a discrete analyser are (a) preparation unit, (b) centrifuge, (c) incubator, (d) automatic colorimeter and printer, and (e) automatic pipettes and dispensers. The samplers and reagents are dispensed or removed by means of the fifth unit. Like the

85

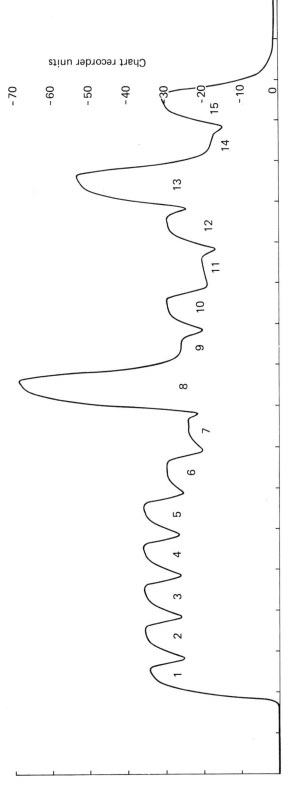

Figure 6.26. Traces from the AA II system showing a typical recording for glucose analysers: 1–5 are 10 mmol/l standards; 6–15 are test samples

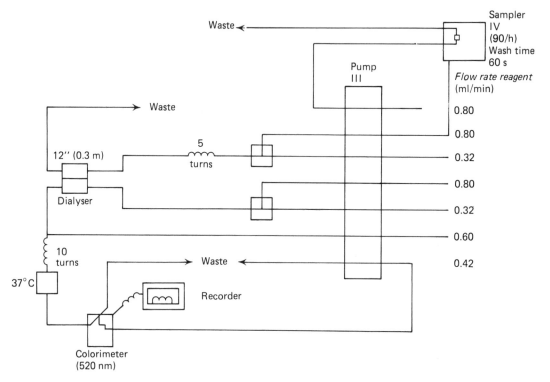

Figure 6.27. AutoAnalyser II flow diagram

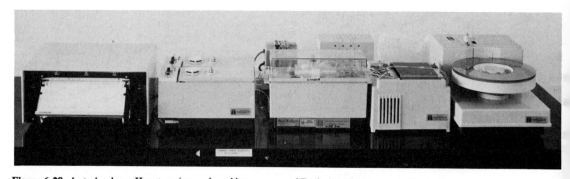

Figure 6.28. AutoAnalyser II system (reproduced by courtesy of Technicon Instruments Co. Ltd)

continuous flow multi-channel analysers, data handling modules are also incorporated into the systems.

Although not all discrete systems are completely based on the above system, some of the available discrete analysers are the Vickers M 300 (now being phased out), Coulter Kem-O-Lab, Greiner Selective Analyser II, Du Pont Automatic Clinical Analyser (ACA) and Astra and centrifugal analysers.

Reaction rate analysers

These are instruments which have been developed for the automatic determination of enzymes under specified conditions. Some of the instruments described above are capable of working as enzyme analysers in the same way as the centrifugal analysers described below. They were originally developed to estimate enzyme activity by kinetic methods under zero order reaction conditions, when the rate of change of absorbance is proportional to the activity of the enzyme.

Centrifugal fast analysers

This is a micro-analytical system, often referred to as parallel fast analysers, the first one being developed in collaboration between the General Medical Sciences Division of the National Institutes of Health and the Atomic Energy Commission, USA, when it was referred to as the GEMSAEC analyser.

These analysers consist of a pipetting station with a separate analysis unit incorporating a microprocessor. The reaction takes place in a multicuvette rotor within the instrument. Mixing occurs by the spinning action, the reactants being held against the outer wall of the cuvette by centrifugal force, and finally absorbance data is taken on spinning by a fixed photometer, with the light path in the majority of instruments perpendicular to the axis of rotation. However, one of the later centrifugal analysers, the Cobas Bio (Roche Products Ltd), has the light path parallel to the axis of rotation, with the pipetting station and analysis

unit is integrated and microprocessor controlled, and once the samples and reagents are added to the appropriate vessels no further manual operation is involved.

The cuvettes are precision-engineered measuring receptacles. The optical system consists of a grating spectrophotometer with an optical range of 285–750 nm; the light intensity source is a long-life xenon flash tube.

The centrifugal analyser can be used to estimate, for example, enzymes, bilirubin, glucose, uric acid, proteins, drugs and enzyme immunoassays; the latter is discussed on p. 80 of this chapter.

Chromatography

Early in the twentieth century a Russian botanist, Tswett, was working on plant pigments and devised

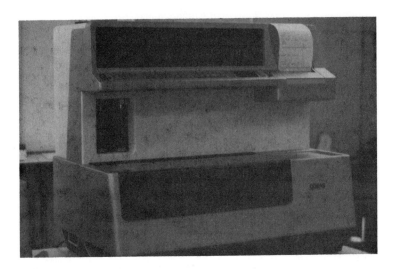

Figure 6.29. Cobas Bio system (reproduced by courtesy of Roche Products Ltd)

microprocessor unit being combined in one instrument.

The Cobas Bio system, shown in *Figure 6.29*, basically consists of a control module, analyser section, rotor, optical system and a data handling unit. The clearly designed control module is used for selecting the tests by using a push button or test number; this then automatically sets all the parameters for the individual test, such as wavelength, reaction time, temperature, reagent volume, etc. The individual programmed methods are stored in a microprocessor. Using this control module, up to 40 tests can be selected at any one time. Ten of the tests can be selected by means of codable push buttons, the remaining tests by entering a test number. The analyser section consists of a sample disc receptor, reagent rack, a pipette for main reagent transfer and a pipette for sample and start reagent transfer, as well as an analyser module with rotor and spectrophotometer. The sample and reagent pipetting

a system very similar to paper chromatography. In his work he was able to separate the various plant pigments on a column of calcium carbonate. Since he worked primarily with coloured solutions, Tswett called this technique chromatography, a term now used today, even though many of the separations commonly used have nothing to do with colour.

General principle

A mixture of substances in solution can be separated when applied to a support medium. This can either be paper (paper chromatography), a thin layer of silica (thin layer chromatography) or a column packed with an adsorbent or ion exchange resin (column chromatography). Tswett adsorbed a mixture of plant pigments on the calcium carbonate and then separated the components into a series of coloured bands by washing or eluting the pigments with solvents. The pigments separated depending upon their solubility in the solvent; if, however, all the pigments were completely soluble in the solvents, there would be no separation.

Terminology

Elution—the use of a solvent to separate components.

Eluate—the solvent containing the component, sometimes called the fraction.

Origin—the point of application of substance to chromatogram.

Loading—the amount of substance applied to the paper or support.

Solvent front—the level at which the elution fluid has reached.

Stationary phase—usually a solid or liquid adsorbent, e.g. paper or water.

Mobile phase—a solvent or gas used to separate the component.

Column—a cylindrical tube usually made of glass for holding either the adsorbent or ion exchange resin.

Polarity—a polar compound is one that is held by the stationary phase, whereas a non-polar compound tends to move forward in the mobile phase.

Adsorption chromatography—when the stationary phase is a solid, while the mobile phase can either be a gas or a liquid.

Paper partition chromatography—when the stationary phase is a liquid, frequently water held onto an inert, porous support (paper), and the mobile phase can either be a liquid or gas. In this type of chromatography more than one solvent is usually present in a liquid mobile phase, since it is always saturated with the stationary phase, thus making the two phases immiscible. Separation occurs between two components of a mixture when one component is more strongly retained than the other by the stationary phase.

Thin layer chromatography—a variant of chromatography in which the support medium is applied to a glass plate or plastic film.

One-dimensional chromatography—when the solvent runs into one direction only.

Two-dimensional chromatography—after the solvent has run into one direction, the paper is dried and turned through 90°, replaced in the tank and developed in the new direction (see *Figure 6.30*).

Multiple development—when the development is re-run a number of times in a solvent system to improve resolution.

Development—the process of allowing the solvent to move along the column or paper.

Resolution—the degree of separation of the component after development.

Location—the detection of the components after development, either by using a specific or general reagent or ultraviolet light.

Tanks—airtight containers in which development takes place.

R_f *value* (relative fraction)—defined as a ratio of the distance the solute has travelled from the point of origin to the distance travelled by the solvent front, i.e.

$$R_f = \frac{\text{Distance solute has moved from origin}}{\text{Distance solvent has moved from origin}}$$
$$= \text{(the value is always less than 1.0)}$$

Sometimes it may be necessary to allow the solvent to run off the support in order to obtain good separation of the components. In this case it is not possible to measure the solvent front, so a standard substance is used and R_g values are obtained in the same way:

$$R_g = \frac{\text{Distance solute has moved from origin}}{\text{Distance standard has moved from origin}}$$

In certain cases the R_f or R_g values are multiplied by 100.

Ion exchange chromatography. An increasing number of laboratories now produce water free from ions, although not all non-electrolytc contaminants may be removed; hence the water is not pyrogen-free. There may also be some extraction of organic impurities from the resins, but under normal circumstances the water obtained by this method is purer than that obtained by distillation. Water purified by ion exchange resins is sometimes called 'conductivity water', as it has such a low electrical conductivity that it is suitable for use in such measurements.

Principles of ion exchange resin. Ion exchange resins are usually crosslinked polymers containing ionic groups as part of their structure. They have

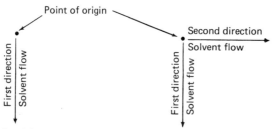

One-dimensional chromatography   Two-dimensional chromatography

Figure 6.30. Directions of flow in chromatography

negligible solubility, but porous enough for ions to diffuse through the resin. During polymerization (manufacture), the polystyrene resins are formed by condensation between the vinyl benzyl (styrene) and small quantities of divinyl benzene to give crosslinked polymer chains. This is important because the amount of crosslinking determines the insolubility of the resin and also the amount of swelling that occurs when the resin is mixed with water and its capacity for exchanging ions.

Ion exchange resins are either (a) anion exchange resins $(R-NH_3)^+OH^-$ which are bases, or (b) cation exchange resins $(R-SO_3)^-H^+$ which are acids. R represents a polystyrene resin. Anion exchangers are usually supplied in the Cl^- form because they are more stable, then they are converted into the OH form which is the exchangeable ion. Cation exchangers are supplied in the H^+ form.

If water containing sodium chloride is passed through a column of cation exchange resin, the Na^+ cations replace the H^+ cations of the resin:

$$(R-SO_3)^-H^+ + Na^+ \rightarrow (R-SO_3)^-Na^+ + H^+$$
(cation exchanger)

The water now contains H^+ ions (obtained from the resin) together with the original Cl^- anions. If the water is passed through an anion exchange resin, the Cl^- replaces the OH^- anion of the resin:

$$(R-NH_3)^+OH^- + Cl^- \rightarrow (R-NH_3)^+Cl^- + OH^-$$
(anion exchanger)

The water now contains H^+ and OH^- ions which combine to form H_2O. In this way the water is prepared ion-free.

Conductivity water is usually produced by passing the water through a 'mixed-bed' de-ionizer, i.e. mixing the two resins together in one column.

Ion exchange resins may be regenerated by passing HCl through the cation resin, followed by washing well with water and passing NaOH through the anion resin, and washing with water. If the resins are of the 'mixed-bed' type, it is necessary to separate the two resins first by passing an upward flow of water through the mixture. The two resins, being of unequal density, will separate out.

Another group of ion exchange resins which are very valuable for protein separations are of the cellulose type. Strongly alkaline cellulose is treated with an acid, chloroacetic acid, which introduces a carboxymethyl group to form carboxymethyl-cellulose (CM-cellulose) a weak cation exchange resin. If 2-chlorotriethylamine is condensed with cellulose, diethyl amino ethyl-cellulose (DEAE-cellulose) is formed which is a weak anion exchanger.

Sephadex is an ion exchanger produced from polymerized dextran. There are many ion exchange resins which are used for a variety of purposes, e.g.

Amberlite for catecholamines, Dowex for amino-acids and Zeocarb for desalting urines prior to chromatography.

Paper partition chromatography

The solvent can either run down the length of the chromatography paper (descending chromatography) or percolate upwards (ascending chromatography). In the descending form the upper end of the paper dips into a narrow trough containing the solvent; the chromatography paper then passes over a glass rod to hang down in the tank (*Figure 6.31*) in which there is also a container with the stationary solvent to keep the atmosphere saturated.

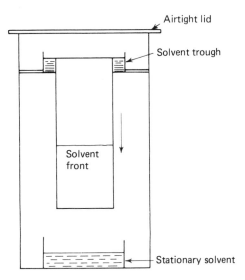

Figure 6.31. Chromatography tank—descending technique

In the ascending technique the solvent is in the bottom of the tank and the paper dips into it. By the side of the trough containing the mobile phase is a small reservoir containing the stationary phase. Chromatography papers vary in size and thickness; the most commonly used in this country are Whatman 1, 4 and 3MM. They should be comparatively free from impurities, which can hinder the resolution and cause irregularities in development.

Technique for one-dimensional chromatography (descending)

1. Take a sheet of Whatman No. 1 chromatography paper of suitable length and width for the tank in use and draw a pencil line parallel to and about 8 cm from one end.
2. 10 μl of test solution is then loaded on the line by allowing the sample to spot the paper several times on the pencil mark (see *Figure 6.32*).

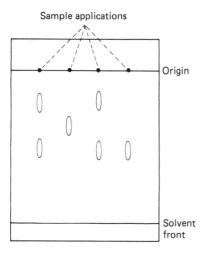

Sample applications

Origin

Solvent
front

Figure 6.32. One-dimensional chromatography—sample applications

3. Always allow the spot to dry at room temperature, or a little above, before adding the next volume. Do not overheat.
4. The smaller the area of application, the more compact will the component be after development.
5. Depending upon the sample being chromatographed, the volumes loaded onto the chromatogram will vary.
6. The standard samples are now applied in the same way.
7. Place the chromatogram in the tank, and align the sheet so that the solvent will run correctly and not irregularly.
8. Replace the lid, run the solvent into the trough and allow development to proceed.
9. The time of development will depend upon the component being investigated, but this can vary from 16 to 36 h.
10. Carefully remove the paper and mark the position of the solvent front if prolonged development has not been used.
11. Hang the paper in a fume-cupboard and blow off the solvent in a stream of cold air, until completely dry.
12. The paper is now ready for locating the position of the separated components.
13. Place the locating reagent in a glass spray or atomizer and spray the area quickly and evenly until the paper is damped.
14. Rehang the paper in the fume-cupboard and allow most of the reagent to dry.
15. It may now be necessary to resuspend the chromatogram in a hot-air oven for a few minutes at 95–100°C.
16. Examine the paper every few minutes until all the individual components can be seen.

17. Overheating can char the paper with particular reagents and therefore the paper must be prevented from 'breaking up'.
18. Compare the spots of the unknown components with that of the standards.
19. Calculate the R_f value if necessary.

Thin layer chromatography

In 1938 two Russian scientists made a great advance in the field of adsorption chromatography by introducing thin layer adsorption chromatography on carrier plates. Approximately 20 years later Stahl in 1958 introduced thin layer chromatography (TLC) and demonstrated its many applications. TLC gives much more rapid results and is a far more sensitive technique. These are only two of the advantages over paper chromatography; on the other hand some separation techniques still require paper chromatography. This technique is now used far more often than paper chromatography and most laboratories have adopted it.

The plates can be made by obtaining the basic equipment for their preparation from the usual commercial organizations or they can be purchased precoated from Merck or Camlab. However, if some laboratories still wish to make their own thin layer plates, the procedure described below can be used quite successfully.

Preparation of home-made thin layer plates

Flat plates of ordinary window glass (2.5 mm) can be used, the size depending upon the airtight tank available. The three usual sizes are $10\,cm^2$, $20\,cm^2$ or $10 \times 20\,cm$.

All plates must be thoroughly cleaned before use, preferably by washing in a good detergent, followed by hot water and finally running in distilled water before drying.

Absorbents

Materials used are generally silica gel, alumina and cellulose. The required quantity of absorbent is mixed with distilled water to form a slurry; 30 g of silica gel and 60 ml of water, shake thoroughly for 1–2 min in a stoppered flask and then use promptly as described below.

Preparation of chromatoplates

The following method of preparing plates has the advantage of being simple, versatile, and plates of various sizes can be coated. After thoroughly cleaning the glass plates, a narrow strip of adhesive tape (Elastoplast) is applied to the edges of the plate. The thickness of the tape determines the thickness of the absorbent coating. To prevent the plates moving during the coating process, the tape is lapped over onto the supporting surface. Sufficient slurry to cover the plate is prepared as described above, then poured along the untaped edge of the plate. Using a thick uniform glass rod, the slurry is drawn along the plate in one continuous glide along the tape. Care should be taken not to roll. If the glass plate is placed on a large piece of filter paper, any excess slurry falling over the edge of the plate is dried immediately and therefore will not creep back onto the plate. After the plate has dried for about 30 min, the tape is carefully removed and the plate activated at 110°C for 30 min. Very small plates can be taped together and coated at the same time.

Application of the sample

The sample is applied with a micropipette to the plate under a stream of warm air (hair drier) on a

line about 2–5 cm from the lower edge of the plate. A plastic spotting plate can be used for the correct spacing of the various samples along the starting line. The distance between spots is usually 1–3 cm; the diameter of the spots should not exceed 8 mm (see *Figure 6.33*). To ensure standard development it is usual to score-mark the plate about 12–15 cm from the bottom; in this way the absorbent is removed from the plate and no more solvent can move about the score line (see *Figure 6.33*).

After evaporation of the solvent in which the sample was applied, the plate is placed in a chromatographic jar containing enough solvent to cover the bottom of the jar, but without reaching the surface of the absorbent.

To obtain rapid equilibrium, one side of the jar should be lined with filter paper, which extends into the solvent at the bottom. When the jar has become saturated with solvent vapours, additional solvent is carefully poured down one side of the jar until about 2 cm of the chromoplate is covered, thus starting the development. When the solvent has completely reached the score line, the plate is removed from the tank and dried.

Visualization

The locating agent is usually sprayed onto the dried plate after development with one of the spray guns available for this purpose. The Shandon spray gun utilizing disposable canisters of propellant is very satisfactory.

Identification

After visualization by spraying with locating agent, the individual components can then be identified by their characteristic colour and R_f value.

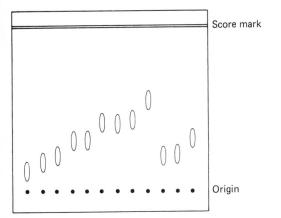

Figure 6.33. Sample applications to a thin layer chromatogram

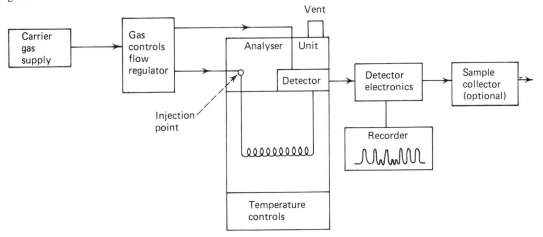

Figure 6.34. Diagrammatic layout of a gas chromatograph

Gas chromatography

In gas chromatography the mobile phase is normally an inert gas, e.g. argon, by which the various compounds in the sample mixture are separated as they pass along a special column containing a stationary phase. The mixture to be separated is introduced at the start of the column, as shown in *Figure 6.34*. The gas stream then carries the sample through the chromatographic column, which is a tube containing a relatively non-volatile material capable of reversibly absorbing the sample. The absorption process results in the sample being retarded in its passage through the column to a degree that depends upon the partition ratio between the stationary and mobile phases. Different components of the sample travel through the column at different speeds and therefore arrive at the end of the column where they pass through a detector. The detector gives an electrical signal related to the varying composition of the gas passing through it. The signal is then amplified in the electronic box, where it is converted into a suitable response so that it can be recorded on chart paper. The recorder draws a curve or chromatogram showing the changes in composition of the gas passing through the detector, thereby illustrating the composition of the sample. The behaviour of each component of a mixture is expressed as the time taken, after injection into the column, for it to reach the detector. This is then referred to as the retention time or, if compared against a reference substance, as the relative retention time.

Detectors

The early form of detector was the katharometer, or thermal conductivity detector. Those now in use are flame ionization, alkaline flame ionization, flame photometric, argon ionization and electron capture detectors. Each of these has its particular advantages.

Support media

The most commonly used support is kieselguhr or diatomaceous earth, such as Chromasorb and Gas-chrom. Other support media are the fluoroethylene polymers such as Teflon and Fluoropak.

Stationary phase

There are over 300 commercially available stationary phases. The most commonly used ones are the silicones, such as SE30 and OV1, which are methyl silicones. By introducing phenyl or fluorinated groups into the silicones, the selectivity of the stationary phase is considerably altered.

Columns

There are two types—packed and capillary. The packed columns contain inert media to support the stationary phase and vary in length from 1.5 to 4 m; the internal diameter is usually about 1.5 mm. Capillary columns can be as long as 700 m, with an internal diameter of about 0.5 mm. In these columns the stationary phase is distributed along the walls of the capillary.

Gas–liquid chromatography (GLC)

This is any method of gas chromatography in which the stationary phase is a liquid distributed on a solid support.

Gas–solid chromatography (GSC)

This is any method of gas chromatography in which the stationary phase is an active solid.

Application of gas chromatography

The application of gas chromatography in clinical chemistry is continuing to grow for steroid assays, drug levels, organic acids and lipids, to name just a few. This methodology has the advantage of high resolution and a greater sensitivity than other chromatographic procedures. The sample is easily applied after an initial preparation step, and if necessary the fractions can be collected at the end of the assay. However, the speed and efficiency of all separations are temperature dependent, so the control of the column oven temperature must be accurate to ensure good precision.

High pressure liquid chromatography

High pressure or high performance liquid chromatography (HPLC) is one of the rapidly expanding methods of analysis of organic materials. In common with other chromatographic procedures it permits the separation, detection and estimation of a wide range of compounds with a high degree of specificity. It is an ideal chromatographic system for clinical laboratories, since the majority of compounds analysed are aqueous soluble, non-volatile and/or thermally unstable. The technique of HPLC involves the separation of the various constituents of a sample followed by their individual detection and measurement. Separation is achieved by a competitive distribution of the sample between two phases, one a mobile liquid and the other a stationary liquid or solid. High separating efficiency is achieved by the column which is the heart of the system where actual chromatography or separation takes place.

The basic apparatus, as shown in *Figure 6.35*, is a solvent reservoir, a pump, a column with an

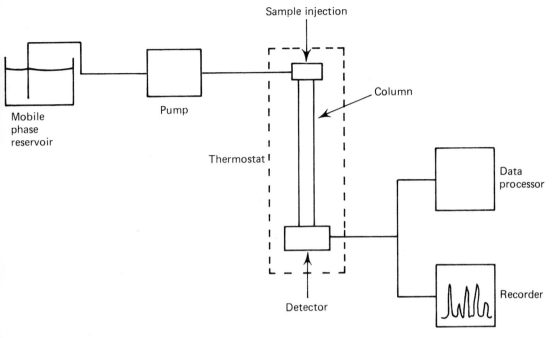

Figure 6.35. Basic layout of a high-pressure liquid chromatograph

injection unit, a detector and a recorder. The mobile phase is forced by the pump through the separating column and then through the detector. As the separated component passes through the detector a change in electrical output is produced which is recorded on a moving chart to give a chromatogram.

The time taken for the substance to pass through the column under fixed conditions is constant and is therefore called the retention time. The substances can be identified by comparing the retention time obtained with a standard solution. The area under each peak of the chromatogram is proportional to the concentration of the components in the sample, thereby enabling quantitative analysis to be used.

Pumps

These are reciprocating pumps which employ small volume chambers with reciprocating pistons to work directly on the solvent or diaphragm, in which a hydraulic fluid transmits the pumping action to the solvent via a flexible diaphragm. Two check valves are synchronized with the piston or diaphragm drive to allow alternate filling and emptying of eluent from the solvent chamber.

Injectors

Sample injection may be by a microsyringe through a septum or by use of an injection loop or valve. Automatic samplers are also available.

Detectors

The most commonly used detector is the ultraviolet detector at a fixed or variable wavelength, but fluorimetric and electrochemical detectors are also available. Besides using the detectors, separate fractions can be collected and analysed by any of the conventional methods such as colorimetry or radioassay.

Columns and packings

Columns are made of stainless steel and usually vary in length from 100 to 250 mm and 4 to 8 mm in internal diameter, thereby enabling high mobile phase pressure. Glass columns are occasionally used. The column packings vary, depending upon the compound to be separated. For example, a bonded phase packing is a packing material in which an organic liquid, octadecyl, is covalently bonded to silica. The octadecyl bonding confers non-polar characteristics to a normally polar (hydrophilic) material. Other types of bonding can also alter the hydrophilic character of the silica or packing to give reversed phase or stationary phased chromatography. Ion exchange chromatography is also available.

The solvent selection and sample preparation are essential for a successful analysis and these will vary depending upon the assay. In clinical chemistry, the HPLC can be used for drug assays, steroid estimations, catecholamines, bile acids, proteins and vitamins. This list is not comprehensive, but many more compounds can be estimated by HPLC than with GLC and the former is now taking the place of GLC in many centres. The reason for this is that HPLC does not suffer from the inherent problems of GLC with regards to decomposition during analysis.

Electrophoresis

Electrophoresis is similar in many ways to chromatography, except that separation is due to the movement of charged particles through an electrolyte (buffer) when subjected to an electric current. If these particles are charged differently they will move in opposite directions, the positively charged particles to the cathode and the negatively charged to the anode. In this separation technique a buffered medium at a fixed pH is essential to ensure that the charge on the particles and therefore the rate of migration is stabilized. One such mixture is protein which contains numerous fractions of similar mobility; therefore, when submitted to electrophoresis, the sharpness of the separation will depend upon the extent to which each fraction is homogeneous in its migration. Each protein carries a net charge which varies with the pH of its environment. Therefore, in a stable pH solution, proteins submitted to an electric current will migrate to the position where the pH is equal to the isoelectric point of the molecules.

The direction and speed of electrophoresis depends upon several factors, the chief one of which is the pH of the buffer solution. When no movement occurs in an electric field, the colloid (protein) is said to be isoelectric to the medium and the corresponding pH is the isoelective point, i.e. the protein is electrically neutral.

The most commonly used pH for protein electrophoresis is pH 8.6, under which conditions most proteins are negative and therefore migrate towards the anode.

Early electrophoresis was carried out for the most part by free movement of ions in solution, in which the moving ions formed a boundary which was detected by measuring charges in the refractive index throughout the solution. This type of electrophoresis was called *moving boundary electrophoresis* and was developed to a high degree by Tiselius in about 1937. This type of separation was very expensive due to the high cost of the apparatus and the complex optical system needed. Electrophoresis can be carried out in a system whereby the solution containing the ions to be separated is supported in a medium such as paper, starch, agar or cellulose acetate. This type of electrophoresis is then known as *zone electrophoresis*.

Paper electrophoresis generally requires up to 18 h to provide relatively diffuse separations with variable degrees of absorption. Besides diffuse separation bands, there are also variable degrees of absorption in the paper and therefore it can be difficult to make transparent. This form of electrophoresis is now rarely used in clinical laboratories.

In 1957, Kohn introduced cellulose acetate, since when it has become a widely used support medium in clinical laboratories. This medium requires less sample than paper, and higher voltages can be used, resulting in quicker separation times and increased resolution. It is stable, non-toxic and can be made almost transparent for more accurate quantitation.

Electrophoresis of serum or urine proteins using cellulose acetate strips

Principle

Electrophoresis is the migration of charged particles in an electric field. At a pH above or below their isoelectric points, proteins carry net negative or positive charges and therefore can be made to migrate under these conditions. At a pH alkaline to its isoelectric point, a protein will carry a net negative charge and therefore migrates to the anode when a current is passed. Different proteins vary markedly in their isoelectric points and therefore differ in electric mobility at any given pH value.

Serum proteins vary in their isoelectric points from 4.7 (albumin) to 7.3 (γ-globulin) and thus each protein will migrate at a different rate when in a buffer of pH 8.6 (*Figure 6.36*).

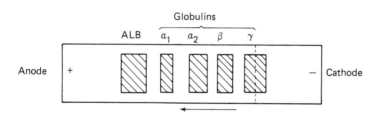

Figure 6.36. Normal electrophoretic pattern in a buffer of pH 8.6

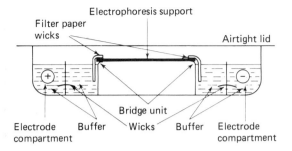

Figure 6.37. Horizontal strip electrophoresis tank

Equipment

1. Electrophoresis tank, e.g. Shandon Electrophoresis Apparatus after Kohn SAE 3225.
2. Polarity controller and safety switch complete with lead for power supply SAE 2692.
3. Power unit—Vokam constant voltage/constant current d.c. supply SAE 2761.

A layout of an electrophoresis apparatus can be seen in *Figure 6.37*.

Reagents

1. Cellulose acetate strips, 12 × 2.5 cm.
2. Barbitone buffer, pH 8.6, ionic strength 0.05: 9.2 g barbitone, 15.5 g sodium barbitone and 23 ml 5% thymol in isopropanol is dissolved in warm distilled water, cooled and diluted to 5 litres.
3. Ponceau S, 0.5% w/v in 5% trichloracetic acid.
4. Acetic acid, 5.0% w/v in water.

Method

1. The cellulose acetate strips are marked in pencil at the point of application of the sample, approximately 4 cm from one end (which will be the cathode end).
2. They are then labelled for later identification and placed lightly on the surface of the buffer in a shallow plastic tray, allowing the buffer to impregnate the strip from below by capillarity before being submerged completely.
3. The impregnated strip is removed from the buffer (using forceps) and lightly blotted between two sheets of filter paper, to remove excess moisture, but ensuring that no opaque, white spots are present. If this happens the strips should be returned to the buffer solution for a short time before being blotted again.
4. The strips are then positioned into the tank, with the point of application on the cathode side, and a wick of filter paper is placed over either end of the strips, dipping into the buffer in the tank.

5. Approximately 5 µl of the same sample is applied to each of two of the strips, slowly, leaving a margin down either side and in as fine a streak as possible along the pencil line. A sheet of Perspex placed on top of the tank helps by providing support for the hand.
6. The lid is replaced on top of the tank and the power supply connected.
7. Switch on the current and adjust it to 0.4 mA per cm width of strip; this usually gives a voltage in the region of 185 V.
8. Leave for 2 h.
9. The strips are removed from the tank and dried.
10. Stain with ponceau S solution for 10 min, again floating the strips on the surface of the dye to ensure complete impregnation before submerging.
11. After staining is complete, the strips are placed in a small tank containing 5% acetic acid.
12. Replace the acid several times to ensure the dye has been removed from the background completely.
13. Dry and Sellotape one strip to the laboratory record card for reference, the second one for dispatch to the ward.
14. The fractions can be eluted from the strip by cutting out the individual fractions and placing the cut strip into a test-tube containing 4.0 ml 10% v/v Teepol in water.
15. The absorbance can then be read at 520 nm.

■ Notes

(a) Reverse direction of the current after each run. (b) If poor separation of the protein fractions is found, check the pH of buffer. (c) Serum from well-clotted unhaemolysed blood must be used. (d) Fresh serum may show an extra band in the α_2 to β region. (e) Strips are run from the cathode to anode. (f) As paper takes 16–18 h for complete separation, using cellulose acetate separation can be achieved in about 20 min. (g) Different stains for identifying the protein can be used. (h) If higher currents are used, a cooling system is usually necessary to prevent the protein becoming denatured.

Starch gel electrophoresis

In 1955, Smithies introduced a major development in electrophoresis by using the remarkable resolving powers of starch gel electrophoresis for serum proteins. Since this medium is not inert it exhibits a molecular sieving as well as an electrophoretic effect. This can increase the number of serum protein bands from fewer than ten to more than 20 and, unless examined by an experienced worker, the resulting patterns can be very difficult to interpret.

Polyacrylamide gel electrophoresis

The introduction of a completely new medium for electrophoresis, polyacrylamide gel, occurred in

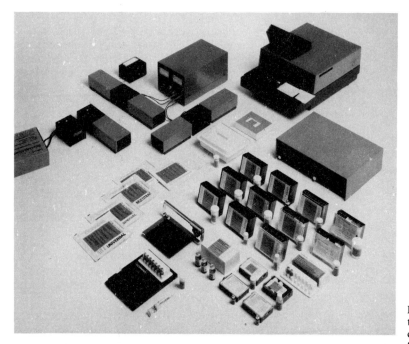

Figure 6.38. Corning agarose electrophoresis system (reproduced by courtesy of Corning Medical and Scientific)

1960. The gels are formed by polymerizing acrylamide monomers in the presence of methylene-bis-acrylamide, which acts as a crosslinking agent. This medium has a far more superior resolving power than starch gel; moreover, the gels are stable and clinically inert over a wide range of chemical and physical conditions. Like starch, this gel has molecular sieving principles and can be used for protein electrophoresis and the separation of different classes of nucleic acids.

Agar gel electrophoresis

This support medium was first used by Consden and colleagues in 1946, when agar was used in the separation of peptides from wool hydrolysates. Proteins were separated by Gordon and colleagues in 1950, but the modern application of this support was by Grabar and Williams in 1953, who used the immunodiffusion methods of Ouchterlony following agar gel electrophoresis to obtain immunoelectrophoretic analysis. Agar is a galactose polymer containing carboxyl and sulphonic groups, which give it a good degree of endosmosis and relatively low absorption of proteins, and therefore sharper zones of separation are obtained.

Agarose gel electrophoresis

Removal of the carboxyl and sulphonic groups from agar results in the product agarose, which has very

little endosmotic effect; it is stable, inert and non-toxic. It is transparent and therefore requires no clearing. It has no absorption effects, is non-fluorescent and does not require presoaking. Agarose is therefore most suitable for protein electrophoresis, immunodiffusion, immunoelectrophoresis and isoenzyme separations, etc.

The prepared agarose universal electrophoresis films, with instructions, are obtainable from Corning and the agarose electrophoresis system is shown in *Figure 6.38*.

Immunoelectrophoresis

This procedure is a combination of electrophoresis and immunological detection. It is a specialized method for the qualitative investigation of complex protein mixtures in biological fluids. Electrophoresis is performed using either agar or agarose as the medium and the sample is placed in a well (*Figure 6.39*) cut into a thin layer of support on a glass slide. After electrophoresis, the various proteins are separated in a linear direction. A trough is then cut in the gel (*Figure 6.39*) in a direction parallel to the electrophoretic migration, but separated from the point of origin. This trough is then filled with antiserum which will then diffuse into the gel towards the antigens (proteins). When an antigen encounters its corresponding antibody, a precipitation arc will form, as shown in *Figure 6.39*. This

Antigen wells

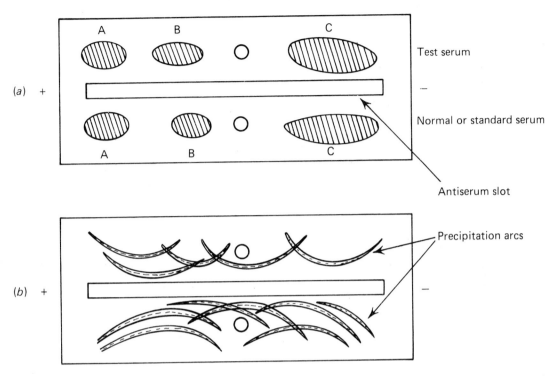

Figure 6.39. Principles of immunoelectrophoresis: (a) areas occupied by the antigens after electrophoresis—A, B and C = antigen areas; (b) precipitation arcs after the addition of antiserum

procedure is used for identifying proteins, particularly those associated with dysproteinaemias, and for typing monoclonal γ-globulin bands with regard to their light and heavy chain structure. Although this technique is satisfactory, a far better procedure is immunofixation.

Immunofixation

In immunofixation techniques, electrophoretically separated proteins are reacted with appropriate antisera. Suitable dilutions of the test serum or preconcentrated urine are prepared using saline as the diluent. Immunofixation is best done near equivalence of antigen and antibody, i.e. a 1:1 ratio of protein antigen to the specific antibody. These dilutions depend on the potency and avidity of the antisera used. High titre antibodies may first be diluted using a special diluent composed of sodium azide, sodium chloride and polyethylene glycol.

A concentration of serum of between 0.2–0.4 g/l for the heavy chains and 0.6–0.8 g/l for the light chains should be aimed for; again this depends on the strength of the antibody used, and adjustment by trial and error may improve the final result.

An agarose gel plate is then inoculated using 1 μl of diluted serum or urine and run in an electrophoretic chamber at 90 V for approximately 30 min in barbitone acetate buffer, pH 8.6 (Corning Electrophoresis System). The strip is then removed and allowed to drain. While the strip is draining, cellulose acetate strips, 25 mm × 5 mm, are impregnated with 20 μl of the appropriate antisera.

These are then placed on the agarose plate in such a position that they cover the zone known to be occupied by the protein under study. Care must be taken to remove air bubbles from beneath the strips and to ensure that adjacent strips containing different antibodies do not touch. The film is then placed in a moist chamber at room temperature for 1 h.

After the incubation, the strip is placed in 0.9% saline and left overnight. This removes unprecipitated protein, leaving the 'fixed band' in place. The strip is then dried in an oven at 50°C (for approximately 30 min) and stained with Coomassie blue. It is then destained with alcoholic destaining fluid until the background is clear.

The dried film is then labelled and commented on.

7

Introduction to clinical chemistry

Introduction

It is important for every medical laboratory scientist to have an intelligent understanding of the laboratory investigations he or she carries out. This can only be accomplished by having a basic knowledge of physiology—the science of bodily functions—and further reading is recommended in the Bibliography at the end of the book.

The human body develops from a single initial cell which grows and reproduces, forming millions of cells which in turn arrange themselves into tissues. The tissues in turn arrange themselves into organs, which form a new being. The cell is described on p. 171. Chemical functions within these organs are taking place all the time, and it is the role of the clinical chemistry department to observe any chemical changes.

Metabolism

This is a general term applied to various changes, whatever their nature, taking place in living cells or in the body. Ceaseless chemical activity takes place within the protoplasm as materials are built up (anabolism) from simple units to complex ones (e.g. the synthesis of protein from amino acids), while simultaneously others are broken down (catabolism) from more complex substances to simple forms, such as the hydrolysis of glycogen to glucose units.

Since both these processes occur side by side it is convenient to use the term metabolism when referring to both processes. When exogenous catabolism takes place it refers to the breakdown of the diet; on the other hand cellular breakdown is described as endogenous catabolism.

Metabolic processes are accompanied by the production of heat and energy, the necessary energy and heat required for the bodily processes being acquired by the metabolic utilization of foodstuffs. Since these chemical reactions are under the control of enzymes, the cells can only survive within certain limits of temperature. If the temperature is too high these organic catalysts are destroyed, while at low temperature reactions are retarded and finally cease.

Metabolic rate

The amount of energy liberated by the catabolism of food in the body is the same as the amount liberated when food is burned outside the body. This finding enabled the physiologists to understand more about the metabolic rate of the body. The output of energy by the body, and the rate of oxygen consumption, depend upon muscular activity, environmental conditions, body temperature and so on.

In order to reduce these factors to a minimum, the metabolism of one individual can be compared with that of another by keeping the subject in bed warm and completely relaxed both mentally and physically for 12–15 h after the last meal. The output of the body under these conditions is then called basal metabolism, which is the amount of energy expenditure of the body at complete rest, assessed from the oxygen consumed in kcal per m^2 of body surface per h. The basal metabolic rate (BMR) was determined by using an indirect form of calorimetry using the Benedict–Roth BMR apparatus. This apparatus is basically an oxygen-filled spirometer and a carbon dioxide absorber. The spirometer bell is connected to a pin which writes on a rotating drum and records the amount of oxygen consumed during the experiment. Nowadays the determination of BMR has been replaced by much more reliable laboratory investigations, such as serum thyroxine, since this hormone from the thyroid gland is concerned with the regulation of the BMR.

Nutrition

In nutrition, the so-called 'calorie' has been replaced by the new SI unit, the joule. Although calorie has been used for many years, there is no such unit and the correct name for the unit used in nutrition and for the calculation of energy is the thermochemical calorie (symbol: cal_{th}, not cal). Contrary to what most textbooks state, the thermochemical calorie has been defined solely in terms of the joule since 1935. The principal objection to using joule alone in nutrition is the fact that the dietary values giving values in joules are as yet not widely available. As an interim measure, values should be quoted on both joules and thermochemical calories.

Regulation of body temperature

In the body, heat is produced by muscular exercise, utilization of foodstuffs and all vital processes that contribute to basal metabolism. It is lost from the body through respiration, by the skin and small amounts are lost in the faeces and urine. The skin is by far the most important regulator of the body temperature.

The balance between heat production and heat loss determines the body temperature which is maintained within very narrow limits.

Normal body temperature

The temperature of the body ranges from 35.8°C to 37.3°C, the mean being 36.7°C with a standard deviation of 0.22°C. Many normal individuals have temperatures differing from 36.7°C by more than 0.56°C and therefore to refer to a normal temperature is clearly illogical. In temperate climates the body temperature is nearly always higher than the environmental temperature, when there is a continuous loss of heat through the skin.

Blood gas analysis

Respiration exchange

Respiration is the term generally used in the interchange of two gases, oxygen and carbon dioxide, between the body and the environment. Two processes are involved: external respiration when the lungs absorb oxygen and remove carbon dioxide from the body, and internal respiration when the uptake of oxygen and the formation and liberation of carbon dioxide by the cells are involved.

In external respiration, air is drawn into the lungs (inspired) by breathing in through the nostrils. This air is drawn down the windpipe or trachea, which divides into two tubes called bronchi, each of which passes into the substance of the lung and divides into a number of smaller bronchioles. Branching of the bronchioles continues until each one ends in a minute air sac, called an alveolus. The walls of the alveoli are covered with a film of water, which because of the constant supply of air is saturated with oxygen. Each alveolus is within, and in close contact with, a meshwork of capillaries. The oxygen diffuses through the alveolar walls into the blood capillaries, first into the plasma and then into the red cells (erythrocytes), where it combines with the haemoglobin to form an unstable compound, oxyhaemoglobin. This is a reversible process because the dissociation of oxyhaemoglobin to release oxygen is dependent upon the tension of the oxygen in the medium surrounding the haemoglobin:

$$Hb + O_2 \rightleftharpoons HbO_2$$

where Hb is the deoxygenated haemoglobin and HbO_2 the oxyhaemoglobin.

Simultaneously, the carbon dioxide in the plasma and red cells diffuses out of the blood capillaries and dissolves in the watery covering of the alveolus. This carbon dioxide now diffuses into the alveolus and it is removed as air is breathed out (expired). In internal respiration the oxygen is transported by the blood from the lungs to the tissues as oxyhaemoglobin, as mentioned above. The red colour of deoxygenated haemoglobin is darker than the bright red colour of oxyhaemoglobin, and this is why arterial blood is always brighter than venous blood. In carbon monoxide poisoning, haemoglobin combines with carbon monoxide to form cherry-red carboxyhaemoglobin. This combination is far more readily carried out than with oxygen, being about 210 times as fast.

The dissociation of oxyhaemoglobin is dependent upon temperature, electrolyte concentration and carbon dioxide concentration.

Carbon dioxide is carried by the blood both in the cells and plasma, but as with oxygen it exists in three main forms: (a) a small amount of carbonic acid; (b) in combination with proteins, mainly haemoglobin, to form carbamino-bound carbon dioxide; and (c) as bicarbonate combined with either sodium or potassium cations.

The amount of carbon dioxide dissolved in the blood is not large, but it is important because any change in its concentration will cause the following reaction to shift from its equilibrium:

$$\downarrow \uparrow CO_2 + H_2O \rightleftharpoons H_2CO_3 \rightleftharpoons H^+ + HCO_3^-$$

The enzyme carbonic anhydrase specifically catalyses the removal of CO_2 from H_2CO_3; however, the reaction is reversible, as the formation of carbonic acid in the tissues from CO_2 and H_2O is accelerated by the enzyme.

It is estimated that in 24 h the lungs remove the equivalent of 20–40 litres of normal acid in the form of carbonic acid. This acidity is transported by the blood with hardly any variation in blood pH, since most of the carbonic acid formed is rapidly converted to bicarbonate:

$$H_2CO_3 \rightleftharpoons H^+ + HCO_3^- + B^+ \rightleftharpoons BHCO_3 + H^+$$

where B^+ represents cations in the blood, principally sodium, Na^+.

Acid–base balance

Buffering system of the blood

The normal venous blood pH is within the range 7.36–7.42. The buffer systems of the blood are so efficient that the pH of venous blood is more acid than arterial blood by only 0.01–0.03 pH units.

These blood buffer systems are the plasma proteins, haemoglobins, the carbonic acid–bicarbonate system and inorganic phosphates.

A small decrease in pH which occurs when CO_2 enters the venous blood at the tissues had the effect of altering the ratio of acid to base in all these buffer anion systems:

$$H^+ + Hb^- \rightleftharpoons HHb \tag{1}$$
$$H^+ + Prot^- \rightleftharpoons HProt \tag{2}$$
$$H^+ + HCO_3^- \rightleftharpoons H_2CO_3 \tag{3}$$
$$H^+ + HPO_4^{2-} \rightleftharpoons H_2PO_4^- \tag{4}$$

where Hb = haemoglobin and Prot = protein. Anions such as bicarbonate which can filter through the glomerulus enter the renal tubules accompanied by cations, especially sodium. Renal tubular cells can actively secrete H^+, the net effect being exchange of one H^+ for one Na^+ from the glomerular filtrate. As the secreted H^+ comes from cellular carbonic acid, HCO_3^- is left behind, thus replenishing buffer anion. Some of the H^+ secreted by the tubular cells combines with filtered bicarbonate to form carbonic acid; this dissociates to water and CO_2, which diffuses back into the tubular cells. Thus the acid is excreted, cations conserved and buffer anion replenished.

In the plasma the phosphate concentration is too low to be a quantitatively important buffer, its significance being in the urinary control of acidity. The urine normally contains little HCO_3^- since it is almost completely reabsorbed by the tubules.

In plasma the ratio of $H_2PO_4:HPO_4^{2-}$ is about 1.5, but in urine it is 9:1 and may rise as high as 50:1 when large amounts of acid have to be eliminated. This is because most of the phosphate in the glomerular filtrate is in the form of monohydrogen phosphate HPO_4^{2-}. This accepts H^+ to become dihydrogen phosphate ($H_2PO_4^-$), which is excreted in the urine accompanied by cations and therefore conserves the valuable HCO_3^-:

$$HPO_4^{2-} + H_2CO_3 \rightarrow H_2PO_4^- + HCO_3^-$$

Blood gas analysis

In the clinical laboratory when blood gases are requested, the estimations usually carried out are pH, pCO_2 and pO_2. From these parameters some idea of acid–base balance and respiration exchange can be obtained.

There are a number of blood gas analysers on the market and some laboratories prefer one particular model to another, but on the whole they are all basically of the same design. When blood gases are requested, an arterial blood specimen collected into a pre-heparinized syringe anaerobically is placed into a vacuum flask containing ice and water for transport to the clinical chemistry laboratory. The blood gas analyser contains three specific electrodes all equilibrated to 37°C. The pH electrode is standardized by using two different buffer solutions, e.g. pH 6.84 and pH 7.38. After standardization, the arterial blood is placed into the pH electrode and three measurements are made, all of which should agree to within 0.01 of a pH unit.

While the pH measurements are being made, the pCO_2 and pO_2 selective electrodes are being equilibrated with known gas mixtures for standardization. When adequate equilibration and standardization is obtained, the gas mixtures which have been 'flowing through' the electrodes are stopped and the pCO_2 and pO_2 content of the arterial blood measured. Three readings are again made and provided they agree between certain limits (depending upon the instrument), the mean value is obtained. From the pH and pCO_2 parameters, the standard bicarbonate and base excess can be calculated:

pH is a measure of hydrogen ion concentration, e.g. pH 7.3
pCO_2 and pO_2 are measured in kilopascals, e.g. 6.0 kPa
Normal arterial pH 7.38–7.45
Normal arterial pCO_2 4.7–6.0 kPa
Normal arterial pO_2 11.3–14.0 kPa

The endocrine system

The endocrine system adjusts and correlates the various activities of the body, making adjustments to the body systems by the changing demands of the external and internal environment. This integration

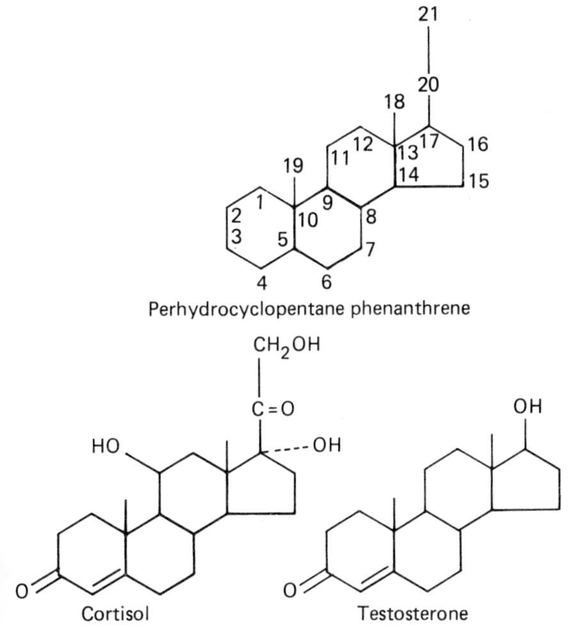

Structurally, they are not always protein in nature; the known hormones include proteins or polypeptides or single amino acids and steroids.

A steroid is a hormone derived from the tetracyclic hydrocarbon perhydrocyclopentane phenanthrene, as shown in *Figure 7.1*, examples of which are cortisol or testosterone. Non-steroid hormones are substances such as adrenaline or thyroxine (*Figure 7.2*).

The most widely recognized hormones are the ones commonly referred to as the 'sex hormones'. However, they represent only a very small fraction of the hormones of interest in clinical chemistry and medicine.

In addition to the ovary and testis, hormones are secreted by the adrenal cortex and medulla, anterior and posterior pituitary, parathyroid, thyroid and the islets of Langerhans in the pancreas. Calcitonin, a calcium-reducing hormone, is generally thought to be produced by cells in the thymus as well as the thyroid and parathyroid, so the thymus should be included in this list. Other tissues such as those of the gastrointestinal tract are known to be concerned with hormone production.

The pituitary gland (often described as the master gland or the leader of the endocrine orchestra) is reddish-grey in colour, roughly oval in shape and is situated in the base of the brain. The gland is attached to the brain by a stalk which is continuous with the part of the brain known as the hypothalamus. The pituitary has three lobes or parts:

1. The anterior lobe or pars anterior.
2. The mid-lobe or pars intermedia.

both of these are also called the adenohypophysis

3. The posterior lobe or neurohypophysis.

Anterior pituitary

The anterior pituitary secretes six separate trophic hormones ('trophic' is derived from the Greek word *trophein*, which means to nourish), each of which have a specific action in the endocrine system.

They are growth hormone (somatotrophic hormone), adrenocorticotrophic hormone (ACTH), thyrotrophic stimulation hormone (TSH), prolactin (lactogenic hormone) and the two pituitary gonadotrophins, follicle stimulating hormone (FSH) and luteinizing hormone (LH) or interstitial cell stimulating hormone (*Figure 7.3*). All these hormones except growth hormone do not generally affect metabolic processes, but normally act on other endocrine glands to stimulate the production or release of secondary hormones; for example, ACTH stimulates the release of cortisol. An increase in concentration of a secondary hormone, whether secreted by the endocrine glands or administered for medical reasons, will depress the secretion of the

Perhydrocyclopentane phenanthrene

Cortisol

Testosterone

Figure 7.1. Steroid hormones

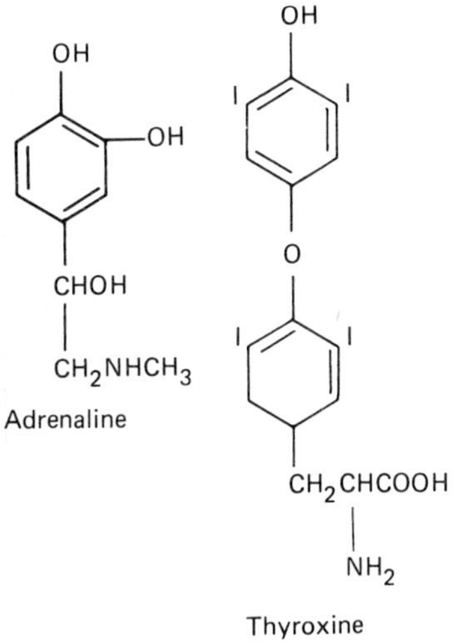

Adrenaline

Thyroxine

Figure 7.2. Non-steroid hormones

is brought about by the secretions of chemical substances directly into the blood stream to regulate the metabolic processes of various 'target' tissues. The organs manufacturing the chemical substances are the endocrine or ductless glands; their secretions, the hormones, have diverse metabolic processes, yet have several characteristics in common:

1. They are only required in very small amounts.
2. They are produced in an organ other than that in which they perform their action.
3. They are secreted into the blood stream prior to use.

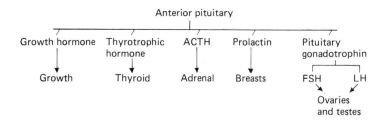

Figure 7.3. Scheme showing the various hormones secreted by the anterior lobe of the pituitary

appropriate trophic hormone; for example, the administration of excess exogenous thyroxine will decrease the secretion of TSH.

Function of hormones

Growth hormone

Growth hormone acts directly on tissue to promote nitrogen retention and growth, probably through the control of protein metabolism. It is an antagonist to insulin, causing hypoglycaemia.

Adrenocorticotrophin

ACTH acts directly on the adrenal cortex to predominantly stimulate the formation of glucocorticoids (hormones involved in carbohydrate metabolism) such as cortisol and adrenal androgens such as dehydroepiandrosterone (androgens stimulate male secondary sexual characteristics). It does also have some effect on aldosterone, a mineralocorticoid concerned with electrolyte balance.

Thyrotrophic stimulating hormone

TSH acts on the thyroid gland to promote the production and release of the thyroid hormones, thyroxine and triiodothyronine. In physiological concentrations thyroxine is a protein anabolizer (build-up) but in excess is a protein catabolizer (breakdown). Excess thyroxine lowers the blood cholesterol and stimulates the breakdown of bone.

Prolactin

In conjunction with other hormones, the lactogenic hormone is responsible for milk formation and mammary (breast) development. A hormone of the placenta also stimulates growth of the mammary glands but inhibits production of prolactin. After delivery of the baby the placental inhibition is removed, prolactin is secreted and the secretory cells are stimulated to secrete milk.

Follicle stimulating hormone

FSH induces growth in the ovarian follicle during the first half of the menstrual cycle and together with

LH stimulates production of oestrogens. In the male it stimulates the production of spermatozoa (male egg cells).

Luteinizing hormone

LH induces ovulation and stimulates the development of cells in the ruptured follicle to form structures called the corpora lutea, which in turn secrete a second ovarian hormone progesterone. In the male, LH stimulates the testes to secrete testosterone, the most potent androgen.

The mid-lobe of the pituitary

The intermediate lobe of the pituitary secretes a hormone called melanocyte stimulating hormone (MSH), which physiologically causes dispersion of the melanin pigment in the skin.

Posterior pituitary

Two hormones are secreted by the posterior lobe, oxytocin or pitocin and antidiuretic hormone or vasopressin. Principally, vasopressin increases the blood pressure and exerts its effect on the kidney tubules by controlling the reabsorption of water (antidiuretic action), while oxytocin stimulates uterine contractions, particularly at the time of labour.

Pineal gland

The pineal gland is a small body situated in the brain below the corpus callosum and posterior to the third ventricle. It is approximately 10 mm in length and its functions are somewhat vague, but it has been reported to be involved in aldosterone secretion.

The placenta

In addition to permitting the exchange of materials between the embryo and mother, the placenta is an endocrine organ of pregnancy producing steroid hormones such as oestrogens and progesterone and the non-steroid hormones, human chorionic gonadotrophin (HCG) and human placental lactogen (HPL). The presence of HCG in early pregnancy is used as the basis of the immunological pregnancy test, but this hormone can also be produced by certain tumours of the uterus and testes.

The adrenal glands

There are two adrenal glands which are situated on each side of the vertebral column on the posterior abdominal wall behind the peritoneum. They are in close association with the kidneys, each being attached to the upper pole of the kidney.

The glands are divided into two distinct parts which differ both in anatomy and in function. The outer part is called the cortex and the inner the medulla.

Function of the adrenal cortex

It secretes a large number of steroids, of which there are three main groups:

1. The mineralocorticoids.
2. The glucocorticoids.
3. The sex hormones.

The sex hormones, androgens and oestrogens, influence both the development and maintenance of the secondary sex characteristics and the utilization and excretion of nitrogen. The glucocorticoids regulate carbohydrate metabolism, in that they are antagonistic to insulin, stimulating gluconeogenesis and decreasing carbohydrate utilization. They are also protein catabolizers. The mineralocorticoids, the most potent of which is aldosterone, have their main effect on the renal tubules by retaining sodium, chloride and water and exchanging potassium, thus maintaining their balance in the body.

The final stage of aldosterone secretion is, however, stimulated by the renin–angiotensin system, renin being produced in the juxtaglomerular cells of the kidney.

Function of the adrenal medulla

The hormones of the adrenal medulla are adrenaline and noradrenaline. Both hormones prepare the body to withstand rapid physiological responses to emergencies such as cold, fatigue, shock, etc., by mobilizing the 'fight and flight' mechanisms of the sympathetic nervous system. In addition the two hormones induce metabolic effects such as glycogenolyis in the liver and skeletal muscle, mobilization of free fatty acids and stimulation of the metabolic rate.

Endocrine function tests

A variety of hormones (or other parameters) are estimated under this classification, ranging from simple hormones such as the steroid cortisol to more complex hormones like prolactin.

Cortisol, a steroid hormone directly related to the adrenal cortex, was estimated by fluorimetry, but like many other steroids is now usually estimated by a radioimmunoassay procedure (see p. 80). A level below normal is usually found in Addison's disease (hypoadrenocortical activity) and elevated values can be found in Cushing's syndrome (hyperadrenocortical activity).

These tests usually give us some idea of the activity of the adrenal cortex and similar tests can be done to assess the activity of other hormones or endocrine glands. Although this may not be as straightforward as a cortisol estimation, most of the hormones can be estimated directly or indirectly; for example, vasopressin by osmolality, the placenta by HPL or oestriol determinations and the parathyroid gland by calcium and phosphate levels.

The thyroid gland

The thyroid gland consists of two lobes, one on each side of the trachea with a connecting portion, the isthmus, making the entire gland more or less H-shaped in appearance. In the adult the gland weighs about 25–30 g.

Function

The principal function of the gland is to secrete two hormones, thyroxine and triiodothyronine, and to store iodine (see also Thyrotrophic stimulating hormone, p. 102).

Thyroid function tests

Serum thyroxine is now measured by radioimmunoassay or by enzyme immunoassay (see p. 80). The antigen–antibody reaction (radioimmunoassay) is a far more common procedure, but due to the availability of commercial kits for immunoassay and their convenience in use these latter are gaining in popularity.

Values below normal are found in hypothyroidism and values above normal are found- in hyperthyroidism.

The parathyroid glands

There are four parathyroid glands, which usually lie on the posterior aspect of the lobes of the thyroid gland and are arranged in two pairs.

Function

The principal function of the parathyroids is to secrete parathormone (PTH), a hormone responsible for the metabolism of calcium in the body, and therefore the maintenance of a constant level of plasma calcium. Besides raising the plasma calcium, PTH also lowers the plasma phosphate. Calcitonin, a hormone which lowers the plasma calcium, is also thought to come from the parathyroids but is primarily of thyroid origin.

Water and body fluids

Water plays an important part in the structure and function of the body. In the healthy adult approximately 60% of the body consists of water; even bone contains approximately one-third and adipose tissue contains a large amount in the connective tissue and in the spaces between the fat cells.

Body fluid is divided into functional compartments, separated from one another by cell membranes. Fluid within these cells is called intracellular fluid (ICF), and fluid outside, extracellular fluid (ECF). Extracellular fluid is further divided into intravascular fluid (plasma water) and interstitial fluid. Interstitial fluid is tissue fluid and includes cerebrospinal fluid (CSF), lymph, amniotic fluid, water in the gastrointestinal tract, aqueous humour, pleural fluid, etc. The ECF is the immediate environment of the organism and the aqueous medium which surrounds the tissue cells is the transport mechanism for nutrient and waste materials. Besides this service it also provides stability of physiochemical conditions such as temperature, osmotic pressure and pH (see *Figure 7.4*).

Measurement of body fluids

The direct measurement of body fluids involves complicated procedures which are not practical in man. Indirect methods are therefore used which involve the administration of substances which are believed to diffuse into the various compartments of the body.

Water loss and balance

A normal subject's intake and output of water is usually in equilibrium. Any minor short-term discrepancies are balanced by an exchange of water from the intracellular pool. During one day a normal adult will lose about 2.6 litres of water, made up approximately as follows:

Sweat	100 ml
Lungs	500 ml
Skin	400 ml
Faeces	200 ml
Urine	1400 ml
	2600 ml

The water intake is therefore approximately 2600 ml, of which about 2000 ml is from moist food and drinks; the remaining 600 ml is manufactured by oxidation during metabolic processes. There are approximately 45 litres of water in the body, 3 litres in the plasma, 12 litres in interstitial fluid and 30

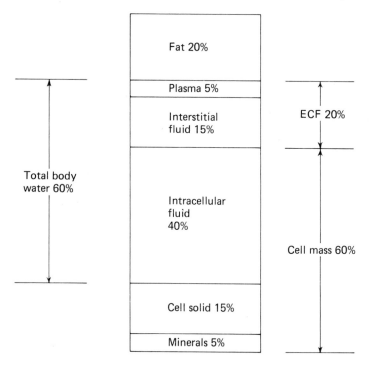

Figure 7.4. Distribution of different phases of body fluids as percentage of body weight

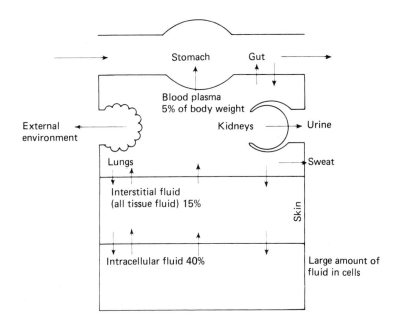

Figure 7.5. Interrelationship of body fluids

litres in the intracellular fluid; therefore, any short-term discrepancies in the water balance will be drawn from this water pool. All body fluids contain electrolytes.

The normal water balance of the body can be upset in various ways. Water depletion is the commonest and disturbances in both water and electrolytes will then occur. When fluid intake is restricted, the plasma sodium concentration rises above normal and the ECF becomes hypertonic. Water passes into the ECF (5 litres) from the ICF (30 litres) by osmosis, but the volume of the ICF is relatively little altered. Water intoxication occurs when large volumes of water are drunk, or when too much hypotonic fluid has been given intravenously, the reverse process will then occur (*Figure 7.5*). Salt depletion is the result of Na^+ (and Cl^-) loss from the ECF in excess of water loss, e.g. diarrhoea, vomiting. Potassium depletion also occurs; this may result from disturbed function of the renal tubule; for example, the effect produced by certain diuretic drugs.

Hormonal control of water output

The hormone involved in water regulation is ADH or antidiuretic hormone released by the posterior pituitary. Its main purpose is to retain water, i.e. reduce the urinary output. This is done in the distal, convoluted and collecting tubules of the kidney. In the presence of ADH, water flows back into the interstitial fluid which is hypertonic until equilibrium has been reached (osmosis). The production of the hormone is stimulated by changes in plasma osmolarity or blood volume, and is released by the hypothalamus, the posterior pituitary acting as a storage centre for ADH. When the blood is diluted by, for example, large amounts of water, the ADH secretion is inhibited, more water is excreted in the distal and collecting tubules and a large volume of dilute urine results. In contrast, when blood becomes more hypertonic and the osmolarity increases, ADH is stimulated and retains more water in the tubules, resulting in concentrated urine of small volume being excreted.

A number of drugs, including alcohol, will suppress ADH and thus increase urine flow.

Electrolyte studies

The direct or indirect measurement of body fluids cannot be carried out on a routine basis. The estimation of electrolytes is the usual alternative, since the control of sodium and water balance are so closely related. Sodium (Na^+) is widely distributed in the body; it is predominantly present outside the cell, while potassium (K^+) is almost intracellular. Salt depletion is the result of Na^+ (and Cl^-) loss from extracellular fluid as in the case of diarrhoea and vomiting. Potassium depletion also occurs from disturbed function of the renal tubules produced by diuretic therapy. Chronic potassium depletion can be accompanied by a high plasma bicarbonate, and disturbed renal tubular function can also be assessed by plasma urea levels.

Electrolyte requests can therefore involve the clinical chemistry department in the estimation of Na^+, K^+, HCO_3^- and urea levels. Chlorides are not usually estimated now except in very special circumstances.

A specimen of heparinized blood is collected with as little stasis as possible and quickly sent to the laboratory to separate the cells from the plasma. Red cells contain a lot of potassium and rapid separation of the cells from the plasma prevents the leakage of potassium into the plasma. Haemolysis must also be avoided.

Sodium and potassium are estimated by flame emission spectroscopy (flame photometry) or by ion-selective electrodes (see p. 76). Urea levels can be determined by any of the methods described in Chapter 10, while plasma bicarbonate can be estimated by a continuous flow system or by the following manual method.

Plasma bicarbonate

The Harleco CO_2 apparatus is a convenient way of measuring carbon dioxide content (bicarbonate) in approximately one minute. The sample is placed into the reaction vessel, and after acidifying with lactic acid the CO_2 liberated is measured in the CO_2 syringe. A sodium bicarbonate standard is used to calibrate the apparatus to the varying atmospheric temperature and pressure under which the test is being performed.

The normal

plasma sodium	ranges from	135 to 146	mmol/l
plasma potassium	ranges from	3.5 to 5.2	mmol/l
plasma bicarbonate	ranges from	23 to 30	mmol/l
plasma urea	ranges from	3.3 to 6.7	mmol/l

8

Gastric and pancreatic function tests

It is important before discussing tests concerned with the digestive and pancreatic system to have an understanding of the nutritional needs of the body. The food we eat is composed largely of animal and plant materials or of products derived from them, and includes the essentials of the diet such as carbohydrates, proteins, fats, vitamins, mineral salts, water and roughage. If the cells of the body are to function efficiently these essential nutrients must be available in the correct proportions.

Most foodstuffs are *ingested* in forms which are unavailable to the body, since they cannot be absorbed from the gastrointestinal tract until broken down to basic units. The breakdown of the naturally occurring foodstuffs into absorbable units is the process of *digestion*, helped by the *secretion* of enzymes and juices in the tract. The products of digestion, along with fluids, minerals and vitamins, cross the mucosa of the intestines and enter the lymph or blood, a process known as *absorption*. Certain constituents of the diet which cannot be digested and absorbed are excreted from the bowel in the form of faeces, a process of *elimination*. These five processes—ingestion, digestion, secretion, absorption and elimination—are all activities of the digestive system.

The diet contains various foods which are classified according to their chemical structure and physical properties.

Carbohydrates

Carbohydrates are found in sugar, jam, cereals, bread, potatoes, fruit, vegetables and milk. They consist of carbon, hydrogen and oxygen, the ratio of hydrogen to oxygen being the same as that in water,

the exception being in the deoxy (one less oxygen) sugars.

The three main dietary carbohydrates are monosaccharides, disaccharides and polysaccharides.

Function

In the body the carbohydrates are utilized to provide energy and heat, and help to maintain the normal blood glucose level. They are stored as glycogen in the liver and muscle, and any excess remaining is converted to fat and stored in the fat depots. There are three main groups:

1. *Monosaccharides*—these are simple sugars which can be directly absorbed from the small intestine.

   Hexoses ($C_6H_{12}O_6$)—the main one is glucose which plays an important role in supplying energy to the cells. Fructose and galactose are further examples.

   Pentoses ($C_5H_{10}O_5$)—are simple sugars, widely distributed in plant material such as fruits and gums, the chief ones being ribose, xylose and arabinose. All animal cells contain ribose and deoxyribose as constituents of nucleic acids.

2. *Disaccharides* ($C_{12}H_{22}O_{11}$)—these cannot be absorbed directly but must be hydrolysed to monosaccharides by their appropriate enzyme (disaccharidase) before absorption can take place. The enzyme is present on the surface of the intestinal cell, where the hydrolysis takes place. Examples of disaccharides are sucrose, found in cane sugar; lactose, found in milk sugar; and maltose, an intermediate product in the breakdown of starch to glucose. From *Table 8.1* it can be seen that the appropriate disaccharide is hydrolysed by its specific enzyme and the

resulting monosaccharide is then absorbed in the usual way.

Table 8.1

Disaccharide	Disaccharidase	Monosaccharide
Lactose	Lactase	Galactose + glucose
Maltose	Maltase	Glucose + glucose
Sucrose	Sucrase	Fructose + glucose

3. *Polysaccharides* $(C_6H_{10}O_5)_x$—their structure is known and a considerable amount of digestion is required before they can be absorbed. The most important polysaccharides are starch, glycogen, inulin and cellulose. Starch and glycogen are hydrolysed by amylase to mainly maltose and glucose; maltase finally breaks it down to glucose before it can be utilized by the body.

Thus it can be seen that although the diet may contain adequate carbohydrate, absorption will depend upon normal pancreatic function (amylase), the presence of disaccharidases and normal mucosal cells for transport across the intestinal wall.

Proteins and nitrogenous foods

Proteins are the chief nitrogenous constituents of the tissues of the body and of the food we eat. They are obtained chiefly from meats, eggs, milk, cheese, fish, cereals and certain vegetables such as peas and beans. Proteins are complex compounds containing carbon, hydrogen, oxygen, nitrogen, sulphur and phosphorus. Before they can be absorbed they are broken down by proteolytic enzymes to their simplest constituents, the amino acids, because it is only as such that protein can be absorbed into the venous capillaries of the villi for transportation to the liver. Normal absorption will therefore depend upon normal pancreatic function to provide the proteolytic enzymes and normal mucosal cells for the transport mechanism. Amino acids are divided into two groups, essential and non-essential. Essential amino acids are those which are not synthesized by the body out of the materials ordinarily available at a speed commensurate with normal growth, e.g. valine, methionine, threonine, leucine, isoleucine, phenylalanine, tryptophan and lysine. They are essential for the repair of body tissue, the maintenance of the osmotic equilibrium between blood and tissue fluids and for providing energy and heat, when there is an insufficient supply of carbohydrate. Non-essential amino acids are those readily synthesized from —NH_2 groups and simple carbon compounds, e.g. glycine, tyrosine, alanine, glutamine, serine, etc.

Proteins are usually classified as (a) simple or (b) conjugated. The simple proteins on hydrolysis yield only amino acids and include albumin, globulin, glutelins and gliadins (plant proteins), scleroproteins, protamines and histones, whereas a conjugated protein is a protein to which is attached a non-protein substance known as a prosthetic group (*Table 8.2*). The classification in the table is arbitrary, but for descriptive purposes is quite convenient.

Table 8.2

Conjugated protein	Prosthetic groups	Example
Chromoproteins	Haem	Haemoglobin
Lipoproteins	Lipid	Chylomicrons
Glycoproteins	Carbohydrate	Pituitary gonadotrophins
Nucleoproteins	Nucleic acid	Viruses

Fats (lipids)

Fat in the diet is important not only for its high energy, but because it contains the fat-soluble vitamins A, D, E and K, and certain essential fatty acids, linoleic and linolenic acid. Fat is also necessary for nerve sheaths, cholesterol in the bile, and to support and cushion certain organs in the body, e.g. the kidneys and eyes.

Dictary fat is digested by the action of pancreatic lipase, partially to glycerol and fatty acids and partially to split products monoglycerides and diglycerides. With the aid of bile salts, these products of digestion enter the mucosal cells of the small intestine where the fats are completely digested by the action of intestinal lipase. The lipid material is eventually converted to chylomicrons, a material which can easily pass through the intestinal cell wall into the lymphatic system.

It can therefore be seen that normal fat absorption will depend upon the presence of bile salts, pancreatic and intestinal lipase and normal intestinal mucosa for the formation of chylomicrons.

Chylomicrons are triglycerides, cholesterol, cholesterol esters and phospholipids coated with a layer of lipoprotein.

Lipids are divided into two groups, animal and vegetable. Animal fat is obtained chiefly from dairy produce such as milk, butter and cheese, from eggs, meat and bacon and from oily fish such as cod, halibut and herring. Vegetable fat is found in margarine, olive oil, groundnuts and hazel nuts.

CH_2OH	$HOOC\ C_3H_7$	$CH_2OCOC_3H_7$
$\|$	$\|$	$\|$
$CHOH$	$HOOC\ C_3H_7$	$CHOCOC_3H_7$
$\|$	$\|$	$\|$
CH_2OH	$HOOC\ C_3H_7$	$CH_2OCOC_3H_7$
Glycerol +	Butyric acid	→ Tributyrin (triglyceride)

Lipids can be divided structurally into (a) simple or (b) compound lipids. The simple lipids are either (1) fats, which are esters of glycerol with fatty acids, e.g. the mono-, di- and triglycerides (the major portion of human depot fat is made up of triglycerides, the minor portion being the mono- and diglycerides); or (2) waxes, which are esters of alcohol other than glycerol, e.g. beeswax, which is an ester of palmitic acid with myricyl alcohol. The compound lipids are (1) the phospholipids (lecithin, cephalin, sphingomyelin) and (2) the glycolipids (cerebrosides, which occur in large amounts in brain tissue).

Cholesterol is a sterol and not a lipid, but it and its esters, being lipid-soluble, are usually considered along with the lipids.

Vitamins

Vitamins are organic compounds essential for life, health and growth. They are not eaten as such in the diet, but are widely dispersed in the food we eat. Their absence causes the so-called 'deficiency' diseases. They are divided into two groups, fat-soluble and water-soluble vitamins. Vitamins A, D, E and K are fat-soluble, while the water-soluble ones are the B group vitamins and vitamin C.

For the absorption of the fat-soluble vitamins it is essential to have a normal bile secretion, while in the absorption of B_{12} the intrinsic factor secreted by the stomach is essential. In the presence of intrinsic factor a complex is formed with B_{12} which can bind to the intestinal wall where it is absorbed. Most of the other water-soluble vitamins are absorbed in the upper small intestine.

Fat-soluble vitamins

Vitamin A

This vitamin is essential for normal mucopolysaccharide synthesis, and a deficiency causes drying up of mucus-secreting epithelium. Rhodopsin, the retinal pigment, which is a protein (opsin) combined with a derivative of vitamin A, is necessary for vision in dim light. It is found in fish oils and animal fats. It can be formed in the body from β-carotene, of which the main dietary sources are green vegetables and carrots.

Vitamin D (calciferol)

Vitamin D is necessary for normal calcium absorption. A deficiency causes rickets in children and osteomalacia in adults, hence the name 'antirachitic' vitamin. Like vitamin A, it is found in fish oils and animal fats. In the skin, the precursor or pro-vitamin, 7-dehydrocholesterol can be converted into active vitamin D_3 (cholecalciferol) by ultraviolet light.

Vitamin E (tocopherol)

In experimental animals a deficiency of vitamin E causes failure in reproduction, but there is no proof that the same holds good for man. Its function is not clearly understood, but the sources of this vitamin are peanuts, lettuce, wheat germ, oil and dairy produce.

Vitamin K

Vitamin K is necessary for prothrombin synthesis in the liver, which in turn is essential for blood coagulation. Other coagulation factors also need vitamin K for their synthesis. It is found in fish, green vegetables, liver and spinach. It cannot be synthesized by man, but it can be formed by the bacterial flora of the colon.

Water-soluble vitamins (the B complex)

Vitamin B_1 (thiamine or aneurine)

Thiamine pyrophosphate is an essential coenzyme in the enzyme system needed for the decarboxylation of α-oxoacids, one of the reactions involved being the conversion of pyruvate to acetyl coenzyme A. Besides being involved in carbohydrate metabolism, it regulates the normal functioning of the nervous system.

Thiamine is present in many plants, and is in particularly high concentration in wheat germ, oatmeal and yeast. Adequate amounts are present in a normal diet, but the deficiency syndrome is still prevalent in rice-eating areas.

Vitamin B_2 (riboflavine)

This vitamin is concerned with biological oxidation systems, necessary for growth and catabolism in all tissues in man and animals. It is a component of flavin adenine dinucleotide (FAD), a coenzyme involved in oxidation–reduction reactions. It is found in yeast and vegetables, such as beans and peas, and in wheat, milk, cheese, eggs, liver and kidney.

Nicotinamide

Nicotinamide is necessary for the metabolism of carbohydrates, being an important constituent in the coenzyme, nicotinamide adenine dinucleotide (NAD) and its phosphate (NADP). Besides being involved in carbohydrate metabolism, it is essential for the normal function of the gastrointestinal tract, and for satisfactory function of the nervous system. It can be formed in the body from nicotinic acid. Both substances are plentiful in animal and plant foods. Nicotinic acid is present in high concentrations in yeast, bran, fresh liver and fish.

Vitamin B$_6$ (pyridoxine)

In the same way as thiamine and nicotinamide, pyridoxine can also be phosphorylated to yield a coenzyme, pyridoxal phosphate, which is a coenzyme for the amino transferases (transaminases) and for the decarboxylation of amino acids. Pyridoxine is found in egg-yolk, beans, peas, yeast and meat. Dietary deficiency is very rare, but the antituberculous drug isoniazid produces a picture of pyridoxine deficiency, probably by competition with it in metabolic pathways.

Pantothenic acid

The B group vitamin is a component of coenzyme A which is essential for carbohydrate and fat metabolism, promoting fatty acid oxidation and the oxidation of pyruvate. It is also used in detoxication mechanisms involving acetylation. It is widely distributed in foodstuffs such as liver, kidney, meat, wheat, bran and peas.

Biotin

Biotin is essential for the growth of many microorganisms and is a coenzyme in carboxylation reactions (i.e. the conversion of pyruvate to oxaloacetate). It is another vitamin belonging to the B group which is found in eggs. A high concentration of uncooked egg-white is toxic to rats and man, causing loss of hair and dermatitis. This is because the protein avidin, present in egg-white, combines with biotin and prevents its absorption.

Folic acid (pteroylglutamic acid)

Folic acid plays an important role in cellular metabolism, especially in the transfer of one carbon unit such as the aldehyde group —CHO. It is necessary for the normal maturation of erythrocytes. It is also included in the B group, and is found in green vegetables and some meats. It is easily destroyed in cooking, but a dietary deficiency is very rare.

Vitamin B$_{12}$

Deficiency of B$_{12}$, like folic acid, causes megaloblastic anaemia, but unlike that of folate it can result also in sub-acute combined degeneration of the spinal cord. Cyanocobalamin is found in beef,

kidney and liver. Fresh milk and dairy produce contain a small amount. A dietary deficiency is very rare, but absorption of the vitamin depends upon its combination with intrinsic factor secreted by the stomach.

Vitamin C

Ascorbic acid is necessary for erythropoiesis, for healthy bones and teeth, for normal collagen formation and for the maintenance of the strength of the walls of the blood capillaries. It is found in fresh fruit, especially blackcurrants and citrus fruits. Green vegetables also contain vitamin C.

Mineral salts

Mineral salts are necessary in the diet for all body processes, and although required in varying quantities, the amount is usually small.

Calcium and magnesium are absorbed in the small intestine with the help of vitamin D, and normal fat absorption. Sodium and potassium, which occur as chlorides and phosphates in body tissues and fluids, are absorbed in the small intestine by an active process in the same way as they are in the renal tubule. Sodium–potassium exchange is also regulated by the hormone aldosterone.

Iron present in haemoglobin is absorbed in the duodenum and upper jejunum, the absorption being stimulated by the presence of anaemia. All the minerals are present in adequate amounts in a normal diet.

Calcium

Calcium is the chief constituent of teeth and bones and is absorbed in the small intestine with the help of vitamin D. It plays an important part in the coagulation of blood, in the contraction of muscles, and in the permeability of cell membranes. It is found principally in milk, cheese, eggs and green vegetables.

Phosphate

Phosphate combines with calcium in the formation of bone and teeth and helps to maintain the normal composition of body fluid. Bone salt is mainly hydroxyapatite $3Ca_3(PO_4)_2.Ca(OH)_2$. Phosphate is found in cheese, liver, kidney and oatmeal.

Sodium

Sodium is present mainly in tissue fluids and therefore plays an important part in cell activity and in the fluid balance of the body. The amount of sodium in our normal diet far exceeds the requirements of the body. It is found in fish, meat, eggs, milk and in table salt, and especially in prepared foods such as bacon and sausages.

Potassium

Potassium is an essential constituent of all cells, and is necessary also for the normal activity of cardiac, skeletal and smooth muscle. It is present mainly in cells. It is widely distributed in all foods.

Iron

Iron is necessary for the formation of the cytochromes which are involved in tissue oxidation and is of course essential for the formation of haemoglobin. It is found in liver, kidney, beef and green vegetables. About 0.012 g are considered to be the average daily requirement.

Iodine

Iodine is essential for the formation of the thyroid hormones, thyroxine and triiodothyronine. It is found in salt-water fish and in vegetables grown in soil containing iodine.

Water

Water has many functions, some of which are the formation of urine and faeces, transport of water-soluble substances, e.g. vitamins, and the dilution of waste products and poisonous substances in the body. It is absorbed passively as in the renal tubule along an osmotic gradient created by the absorption of sodium and other solutes. Any water remaining for absorption after passing through the osmotic gradient, will be absorbed in the colon. Many foods contain at least 75% by weight of water. Some water is taken also in the diet as liquid and some is derived from the oxidation of foods.

Roughage

Roughage gives bulk to the diet and stimulates peristalsis and bowel movement and is the undigested part of the diet.

In addition to providing all the above-mentioned components, the diet must altogether provide a sufficient number of calories for the energy needs of the body, otherwise the body's protoplasm is utilized to provide energy, the body weight falls and the tissues waste, as may happen during a period of illness.

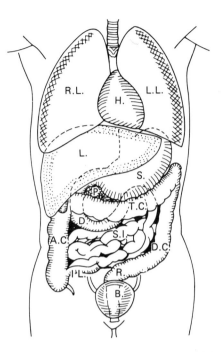

Figure 8.1. Diagram showing the position of the main organs of the body, including the alimentary tract (R.L., right lung; L.L., left lung; H, heart; L, liver; S, stomach; P, pancreas; D, duodenum; S.I., small intestine; A.C., ascending colon; T.C., transverse colon; D.C., descending colon; B, bladder; R, rectum)

Alimentary tract

The alimentary tract (*Figure 8.1*) is a convoluted tube where the food is ingested, digested, absorbed and eliminated. It extends from the mouth to the anus and consists of the mouth, pharynx, oesophagus, stomach, small intestine and large intestine, including the rectum and anus. Various secretions are poured into the alimentary tract, some by the lining membranes of the organs mentioned and some by glands situated outside the tract. The accessory organs are the salivary glands, pancreas, liver and biliary tract, their secretions being poured into the tract through various ducts.

Digestion

Digestion starts in the mouth where the lips, cheeks, muscles and teeth are all involved in the ingestion and mastication of food. The food is moistened by saliva, the secretion from the salivary glands, to form a bolus or soft mass of food ready for deglutition or swallowing. The three pairs of salivary glands, two parotid, two submandibular and two sublingual, secrete about 1500 ml of serous fluid rich in enzyme into the oral cavity per day, the only stimulus for its secretion being the sight and smell of food. Saliva consists of water, mucin, mineral salts and the enzyme α-amylase or ptyalin, which starts the digestion of starch to maltose.

This digestive action is of secondary nature since food remains in the mouth for only a short time. Mucin, a glycoprotein, lubricates the food, and the saliva, besides keeping the mouth and teeth clean, may also have some antibacterial action. When mastication is complete and the bolus formed it is pushed backward into the pharynx by the upward movement of the tongue. The pharynx, the cavity between the mouth and tongue, is divided into three parts, the nasopharynx, the oropharynx and the laryngopharynx, which is then connected to the oesophagus, the narrowest part of the tract. The bolus is then carried down the gullet or oesophagus by peristalsis, which propels the food through the cardiac orifice into the stomach. The stomach is a J-shaped dilated portion of the alimentary tract; its size and shape varies with each individual and with its contents. From *Figure 8.2* it can be seen that it is divided into the fundus, body and pyloric antrum. It has three layers of muscle tissue: an outer longitudinal layer, a layer with circular fibres and an inner layer of oblique fibres. This arrangement allows for the churning motion characteristic of gastric activity.

The stomach is lined with a mucosal layer which is fairly flexible, called the gastric mucosa. When the stomach is in a state of contraction, the mucous membrane lining is thrown into longitudinal folds or rugae, and when the stomach is dilated the lining is smooth and velvety. The gastric mucosa contains many deep glands; in the pyloric and cardiac region the glands secrete mucus, while in the fundus and body of the stomach the glands contain the parietal or oxyntic cells, which secrete hydrochloric acid, and chief or peptic cells, which secrete pepsinogens.

Besides these secretions, gastric juice will also contain the intrinsic factor secreted by the gastric mucosa, gastric lipase and possibly rennin. The hormone *gastrin*, normally produced by the pyloric glands, in response to the presence of food, is carried by the blood stream to the stomach, where it stimulates the secretion of gastric acid and pepsin. The upper two-thirds of the stomach act as a reservoir, in that it holds the food for a sufficient period of time to allow thorough mixing with the gastric juice, so that the HCl and pepsinogen can act on the constituents of food. The time the food is held will depend upon its nature and consistency, but it is normally for 2–2½ h. The lower one-third of the stomach churns the food to a semi-fluid mass of uniform consistency called chyme, which is slowly passed through into the duodenum in small jets when the pyloric sphincter relaxes and the muscular walls of the stomach contract. Although the main digestive processes begin in the duodenum, food will be digested by salivary amylase until it is stopped by the concentration of hydrochloric acid, while proteins are broken down to proteases and peptones by the action of pepsin. Hydrochloric acid also limits the growth of micro-organisms entering the stomach.

The duodenum is part of the small intestine, which starts at the pyloric sphincter and leads into the large intestine at the ileocolic valve, the other two sections being the jejunum and ileum. The duodenum is the C-shaped section of the gut, which goes round the head of the pancreas and contains the ampulla of the bile duct where the pancreatic duct joins the bile duct, the opening of which is controlled by the sphincter of Oddi. It is through the sphincter of Oddi that the pancreatic juice and bile enter the duodenum to continue the digestion of food. The partially digested food is gradually

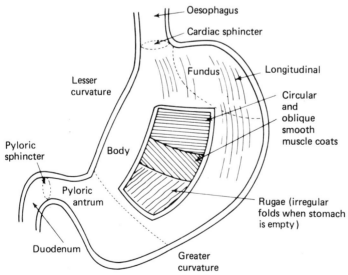

Figure 8.2. The stomach

transferred from the duodenum into the second part of the small intestine, the jejunum and then into the ileum, the latter part of the small intestine, by muscular contractions known as peristalsis. The ileocolic valve controls the flow of the contents of the ileum into the large intestine and also prevents the backflow of contents from the large intestine. During its passage through the small intestine the acid chyme comes in contact first with the alkaline pancreatic juice and bile, then with intestinal juice, secreted by glands in the mucosa of small intestine induced by the hormone enterocrinin. It is this juice which completes the digestion of nutritional materials after the pancreatic juice and bile have had their effect. Carbohydrates, proteins and fats in their undigested or partly digested state cannot pass through the mucosa of the gut into the body, but in the form of glucose, amino acids and fatty acids they can permeate through the minute projections in the wall of the small intestine, called villi (see *Figure 8.3*). The villi create an enormous surface area for

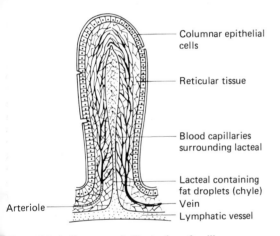

Columnar epithelial cells

Reticular tissue

Blood capillaries surrounding lacteal

Lacteal containing fat droplets (chyle)

Vein

Arteriole

Lymphatic vessel

Figure 8.3. A diagrammatic illustration of a villus

absorption which is said to be about five times that of the skin surface of the body. Glucose and amino acids are absorbed into the blood capillaries, fatty acids and glycerol are absorbed into the lacteals. Other nutritional materials such as vitamins, minerals and water, are absorbed from the small intestine into the blood capillaries. The ileum leads into the large intestine, the terminal part of the alimentary tract which commences at the caecum and terminates at the anal canal. It is divided into the caecum, the ascending, transverse, descending and pelvic colons, rectum and anal canal. When the contents of the ileum pass through the ileocolic valve into the caecum they are fluid, even though some water has been absorbed in the small intestine. Water absorption therefore continues in the colon, along with the absorption of glucose, some minerals and

drugs. Mucin and certain minerals such as calcium, copper, iron, in excess of body needs, are secreted.

Cellulose is broken down by bacterial action, mainly in the caecum, and micro-organisms present in the large intestine have the ability to synthesize some vitamins, for example vitamins D and K. The elimination of all the waste solidified matter, called faeces, is carried out by the muscular action of the rectum.

Intestinal juice or succus entericus

This is the digestive juice which completes the digestion of the nutritional materials. It is difficult to obtain uncontaminated juice, but it is basically alkaline in pH and consists of water, mineral salts, mucus and the enzymes, enterokinase, peptidase, lipase, sucrase, maltase and lactase.

Accessory organs and juices in digestion

Besides the salivary glands, the other organs are the pancreas, liver and biliary tract.

The gall bladder and bile duct

Bile from the liver flows through the right and left hepatic ducts to join up to form the hepatic duct (see *Figure 8.4*). The hepatic duct passes downwards where it is joined at an acute angle by the cystic duct from the gall bladder. The cystic and hepatic ducts join together to form the bile duct, which passes downwards to the head of the pancreas to be joined by the pancreatic duct at the ampulla of the bile duct. The two together open into the duodenum at the sphincter of Oddi.

The gall bladder is a pear-shaped sac, which acts as a reservoir for the bile before it is discharged into the duodenum. It is divided into a fundus, body and neck.

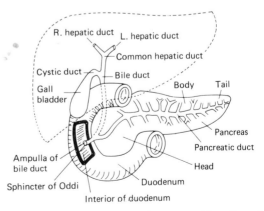

R. hepatic duct   L. hepatic duct

Common hepatic duct

Cystic duct

Bile duct

Gall bladder

Body   Tail

Pancreas

Pancreatic duct

Ampulla of bile duct

Head

Sphincter of Oddi

Duodenum

Interior of duodenum

Figure 8.4. The gall bladder and pancreas with outlines of the liver

Functions of the gall bladder

Besides being a reservoir for bile it concentrates the bile and regulates its discharge into the duodenum. During its stay in the gall bladder the bile is concentrated by absorption of water and at the same time its viscosity is increased by the secretion of mucus from the epithelial cells of the wall of the gall bladder. The contraction of the muscular walls of the gall bladder and the relaxation of its sphincter is initiated by the hormone cholecystokinin. Cholecystokinin is secreted by the mucosa of the upper intestine in response to the presence of food, mainly meats and fats, in the duodenum.

The pancreas

The adult pancreas is a pale yellowish gland about 20–25 cm long and weighs between 60 and 160 g. It is situated in the epigastric and the left hypochondriac region of the abdominal cavity. It is divided into a broad head which lies in the curve of the duodenum, a body which lies behind the body of the stomach, and a narrow tail which lies in front of the left kidney and which just reaches the spleen. It is a dual organ, having both endocrine (internal) and exocrine (external) secretions or functions.

Exocrine functions

The gland consists of a number of lobules which are made up of small alveoli lined with secretory cells. The secretion from each cell is drained by a tiny duct which unites with other ducts and joins the main pancreatic duct. The main duct passes the whole length of the organ to open into the duodenum about 10 cm from the pyloric sphincter. Just before entering the duodenum the main duct joins with the bile duct at the ampulla of the bile duct and discharges the secretion into the duodenum through the sphincter of Oddi. The secretion is formed by the cells of the pancreatic acini and cells of the intralobular ducts and its composition is divided into organic and inorganic constituents, both of which assist in the digestive processes of the tract.

Pancreatic juice

The inorganic constituent is the alkaline juice of pH 7.5–8.0 or higher, which is mainly bicarbonate used to render the acid chyme entering the duodenum alkaline. The chloride content rises and falls inversely with the bicarbonate level, while the sodium and potassium levels are almost identical with the levels found in plasma. The alkaline reaction is also necessary for the effective function of the pancreatic enzymes which are the organic constituents of the juice. Some of the pancreatic

enzymes are trypsin, chymotrypsin, carboxypeptidase, amylase and lipase. Trypsinogen, an inactive enzyme, is activated to trypsin by enterokinase, an enzyme secreted by the duodenal mucosa. Trypsin also converts chymotrypsinogen into chymotrypsin. This powerful protein-splitting enzyme (proteolytic) eventually converts all the proteins and proteoses into peptides. Carboxypeptidase, which is secreted as procarboxypeptidase but activated by trypsin, splits peptide bonds located at the lower end of the polypeptide chains into free amino acids when as such they are absorbed by the intestinal mucosa. Pancreatic amylase, an enzyme identical with salivary amylase, converts all starches not affected by the salivary amylase into maltose and maltase completes the breakdown to glucose. Some pancreatic amylase is absorbed into the blood and excreted into the urine, therefore possessing diastatic properties. Lipase is a powerful enzyme which hydrolyses fat into a mixture of lower glycerides and fatty acids. Bile salts emulsify the fats and therefore assist in the breakdown.

Secretion of pancreatic juice

The sight, smell and thought of food stimulates the production of pancreatic juice via the vagus, but this nervous phase is a minor one compared to the humoral control. The presence of acid chyme from the stomach activates the duodenum to produce secretin, a hormone which stimulates the production by the pancreas of a thin, watery fluid, high in bicarbonate but low in enzymes. The upper jejunum produces a hormone, pancreozymin, which stimulates the production of a viscous fluid low in bicarbonate but high in enzyme content. While the acid chyme stimulates the secretion of secretin, the products of digestion, particularly protein, are the stimulus for pancreozymin production.

Endocrine function

The pancreatic islet tissue, first described by Langerhans, consists of a large number of discrete cells widely distributed throughout the pancreas. The islet tissue cells function independently of the acini and are of two types, α-cells and β-cells, each producing a hormone which affects carbohydrate metabolism. The islet of Langerhans makes up 1–2% of the pancreatic tissue. The α-cells (25% of islets) secrete glucagon directly into the circulating blood to promote glycogen breakdown (glycogenolysis), which increases the blood glucose and utilization of glucose by the tissues. Besides the rapid mobilization of hepatic glucose it also utilizes to a lesser extent fatty acids from adipose tissue. The effects of glucagon are overshadowed by the β-cells (50–75% of islets) which also secrete insulin directly into the circulating blood. Insulin increases the permeability of cells to glucose, accelerates carbohydrate oxidation, and at the same time gluconeogenesis (formation of glucose or glycogen from non-carbohydrate sources) is depressed and the conversion of glucose to fat is increased. Glucagon is therefore a hyperglycaemic agent (elevates blood glucose), while insulin is the hypoglycaemic hormone. In spite of the irregular intake and uneven utilization of carbohydrates, the level of blood and tissue glucose is maintained at a fairly constant level by these two hormones, the most important of which is insulin. Other hormones concerned in the regulation of blood glucose but not secreted by the pancreas are: cortisol (adrenal cortex), adrenaline (adrenal medulla), thyroxine (thyroid) and ACTH (anterior pituitary).

Diabetes mellitus in man is due to a deficiency of insulin, which is characterized by hyperglycaemia and glycosuria (glucose in the urine), while insulinoma (hypoglycaemia) is caused by a functioning β-cell tumour of the islets producing too much insulin.

Gastric function tests

The stomach is an organ of digestion and gastric juice is secreted by the cells in the walls of the stomach in response to (1) gastrin, a hormone secreted by the gastric antrum mucosa when food is in the stomach; (2) psychic factors (sight, taste or smell of food); and (3) the presence of some products of digestion in the intestine. One of the commonest investigations, until quite recently, for gastric function, was the collection of gastric juice before and after drinking a pint of oatmeal gruel. This has now been replaced by histamine and pentagastrin stimulation tests. This direct method of gastric analysis is carried out by removing the gastric contents by intubation, but there is an indirect method, which involves the use of diagnex blue and collecting urine samples.

Composition of normal gastric juice

Volume: 2–4 litres per day, but there is always a small quantity (about 50 ml) present in the stomach even when it contains no food.
Appearance: colourless-grey fluid.
pH: 1.0–1.5 due to the hydrochloric acid produced by the parietal cells.
Water content: about 97–99%.
Inorganic constituents: sodium, potassium, chloride, calcium, magnesium, phosphate and sulphate.
Organic constituents: pepsins, mucin, intrinsic factor, rennin (said to be absent from stomach of the adult), gastric lipase, albumin and globulin.

The composition may vary considerably, depending upon the physiological state of the stomach.

Stimulants of gastric juice secretion

1. Tea and toast.
2. 1 pint (568 ml) of oatmeal gruel.
3. Alcohol—100 ml 7% alcohol plus methylene blue used as an indicator for the emptying time of the stomach.
4. Histamine, given subcutaneously, 0.01 mg per kg body weight.
5. Pentagastrin, given intramuscularly 6 µg per kg body weight.

Anything entering the stomach can constitute a humoral agent, but some meals act as a greater stimulus than others. If a meal is given, there are two variables, one being the rate of emptying of the stomach and the other being the rate of secretion of stomach juices. This is why the older forms of test meals (oatmeal, alcohol) have now been dropped in favour of other stimulants.

Direct stimulation of parietal cells

(a) Histamine

Histamine, produced by the decarboxylation of the amino acid, histidine, acts directly on the parietal cells and stimulates the secretion of gastric juice. It has undesirable side effects and, therefore, should be given with anti-histamine cover, which does not block the gastric stimulating effect of histamine. Anti-histamine does, however, cause drowsiness.

(b) Pentagastrin

Pentagastrin is a synthetically produced pentapeptide consisting of the physiologically active part of the gastrin molecule. It is used in the same way as histamine but in smaller doses. Although it has fewer side effects compared with histamine it is expensive to use.

Augmented histamine test

In the 'augmented' histamine test much larger doses of histamine are given, thereby providing a more reliable proof of an ability to secrete acid. The test has two purposes: first to show the inability to secrete acid, and secondly to assess the maximum possible acid secretion as a diagnostic aid to surgical treatment.

1. Prepare the patient by fasting for 12 h, to ensure the stomach is completely emptied.
2. Pass a number 14 Ryle's tube pernasally into the stomach (preferably under X-ray control) until it lies in the pyloric antrum. The tube has markings on it to indicate how far the tube has been swallowed. The position of the tube is maintained by strapping it to the cheek with plaster and insisting that the patient does not alter his or her posture until completion of the test.

3. 8.00 a.m. All the gastric juice is aspirated from the stomach by means of a syringe attached to the end of the Ryle's tube and placed in a bottle marked 'Resting Juice'.
4. 8.00–9.00 a.m. Aspirate all the gastric juice at 15-min intervals for the next 60-min period and place in the bottle marked 'Basal Secretion'. (Sometimes the basal secretions are divided into pre- and post-Anthisan collections.)
5. 100 mg mepyramine (Anthisan) is given by *intramuscular* injection half-way through the basal collection period at 8.30 a.m.
6. 9.00 a.m. Inject 2 mg histamine acid phosphate (average adult dose) *subcutaneously* 30 min after the Anthisan injection.

7. 9.00–9.15 a.m.⎫ Aspirate gastric juice at 15-
   9.15–9.30 a.m.⎪ min intervals for 60 min and
   9.30–9.45 a.m.⎬ place in bottles marked with
   9.45–10.00 a.m.⎭ the appropriate times, thereby obtaining four 15-min samples. Alternatively, three 20-min samples may be used.

(Since the stomach juices are equivalent to the secretion by the glands, the secretory rate can be determined.)

8. All specimens are sent to the laboratory for analysis.

Laboratory procedure

1. Measure and record the volume of each collection.
2. Examine visually for blood, mucus and bile.
3. Measure the pH of each specimen using a pH meter.
4. Determine the titratable acidity of each collection by titration with standardized sodium hydroxide to pH 7.4 (blood pH) electrometrically or with phenol red as indicator.
5. Express the results as total acid concentration (titratable acidity) per specimen in mmol/l and also as hydrogen ion concentration in mmol per specimen and total hydrogen ion concentration in mmol per basal hour and post-histamine hour.

Estimation of titratable acidity

Reagents

(a) Phenol red indicator—0.1 g phenol red, 5.7 ml 0.05M NaOH diluted to 250 ml with distilled water.
(b) 0.02M sodium hydroxide solution—prepare fresh for use by diluting 20.0 ml stock solution of 0.1 mol sodium hydroxide to 100 ml with distilled water in a volumetric flask. Standardize before use on each occasion.

Method

Some laboratories will be in the position of determining the titratable acidity by using an automatic burette and pH meter, a method which will not be dealt with in this book. If the pH is greater than 7.4 no further examination is necessary. All specimens with a pH less than 7.0 are treated as follows:

1. Centrifuge or filter the gastric contents.
2. Pipette 1.0 ml or 2.0 ml of clear gastric juice into a 50 ml conical flask, add about 5 ml distilled water and 2–3 drops of phenol red indicator.
3. As a control for end-point determination use 1.0 ml or 2.0 ml of pH 7.4 buffer instead of the gastric contents.
4. Titrate each specimen carefully with 0.02M standardized NaOH from a 10 ml burette until a faint pink end point is obtained.
5. Note the titre and record the result.

■ Notes

(a) *Titratable acidity* is the sum of the hydrogen ion concentration and un-ionized hydrogen ion concentration. This is now used instead of the obsolete terminology, total acidity, which was the free acidity plus combined acidity (determined by using Topfer's reagent and phenolphthalein; this method should be discontinued).
(b) *Hydrogen ion concentration* as measured by pH is not the same as titratable acidity, for example, 0.1M HCl has a pH of 1.00 and 0.1M CH_3COOH has a pH of 2.6, but these two acid solutions are of identical titratable acidity, 100 mmol/l.

Calculation

0.02M NaOH contains 20 mmol/l. Therefore 1.0 ml 0.02M NaOH is equivalent to 20 mmol/l. Let x = titre of gastric juice, y = volume of sample taken and Y = volume of specimen collection:

$$\text{Titratable acidity} = \frac{x \times 20}{y} \text{ in mmol/l}$$

Hydrogen ion concentration per specimen

$$\frac{\text{mmol/l} \times Y}{1000} \text{ in mmol}$$

For example:

$$x = 4.3 \text{ ml} \qquad y = 1.0 \text{ ml} \qquad Y = 24 \text{ ml}$$

$$\text{Titratable acidity} = \frac{4.3 \times 20}{1.0} = 86.0 \text{ mmol/l}$$

Hydrogen ion concentration per specimen

$$\frac{86.0 \times 24}{1000} = 2.064 \text{ mmol}$$

During an augmented histamine test the result shown in *Table 8.3* were obtained when 1.0 ml of gastric juice was titrated. The hydrogen ion concentration per specimen was:

Table 8.3

	Time (a.m.)	Volume (ml)	pH	Titre	Titratable acidity	Comments
1. Basal secretion	8.00–9.00	40.0	6.0	0.4	8.0	
2. Post-histamine	9.00–9.15	47.0	2.5	1.2	24.0	bile present
3. Post-histamine	9.15–9.30	97.0	1.5	4.5	90.0	bile present
4. Post-histamine	9.30–9.45	88.0	1.2	5.8	116.0	
5. Post-histamine	9.45–10.00	82.0	1.3	5.7	114.0	flecks of blood present

1. $\dfrac{8.0 \times 40}{1000} = 0.32$ mmol

2. $\dfrac{24.0 \times 47}{1000} = 1.13$ mmol

3. $\dfrac{90 \times 97}{1000} = 8.73$ mmol

4. $\dfrac{116 \times 88}{1000} = 10.2$ mmol

5. $\dfrac{114 \times 82}{1000} = 9.35$ mmol

The sum of the hydrogen ion concentration in samples 2–5 will be total hydrogen ion concentration per post-histamine hour = 29.41 mmol

Notes

1. *Resting juice* is of little significance clinically.
2. *Basal secretion* is used for the fasting gastric secretion and is helpful in diagnosing duodenal ulcer, since about one-quarter of patients have a significantly high output. The basal secretion has a poor repeatability.
3. *Maximum secretions* are of excellent repeatability and this is why the augmented histamine test has completely replaced the fractional test meal.
4. *Bile* staining usually invalidates the tests unless the specimen has a pH of less than 3.5. When found in the gastric contents it is usually due to regurgitation from the duodenum into the stomach, or the Ryle's tube was in the duodenum.
5. *Blood* should not be present. Small amounts of bright red flecks of blood usually indicate trauma during aspiration. Quantities of altered blood which is usually brown or reddish-brown in colour (HCl in the gastric contents plus red cells are haemolysed to form acid haematin) are usually found in gastric ulcer or gastric carcinoma.
6. *Mucus* is normally only present in small amounts, but can be increased in gastric carcinoma.

Normal values

The normal values for the augmented histamine test depend upon age and sex.

Post-histamine hour values:

Normal males
(All ages)   less than 30 yr   greater than 30 yr
0.1–42.1   14.1–42.1   0.1–33.3
Normal females
(All ages)
0.3–28.2   12.6–28.2   0.3–10.8

expressed as total hydrogen ion concentration in mmol.

The acidity of the gastric contents yields valuable diagnostic information.

Hypersecretion of gastric juice may be associated with duodenal ulcers. Acid secretion by the stomach is very high.

Hyposecretion of gastric juice occurs in pernicious anaemia and the achlorhydria is usually 'histamine fast'. Gastric carcinoma and chronic gastritis may also fall into this group.

Hyperchlorhydria—excessive secretion of hydrochloric acid.

Achlorhydria—a complete absence of hydrochloric acid.

Pentagastrin test

This is carried out in a similar manner to the augmented histamine test, except that 6 µg/kg body weight is injected intramuscularly. Histamine is gradually being replaced by the synthetically produced pentapeptide.

Faeces

Occult blood

Blood or its breakdown products may be present in the faeces, and its detection is another test used in the investigation of the gastrointestinal tract.

It can be found in the faeces from patients with carcinoma of the stomach, or an ulcer of the alimentary tract. Rectal or menstrual bleeding may contaminate the surface of the specimen with fresh blood; if this is seen, a report is issued stating that blood was detected macroscopically. Minute quantities may not be visible to the naked eye and the blood is said to be 'occult' or hidden. It may be detected by chemical means and microscopical examination may reveal intact red cells.

In 1969 the Department of Health issued two circulars, HM(69)57 and HM(69)74, directing laboratory and clinical hospital staff to the implications of using solutions containing amines controlled or prohibited under the Carcinogenic Substances Regulation 1967: SI No. 879. Owing to the carcinogenic properties of benzidine and orthotolidine, routine laboratory procedures for occult blood testing now use a non-carcinogenic chromogen, such as guaiacum, although reduced phenolphthalein and dichlorophenol-indophenol can be used. The Okokit (Hughes and Hughes Ltd), a tablet test for occult blood, also contains a non-carcinogenic chromogen, and appears to be generally used throughout the UK when the 'faecal smear' method is not available.

Preparation of patient

It used to be essential for the patient to be kept on a meat-free diet for three days prior to the examination of the faeces for occult blood, but nowadays the sensitivity of the tests are adjusted so this restriction is unnecessary, although foods such as liver and black puddings should be avoided. The sensitivity of the test should indicate blood loss greater than 2.5–4.5 ml per day and should be strongly positive for the characteristic black and glistening tarry specimen.

Irrespective of whether a meat-free diet is adhered to or the sensitivity of the tests adjusted, it is usual to examine three daily specimens before the presence or absence of occult blood is confirmed.

(a) The Okokit

Principle

The peroxidase activity of haemoglobin and its iron-containing derivative catalyse the oxidation of the non-carcinogenic chromogen (nature not stated) to form a blue colour in the presence of hydrogen peroxide. Other peroxidases in the faeces with a similar action can be destroyed by heat. Boiling and heating may denature some of the peroxidases of the haemoglobin as well as that of the bacterial and plant origin.

Materials supplied in the kit are (1) the diluent, (2) Okokit tablets, and (3) test papers.

Method (modified April 1972)
1. A small amount of the sample to be tested (faeces, boiled faeces, urine, etc.) is placed in the centre of the test paper, as a thin smear.
2. One Okokit tablet is then placed in the centre of the smear.
3. Three drops of diluent are then applied onto the tablet.
4. After 2 min add a further three drops of diluent.
5. Read after 5½ min.

Results

Positive—A specimen of faeces containing blood will show a blue reaction around the tablet. The intensity of the reaction will be proportional to the concentration of blood in the specimen.
Trace—For trace amounts it is advisable to read the reverse side of the test paper held up to a direct light.

Negative—A specimen of faeces containing no blood will show no reaction around the tablet.

■ Notes

1. The present form of the Okokit is sensitive to a 1 in 40 000 dilution of whole blood (manufacturer's comments), but a subjective element is inherent in any test which depends upon the judgement of the colour developed. It is therefore important that intending users should determine for themselves whether the test fulfils their requirements.
2. Check each time by using a positive control of a 1 in 40 000 dilution of whole blood.
3. When stored at 5–15°C, the kit is stable for a minimum of two years.

(b) Faecal smear method (Haemoccult*)

Principle

The filter paper envelopes are impregnated with long-life guaiac resin. The filter paper is smeared with faeces and on the addition of a stabilized solution of hydrogen peroxide, haemoglobin or iron degradation products liberate oxygen on contact with the peroxide, which oxidizes the colour indicator guaiac—resulting in the coloration.

Preparation of the patient

The sensitivity of this test has been adjusted so that dietary restrictions are unnecessary. It is advisable for the patient to take a high-bulk diet for three days before commencing the test and throughout the test period, since a restricted diet may conceal any lesions present. As high levels of vitamin C may give false negative results, this treatment should be avoided.

Test

(a) *Patient.* The patient receives three test envelopes. On three consecutive days (using the applicators supplied) spread a thin smear of faeces taken from two parts of the stool onto the two red-frame openings inside the test envelope. The envelope is then closed, labelled and sent to the laboratory.

(b) *Laboratory.* The specimens are allowed to dry for 24 h before completing the development. After 24 h open the back of the test envelope, avoiding contact with the faeces, and then add 2 drops of the developer solution to each of the two faecal smears covered by the reagent paper. Read the test exactly 30 s after applying the developer solution, at which time the blue coloration is most intense. This timing

*Haemoccult is the trademark of Smith, Kline and French Laboratories. It is marketed by Eaton Laboratories, Reagent House, The Broadway, Woking, Surrey GU21 5AP

is critical as both an earlier or later evaluation may lead to false (negative) results.

Any blue around the specimen, irrespective of intensity, is positive. Even one positive smear from the six is taken as a positive result.

◀ Notes

1. The Haemoccult has detected blood *in vitro* to a dilution of 1 in 5000.
2. If the time lag between collecting the specimen and its evaluation exceeds 12 days, the sensitivity of the test is reduced.
3. This test can be used by the patient at home and in the ward, as easily understood instructions are issued with the test envelopes.

Pancreatic function tests

Tests of exocrine function

Changes in the external secretion of the pancreas can be studied by either direct or indirect procedures. The *direct* studies are usually the quantitative estimation of the various enzymes of pancreatic juice, bilirubin, bicarbonates and fluid volume obtained by duodenal intubation following pancreatic stimulation with pancreazymin and secretin. As this procedure is beyond the scope of this book, we will be mainly concerned with some of the *indirect* studies, but a brief résumé of the most common and serious diseases of the pancreas—acute and chronic pancreatitis—is included.

Pancreatitis

This is a condition in which there is a premature activation of pancreatic enzymes leading to self-digestion of the gland.

In *chronic pancreatitis*, there is a gradual necrosis of the glandular tissue which leads to pancreatic insufficiency. *Acute pancreatitis*, on the other hand, when biliary tract disease is the most common cause, eventually leads to recovery from the inflammatory state with the restoration of normal organ function. The indirect studies can be divided into the following groups:

1. *Serum enzymes.* The determination of lipase and α-amylase in serum plays an important role in the laboratory diagnosis of pancreatic disease; however, α-amylase is the far more common parameter. Tests of pancreatic function are not very satisfactory as serum amylase levels usually show little change from normal in pancreatic disease, except in acute pancreatitis, when they may be raised. Serum lipase levels are not estimated routinely, but they can be of some value in that in acute pancreatitis lipase shows

the greatest increase, but its estimation alone is not sufficiently accurate to establish a diagnosis of acute pancreatitis. In chronic pancreatitis, the assays of lipase and α-amylase are of less value, since parenchymal destruction leads to a substantial depression of the pancreatic enzyme production, resulting in low levels of both enzymes in the blood.

2. *Serum amylase.* There are two main types of methods available for estimating amylase activity, saccharogenic and amyloclastic. The saccharogenic methods determine the increase in reducing sugars released by the enzyme from the starch molecule. Amyloclastic methods measure the decrease in blue colour given when iodine is added to starch after digestion by the enzyme.

Methods are now available, often in kit form, which use dye-marked starches, which on hydrolysis release the dye fragments from the substrate; they are simple to use and follow zero-order kinetics over a wide range of enzyme activity. A variety of these dye-marked substrates are on the market in a kit form, two of which are the Phadebas (Pharmacia) and Amylochrome (Roche), both of which are very satisfactory.

Two methods will be mentioned, an amyloclastic and a dye-marked substrate procedure. The amyloclastic method is still used in some laboratories and is a very good practical exercise. On the other hand, the Phadebas procedure is just one example of a zero-order kinetics reaction.

1. Amyloclastic

Principle

A small amount of plasma or serum is incubated at 37°C with a solution containing 0.4 mg of starch. The loss of blue colour which the starch gives with iodine solution is taken as a measure of the extent to which the starch has been digested by the amylase.

Reagents

1. Buffered starch substrate (pH 7.0). Dissolve 13.3 g of dry anhydrous disodium hydrogen phosphate (or 33.5 g $Na_2HPO_4.12H_2O$) and 4.3 g benzoic acid in 250 ml of water. Bring to boil. Mix 0.2 g of soluble starch in 5–10 ml of cold water in a beaker and add it all to the boiling mixture, rinsing the beaker out with additional cold water. Continue boiling for 1 min, then cool to room temperature and dilute to 500 ml. Keep the solution at 4°C and prepare freshly each month.

2. Stock iodine solution. Dissolve 13.5 g of pure sublimed iodine in a solution of 24 g of potassium iodide in about 100 ml of water and make to 1 litre with water.

3. Working iodine solution. Dissolve 50 g of potassium iodide in a little water, add 100 ml of stock iodine solution, and dilute to 1 litre with water.

4. 0.9% sodium chloride.

Method

Test:

1. Serum or plasma is diluted 1 in 10 with 0.9% sodium chloride solution.
2. Add 1.0 ml of buffered substrate to a 150 × 15 mm test-tube and place in a 37°C water bath for 2 min.
3. 0.1 ml of diluted serum is added, mixed and kept at 37°C for 15 min.
4. The tube is removed, cooled and 8.5 ml of water is added.
5. 0.4 ml of dilute iodine is now added and the solution mixed.
6. A blank is prepared similarly to the test, except that the 0.1 ml of diluted serum is added last, i.e. after the addition of the dilute iodine solution.
7. The absorbances of the test and blank are read within 5 min at 660 nm, zeroing the spectrophotometer with distilled water.

Calculation: A Somogyi amylase unit is the amount of amylase which will destroy 5 mg starch in 15 min.

Since 1 ml of buffered substrate contains 0.4 mg starch and 0.1 ml of diluted serum is equivalent to 0.01 ml of undiluted serum, then

$$\frac{A \text{ of blank} - A \text{ of test}}{A \text{ of blank}}$$

(where A = absorbance) is equivalent to the amount of starch digested by 0.01 ml of serum in 15 min, and as 1 amylase unit will destroy 5 mg of starch (but only 0.04 mg of starch was used):

$$\frac{A \text{ of blank} - A \text{ of test}}{A \text{ of blank}} \times \frac{0.4}{5.0} \times \frac{100}{0.01}$$
$$= \text{amylase units per 100 ml serum}$$

or

$$\frac{A \text{ of blank} - A \text{ of test}}{A \text{ of blank}} \times 800$$
$$= \text{amylase units per 100 ml serum}$$

To convert the Somogyi amylase unit into U/l use the following assumption. One mg of glucose liberated under defined conditions corresponds to the formation of 0.185 μmol of reducing group per min. Therefore, 1 Somogyi unit/100 ml equals 1.85 U/l. This is only an arbitrary conversion since reducing groups of different oligosaccharides do not react in the same way.

Results

Somogyi quoted values of between 80 and 180 Somogyi units per 100 ml or 148–333 U/l, but this can vary from method to method, so it is best to establish your own reference range.

In acute pancreatitis, values over 1000 Somogyi units (1850 U/l) can be expected.

■ Notes

(a) As salivary amylase will invalidate the results, contamination from saliva must be avoided.
(b) When values over 350 units (555 U/l) are obtained, the determination should be repeated with a higher dilution of serum.

2. Phadebas

Principle

The substrate is a water-insoluble crosslinked starch polymer carrying a blue dye. During hydrolysis by amylase, water-soluble blue fragments are found. The absorbance of the blue solution is therefore a function of the amylase activity in the sample. A calibration curve is constructed from Phadebas ACR serum which is assayed by the manufacturer using a saccharogenic method as the reference method.

Reagents, test procedure and precautions

Refer to the manufacturer's instructions supplied with the kit package.

Results

Ranges from 70 to 300 U/l are quoted, the mean value being 170 U/l.

Faecal studies

In severe pancreatic disease, evidence of impaired digestion of foodstuffs can be obtained by a microscopical examination of the faeces, and in cases of pancreatic obstruction and/or in fibrocystic disease of the pancreas in infants, trypsin activity may be of importance. In fibrocystic disease of the pancreas a sweat test is a better laboratory procedure to use; this will be discussed later.

Microscopical examination

Faeces contain various crystals, cells, bacteria and foreign bodies such as hairs. Also present are the various food residues, both digested and undigested. These include fats, muscle fibres, starch granules and cellulose structures. For a description of the various crystals, cells, ova and parasites, other works should be consulted. Only fats and the various food residues will be considered.

Preparation of slide

1. On one end of a microscope slide place 1 drop of saline solution. At the other end place 1 drop of Lugol's iodine (see p. 251) solution.
2. Using a swab stick, first emulsify a small portion of fresh faeces in the saline solution, and another portion in the iodine.
3. With a little experience it is easy to avoid making a suspension either too thick or too thin.
4. Carefully apply a coverslip to each drop.
5. Using the 16 mm objective examine the saline suspension to obtain a general impression of the specimen.
6. Use the 4 mm objective to obtain a detailed view of the various constituents.
7. Now examine the iodine preparation. Confirm whether any structures thought to be starch granules in saline preparation have stained blue in the presence of the iodine and have stained cells and muscle fibres, etc., brown.

Microscopical appearance

Cellulose structures

These structures form the skeletal wall of plant cells. As cellulose is not usually digested, it tends to be excreted intact, and appears in some bizarre forms. Cellulose appears as a clear structure with a sharply defined wall. Some of the forms seen are illustrated in *Figure 8.5*.

Starch granules

These granules, when found intact and undigested, are usually seen within a cellulose sac (*Figure 8.5*).

The intake of raw vegetables results in more starch granules in faeces than when the vegetables are eaten cooked, as this softens the cellulose, releasing the starch granules which become digested. Under ordinary conditions starch granules are uncommon in the faeces of adults, but are more often seen in the faeces of infants. The most important cause of an increased quantity of starch in faeces is because of the increased rate of passage through the intestine.

Muscle fibres

Muscle fibres, which are derived from meat, are stained yellow-brown by faecal stercobilin. They are normally excreted fully or partially digested. The presence of undigested fibres indicates digestive impairment, for example pancreatic disease. The various stages of muscle digestion are as follows, but it must be realized that there is no sharp demarcation between the types; it is a gradual transition.

Undigested muscle fibres as seen in the faeces are shown in *Figure 8.6(a)*. They have irregular ends, nuclei and transverse striations; an isolated undigested fibre is seen in *Figure 8.6(b)*. Note the irregular ends and transverse striations. When acted upon by the digestive juices, the nuclei disappear first and then the ends become rounded. This partially digested fibre can be seen in *Figure 8.6(c)*. In *Figure 8.6(d)* the muscle fibre has been further digested when it can be seen that the ends are still

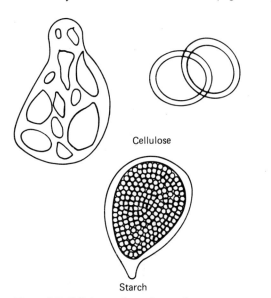

Cellulose

Starch

Figure 8.5. Cellulose and starch granules

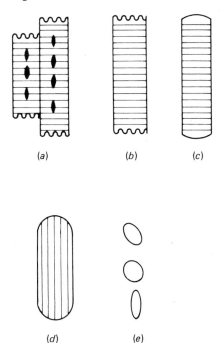

(a) (b) (c)

(d) (e)

Figure 8.6. Muscle fibres showing various stages of digestion

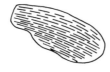

Figure 8.7. Various forms of soap plaques

round, but now it has longitudinal striations. *Figure 8.6(e)* shows fragments of fibres free from striations with rounded ends, the digestion being more complete than in *Figure 8.6(d)*.

Soaps

These appear as plaques with rolled-over edges or as masses of needle-shaped crystals (*Figure 8.7*) and are often seen as a mass of soap crystals. They are insoluble in ether and ethanol, whereas fats and fatty acids are solubles. A simple method of identification consists of making a suspension of the faeces in a few drops of saturated copper nitrate on a slide, covering with a coverslip and examining after a few minutes. Soaps are stained green owing to their conversion to copper soaps. Fatty acid crystals are not stained. In a normal specimen of faeces an occasional soap plaque may be seen. Excessive amounts of soaps indicate defective absorption.

Fat globules

These tend to rise to the surface of the preparation. They are called neutral fats and vary in size, are highly refractable and look oily. But before deciding that the oil globules are neutral fat (stearin, palmitin and olein) it is important to make sure the patient is not receiving liquid paraffin or other oily drugs (*Figure 8.8*).

Fatty acid crystals

These appear as colourless needle-shaped crystals. They are longer than bacilli and are often slightly curved. Usually, they are seen in groups of two, three or more. They are unaffected by aqueous copper nitrate, but are soluble in ether and ethanol.

Pancreatic enzymes in faeces

As trypsin and chymotrypsin are normally found in faeces, an inadequate secretion of pancreatic enzymes should affect their faecal excretion. If the excretion of these proteolytic enzymes in faeces is investigated it may be a useful guide in the diagnosis of pancreatic insufficiency. Trypsin, the main enzyme present, is of little value in the diagnosis of chronic pancreatic disease in adults, as the ranges found in the normal are very wide. Chymotrypsin excretion has proved to be more reliable than that of trypsin and, in minor cases of impaired excretion, the detection of chymotrypsin in a 'timed' specimen of faeces can help even more. In cases of fibrocystic disease of the pancreas in infants, these two enzymes are reduced or completely absent when a fresh specimen of faeces is examined. Trypsin and chymotrypsin will liquefy gelatin, they are active at an alkaline pH and, as the test must be carried out on freshly passed faeces, specimens more than 1 h old are unsuitable. Although gelatin can be used as a substrate for the two enzymes, there are now specific substrates available to study the two enzymes separately, benzoylarginine-*p*-nitroanilide and *N*-(3-carboxylpropionyl)-phenylalanine-*p*-nitroanilide, for trypsin and chymotrypsin, respectively. BCL have now made use of the latter substrate for the estimation of chymotrypsin in faeces. Hydrolysis of the substrates by both enzymes liberates *p*-nitroanilide which is then measured spectrophotometrically.

Proteolytic activity

Principle

Gelatin is incubated with several dilutions of the faeces in sodium hydrogen carbonate. If trypsin is

Neutral fat

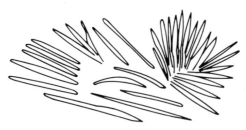
Fatty acid crystals

Figure 8.8. Neutral fat and fatty acid crystals

present the gelatin is digested to water-soluble products, causing liquefaction of the gelatin. The more enzyme there is in the faeces, the higher the dilution at which liquefaction takes place.

Reagents

1. 5% sodium hydrogen carbonate.
2. 7.5% gelatin solution. Prepare by dissolving the gelatin in warm water, then diluting with distilled water to 100 ml. Store in the refrigerator and warm to about 40°C to liquefy when required for the test.

Method

1. Prepare a 1 in 10 dilution of faeces. Place 9 ml of the sodium hydrogen carbonate solution into a tube marked at 10 ml, then add faeces to the mark and emulsify with a glass rod.
2. To a series of 10 tubes add 5 ml of the sodium hydrogen carbonate solution.
3. Add 5 ml of the 1 in 10 faecal suspension to the first tube, mix and deliver 5 ml of this to the next tube.
4. Repeat the doubling dilutions until the ninth tube, then discard this 5 ml (approximately 1 in 2560), leaving the last tube containing sodium hydrogen carbonate alone to act as a control.
5. Add 2 ml of the warmed gelatin to each tube and mix well.
6. Place in the 37°C water bath for 1 h.
7. Remove the rack from the water bath and place it in the refrigerator overnight.

Results

The presence of trypsin is indicated by the liquefaction of the gelatin, so record the highest dilution at which the gelatin is liquefied. Check that the control tube is still a complete gel; if not, discard the test.

X-ray film method

It is also possible to use undeveloped, unfixed X-ray film as the substitute for this test. Simply cut a piece of film to fit a petri dish containing damp filter paper, and continue as follows:

1. Beginning with the highest dilution of faeces, place one drop from each tube on the film. Add one drop of sodium hydrogen carbonate to act as control.
2. Close the lid of the dish and incubate at 37°C for 30 min to allow any trypsin present to digest the gelatin off the film.
3. Place the dish in the refrigerator for about 10 min to harden the gelatin.
4. Carefully wash the film in cold water.

Results

Digestion of the film emulsion, shown by a clear area, indicates the presence of trypsin. Where the surface of the film is merely crinkled, as with the control, there has been no proteolytic activity.

Note the highest dilution of faeces which contained trypsin.

After the first three days of life, the faeces of babies and young children have a high proteolytic activity. By the age of 12 years, the activity has decreased markedly. It has been shown that the faeces of most normal babies digest gelatin at a dilution of 1 in 100 or greater, whereas infants with fibrocystic disease of the pancreas digest it only with a dilution of less than 1 in 50.

Fibrocystic disease of the pancreas (cystic fibrosis: mucoviscidosis)

This disease of the pancreas is the commonest inborn error of metabolism, usually presenting in earlier childhood, and is a general dysfunction of the exocrine glands. The pancreatic and bronchial secretions are viscid, which block the pancreatic ducts and bronchi, causing obstructions of these organs. Sweat glands are also affected and the diagnostic feature is a high content of sodium and chloride in the sweat, often to about twice the normal level.

Although pancreatic trypsin is deficient it is not always diagnostic, and therefore the analysis of electrolytes in sweat is the most valuable investigation. Sweat can be collected in a number of ways, some of which are described below, but careful consideration must be given as without care, experience and scrupulous attention to detail, errors may occur giving rise to misleading results.

Collection of sweat

A. Local stimulation using methacholine chloride

This procedure should be carried out by a registered medical practitioner. By a subcutaneous injection of 2 mg methacholine chloride in the forearm, covering the area around the injection with filter paper, up to 100–300 mg of sweat can be collected. The sodium chloride content is then estimated by the usual methods. This method is very rarely used nowadays and has been replaced by a pilocarpine stimulation procedure.

B. Pilocarpine iontophoresis

A direct current of 1.5 mA is passed for 25–35 min between two electrodes. The positive electrode is filled with 0.5% aqueous pilocarpine nitrate solution and the negative with 1% aqueous sodium nitrate solution. Under the surface of the positive electrode is a circle of ashless filter paper saturated with pilocarpine nitrate, and the negative electrode with a gauze saturated in the sodium nitrate solution. The positive electrode is strapped to the flexor surface and the negative electrode on the extensor surface of the forearm.

After 5 min the area covered by the positive electrode is washed with distilled water and covered with a Whatman No. 40 filter paper of known weight. The paper is carefully handled with forceps, covered with parafilm and the sweat collected for 25–35 min. After this the paper is removed, weighed, placed in a flask and the electrolytes eluted with 10 ml distilled water. The sodium and chloride concentrations are measured by any of the methods described in Chapter 6.

C. Cystic fibrosis analyser

This is an instrument produced commercially by Advanced Instruments, of Massachusetts, USA, and marketed by MSE Scientific Instruments, which induces sweat by a pilocarpine iontophoresis method and then measures the sweat electrolytes concentration by a conductivity meter. The difference between the collection of sweat by this method compared with method B is that a specially designed collection cup is applied to the area around the forearm, into which the sweat is collected. A capillary tube is then used to fill the sample holder (2 µl size) which is then plugged into the instrument. The concentration of the electrolytes are read on the meter in mmol/l, after first of all calibrating the instrument. Because of this instrument's dual function as an iontophoresor and analyser, a second patient can be iontophoresed while collecting sweat from the first patient.

D. Wescar sweat collection system

This is a new method of sweat collection using pilocarpine iontophoresis and a unique collection device—a heated cup which reduces evaporation and condensation errors. Sweat electrolytes are then measured by the usual methods and sweat osmolality by using a Wescar (Chem Lab Instruments Ltd) vapour pressure osmometer.

E. Pilocarpine iontophoresis

Another method is available which uses pilocarpine iontophoresis followed by *in situ* measurement of sweat chloride using an ion-specific electrode (Orion Research*).

*Marketed by MSE Scientific Instruments, Manor Royal, Crawley, West Sussex.

Results

In normal children, the upper limit for sweat sodium is 70 mmol/l, while the upper limit for chloride is 65 mmol/l. In adults, the sodium concentration may exceed 90 mmol/l.

In fibrocystic disease, the values for sweat sodium can vary from 80 to 150 mmol/l and for chloride from 70 to 140 mmol/l. The distinction between normal and fibrocystic subjects is very good in young children.

The correlation between sodium and osmolality in sweat collections shows a very close relationship, but it is better to use the two parameters in order to achieve a better form of discrimination. Sweat osmolality in normal children ranges from 65 to 180 mmol/kg, while in cystic fibrosis values from 180 to 420 mmol/kg have been obtained.

Tests of endocrine function

Changes in the internal secretions of the pancreas are usually assessed by estimating the blood glucose (sugar), or for diagnostic purposes a glucose tolerance test is of greater value. In the blood, in addition to glucose, there are small amounts of other sugars such as lactose, fructose, pentoses and a negligible amount of galactose. Urine contains very small amounts of glucose, lactose, fructose, galactose and sucrose.

Blood glucose and blood sugar

The estimation of carbohydrates in the blood can be divided into two steps, the estimation of (1) blood glucose and (2) blood sugar. As the main carbohydrate present in the blood is glucose, the term 'blood sugar' is loosely used to include glucose, other sugars, and other reducing substances which may be present in the blood (glutathione). The vast majority of methods for sugar analysis until recently depended upon the reducing power of glucose and involved using reagents such as copper and ferricyanide in an alkaline medium. The specific procedures for the estimation of blood glucose using the enzyme glucose oxidase, gives results up to 2 mmol/l lower than techniques which estimate blood sugar. On the other hand there are methods available for estimating 'true' glucose values which eliminate the non-specific reduction and measure only that due to sugars. In the latter methods the 'true' glucose values are approximately 0.25 mmol/l higher than the specific glucose methods.

It is therefore important to report blood levels as 'glucose', 'true glucose' or 'sugar' depending upon the method used.

Glycolysis

Glucose disappears from whole blood on standing as a result of glycolysis due to its conversion into lactic acid:

$$C_6H_{12}O_6 \rightarrow 2C_3H_6O_3$$

It is an enzymatic reaction; the rate decreases with respect to temperature. At 37°C the loss of glucose is about 1.0 mmol/l per h, while at 4°C the decrease is about 0.25 mmol/l per h. Glycolysis can be prevented by using preservatives, the commonest being sodium fluoride, used in combination with the anticoagulant potassium oxalate; 2 mg sodium fluoride and 6 mg of potassium oxalate per ml of blood will act as a preservative and anticoagulant for 2–3 days. Although fluoride is an enzyme poison, it can be used for glucose oxidase methods up to a concentration of 5 mg sodium fluoride per ml of blood. Fluoride is an inhibitor of both erythrocyte metabolism and of bacterial growth. In erythrocyte metabolism it inhibits the enzyme enolase involved in the glycolytic pathway, but has less effect on the bacterial growth. Saturated benzoic acid used in the preparation of glucose solutions is more effective as a bactericide, but is not necessary for preserving blood samples.

Estimation of blood glucose and blood sugar

There are three main methods for estimating the 'sugar' content of body fluids: (a) the reduction of cupric to cuprous salts; (b) reduction of ferricyanide to ferrocyanide; and (c) glucose oxidase methods. Of these three methods only (a) and (c) will be described here. Blood glucose test strips are available for the semi-quantitative estimation of blood glucose. Both Ames and BCL supply meters for use with either *Dextrostix* (Ames) or the *Reflotest* (BCL). However, it is better to use a conventional blood glucose method, the reagent strips usually being used by diabetics in their own homes.

Determination of 'true glucose'

Although not commonly used, this method has been retained, as some laboratories have difficulty in obtaining enzyme preparations.

Principle

After protein precipitation with copper tungstate, the supernatant is heated with alkaline tartrate reagent, under standard conditions. The cuprous oxide so formed is then estimated by the blue-green compound produced upon the addition of arseno-molybdate solution. This colour is measured in the absorptiometer or spectrophotometer against standard glucose solutions treated in a similar way.

Reagents

1. Isotonic sodium sulphate–copper sulphate solution—mix 320 ml of 3% sodium sulphate ($Na_2SO_4.10H_2O$) with 30 ml 7% copper sulphate ($CuSO_4.5H_2O$).
2. Sodium tungstate—10 g per 100 ml distilled water.
3. Alkaline tartrate reagent—25 g sodium hydrogen carbonate are dissolved in a minimum amount of distilled water (about 300 ml). When in solution add 20 g anhydrous sodium sulphate with constant stirring. After the carbonate has dissolved, a solution of 18.4 g potassium oxalate in 60 ml warm distilled water is added. Finally add 12 g sodium potassium tartrate dissolved in about 50 ml distilled water. Dilute to 1 litre and mix well.
4. Arsenomolybdate solution—25 g ammonium molybdate are dissolved in 450 ml of distilled water, 21 ml concentrated sulphuric acid are added slowly, mixed and then followed by 3 g sodium arsenate ($Na_2HASO_4.7H_2O$) dissolved in 25 ml water. Mix and keep at 37°C for 2 days. If the reagent is needed quickly the mixture can be heated to 55°C but should be stirred well to prevent local overheating. It is better to keep at 37°C for 2 days. Keep in a dark bottle. For use, dilute 1 volume of this reagent with 2 vol of water.
5. Stock standard glucose solution—100 mg glucose dissolved in saturated benzoic acid (0.3%) and made up to 100 ml. Store at 4°C. The stock solution should be prepared 24 h before use to allow for equilibrium between mixtures of α- and β-glucose to be attained. Solid glucose is usually predominantly the α form in commercial preparations. This is important when using glucose oxidase (see p. 126).
6. Working standard glucose solutions—prepared by diluting 1.0 ml, 2.5 ml and 5.0 ml of stock standard to 100 ml with isotonic sodium sulphate–copper sulphate solution (equivalent to 0.01, 0.025 and 0.05 mg glucose per ml). Store at 4°C.

Method

1. Pipette 0.05 ml blood or plasma into a centrifuge tube containing 3.9 ml isotonic sodium sulphate–copper sulphate solution.
2. To ensure accurate measurement of blood, wipe the outside of the blood pipette carefully. Allow the blood to run out of the pipette at the bottom of the tube. Raise the pipette to the top of the

diluent and rinse out the pipette well with the clean diluent.
3. Add 0.05 ml sodium tungstate solution.
4. Mix well and centrifuge at 2500 rpm for 5 min.
5. Into suitably labelled boiling tubes (150 × 25 mm, pipette the following:

	Test	Blank	Standard
Supernatant	2.0 ml	—	—
Isotonic $Na_2SO_4.CuSO_4$ solution	—	2.0 ml	—
Standards	—	—	2.0 ml
Alkaline tartrate	2.0 ml	2.0 ml	2.0 ml

6. Mix well, stopper with cotton wool and place in the boiling water bath for 10 min.
7. Remove from bath and cool immediately.
8. Add 6.0 ml arsenomolybdate to each tube, mix well and then
9. Add 5.0 ml of distilled water to all tubes.
10. Mix well and read absorbance at 680 nm (red filter) in a spectrophotometer or absorptiometer.

Calculation

The calculation can be worked out in two ways:

(a) Draw a calibration curve (see p. 68) using the three standards, which will also confirm that Beer's law is obeyed, and from this the concentration of glucose in the test sample is found. This is the correct approach and should be done every time, and more especially when a new reagent has been prepared.
Let x = concentration of glucose in test, then 2.0 ml of supernatant (= 0.025 ml of whole blood) will contain x mg of glucose. Therefore

$$x = \frac{100}{0.025} = \text{mg glucose per 100 ml}$$

or

$$x \times 4000 = \text{mg glucose per 100 ml}$$

(b) If the first method is not used, then it is most important that two standards are carried through the test procedure. Then the standard which gives an absorbance nearest to the test sample is used in the calculation. Subtract the blank reading from both the test and standard absorbances.
Let Y = the concentration of standard in mg per ml, then as 2 ml of supernatant will contain the equivalent of 0.025 ml of whole blood or plasma, let A = absorbance; then

$$\frac{A \text{ of unknown}}{A \text{ of standard}} \times \frac{100}{0.025} \times Y = \frac{\text{mg glucose}}{\text{per 100 ml}}$$

e.g. let A of test (T) = 0.32
A of blank (B) = 0.02
A of standard (S) = 0.42
Standard concentration = 0.025 mg/ml

Then

$$\frac{T - B}{S - B} \times \frac{100}{0.025} \times 0.025 = \text{mg glucose per 100 ml}$$

or

$$\frac{0.32 - 0.02}{0.42 - 0.02} \times \frac{100}{0.025} \times 0.025 = \frac{\text{mg glucose per}}{100 \text{ ml}}$$

$$\frac{0.30}{0.40} \times 100 = 75 \text{ mg glucose per 100 ml}$$

■ Notes

1. If the results are higher than 350 mg per 100 ml repeat the test using less supernatant, i.e. 1.0 ml supernatant and 1.0 ml isotonic sodium sulphate–copper sulphate. Do not forget to include a factor of 2 in the calculation.
2. The use of an isotonic sodium sulphate–copper sulphate solution for protein precipitation has enabled a 'true glucose' to be estimated.
3. SI units are now used in clinical chemistry and therefore all mg glucose per 100 ml must be converted into mmol per litre as follows:

$$\text{mg per 100 ml} \times \frac{1}{18} = \text{mmol per litre}$$

Determination of glucose

The method mentioned above is not specific for glucose, but greater specificity can be obtained by using an enzyme, glucose oxidase. This enzyme, which is specific, oxidizes glucose to gluconic acid. It acts on β-D-glucose, but has a negligible effect on α-D-glucose. The two isomers exist in solution in equilibrium with the chain form (*Figure 8.9*) and the shift from one to the other in solution is called mutorotation. Mutorotation is important, as it must be complete during the oxidation of glucose in the sample. This step can be speeded up in the presence of the enzyme glucomutarotase, which is present in most commercial glucose oxidase preparations.
In the estimation of glucose using the enzyme oxidase it is important that the stock standard glucose solution is prepared at least 24 h before use (to allow for equilibration between mixtures of α- and β-glucose to be attained) as solid glucose is usually predominantly the α-form in commercial preparations. Since glucose oxidase reacts only with β-glucose, a freshly prepared solution will not go to completion, as shown in equation (1), if there should be insufficient glucomutarotase in the sample of glucose oxidase used:

$$\text{Glucose} + O_2 + \xrightarrow[\text{oxidase}]{\text{glucose}} \text{gluconic acid} + H_2O_2 \quad (1)$$

Various procedures can be used to estimate glucose using glucose oxidase. One method makes use of the glucose analyser, as described in Chapter 6. In this type of estimation the maximum rate at which the

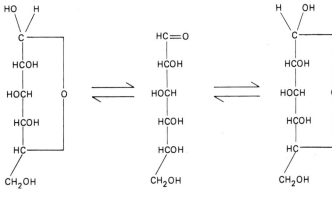

Figure 8.9. Mutorotation of glucose

$\beta-D-glucose$ · · · · · · Chain form · · · · · · $\alpha-D-glucose$

oxygen concentration in the diluted sample decreases is measured polarographically, which is directly proportional to the glucose concentration in the sample as shown in equation (1).

In the YSI glucose analyser a probe oxidizes a constant preparation of hydrogen peroxide at the platinum anode, as follows:

$$H_2O_2 \rightarrow 2H^+ + O_2 + 2e^- \qquad (2)$$

The current so produced is directly proportional to the glucose level in the diluted sample.

An enzymatic colorimetric method can also be adopted by using the following reactions:

$$\text{Glucose} + O_2 + H_2O \xrightarrow[\text{oxidase}]{\text{glucose}} \text{gluconate} + H_2O_2 \qquad (3)$$

$$H_2O_2 + \text{4-aminophenazone} + \text{phenol} \xrightarrow{\text{peroxidase}}$$
4-(*p*-benzoquinone-mono-imino)phenazone + $4H_2O$ (4)

Instead of using 4-aminophenazone as the oxygen acceptor, 2,6-dichlorophenolindophenol, guaiacum, and perid (2'2-diazo-di(3-ethylbenzthiazoline-6-sulphonic acid)) can be used. Most methods use either perid or 4-aminophenazone: the latter procedure will be described.

Blood glucose method

Principle

Phenol in the presence of an oxidizing agent, in this case hydrogen peroxide, gives a pink colour with aminophenazone. Two solutions are used: a protein precipitant (phosphotungstic acid containing phenol) and the enzyme solution (glucose oxidase, peroxidase) containing the 4-aminophenazone.

Reagents

Use AR reagents wherever possible:

1. Protein precipitant—10 g sodium tungstate, 10 g disodium hydrogen phosphate (Na_2HPO_4) and

9 g sodium chloride are dissolved in 800 ml distilled water. Add 125 ml 1.0M HCl to bring the pH to 3.0 (check with narrow range indicator paper). Add 1 g phenol and dilute to 1 litre with distilled water. Keeps indefinitely at 4°C.
2. Colour reagent—to 75 ml of 4% disodium hydrogen phosphate (Na_2HPO_4) add 215 ml distilled water, 5 ml Fermcozyme 653AM glucose oxidase (Hughes and Hughes Ltd), 5 ml 0.1% peroxidase RZ (Hughes and Hughes Ltd). Mix well, then add 300 mg sodium azide and 100 mg 4-aminophenazone. Mix again and store at 4°C. Keeps for at least 2 months.
3. Standard glucose solution 10 mmol/l—1.80 g of glucose is dissolved in and made up to 1 litre with saturated benzoic acid (0.3%). Prepare at least 24 h before use.

Method

1. Into suitably labelled centrifuge tubes add the following:

	Test	Standards
Protein precipitant	2.9 ml	2.9 ml
Working standard	—	0.1 ml
Blood or plasma	0.1 ml	—

2. Mix well and centrifuge at 2500 rpm for 5 min.
3. Transfer 1.0 ml supernatant to another test-tube and add 3.0 ml colour reagent.
4. Use 1.0 ml protein precipitant and 3.0 ml colour reagent for the blank.
5. Mix well and incubate all tubes at 37°C for 10 min, shaking occasionally to ensure adequate aeration.
6. Remove from water bath, cool and measure the absorbances against the blank at 515 nm (green filter) in 1 cm cells.

Calculation

Blood glucose:

$$\frac{\text{Ab of unknown}}{\text{Ab of standard}} \times 10 = \text{mmol/l}$$

A calibration curve can be prepared in the following manner:

Blood glucose (mmol/l)	0	5.0	10.0	15.0	20.0	25.0
Standard solution (ml)	0	0.10	0.20	0.30	0.40	0.50
Protein precipitant (ml)	6.00	5.90	5.80	5.70	5.60	5.50

Mix well, remove 1.0 ml of each and add 3.0 ml of colour reagent; mix well and proceed as for 5 and 6 in the above method.

■ **Notes**

1. Beer's law is obeyed up to about 25 mmol/l.
2. The colour is stable for at least 30 min.
3. 5 mg sodium fluoride per ml of blood has no effect on glucose values.
4. For CSF glucose use 0.2 ml CSF and 1.8 ml protein precipitant; this will give a three-fold increase in sensitivity.

Results

The normal range of fasting venous blood glucose taken not less than 3–4 h after the last meal usually lies between 3.0 and 5.3 mmol/l, but values outside this range are occasionally found. In capillary blood the value is usually about 0.3 mmol/l higher. The range for children and infants is the same as for adults. In methods which estimate blood sugar the normal range can vary between 4.2 and 6.7 mmol/l.

Fasting hyperglycaemia is defined as a blood glucose value above 5.5 mmol/l or more than 6.7 mmol/l for other methods. The diagnosis of diabetes mellitus cannot be confirmed on a single estimation, but further investigations such as a glucose tolerance curve have to be carried out.

Fasting hypoglycaemia is defined as a blood glucose value below 2.8 mmol/l. A value 0.5–1.7 mmol/l higher would be obtained with blood sugar methods. As in the case of hyperglycaemia, a single value does not diagnose hypoglycaemia; further tests are required.

Blood glucose values after meals

A rise and fall in blood glucose values occurs after having a meal containing carbohydrates in any form. The increase in blood glucose will depend upon the amount of glucose produced as a result of carbohydrate digestion, the rate of digestion, the rate of absorption and with the rate of removal of glucose from the circulating blood.

It is therefore important to state the time the blood was taken for glucose estimation on the report form, along with the time the last meal was taken.

Standard oral glucose tolerance test

As mentioned above, there is a temporary rise in blood glucose when a subject ingests glucose, or a meal containing carbohydrate; the extent and duration of rise will depend upon the type of food taken. This effect of ingested carbohydrate, when studied under standard conditions, is the basis of the glucose tolerance test. It is used for investigating abnormalities of carbohydrate metabolism and in cases where glycosuria has been found.

The response to a carbohydrate load depends upon the previous carbohydrate diet and on the amount of glucose ingested. It is important therefore that the subject is placed on a normal carbohydrate diet for about 3 days before the test is carried out. When the subject is placed on a low carbohydrate diet for some time before the test, an impaired glucose tolerance test can be obtained (the blood glucose level rises higher than normal and the rise is more prolonged). Conversely, if placed on a very high carbohydrate diet (or non-fasting before the test) there can be an enhanced glucose tolerance (diminished rise in blood glucose level).

The changes in glucose tolerance with alteration of the diet are probably caused by alteration in tissue oxidation of glucose, changes in insulin and growth hormone secretions and in liver glycogen metabolism.

Method

1. The subject must be on a normal hospital diet for about 3 days prior to the test.
2. The patient has nothing to eat after supper and no breakfast is given.
3. In the morning, urine is collected before commencing the test.
4. Take a fasting sample of blood for glucose estimation and then give 50 g of glucose dissolved in 150–200 ml water by mouth. (For children the dose is usually 1 g of glucose per kg body weight up to a maximum of 50 g.)
5. Take further samples of blood at 30-min intervals for 2½ h.
6. Urine samples are taken at intervals during the test. Some workers collect half-hourly, but this is not always possible.
7. Two specimens 1 h and 2 h after taking the glucose can usually be obtained.
8. Estimate the blood glucose levels of each specimen using the methods previously described, and test the urines for the presence of glucose by the method described on p. 127.

The World Health Organisation (WHO) has proposed certain changes in the diagnosis of diabetes mellitus and these have also been recommended by the British Diabetic Association:

(a) If symptoms of diabetes are present, the diagnosis is confirmed by elevated blood glucose

values found on more than one occasion without an oral glucose tolerance test.
(b) If blood glucose levels are less markedly elevated, blood glucose values should be measured 2 h after an oral glucose load.
(c) In the absence of symptoms of diabetes, at least one additional abnormal blood glucose value is essential to confirm the diagnosis, i.e. 1 h and 2 h after a glucose load.

WHO recommended oral glucose tolerance test

The patient should fast as above for 10–14 h (overnight) and have nothing by mouth other than water. The patient should also remain seated throughout the test and should not smoke until the test is completed.

1. Take a fasting sample for blood glucose and collect a urine sample.
2. Give the patient 75 g glucose dissolved in 250–350 ml of water to drink (for children 1.75 g per kg body weight to a maximum of 75 g). As an alternative, a 105 ml lemon-flavoured glucose syrup called Hycal (Beecham Research Laboratories), diluted to 250–350 ml with water, can be given; this dose only applies to adults, for children the pharmacy will supply the appropriate dose on request.
3. After 1 h take a sample for blood glucose; a urine sample is also collected.
4. After 2 h take a further sample for blood glucose and collect the final urine sample.
5. Estimate the blood glucose levels of each specimen, and test the urines for the presence of glucose.

Results

Standard method: normal response. A typical normal response is shown in *Figure 8.10*, when the fasting level is within the normal limits; at no stage of the test should the level exceed 7.8 mmol/l, and it usually returns to the fasting level within 2 h of drinking the glucose solution. Glucose is not found in the urine.

Standard method: diabetic response. In diabetes mellitus, the fasting level and the peak of the curve may be well above normal limits. In severe diabetes, the peak glucose level can be as high as 19 mmol/l and a considerably longer time may elapse before the blood glucose returns to the fasting level (*Figure 8.10*). Glucose may be found in one or more of the urine specimens (glycosuria).

WHO method: normal response. The fasting blood glucose should be below 5.5 mmol/l and the two-hour level below 7.0 mmol/l.

WHO method: diabetic response. The fasting level should be greater than 7.0 mmol/l and the two-hour level greater than 10 mmol/l.

Effect of age

Blood glucose values rise with increasing age. In old people the maximum glucose value may exceed 10 mmol/l in a normal response.

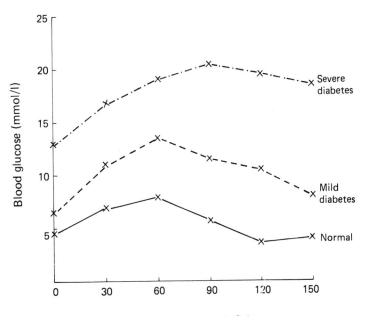

Figure 8.10. Glucose tolerance curves

Min after a 50 g load of glucose

Venous blood

While there may be no difference between arterial and venous blood glucose values at fasting levels, the arterial blood glucose and hence the capillary value can be about 1.0–2.0 mmol/l higher than the venous sample, since there is an increased carbohydrate utilization at that time.

Renal threshold for glucose

Renal threshold for glucose is the highest level the blood glucose reaches before glucose appears in the urine and is detectable by routine laboratory tests.

In normal persons, provided there is normal renal function, the renal threshold for blood glucose is about 10 mmol/l. This is because the renal tubules are able to absorb all glucose passed through the glomeruli. At higher blood levels tubular reabsorption may not be sufficiently rapid, and glucose may appear in the urine. The renal threshold may be somewhat lower than 10 mmol/l in some subjects. In such cases glucose may be found in the urine whenever the blood glucose levels exceed the low threshold value; that is, glycosuria may occur without the blood glucose level rising to abnormal heights. This condition is known as 'renal glycosuria', and it can be distinguished from diabetes mellitus by examination of a glucose tolerance curve.

During a glucose tolerance test, because of the delay in urine reaching the bladder, maximum glycosuria is found in the next specimen after the highest blood glucose concentration is reached.

9

Liver function tests

The liver is the largest organ in the body and from a metabolic standpoint is the most complex. Tests of its many functions have been devised in the hope that they will serve as diagnostic aids when a metabolic process has been disturbed. Unfortunately, these liver function tests differ in sensitivity and many give normal results, even when only about 15% of the liver parenchyma are functioning. The only liver function tests described here are those for the detection of urinary bilirubin and its derivatives, together with the estimation of bilirubin in serum or plasma.

Gross structure

The adult liver weighs about 1500 g and is situated underneath the diaphragm (*Figure 9.1*). It has four lobes. The right lobe is the largest, the left lobe is smaller and wedge-shaped, the quadrate lobe is nearly square in outline and the caudate lobe has a tail-like appearance. The latter two lobes are very small and can only be distinguished on the undersurface of the liver. Attached to the undersurface of the liver by connective tissue is a pear-shaped sac, the gall bladder, which acts as a reservoir for the bile before it is discharged into the duodenum.

The portal fissure is the name given to a cleft on the undersurface of the liver where various structures enter and leave the organ. Entering the liver is the portal vein carrying blood from the stomach, spleen, pancreas and intestines, and the hepatic artery carry arterial blood. Leaving the liver are the hepatic veins carrying blood to the inferior vena cava, and the right and left hepatic ducts carrying bile to the gall bladder (see *Figure 8.4*).

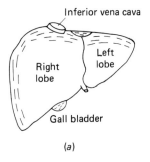

(a)

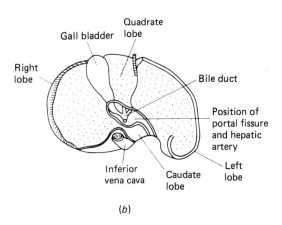

(b)

Figure 9.1. (a) Liver showing the right and left lobes. (b) The undersurface of the liver

Anatomic structure

The basic structure is the hepatic lobule, which is hexagonal in outline and formed by cords of cells arranged in columns which radiate from a central vein. Between the column of cells run the sinusoids (a system of capillaries and open spaces) containing blood derived from the portal vein and hepatic artery. In this way each hepatic cell is provided with an adequate amount of blood containing essential nutrients. After the blood has been in contact with these cells it drains into the central vein and eventually into the hepatic vein.

Bile secretion

Bile is secreted by the cells of the lobules into the biliary canaliculi which in turn drain eventually into the right and left hepatic ducts. Between meals the sphincter of Oddi (see *Figure 8.4*) is closed and bile is therefore stored and concentrated in the gall bladder. The sphincter, at the sight, taste or smell of food, relaxes and when the gastric contents enter the duodenum, cholecystokinin, a hormone secreted by the intestinal mucosa, causes the gall bladder to contract and bile enters the duodenum.

Composition and functions of bile

There is a slight difference between the composition of bile produced by the liver and that entering the duodenum. In the gall bladder the liquid is slightly alkaline (pH 7.0–7.6), viscous and golden yellow or greenish in colour. As it acts as a transport medium for the biliary constituents during excretion from the body, its composition varies from time to time. In the main, bile contains mucus, bile salts, bile pigments, cholesterol, fatty acids, fats and inorganic salts. It can also contain drugs, toxins, dyes and heavy metals removed from the blood stream by the liver cells. The bile salts are the sodium and potassium salts of bile acids conjugated by the liver with glycine or taurine. In this form the bile acids are water-soluble and the four found in human bile are cholic, deoxycholic, chenodeoxycholic and lithocholic acids. Deoxycholic acid is the main bile acid found in the faeces of a normal adult. Conjugation of cholic acid with glycine or taurine will form glycholic and taurocholic acids, respectively. Bile salts react with water-insoluble substances such as stearic acid (fatty acid), cholesterol and fat-soluble vitamins (A, D, E and K) to form water-soluble complexes, sometimes called micelles. This hydrotrophic power of bile salts is important in promoting absorption of water-insoluble substances, and because they reduce surface tension their emulsifying action within the intestines helps in the digestion of fats. Lipases are also activated by bile salts and when bile is excluded from the intestines as much as 25% of the ingested fat appears in the faeces.

Bile, because of its alkalinity, helps also to neutralize the acid chyme from the stomach.

Functions of the liver

These are numerous but for convenience may be classified into seven main groups.

1. Excretion

This is basically the production and excretion of bile into the intestine.

2. Carbohydrate metabolism

In periods of availability, the principal monosaccharides resulting from the digestive processes (see p. 107) are synthesized to glycogen and stored in the liver. During a fast, blood glucose levels are maintained within normal limits by breakdown of stored glycogen (glycogenolysis), while non-carbohydrates (amino acids and fats) are converted into glucose (gluconeogenesis).

3. Lipid metabolism

Besides the esterification of cholesterol, the synthesis of cholesterol, phospholipids, endogenous triglycerides and lipoproteins occurs mainly, but not exclusively, in the liver.

4. Protein synthesis

Many of the plasma proteins, but not the γ-globulins, are synthesized in the liver. Many of the coagulation factors, fibrinogen, prothrombin, factors V, VII, IX, X, XI and XII, are also manufactured there. Vitamin K is required for the production of prothrombin, factors VII, IX and X. The liver contains a little heparin, most of the heparin being found in the granules of circulatory basophils and in the granules of mast cells.

5. Storage

In addition to glycogen and many vitamins, the liver is the main storage site for iron.

6. Detoxication and protective function

Drugs and toxic substances are detoxicated by conjugation, methylation, oxidation or reduction. Ammonia derived from amino acids and protein metabolism, or produced in the gut by bacteria, is converted to urea and rendered non-toxic.

7. Haematopoiesis

The Kupffer cells lining the sinusoids form part of the reticulo-endothelial system and are involved in the normal destruction of erythrocytes.

Bile pigment metabolism

Erythrocytes at the end of their life span, which is usually about 120 days, are removed from the circulation by the reticulo-endothelial system (RES). The protoporphyrin ring of the haem group of haemoglobin is opened up and the resulting bilirubin–iron complex (choleglobin) is formed. The protein and iron are then removed; the former is catabolized to amino acids which enter into new protein synthesis, while the latter is used for the synthesis of new haemoglobins and is retained in the RES in the form of haemosiderin and ferritin. Ferritin is a soluble iron–protein complex, while haemosiderin is an insoluble iron storage complex which gives an intense blue colour with potassium ferricyanide (Prussian blue reaction). After the removal of the protein and iron, the remaining green pigment, biliverdin, is reduced by the tissue enzymes to a yellow pigment, bilirubin. Bilirubin, a water-soluble substance, enters the plasma and is bound to plasma albumin, which on passing into the parenchymal cells of the liver is conjugated principally with glucuronic acid to form the water-soluble mono- and diglucuronides of bilirubin. This conjugation takes place under the influence of uridyl diphosphate glucuronyl transferase. Conjugated bilirubin may enter the circulation and is then also bound to albumin, but principally is transported out of the liver cell into the bile canaliculi and excreted

in the bile. The two conjugated forms of bilirubin are present in normal plasma and are responsible for a normal bilirubin level of up to 17 μmol/l. In the majority of normal persons, much lower levels will be found. The unconjugated bilirubin (water-insoluble) is also present in plasma during jaundice.

After passing into the gall bladder, the bilirubin glucuronides may be re-oxidized to biliverdin, thus giving rise to the green colour of gall bladder bile. From the gall bladder the bilirubin passes via the bile duct into the small intestine where it is ultimately reduced by bacterial enzymes to a colourless compound, stercobilinogen (faecal urobilinogen). This colourless compound is then oxidized to a brown pigment, stercobilin, the chief pigment of faeces. A small amount of stercobilinogen is reabsorbed and passes via the portal vein to the liver, where it is re-excreted in the bile. A small amount escapes removal from the blood by the liver and is excreted by the kidney. The urinary excretory product, although identical to stercobilinogen, is called urobilinogen and when exposed to air is oxidized to urobilin, which is identical to the stercobilin of faeces. *Figure 9.2* shows the schematic formation of bilirubin and its derivatives. A normal adult may excrete up to 6.8 μmol of urobilinogen per day in the urine, while the faecal excretion of the pigment may be up to 420 μmol per day.

Bile salts

Bile salts enter the duodenum with the bile and are normally found in the faeces in small amounts, but a normal urine should contain very little. During the process of absorption from the intestine, the bile salts are almost completely reabsorbed via the portal vein, removed by the liver and re-excreted in the

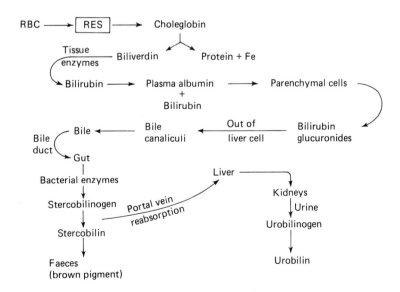

Figure 9.2. Schematic formation of bilirubin and its derivatives

bile. Bile salts are usually present along with bile pigments in the urine in obstructive jaundice, but they can be absent when pigments are still present, during recovery.

Jaundice

Bilirubin is normally present in the plasma and is partly responsible for the yellow colour. In certain conditions, the concentration of pigment increases and causes jaundice (icterus) when the skin, sclera of the eye and the body fluids become pigmented (yellow). Some of the causes of jaundice are:

1. An obstruction in the bile duct by either a gall stone within the lumen or by a tumour (usually pancreatic) exerting pressure from outside. In these disorders there is an increase usually of the conjugated bilirubin.
2. An excessive breakdown of erythrocytes as in haemolytic anaemia, giving an increase mainly in unconjugated bilirubin.
3. Diminished function of the liver cells, as in hepatocellular or toxic jaundice, giving an increase of both types of bilirubin.

Jaundice, when present, results not only in a raised plasma or serum bilirubin level, but in the excretion of bilirubin and/or its derivatives in the urine in a greater concentration than that normally present. *Table 9.1* indicates the type of pigment found in the urine in the three causes of jaundice listed above. In haemolytic jaundice the unconjugated bilirubin is absent from the urine because the bilirubin–albumin complex does not pass through the glomeruli.

alkaline pH, when it is blue. The latter is measured at 600 nm.

The estimation of serum bilirubin by the Malloy and Evelyn (1937) method has been used for many years. In this method serum is diluted with water, diazotized with sulphanilic acid and then methanol is added in an amount insufficient to precipitate the proteins, but at the right concentration to allow all the bilirubin to react with the diazo reagent. The red azo bilirubin is then measured at 450 nm. In recent years, a method of Jendrassik and Grof has gained increasing popularity and is now the method of choice by many scientific workers.

Estimation of serum bilirubin

Principle

Serum is diluted with water and diazotized with sulphanilic acid in the presence of diphylline as an accelerating agent. Ascorbic acid is added to stop the reaction and to prevent haemoglobin from interfering with the azo-coupling. The azo bilirubin so formed is then measured at an alkaline pH.

Reagents

1. Diazo solution A: sulphanilic acid. To about 600 ml of warm water add 5 g sulphanilic acid, and when dissolved add 15 ml concentrated hydrochloric acid. Cool and dilute 1 litre.
2. Diazo solution B: sodium nitrate. Dissolve 5 g sodium nitrate in about 90 ml of water and dilute to 100 ml. Prepare fresh each month.

Table 9.1. Increased amounts of pigments found in urine during jaundice

Cause	Bile salts	Pigments	Urobilin	Urobilinogen
Haemolytic jaundice	−	−	+	+
Obstructive jaundice	+	+	−	−
Hepatic or toxic jaundice	±	+	+	+

Detection of bilirubin and its derivatives

1. Bile pigments (bilirubin)

Serum or plasma

Bilirubin in the serum has been determined for many years by using the Van den Bergh diazo reaction. This involves treating the serum with diazotized sulphanilic acid. The azobilirubin complex so formed is estimated quantitatively in the spectrophotometer against a suitable standard either in an acid medium at 540 nm, when it is red, or at an

3. Diazo reagent. Prepare fresh prior to use by mixing 10 ml of solution A with 0.25 ml of solution B.
4. Ascorbic acid solution, 4 g per 100 ml. Prepare a small volume daily.
5. Dyphylline solution. 5 g dyphylline is dissolved in about 70 ml of water at 40°C; when dissolved add 12.5 g sodium acetate trihydrate and 0.1 g EDTA. Cool and dilute to 100 ml with water.
6. Alkaline tartrate solution. Dissolve 100 g sodium hydroxide pellets and 350 g sodium potassium tartrate in about 800 ml of water and make up to 1 litre with water.
7. Standard bilirubin solution, 200 μmol/l. Prepare a

pool of non-icteric human serum which has been frozen within 12 h of collection (ensuring that it is free from Australia antigen (AuSH)). Thaw, mix well and filter through glass wool to remove debris. Weigh out 11.7 mg of pure bilirubin (an acceptable standard is one which conforms to a molar extinction of 60700 ± 800 (BDH) and which has been dried for several days in a desiccator) and transfer to a 100 ml stoppered flask, by using 4 ml dimethylsulphoxide. Warm to about 35°C and dissolve by shaking, at the same time keeping out of the bright sunlight. When dissolved, dilute to 100 ml with the pool of non-icteric human serum. The standard can then be dispensed into small containers (approximately 1 ml) and deep frozen until required.

Method

Into five test-tubes labelled S (standard), SB (standard blank), B (blank), TB (total bilirubin) and CB (conjugated bilirubin). Mix after each addition:

TB. To 0.2 ml serum add 0.8 ml water, then add 0.5 ml diazo reagent, followed by 2 ml dyphylline. Stand for 10 min, then add 0.1 ml ascorbic acid.

CB. To 0.2 ml serum add 0.8 ml water, followed by 0.5 ml diazo reagent. Stand for 10 min, then add 0.1 ml ascorbic acid, followed immediately by 2 ml dyphylline.

S. To 0.2 ml standard (200 μmol) add 0.8 ml water, then add 0.5 ml diazo reagent, followed by 2 ml dyphylline. Stand for 10 min, then add 0.1 ml ascorbic acid.

SB. To 0.8 ml water add 0.1 ml ascorbic acid and 0.5 ml diazo reagent, followed immediately by 0.2 ml standard and 2 ml dyphylline.

B. To 0.8 ml water add 0.1 ml ascorbic acid and 0.5 ml diazo reagent, followed immediately by 0.2 ml serum and 2 ml dyphylline.

To all tubes add 1.5 ml alkaline tartrate and read the absorbance at 600 nm, zeroing the instrument with water. This should be done soon after adding the tartrate.

Calculation

Serum bilirubin in μmol/l =

$$\frac{\text{Absorbance of TB (or CB)} - \text{Absorbance of B}}{\text{Absorbance of S} - \text{Absorbance of SB}} \times 200$$

Notes

1. If the serum value is over about 250 μmol/l, dilute the specimen 1 in 2 or, if a low value, use 0.4 ml serum and less water, always remembering to adjust the calculation accordingly.
2. The serum should be assayed as soon as possible after collection.

Results

Normal serum has very little conjugated bilirubin, if any at all. The upper limit for total bilirubin is up to 17 μmol/l, but in the majority of normal persons the upper range may only be 10 μmol/l. In jaundice, the total bilirubin increases when conjugated bilirubin may also be increased.

Urine

Unconjugated bilirubin is unable to pass through the glomerulus and therefore does not appear in the urine. This is generally true with normal and elevated amounts of plasma unconjugated bilirubin, whereas the conjugated bilirubin is filtered at the glomerulus and is not, when the plasma levels are raised, reabsorbed fully by the tubules. The detection of bilirubin in the urine indicates that excess conjugated bilirubin is present in the plasma.

It is advisable to see the notes on urine testing on p. 142, before carrying out these tests.

Fouchet's test

Principle

Barium chloride reacts with the sulphate radicals in the urine to form a precipitate of barium sulphate. Any bile pigment present adheres to the precipitate and is detected by the oxidation of bilirubin (yellow) to biliverdin (green) on treatment with ferric chloride in the presence of trichloracetic acid. A blue colour is given by bilicyanin.

Reagents

1. 10% barium chloride.
2. Fouchet's reagent:

Trichloroacetic acid	25 g
Distilled water	50 ml
10% ferric chloride	10 ml
Dilute to 100 ml with distilled water	

Method

1. Test the reaction of the urine, and if alkaline, acidify with 33% acetic acid.
2. Add 5 ml of 10% barium chloride to 10 ml of urine and mix well. If the precipitate formed is insufficient, add a drop of dilute sulphuric acid or ammonium sulphate solution.
3. Filter through Whatman No. 1 filter paper.
4. Carefully unfold the filter paper and place on top of another dry filter paper, and add 1 drop of Fouchet's reagent onto the precipitate in the centre of the paper. If bile is present, a green or blue colour develops, the colour intensity being proportional to the amount of bile pigment present.

Ictotest (reagent tablets)

These reagent tablets (Ames Co.) are quick, simple, standardized colour tests for bilirubin in urine, based on a diazo reaction (see below on the procedures to be adopted using impregnated strips or tablets).

Composition

The tablet contains *p*-nitrobenzene diazonium *p*-toluene sulphonate, salicylsulphonic acid and sodium hydrogen carbonate.

Principle

When urine is placed on the special mat, bilirubin is adsorbed on its surface. The slight effervescent properties of the tablet partially disintegrate it and cause the reagent to wash onto the surface of the mat, where the bilirubin couples with the diazo compound in the presence of salicylsulphonic acid, forming a bluish-purple compound.

Directions

1. Place 5 drops of urine on square of special test mat provided.
2. Place a tablet in middle of moist area.
3. Flow 2 drops of water over tablet.
4. Observe colour of mat around tablet exactly 30 s later.

Results

Negative: The mat around the tablet remains unchanged at 30 s or turns slightly red or pink.
Positive: The mat around the tablet turns a bluish-purple within 30 s. The concentration of bilirubin is roughly proportional to the intensity of the bluish-purple colour and to the speed with which it develops.

Precautions

1. Make sure that the container for the urine is absolutely clean and free from contaminants, for example disinfectants, detergents.
2. Recap the Ictotest bottle tightly as soon as the tablet has been removed, to avoid uptake of moisture.

Sensitivity

These reagent tablets are very sensitive and can detect 0.8–1.7 µmol bilirubin/l of urine (0.05–0.1 mg/100 ml), which coincides with the lower limit of accepted pathological significance.

Specificity

Bilirubin is the only substance known to give the characteristic bluish-purple colour with the reagent tablets.

Commercial test strips

Several years ago Ames introduced the Ictostix strip which was a test area of cellulose impregnated with stabilized, diazotized 2,4-dichloraniline. In the presence of bilirubin the strip changed from a pale yellow (moist) to various shades of brown. This test strip is no longer available, but the test area is incorporated into the multiple test strips Bili-Labstix and Multistix.

BCL's similar product was the Bilur test: this has a test area which contains the fluoroborate of diazotized 2,6-dichloraniline. In the presence of bilirubin there is a red-violet coloration which is compared with the colour blocks. This commercial test for bilirubin is now only obtainable in combination with a test for urobilinogen (Bilugen test) or as part of the multiple test strips, BM-Test 7 and Combur 8 test. The sensitivity of these test strips is probably similar to the Ictotest.

Faecal bilirubin

Meconium, the material excreted during the first few days of life, contains biliverdin. The faeces of very young infants generally contain unaltered bilirubin, but with the development of the bacterial flora bilirubin is gradually reduced to stercobilin. In adults all bilirubin reaching the intestine is reduced to stercobilin unless there is a rapid intestinal movement, when bilirubin may be excreted. Bilirubin can also be found in the faeces of patients receiving antibiotics such as neomycin, which sterilizes the gut. Biliverdin is oxidized to bilirubin on exposure to air. Bilirubin can be detected by emulsifying a portion of the faeces in distilled water, about 1 in 20 suspension. Treat this with an increasing amount of Fouchet's reagent, but not more than an equal volume is required and usually much less. Bilirubin is oxidized quite rapidly to green biliverdin or blue bilicyanin.

2. Urine urobilinogen

As can be seen from *Table 9.1*, alterations in urobilinogen excretion can be of some value in assessing jaundice or monitoring its progress.

Freshly passed urine contains a trace of urobilinogen which is colourless, but on standing this is oxidized to urobilin, an orange-yellow pigment. This pigment, along with urochrome, contributes to the normal colour of urine, but when there is an excess of the urobilin pigment, the urine is orange-yellow in appearance.

Qualitative test for urobilinogen (Wallace and Diamond reaction)

Principle

Urobilinogen is detected by the red colour it gives with Ehrlich's reagent; porphobilinogen also gives the same colour reaction. Urobilin will not give a colour with this reagent.

Reagents

1. Ehrlich's reagent:

4-dimethylaminobenzaldehyde	2.0 g
Concentrated hydrochloric acid	20 ml
Distilled water	80 ml

2. 20% v/v hydrochloric acid.

Method

Urine samples must be freshly voided:

1. To 10 ml of urine add 1 ml Ehrlich's reagent.
2. To another 10 ml of urine add 20% hydrochloric acid (control).
3. Mix by inversion and stand for 3–5 min at room temperature.
4. Note the colour produced and warm to 50°C if no colour develops at room temperature.

Results

Normal urines should give a faint red colour with Ehrlich's reagent but not with 20% HCl.

A similar colour is also given by porphobilinogen (see p. 139), and other substances may produce colours ranging from yellow to orange-pink (e.g. *p*-aminosalicylic acid). A red colour with 20% HCl is probably due to a dye such as methyl red.

	Room temperature	50°C
Urobilinogen absent	No red colour	No red colour
Urobilinogen in normal amounts	Faint red colour	colour
Urobilinogen in excess	Distinct red colour	

When the urobilinogen is present in excess, dilute the urine from 1 in 10, in steps of 10 up to and beyond 1 in 100 if necessary. Repeat the test on 10 ml aliquots of these dilutions until the last dilution showing the faintest red colour is found.

Normal urine will give no colour at room temperature at a dilution of 1 in 20. Abnormal concentrations may give positive results up to and beyond 1 in 100 dilution.

Bilirubin, if present, must be removed before carrying out Ehrlich's test. Use either the filtrate from Fouchet's test or add 1 volume of 10% calcium chloride to 5 vol of urine. Mix well and filter through Whatman No. 1 filter paper. Use the clear filtrate for the test. The bilirubin is adsorbed onto calcium phosphate in the same way as it adheres to barium sulphate in Fouchet's test.

Commercial reagent test strips

These have been introduced by Ames and BCL, and should be used on freshly voided urine.

Urobilistix reagent strips for urobilinogen

These reagent strips (Ames Co.) are firm plastic strips with the reagent impregnated into an absorbent area at the tip of the strip to provide a rapid, convenient test for urinary urobilinogen.

Composition and principle

The reagent, 4-dimethylaminobenzaldehyde, is stabilized in an acid buffer resulting in the formation of a *brown* colour with urobilinogen.

Directions

1. Dip reagent area of strip in fresh, well-mixed freshly voided uncentrifuged urine.
2. Remove strip from urine. Tap edge of strip against urine container to remove excess urine.
3. Allow reaction to continue for exactly 60 s from dipping.
4. Immediately compare colour of reagent area with colour chart, holding reagent area close to the chart. Interpolate if colour produced falls between two colour blocks. Avoid glare.

Results

The test is read in Ehrlich units per 100 ml, the colour varying from yellow to more intense shades of brown with increasing concentrations of urobilinogen. Colour blocks representing 0.1, 1, 4, 8 and 12 Ehrlich units are provided. 1 Ehrlich unit is equivalent to about 1.7 μmol urobilinogen. Values up to 1 Ehrlich unit should be considered marginal and must be left to the clinician to interpret in the light of clinical evidence.

Sensitivity

Urobilistix reagent strips will detect urobilinogen in concentrations of approximately 0.1 Ehrlich unit per 100 ml urine. The absence of urobilinogen cannot be determined with the product. No substances are known to inhibit the reaction of the reagent strips.

Specificity

The reagent strips are not specific for urobilinogen.

They will react with some of the substances known to react with Ehrlich's reagent, e.g. *p*-aminosalicylic acid, but not with porphobilinogen or haemoglobin. This test strip is also incorporated in the multiple test strips Multistix and N-Multistix.

Bilugen (BCL)

Composition and principle

This test strip is a combined one with bilirubin, the urobilinogen part of the strip relies on the coupling of *p*-methoxy benzene diazonium fluoroborate at an acid pH which, in the presence of urobilinogen, gives a red azo-dye complex.

Directions

These are the same as for the Urobilistix, except that the reaction is read 10 s after dipping in the urine. Colour changes after 30 s are of no importance.

Results

The colour blocks correspond to 1, 4, 8 and 12 mg/100 ml urobilinogen. Normal urines usually contain up to 1 mg/100 ml.*

Specificity

The strip is said to be specific for urobilinogen and the only interference with the reaction is due to drugs such as phenazopyridine, which become red in acid. The test area is also incorporated into the multiple test strips, BM-Test 7 and Combur 8 test.

3. Urine urobilin (Schlesinger's test)

Principle

After first oxidizing any urobilinogen present to urobilin, a greenish-yellow fluorescent compound of zinc urobilin is formed, the fluorescence of which is more definite in ultraviolet light than daylight.

Reagents

1. Absolute ethanol.
2. Zinc acetate (powdered).
3. Tincture of iodine.

Method

1. To 10 ml of urine in a test-tube add a few drops of tincture of iodine to oxidize the urobilinogen to

urobilin. Bilirubin must be removed beforehand, as for urobilinogen.
2. Into another test-tube place about 10 ml of ethanol and add approximately 1 g of powdered zinc acetate.
3. Pass the solutions backwards and forwards from one tube to the other, until nearly all the powder is dissolved.
4. Filter the mixture through Whatman No. 1 filter paper into a clean test-tube.
5. View the filtrate from above. It is better to examine by using reflected light with the tube held against a black background. A greenish-yellow fluorescence is present if the urobilin is present. Examine under an ultraviolet light when the fluorescence is more noticeable. Next examine with a direct-vision spectroscope. Zinc urobilin shows an absorption band in the green portion of the spectrum centred at 506.5 nm. Urobilin itself, in acid urine, also exhibits an absorption band, centred at 490 nm (green blue), but this band is more diffuse and less easy to identify than the zinc urobilin absorption band.

Results

Normal urine should give no more than a barely detectable amount of fluorescence.

Faecal urobilin

1. Extract a portion of faeces with a mixture of 20 vol of ethanol and 1 vol of concentrated hydrochloric acid.
2. Mix thoroughly and allow to stand overnight or for several hours.
3. Examine extract spectroscopically and then carry out a Schlesinger's test.
4. Neutralize the extract with concentrated ammonia or with 40% sodium hydroxide. It is preferable to use the latter.
5. When neutralized, mix with an equal volume of ethanolic zinc acetate and proceed as above.

Urine

Detection of bile salts

Bile salts lower the surface tension and can be responsible for increased foaming when urine is shaken. The reduction of surface tension is used in their detection.

Hay's test

Reagents

Flowers of sulphur.

*These are the units used by the commercial organization.

Method

Place some fresh clear urine in a small beaker at room temperature. Sprinkle a little finely powdered flowers of sulphur onto the surface. Sulphur particles sink in the presence of bile salts, but remain on the surface of the urine if absent. Urines preserved with thymol may give a false positive.

Modification

Into a clean beaker place some distilled water and carefully sprinkle some flowers of sulphur on top of the surface in the centre of the beaker. With a clean Pasteur pipette add a drop of urine to the centre of the sulphur. If bile salts are present, the sulphur will be dispersed towards the side of the beaker. In the absence of bile salts, the sulphur will remain in the centre of the beaker.

Treat a normal urine in a similar manner for both methods.

It has been suggested that this test is of little diagnostic value.

Detection of porphobilinogen

In acute intermittent porphyria, porphobilinogen, a colourless compound and an intermediate product in the biosynthesis of haem, is found in the urine. Porphobilinogen, like urobilinogen, gives a red colour with Ehrlich's reagent and the two compounds must be differentiated from each other.

Test for porphobilinogen

Principle

Urine is treated with Ehrlich's reagent, when a red colour is given by porphobilinogen. To distinguish this colour from that given by urobilinogen, the addition of saturated sodium acetate solution, which alters the pH, intensifies the colour given by urobilinogen but not that by porphobilinogen and makes the urobilinogen more soluble in the extracting solvent.

Reagents

1. Ehrlich's reagent:

4-dimethylaminobenzaldehyde	0.7 g
Concentrated hydrochloric acid	150 ml
Distilled water	100 ml

2. Saturated sodium acetate:

Hydrated sodium acetate about	100 g
Distilled water	100 ml

3. Chloroform or amyl alcohol:benzyl alcohol mixture (3:1 v/v).

Method

Urine samples must be freshly voided.

1. To 5 ml of urine add 5 ml of Ehrlich's reagent, mix and allow to stand for 3–5 min.
2. Add 10 ml saturated sodium acetate solution, mix and leave for a few minutes.
3. Add 2 ml of chloroform or amyl alcohol:benzyl alcohol mixture and shake thoroughly. Allow the two layers to separate.

Results

Urobilinogen is soluble in the organic layer, so any red colour remaining in the aqueous phase after extraction constitutes a positive test for porphobilinogen.

Rimington found that the amyl alcohol:benzyl alcohol mixture gave a more complete removal of the coloured complex formed by urobilinogen from the aqueous phase than did chloroform.

It may therefore be necessary to repeat the extraction with chloroform to confirm a positive test for porphobilinogen.

10

Renal function tests

The kidneys are the primary organs involved in the excretion of waste products, the other organs involved being the lungs, skin and intestines. In the urinary system there are two kidneys which form and secrete urine by peristalsis; it is conveyed from each kidney through a ureter to the urinary bladder. The bladder provides temporary storage for about 300 ml urine, which is eventually voided through the urethra to the exterior. The kidneys are situated at the posterior of the abdomen, one on either side of the vertebral column, the right kidney a little lower than the left, due to the space occupied by the liver.

Each kidney, which is bean-shaped, is enclosed in a capsule of fibrous tissue, which is easily stripped off. Underneath the capsule lies the cortex, followed by the medulla, which is made up of renal pyramids, then the hilum, where the renal arteries and nerves enter, and the renal vein and ureter leave the kidney.

The microscopical structure of the kidney is composed of nephrons and collecting tubules. There are approximately one million nephrons to each kidney, this being the functional unit. The nephron consists of the glomerular or Bowman's capsule, proximal convoluted tubule, loop of Henle and the distal convoluted tubule (*Figure 10.1*).

Functions of the kidney

1. Maintenance of water and electrolyte balance of the body

When the amounts of water and/or electrolytes in the body fluctuate, their excretion is regulated by the kidney with the help of antidiuretic hormone and aldosterone, so that the body fluids are restored to their normal composition and volume. This is best

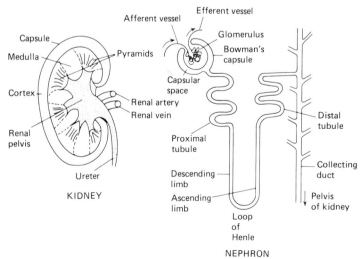

Figure 10.1. The kidney and nephron

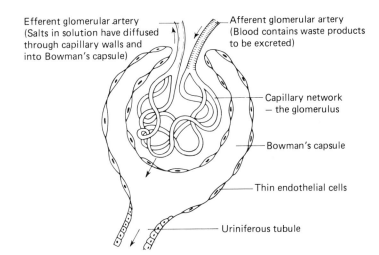

Efferent glomerular artery
(Salts in solution have diffused
through capillary walls and
into Bowman's capsule)

Afferent glomerular artery
(Blood contains waste products
to be excreted)

Capillary network
— the glomerulus

Bowman's capsule

Thin endothelial cells

Uriniferous tubule

Figure 10.2. Diagram of a glomerulus

explained by referring to the osmotic pressure of plasma. Under normal conditions, the osmolarity of the plasma varies only slightly, despite wide variations of the fluid and electrolyte intake of the body. When an excess of water is taken, it will tend to dilute the plasma and reduce its osmotic pressure, producing a renal response which results in the excretion of an increased volume of urine with an osmolarity less than that of the plasma. By excreting water in excess of the solutes, the kidney maintains the water balance of the body. On the other hand, on restricted fluids an increase in plasma osmolarity will be corrected by the excretion of a 'concentrated' urine with an osmolarity higher than that of plasma, showing that the solutes are being excreted in excess of water (see Selective reabsorption, below).

2. Maintenance of pH of the blood

The normal pH of blood in health is slightly on the alkaline side, pH 7.36–7.42, and the kidneys are responsible for removing substances which cause it to become acid or more alkaline. Substances of acid reaction are the waste products of protein metabolism—urea, uric acid and creatinine—which are constantly being formed and therefore must be excreted. Salts of sodium, potassium, calcium, magnesium and phosphorus are alkaline in reaction, and therefore must be excreted if their concentration reaches too high a level in the blood.

3. Excretion of drugs and toxins

Drugs, after completing their action in the body, leave waste products which are excreted by the kidneys. If the drugs are not metabolized they themselves are excreted. Toxins in the body are rendered harmless by detoxification in the liver, and the conjugated compounds so formed excreted in the urine.

Formation of urine

Urine is formed in the nephrons by a combination of two processes, simple filtration and selective reabsorption.

Simple filtration

This process takes place between the glomerulus and glomerular capsule. The blood supply to the kidneys averages 1200 ml per min (25% of the heart's output per min). A higher pressure in the glomerulus meets negligible pressure in the Bowman's capsule, resulting in the passage of substances in solution through the semi-permeable membrane at the rate of about 120 ml per min (glomerular filtrate rate). The filtrate contains salts, glucose, urea, uric acid and other substances of small molecular size. Cells and plasma proteins which have a large molecular size do not pass through the semi-permeable membrane (*Figure 10.2*).

Selective reabsorption

When the filtrate enters the tubule, the tubular epithelium reabsorbs water and selected essential substances into the peritubular capillaries. By passive and active reabsorption the cells adjust the composition of urine to meet the body requirements. Approximately 80% of the water and sodium chloride content, together with glucose, phosphate and amino acids, are absorbed in the proximal tubule. About 20% of the tubular fluid enters the loop of Henle where water is passively absorbed; 6 ml per min of concentrated tubular fluid now enters the distal tubule, where there is an active reabsorption of sodium. The fluid leaves the distal tubule at the rate of approximately 1 ml per min, passing into the collecting ducts in the form of urine. Over a period of 24 h this will give a urine volume of 1–1½ litres.

Renal threshold

The constituents of the glomerular filtrate have either a high, medium, low or no-threshold value. This means that the threshold of a given substance in the plasma is the highest level at which the constituent is present in the blood before it appears in the urine. Glucose, a high threshold substance, is completely reabsorbed from the filtrate and only appears in the urine when the blood level is about 8.33 mmol/l, this being the normal threshold value. Urea has a threshold value of zero, because only small amounts of it are reabsorbed in the tubules, and it is always present in the urine no matter what the blood level happens to be. Finally, creatinine is a no-threshold substance, as it is not reabsorbed and is always present in the urine. (Tubular cells can also secrete some creatinine into the filtrate.) The threshold of any substance can be altered by impaired renal function.

Urine analysis

Composition

Urine is water containing the water-soluble waste products removed from the blood stream via the kidneys. Normal urine consists of approximately 95% water, the remainder being made up of urea, uric acid, creatinine, sodium, potassium, chloride, calcium, phosphate, etc. The composition varies widely from day to day, depending upon the food and fluid intake.

Microscopical and chemical examination of urine may yield useful information in many abnormal conditions. Infections of the kidneys, ureters, bladder and urethra may result in the presence of pus, red blood cells and organisms in the urine. When the kidneys become inflamed various casts may appear in the urine (see p. 145). Reducing substances, ketones, bile and protein can be found in a variety of pathological conditions.

Volume

Of the 75–150 litres of glomerular filtrate produced by the normal adult kidney, tubular reabsorption reduces this volume to between 1 and 2 litres per day. This varies with fluid intake and diet, as well as other physiological factors. As already mentioned, copious drinking will increase the volume of urine passed, while excessive perspiration will decrease the volume. In certain pathological conditions, the output will differ considerably from the normal volume. An increased output (polyuria) can be found in diabetes mellitus, and also in diabetes insipidus, when 10–20 litres may be excreted. A reduced output (oliguria) may be found in acute nephritis or fevers, while a complete suppression (anuria) can be occasionally encountered in blood transfusion reactions.

Appearance

Urine is normally clear and pale yellow in colour, due to a pigment, urochrome, said to be a compound of urobilin, urobilinogen and a peptide substance. Urochrome is a product of endogenous metabolism, and is fairly constant in amount from day to day. In concentrated urines there is the same amount of urochrome, thereby giving a much darker appearance, ranging from dark yellow to brown red in colour.

Table 10.1 Abnormalities of urine

Colour of urine	Cause	Conditions
Milky	Fat globules	Chyluria
	Pus	Infection of the urinary tract
Greenish-yellow Greenish-brown Dark brown	Bile pigments	Jaundice
Orange yellow	Excess urobilin	Jaundice
Red or reddish	Haemoglobin	Haemoglobinuria
	Myoglobin	Trauma
	Porphyrins	Porphyria
	Beetroot	
Brown to brown-black	Haematin	Haemorrhages
	Methaemo-globin	Methaemoglobinuria
	Melanin	Melanotic tumours

Urines may be abnormally pigmented by dyes; for example, the administration of methylene blue by mouth results in a greenish-blue urine, phenols cause a dark, almost black urine, and certain foods and drugs can result in various colours and odours in the urine (*Table 10.1*).

Odour

Freshly passed urine has a characteristic aromatic odour, said to be due to volatile organic acids. When the urine is allowed to stand, decomposition of urea by bacteria occurs, and ammonia is evolved.

Reaction

Freshly passed normal urine is usually slightly acid with a pH about 6.0 and a range of 4.8–6.8. Due to alkaline fermentation cloudiness occurs and phosphates are precipitated; amorphous urates may also be deposited on standing. The urates are insoluble in dilute hydrochloric acid, while the phosphates are soluble.

It is usually sufficient to indicate whether the urine is acid or alkaline by using indicator papers. BDH Chemical plc supply indicator papers in reel dispensers suitable for this purpose. These cover the range for urine pH being from pH 4–6, 6–8 and 8–10. Other pH ranges covered are from pH 1–4, 10–12 and 12–14. A full range indicator from pH 1–14 is also available. The pH is then determined by simply dipping the indicator strips into the urine and then comparing the change of colour of the strip against the colour guide supplied with the indicator papers.

For a more accurate determination of pH, a pH meter should be used. Alternatively a colorimetric method can be used, similar to the determination of pH when preparing media.

Specific gravity

The specific gravity (sp. gr.) of a normal urine is within the range of 1.016 to 1.025. It is subject to wide fluctuations. For example, after drinking a large quantity of water, the sp. gr. may be as low as 1.001, while it can reach 1.040 after excessive perspiration. In diabetes mellitus, due to high concentrations of glucose, the sp. gr. may be as high as 1.040. The presence of protein in large amounts will also increase the sp. gr. A high sp. gr. is found in acute nephritis due to the concentrated urine, whereas in chronic nephritis the reverse is obtained.

Measurement of specific gravity

Specific gravity is the relative proportion of the weight of a volume of urine to that of an equal volume of distilled water, water being a standard unit, i.e.

$$\text{Sp. gr.} = \frac{\text{Weight of urine}}{\text{Weight of same volume of distilled water}}$$

The standard method for determining sp. gr. is by using the specific gravity bottle, or by weighing. The urinometer technique is not as accurate.

A. *Specific gravity bottles.* Specific gravity bottles (density bottles) can be supplied in sizes varying between 10 and 100 ml. They are designed to allow identical volumes to be weighed.

Technique for using the specific gravity bottle
1. Weigh the clean, dry, stoppered bottle accurately.
2. Fill the bottle with the test liquid.
3. Carefully insert the ground-glass stopper. The excess liquid is ejected from the central hole in the stopper.
4. With a clean tissue remove all traces of liquid from the outside of the bottle, and wipe carefully across the top of the stopper. Make sure that there is no air underneath the stopper, or in its capillary.
5. Weigh the bottle of test liquid.

6. Empty the bottle, and rinse it out several times with distilled water.
7. Fill the bottle with distilled water and replace the stopper as before, then wipe the outside and weigh.
8. Subtract the weight of the empty stoppered bottle from both total weights, and divide the weight of the test liquid by that of the distilled water. Both liquids should be at the same temperature, as volume is altered by temperature variations.

B. *Weighing.* If there is only a small volume of urine weigh a known quantity of urine; by using a volumetric pipette and using the same pipette, weigh the same volume of distilled water.

C. *Urinometers.* Urinometers are designed for estimations of specific gravity. Their use in medical laboratories is mainly confined to measurement of the specific gravity of urine. The urinometer is so calibrated that it sinks in distilled water, until the '0' mark on the stem is level with the surface of the water. This denotes a specific gravity of 1.000. In urine, which is more dense than water, the instrument is more buoyant, and the specific gravity is read off the scale at the level of the surface of the urine.

Precautions when using the urinometer

1. Make absolutely certain that the instrument floats centrally in the liquid by rotating it, and that it is not in contact with the bottom or sides of the container.
2. Take readings at the lowest point of the meniscus, which should be viewed at eye-level. Errors will result if this is not done.
3. Always check the accuracy of new urinometers in distilled water. Sometimes a correction factor is necessary; for example, if the reading in distilled water is 1.004, then 0.004 must be subtracted from test readings.
4. As these instruments are usually calibrated at 15°C, one must add 0.001 for every 3°C above 15°C, and subtract 0.001 for every 3°C below 15°C. For every 10 g/l albumin present, subtract 0.003.

D. *Osmometry* A newer technique introduced in the laboratory is that of osmometry, which tends to replace the specific gravity procedures. It is a technique in which the total solute content of body fluids is measured by using instruments called osmometers (see p. 82). In body fluids the osmotic pressure is of significance and this depends upon the total concentration of molecules and ions in solution (solutes). This concentration cannot be expressed in mmol/l, but the unit in which the concentration is expressed is the osmol. An osmol is the amount of substance in 1 litre of solution which under ideal conditions exerts an osmotic pressure of $\simeq 2262\,kPa$ (22.4 atmospheres) and will therefore depress the freezing point by 1.86°C.

The measurement of the depression of freezing point below that of pure water by the total solutes is therefore a measure of the total osmotic pressure of the body fluids.

The osmol is a very large number and to avoid the use of fractions, a milliosmol is used (mosmol), which is one-thousandth of an osmol and is equivalent to a freezing point depression of 0.00186°C.

Osmolarity is the osmotic pressure of $\simeq 2262\,kPa$ exerted by 1 mole per litre of un-ionized substance, while osmolality is the osmotic pressure of $\simeq 2262\,kPa$ exerted by 1 gram-molecule per kg of un-ionized substance—the latter is preferred.

Normally the urine osmolality varies between 700 and 1500 mosmol per kg, but this depends upon the diet taken.

Osmolality is usually affected in disease, as is specific gravity, but because of the variation in the nature of the solutes, one cannot be calculated from the other. For example, a urine with a specific gravity of 1.016 can give values of between 550 and 910 mosmol per kg.

Collection of urine

Sterile specimens of urine are not necessary for biochemical analysis, but the urine should be collected in a clean dry bottle. If a timed specimen is required, the patient should empty the bladder at, for example, 8.0 a.m., this urine being discarded. All the urine passed up to and at 8.0 a.m. the following morning is saved and placed in a labelled bottle. This collection will then be a 24-h sample. The same procedure applies for a 2-, 4- or 6-h specimen of urine. If the patient wishes to defaecate during the collection period, the bladder should be emptied beforehand, to avoid losses of urine. The collection of timed urine specimens is very important and it is surprising how badly this is often done.

Preservatives

Sometimes it may be necessary to keep the urine for 24–48 h before the analysis can be carried out, or bacterial action during the collection period may affect the constituent to be analysed. However, if the urine is collected into a clean, dry container, little change will take place in a 24-h specimen by the time it is received in the laboratory. Keeping the urine container cool and stoppered during collection will also help to preserve the urine. Urea is the most labile constituent in urine, as bacteria will convert it to ammonium carbonate; the ammoniacal odour of grossly bacterially contaminated urine is well

known. Because of bacterial action, the urine would be unsuitable for the determination of pH, urea and ammonia.

The choice of preservative is often influenced by the estimation required on the urine. As a rule acid is quite satisfactory, when 20 ml 2M hydrochloric acid can be added to the container prior to the collection; 8 g boric acid powder or crystals can also be used for certain investigations. This is a very convenient preservative for out-patients, who have to collect 24-h urine samples. Urines preserved in this manner are suitable for the estimation of urea, ammonia and calcium.

Chloroform, toluene, thymol and sodium azide have also been used. A few crystals of thymol will preserve the urine quite satisfactorily for the estimation of sodium, potassium, chloride, urea, protein, reducing substances and amylase.

Microscopic examination

Urine should be examined as soon as possible after it has been voided. Delay may result in disintegration of cells, and the deposition of amorphous urates or phosphates.

Method

1. Centrifuge approximately 10 ml of urine, and decant the supernatant fluid.
2. Tap the bottom of the centrifuge tube to loosen the deposit, and place one small drop on a clean slide.
3. Apply a coverslip, avoiding the formation of air bubbles.
4. Examine the field with the 16 mm objective to obtain a general impression of the deposit, then use the 4 mm objective to identify all the constituents. (Illumination of the field should not be too bright, as casts and other structures may not be seen.)

Method of reporting deposits

■ **Note**

The best way of learning to identify urinary deposits is to seek constant guidance from an experienced scientist. Many extraneous inclusions may be mistaken for casts by the beginner, for example, cotton wool, hair and scratches on the slide or coverslip. Oil or air bubbles may be mistaken for red blood cells (*Figure 10.3*). Sometimes the entire deposit may be missed through incorrect focusing of the microscope.

Deposits may be divided into two main groups—organized deposit and unorganized deposit—as follows:

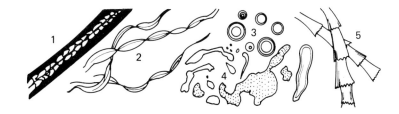

Figure 10.3. Some miscellaneous inclusions: (1) hair, (2) cotton wool, (3) oil droplets, (4) air bubbles, (5) feather barbs

Organized deposit

Cells

1. Epithelial cells of the squamous type are present in many normal urine specimens, especially in non-catheter samples from female patients (*Figure 10.4*).
2. Red blood cells are not present in the urine of normal males. In samples from female patients they may be of menstrual origin. Red cells may be normal, crenated or swollen, depending on whether the urine is isotonic, hypertonic or hypotonic (*Figure 10.4*).
3. Leucocytes in normal urine are found only occasionally, generally not more than 2 per field using the 4 mm objective. Depending on the tonicity of the urine, they may be normal, swollen or shrunken in size. When degenerate, they are sometimes called 'pus cells' (*Figure 10.4*).

Casts

Casts of the renal tubules are not present in normal urine. They indicate renal dysfunction, and are usually associated with albuminuria. The sides of a cast are parallel, and the end may be either rounded or broken off (*Figure 10.4*). They are of three main types, but these are not necessarily clearly defined; for example, a hyaline cast may have cellular inclusions:

1. Hyaline casts are transparent and homogeneous.

2. Cellular casts are partially or wholly composed of pus, epithelial or red blood cells.
3. Granular casts are degenerated cellular casts, and are granular in appearance.

Organisms

Organisms are of no significance when they are found in urine samples that have been standing overnight. The presence of bacteria and pus cells in freshly voided urine is indicative of infection and the findings should be reported.

Spermatozoa

Spermatozoa (*Figure 10.4*) should be reported when present in large numbers, which may suggest a lesion in the genito-urinary tract.

Mucus

Mucus is derived from the mucous glands of the urinary tract, and appears as long translucent shreds. The presence of small amounts of mucus is considered normal.

Unorganized deposit

A knowledge of the reaction of urine samples is of great assistance in identification of deposits. In samples with an acid reaction, the commonest crystalline deposits likely to occur may be calcium oxalate, sodium urate or uric acid. In alkaline

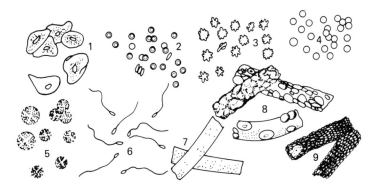

Figure 10.4. Cells and casts. (1) Epithelial cells. (2) Normal red blood cells. (3) Crenated red blood cells. (4) Swollen red blood cells. (5) Leucocytes. (6) Spermatozoa. (7) Hyaline casts. (8) Cellular casts. (9) Granular casts

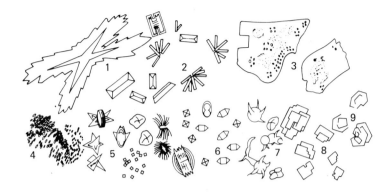

Figure 10.5. Various crystals. (1) Triple phosphate (ammonium magnesium phosphate). (2) Stellar phosphate (calcium phosphate). (3) Calcium phosphate (plate form). (4) Amorphous phosphates. (5) Uric acid (various forms). (6) Calcium oxalate. (7) Ammonium and sodium urate. (8) Cholesterol. (9) Cystine

specimens, deposits are more likely to be phosphates, calcium carbonate or ammonium urate (*Figure 10.5*).

Blood

In some kidney diseases, or if the urinary tract is damaged, blood can be passed into the urine (haematuria). This can often be detected macroscopically, or, if the condition is only slight, microscopical examination will reveal intact blood cells. In intravascular haemolysis, which can occur after an incompatible blood transfusion or in haemolytic anaemia, there are no intact red cells, but free haemoglobin is present (haemoglobinuria). Microscopic detection of red blood corpuscles is not as sensitive as the chemical method. The techniques given on p. 144 can be used.

Protein

Proteins are one of the most important, as well as the most complicated, groups of biological substances. They are built up of amino acid units which can be liberated during acid and basic hydrolysis. Twenty-two different amino acids can be identified in such a way:

$$\begin{array}{c} H \\ | \\ R-C-COOH \\ | \\ NH_2 \end{array} \quad \text{amino acid}$$

When the carboxyl group of one amino acid reacts with the amino group of another amino acid, a peptide is formed. The linkage joining the amino acids together —CO—NH— is known as a peptide bond, and this bond is important when proteins are estimated quantitatively by the biuret reaction:

$$\underset{\text{glycine}}{NH_2-\underset{|}{\underset{H}{CH}}-COOH} + \underset{\text{alanine}}{NH_2-\underset{|}{\underset{CH_3}{CH}}-COOH} \rightarrow$$

$$\underset{\text{glycylalanine}}{NH_2-\underset{|}{\underset{H}{CH}}-CO-NH-\underset{|}{\underset{CH_3}{CH}}-COOH} + H_2O$$

Normal urine contains traces of protein material, but the amount is so slight that it escapes detection by any of the simple laboratory tests. In various pathological conditions, when protein is found in the urine (proteinuria) it may be derived from plasma albumin, plasma globulin, haemoglobin, and related products from red cells. Bence-Jones protein and protein from pus and mucus (from urinary tract lesions) may also be present. Semen and vaginal secretions can also give rise to proteinuria. Contamination of urine samples, for example, by vaginal discharge or faeces must be avoided. To prevent this, catheterization may be essential in the female patient; a mid-stream specimen from the male is satisfactory.

Qualitative tests

1. Boiling test

Principle

Proteins are coagulated and denatured by heat.

Reagent

33% acetic acid.

Method

1. If the urine is alkaline, make slightly acid with 33% acetic acid.

2. Filter or centrifuge if not clear, and fill a test-tube three-quarters full with the urine.
3. Hold the tube at an angle and heat the upper layer of urine.
4. Protein, if present, is coagulated and turbidity occurs.
5. Add several drops of 33% acetic acid and boil again.
6. When protein is present, the turbidity remains; if it disappears on adding acetic acid, it is due to the precipitation of phosphates.
7. During heating of the urine, carbon dioxide is driven off, so that the degree of alkalinity increases with resultant precipitation of phosphates. Acidification reverses this reaction.
8. It is a good policy to add acetic acid after boiling, even when there is no turbidity, because sometimes an alkaline urine will give a turbidity on the addition of acid. This is due to metaprotein, which in alkaline solution is uncoagulable, but when the pH is altered to neutral or slightly acid, the metaprotein is precipitated and immediately coagulated by heat. Excess acid must be avoided, as this keeps the protein in solution, preventing its coagulation.

◀ **Notes**

1. The boiling test is for heat-coagulable protein, such as albumins and globulins. It is not a quantitative test, but the amount of protein may be roughly assessed. Protein can be reported as a trace, +, ++ and +++, depending on the amount of precipitate produced.
2. This test is sensitive to about ·0.05 g protein per litre, and is a more reliable method than the sulphosalicyclic acid test. However, most laboratories appear to use the Albustix method, which can give both false positive and negative results (see below).

2. Sulphosalicylic acid test (SSA)

Principle

Sulphosalicylic acid is an anionic precipitant, and therefore the neutralization of the protein cation results in the precipitation of the protein.

Reagents

25% sulphosalicylic acid in distilled water.

Method

To 5 ml of clear urine add 0.5 ml sulphosalicylic acid. In the presence of protein a white precipitate appears, the turbidity being proportional to the amount of protein present. Compare against untreated urine.

This test is sensitive to as little as 0.1 g per litre of protein; although uric acid may give a positive reaction, the turbidity will disappear on warming the tube. Radio-opaque substances also give false positive reactions with the reagent (see p. 148).

3. Commercial test strips

Albustix

There are two main organizations which supply test strips for detecting albumin—Ames and BCL. The principle of both tests is basically the same.

Albustix reagent strips (Ames Division, Miles Laboratories Ltd) are firm, plastic strips with the reagent system at one end. The reagent is an indicator system and a citrate buffer.

Principle

Tetrabromophenol blue, at pH 3, is yellow, but in the presence of protein and at the same pH, the indicator changes to a shade of green.

Method

Dip the test end into freshly passed uncentrifuged urine for about a second, remove excess urine by tapping the edge against the container. Compare the colour of the strip with the colour chart within 60 s. If the test end remains yellow, the urine contains no protein.

Albym-Test

Albym-Test (BCL) is a plastic reagent strip, at one end of which is an absorbent paper area covered by a nylon mesh.

Principle

The indicator was originally tetrabromophenolphthalein ethyl ester, but this has now been modified to produce green colours with more sensitivity at the lower protein concentrations.

Method

Dip the test strip into the freshly passed uncentrifuged urine for about a second, remove excess urine by tapping the edge against the container. Compare the colour with the test chart 30–60 s later.

Precautions

1. Make sure that the container for urine is absolutely clean and free from contaminants, particularly disinfectants and detergents, including quaternary ammonium compounds. Acid used as a preservative reduces the sensitivity.
2. Do not touch test end of strip.

3. Recap bottle tightly as soon as strip has been removed.
4. Do not leave strip in urine, or hold in or pass through urine stream, to avoid risk of dissolving out reagents.
5. Read strip in a bright white light; coloured fluorescent lighting may interfere with readings. Hold strip very near to colour chart when making readings.

Sensitivity

Positive results are obtained with albumin, globulin, haemoglobin, Bence-Jones protein and glycoproteins. Both test strips are most sensitive to albumin, while the other proteins are less readily detected. With both strips a + colour block represents approximately 0.03 g/l of albumin. Smaller concentrations of protein than this are detectable, as indicated by the presence of the trace colour block. Markedly alkaline urines (pH 9.0 or higher) can give false positive results, while false negative results are likely if the urine is acidified or the protein is not albumin.

Specificity

The strips are unaffected by urine turbidity, X-ray contrast media, most drugs and their metabolites, and urinary preservatives which may affect other tests.

Quaternary ammonium compounds (e.g. cetavalon) will give false positive results.

Differentiation between protein and a radio-opaque substance

In X-rays of the urinary tract, a radio-opaque substance such as uroselectan is used, and if urine is collected following this test a false positive reaction (pseudo-albuminuria) will be given by the sulphosalicylic acid. *Table 10.2* shows how the two substances can be distinguished from each other.

Table 10.2 Differentiation of pseudo-albuminuria

	Boiling test	Sulpho-salicylic acid	Albustix	Albym test
Protein	+	+	+	+
Radio-opaque substance	–	+	–	–

Bence-Jones protein

In multiple myeloma, abnormal proteins are formed in the bone-marrow; these proteins may be found in the plasma and can be excreted in the urine. The most important member of this group of proteins is Bence-Jones protein, and the recognition of its presence is an important aid to the diagnosis of this disease. Bence-Jones protein can be distinguished from the proteins generally found in the urine by its behaviour on heating. It will precipitate at temperatures between 40 and 60°C, whereas the other proteins precipitate between 60 and 70°C. On raising the temperature to boiling, Bence-Jones protein will redissolve, but the other proteins will not. On cooling to 60°C from boiling, Bence-Jones protein reprecipitates. Bence-Jones protein gives a positive reaction with the sulphosalicylic acid reaction, but can be missed with the boiling test.

Tests for Bence-Jones protein

The urine should be an early morning specimen or a mid-stream specimen and a few grains of sodium azide should be added as a preservative.

1. Bradshaw's test

This is the most useful screening test and is more reliable than the heating method:

1. Into a test-tube place a few ml of concentrated hydrochloric acid.
2. Carefully add down the side of the tube a few ml of urine, so as to preserve a sharp junction between the two liquids.
3. If Bence-Jones protein is present a white 'curdy' precipitate occurs at the interface.
4. The test may be positive if other proteins are present in considerable amounts, but if the urine is diluted with distilled water, a true Bence-Jones protein often remains positive.

■ Note

Urines which contain more than 50 g/l of Bence-Jones protein should be detected by Bradshaw's test. However, the only really satisfactory method is that of electrophoresis, which does require the urine to be concentrated.

2. Electrophoresis method

This more complex test should be used before excluding Bence-Jones protein.

As there is usually insufficient protein in the urine for detection by this technique, the urine must be concentrated beforehand. This can be achieved by using either *Lyphogel** or *Minicon-B* clinical sample concentrator (Amicon Ltd).

*Gelman Instrument Co.; sold by Anachem Ltd, 20a North St., Luton, Beds. LU2 7QE

(a) Lyphogel method

Lyphogel is a polyacrylamide hydrogel which will concentrate biological fluids in 5 h. Each Lyphogel pellet expands, in aqueous solutions, to five times its own weight of water, and in low-molecular-weight substances such as salt, while excluding protein and other substances with a molecular weight of 2000 or more.

Concentration of urine

1. To 10 ml urine in a test-tube, add 1.48 g Lyphogel.
2. Cover the test-tube with parafilm and leave for 5 h or more.
3. Remove the gel pellets from the solution with forceps.
4. Any fluid still adhering to the swollen cylinders should be drained back into the concentrate by touching them to the side of the tube.
5. As 1 g of Lyphogel absorbs 5 ml water, this technique will remove 8 ml water.

(b) Minicon method

This is a specially prepared ultrafiltration membrane separating chamber which will hold up to 5 ml of urine and concentrate the urine from 5 to 100 times. The inner surface of the chamber is a membrane of selective permeability, backed in turn by absorbent pads which remove water and permeating substances. The retained constituents are progressively concentrated in the chambers as the sample volume decreases. The cut-off point is for a mol. wt of approximately 15 000.

Concentration of urine

1. The urine should be filtered beforehand using a Whatman No. 1 paper.
2. Place the sample to the fill line through the hole in the top of the chamber, using a Pasteur pipette.
3. The sample volume will decrease unattended up to ×100 in 2–4 h.
4. Concentrate the urine between 100 and 200 times, depending upon the protein content, by refilling the chamber with more urine.

Electrophoresis

1. Apply the concentrate to an agarose electrophoresis strip, as described in Chapter 6, p. 96, along with a fresh specimen of patient's serum if possible.
2. If Bence-Jones protein is present, the abnormal sharp protein band will, on electrophoretic analysis, migrate between the β- and γ-globulin

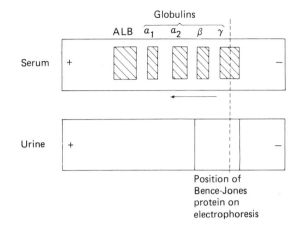

Figure 10.6. Position of proteins on electrophoresis

positions (*Figure 10.6*). Any abnormal bands are then classified by immunofixation (Chapter 6).

Proteinuria

It is generally thought that the glomerular filtrate contains a small amount of protein and the tubular cells reabsorb most of this protein, so that in the normal individual the kidneys may excrete up to 0.05 g of protein per day. Pathological proteinuria (a common finding in renal disease) usually implies glomerular damage causing increased filtration of protein, but it may be due to defective tubular reabsorption. However, proteinuria is sometimes found when there is no renal disease. Increased pressure on the renal veins accounts for proteinuria in 5% of young healthy adults and also in pregnancy.

Reducing substances

A reducing substance is one which will reduce blue alkaline cupric sulphate to red cuprous oxide. The most important substances are the carbohydrates glucose, lactose, fructose, galactose and pentoses (e.g. ribose, xylose and arabinose).

Alkaline cupric sulphate can also be reduced by substances which are not carbohydrates, such as glucuronic acid, salicyluric acid, uric acid, creatinine and homogentisic acid, if present in the urine in sufficiently large concentration. Sucrose will not reduce the alkaline copper reagent. Normal urine contains small amounts of reducing substances, but the concentration is too small to be detected by Benedict's qualitative reagent.

Detection of reducing substances

Benedict's qualitative test

Principle

The aldehyde or ketone group of the carbohydrates reduces blue cupric hydroxide to an insoluble yellow or red cuprous oxide. If no carbohydrate is present in the urine, the cupric hydroxide when heated is converted to an insoluble black cupric oxide, but the presence of sodium citrate in the reagent prevents this spontaneous reduction:

$$Cu\!\!\begin{array}{c} \diagup OH \\ \diagdown OH \end{array} \rightarrow CuO + H_2O$$
cupric oxide
(black)

cupric hydroxide
(blue)

Reaction in absence of reducing agent

$$2Cu\!\!\begin{array}{c} \diagup OH \\ \diagdown OH \end{array} \rightarrow Cu_2O + 2H_2O + O$$
cuprous oxide
(yellow red)

Reaction in presence of reducing agent

Reagent

(A) Dissolve by heat 173 g sodium citrate and 100 g anhydrous sodium carbonate in about 600 ml distilled water. (B) 17.3 g copper sulphate ($CuSO_4.5H_2O$) are dissolved in about 100 ml of distilled water and then added slowly, with stirring, to solution (A). When cool, transfer to a 1 litre volumetric flask and dilute to the mark with distilled water.

Method

Into a test-tube place 0.5 ml urine, followed by 5 ml of Benedict's reagent. Mix well and place in boiling water bath for 5 min. Allow to cool, then observe any colour change due to precipitation of cuprous oxide. Phosphate precipitation may produce a white, turbid appearance, which may be ignored.

If the solution appears green, due to the suspension of a yellow precipitate in a blue solution, report reducing substances present as 'a trace'. If the solution shows a yellow tinge, report result as +, an orange precipitate as + +, and a brick-red precipitate as + + +.

■ **Notes**

1. Benedict's quantitative reagent must not be used in place of the qualitative reagent above.
2. Other reducible reagents have been devised, for example, those containing bismuth, but these are not widely used.
3. Benedict's copper reduction method has been adapted for use by the diabetic patient in his own home. Using a standard dropper, 5 drops of urine, 10 drops of water, and a tablet containing copper sulphate and NaOH are added to a test-tube. The heat evolved by the solution of the caustic soda boils the mixture and any glucose present reduces the copper sulphate to cuprous oxide, the colour of which is compared with a standard colour chart. This is known as the Clinitest.

Identification of reducing substances

Benedict's qualitative reagent will reveal the presence of a number of reducing substances, and it is important to identify the reducing substance.

1. Commercial test strips

There are two main organizations which supply test strips for detecting glucose—Ames and BCL—the principle of both tests being basically similar.

Clinistix reagent strips (Ames)

These reagent strips are a quick, simple, qualitative colour test to detect the presence of glucose only in urine.

Composition

A strip of firm plastic, one end of which is the reagent system, a buffered enzyme preparation and a chromogen system.

Principle

1. Glucose is oxidized by atmospheric oxygen in the presence of glucose oxidase to gluconic acid and hydrogen peroxide.
2. Hydrogen peroxide in the presence of peroxidase oxidizes the chromogen to shades of purple.

Directions

1. Dip test end of the reagent strip in fresh urine and remove immediately or pass briefly through urine stream.
2. 10 s after wetting, compare colour of test area with colour chart. Read the test carefully, in good light and with strip near to colour chart. *Ignore any colour developing after 10 s.*

Interpretation of colour reaction

1. Test end turns purple within 10 s—glucose present.
2. Test end remains cream after 10 s—glucose absent.

Sensitivity

The smallest concentration of glucose in urine which can be detected with the reagent strips ranges from 0.1 to 1 g/litre owing to variations in urinary constituents and pH in different specimens. Ascorbic acid (vitamin C) may decrease the sensitivity of the test. This should be borne in mind when testing the urine of patients receiving therapeutic doses of this vitamin, or parenteral preparations in which ascorbic acid is incorporated as antioxidant, for example, tetracyclines.

Specificity

Glucose oxidase is a specific enzyme for glucose. Thus no substance excreted in urine other than glucose gives a positive result with these reagent strips. In particular, they do not react with other reducing sugars, for example lactose, galactose and fructose, or reducing metabolites of some drugs (e.g. salicylates), as copper reduction methods do. Oxidizing agents such as hydrogen peroxide will give false positive results.

Alternative procedure for use with napkins

The technique is to press the test end of the strip against a freshly wet napkin, remove it when thoroughly wetted, and observe it exactly 1 min later. The result is interpreted as described above.

Test only a really wet napkin, and avoid using one which is contaminated with faeces. Do not leave the strip in contact with the napkin, because of risk of the reagents being dissolved out and because oxygen from the air is necessary to the reaction.

BM-test (glucose) (BCL)

Composition

The test strip has an area impregnated with enzymes, an unstated chromogen and a yellow background dye.

Principle

The same principle applies as for Clinistix.

Directions

1. Dip the test end of the reagent strip in fresh urine and remove immediately.
2. 30–60 s after dipping into the urine, a positive reaction varies from a faint green to a deep blue green, depending upon the concentration of glucose in the urine.

Sensitivity

The smallest concentration of glucose in urine which can be detected with the reagent strips ranges from about 0.6 to 5.5 mmol/l owing to variations in urinary constituents and pH in different specimens. Ascorbic acid (vitamin C) may decrease the sensitivity of the test. This should be borne in mind when testing the urine of patients receiving therapeutic doses of this vitamin, or parenteral preparations in which ascorbic acid is incorporated as anti-oxidant, for example, tetracyclines.

Specificity

The same as for Clinistix.

Alternative procedure for use with napkins

The same as for Clinistix.

Precautions

These apply to both tests:

1. Make sure the container for urine is absolutely clean and free from contaminants, particularly disinfectants and detergents containing oxidizing substances such as hypochlorites and peroxides.
2. Do not touch test end of strip.
3. Recap bottle tightly, as soon as strip has been removed, to avoid uptake of moisture.

2. Seliwanoff's test for fructose

Principle

Fructose, when boiled in the presence of hydrochloric acid, yields a derivative of furfuraldehyde which condenses with resorcinol to form a red coloured compound.

Reagent

Resorcinol	0.05g
Concentrated hydrochloric acid	33 ml
Distilled water	to 100 ml
Stable for about 6 weeks	

Method

Add 0.5 ml urine to 5 ml of the reagent in a test-tube. Mix well and bring to the boil. Treat a normal and positive control urine in the same way.

Results

Fructose gives a red colour in about 30 s. The test is sensitive to 5.5 mmol/l fructose if glucose is absent, but if more than 100 mmol/l of glucose is present, this will also give a red colour on further boiling. Interpretation should therefore be based on colour development time.

3. Bial's test for pentose

Principle

Pentoses, when boiled in the presence of hydrochloric acid, yield aldehydes of furfural type, which in the presence of orcinol condense to form green-coloured compounds.

Reagent

Dissolve 300 mg of orcinol (*m*-dihydroxytoluene) in 100 ml concentrated HCl to which is added 5 drops of 10% ferric chloride. Stable for up to 1 week.

Method

Add 0.5 ml of urine to 5 ml of the reagent in a test-tube. Mix well and place in boiling water bath until liquid begins to boil.

Results

Pentoses give a green colour, with a sensitivity of 6.7 mmol/l. Considerable quantities of pentoses will give a blue/green precipitate. Glucuronates give a similar greenish colour if the boiling is prolonged. Fructose gives a red colour.

4. Fearon's methylamine test for lactose

Principle

Alkaline hydrolysis opens the carbohydrate ring, exposes either the ketone or aldehyde group which is rearranged to form an enediol. Enediol then reacts with the methylamine hydrochloride to form a red-coloured product.

Reagents

0.2% methylamine hydrochloride.
10% sodium hydroxide.

Method

1. To 5 ml urine add 1 ml methylamine solution and 0.2 ml sodium hydroxide solution.
2. Mix by inversion and place tube in a 56°C water bath for 30 min (boiling for 5 min can also be used).
3. Remove tube from bath and allow to cool to room temperature.
4. Compare colour with a 'blank' consisting of the reagents and unheated urine, and a control tube containing water instead of methylamine hydrochloride.

Results

14.6 mmol/l will give an intense red colour in less than 30 min at 56°C, 1.5 mmol/l lactose a slight but definite red colour after standing at room temperature for 20 min. Glucose, fructose, galactose, xylose and sucrose in large amounts give a yellow colour. The only sugars which give a red colour are the reducing disaccharides, lactose and maltose—maltose is not usually found in urine.

Chromatographic identification of urinary sugars

Galactose is found in the urine only very rarely, and the only satisfactory means of confirming its presence is by chromatographic analysis. While paper chromatography can give satisfactory results, thin layer chromatography is quicker and more sensitive.

Thin layer chromatography of sugars

Reagents

1. Solvent mixture *n*-butanol–acetic acid–water 75/25/6, v/v.
2. Aniline–diphenylamine locating agent.
   Solution 1: 1% aniline v/v and 1% diphenylamine w/v in acetone.
   Solution 2: 85% phosphoric acid.
   Before use mix 10 volumes of solution 1 with 1 volume of solution 2.
3. Standards. Prepare standard solutions in 10% aqueous isopropanol so that 5 µl contains 5 µg of sugar. Solutions of glucose, lactose, fructose, galactose and xylose are suggested. After several runs it will be possible for a mixture of the glucose, galactose and lactose to be used as a routine.
4. Silica gel G.
   Purchase precoated 250 µm 20 × 10 cm plates from Merck or Camlab.

Technique

Determine the amount of reducing substance present (see p. 150) and calculate the volume required to be added so that the sample will contain 5–10 µg sugar (usually 2–5 µl).

Apply the required volumes along the point of application at 1 cm intervals, with standards either side of the urine spots. It is not necessary to desalt the urine.

Place the plate in an airtight tank and allow the solvent front to rise 12–15 cm; this usually requires

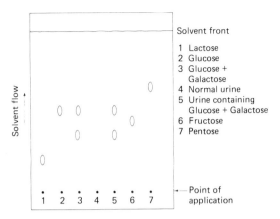

Solvent front
1 Lactose
2 Glucose
3 Glucose + Galactose
4 Normal urine
5 Urine containing Glucose + Galactose
6 Fructose
7 Pentose

Solvent flow

Point of application

1 2 3 4 5 6 7

Figure 10.7. TLC of various sugars

Table 10.3 Approximate R_f values for some sugars

Sugar	Characteristic colour	Approx. R_f
Lactose	grey	0.14
Galactose	grey	0.34
Fructose	pink	0.39
Glucose	grey	0.42
Pentoses	grey brown	>0.5

Table 10.4 Identification of reducing substances

Sugar	Benedict's qualitative reagent	Clinistix or BM-Test (glucose)	Seliwa-noff	Methyl-amine	Bial
Glucose	+	+	−	−	−
Lactose	+	−	−	+	−
Fructose	+	−	+	−	−
Pentose	+	−	−	−	+
Galactose	+	Confirm by chromatography			

2–3 h. Remove the plate from the tank and allow the chromatogram to dry in a fume-cupboard under hot air. Spray with the locating agent and heat for 5 min at 120°C in hot-air oven.

Figure 10.7 shows the position of various sugars and *Table 10.3* shows the approximate R_f values (see p. 88) and characteristic colours obtained with the locating agent. The sensitivity of the method is in the order of 0.1 µg of glucose and it will occasionally detect glucose in normal urine.

The above tests can now be tabulated and the results obtained will be shown in *Table 10.4*.

Glycosuria

Although glucose (and other carbohydrates) is freely filtered through the glomeruli in the kidney, it is almost completely reabsorbed by the renal tubules. The capacity of the tubules to reabsorb glucose is, however, limited, and when the blood glucose concentration rises above about 10.0 mmol/l (renal threshold) the tubules cannot reabsorb all the glucose and therefore glycosuria occurs. The reabsorptive capacity of the tubules varies from person to person and with age.

Glucose (glycosuria)

With rare exceptions, glucose is the only carbohydrate found in the urine in pathological conditions. The most important of these is diabetes mellitus, when as much as 280 mmol/l of glucose can be found in the urine. Glycosuria can also occur in endocrine hyperactivity and severe liver disease.

Lactose (lactosuria)

This is sometimes found in the urine towards the end of pregnancy and during lactation. The condition is harmless and it is important that a positive test for reducing substances during pregnancy is further investigated to ensure it is lactose and not glucose.

Fructose (fructosuria)

Found in the urine after eating fruits, honey, jams. If glucose is found as well, it is indicative of diabetes. Fructose can also be found in the urine in a rare metabolic condition, due to a congenital defect—'essential fructosuria'. Fructosuria is a harmless condition, but it must be identified and not wrongly classified as diabetes.

Galactose (galactosuria)

This is a very rare condition occurring in infants, due to a deficiency of an enzyme, galactose-1-phosphate uridyl transferase, which catalyses the conversion of galactose-1-phosphate to glucose-1-phosphate. It is important that galactose is identified as quickly as possible after birth, as the child must be placed on a galactose-free diet. The accumulation of galactose in brain tissue will mentally retard the infant.

Galactose can also be found in the urine after taking large amounts of galactose or lactose; in this case galactosuria is harmless.

Pentose (pentosuria)

Occurs under similar conditions to fructose.

Sucrose (sucrosuria)

Sucrose can be found in the urine of some infants, usually with gastrointestinal disorders, or adults with pancreatitis. Sucrose does not reduce Benedict's solution, but acid hydrolysis of sucrose will convert it into glucose and fructose, both of which will give a positive test for reducing substances.

Precautions to be adopted when using commercial test strips or reagent tablets

1. Accurate and reliable results are dependent upon strict observance of the manufacturers' directions and careful following of recommended procedures for handling and testing.
2. The specimen container must be absolutely clean and free from contaminants, e.g. antiseptics or detergents.
3. Do not acidify the specimen prior to using strips or reagents.
4. Fresh specimens of urine should be tested whenever possible because chemical changes may take place on storage. Please note the remarks on preservatives given for individual tests.
5. Remember that when using test strips they should be dipped into the urine cleanly and quickly and, where applicable, they must be compared with the colour blocks provided at the times stated.
6. All commercial test strips or reagent tablets involve colour reactions and it is not necessary to filter the urine before testing. Always replace the cap tightly immediately after use and keep away from excessive heat and moisture. Keep at room temperature. Do not store in a refrigerator or above 30°C.
7. Deterioration of reagent strips results in a brownish discoloration of the test area. When this occurs the strips should not be used.

Before commencing examination of the specimen, the following points should be noted:

Appearance

Note colour of specimen	e.g. straw, amber, red, black, etc.
Note nature of deposit	e.g. pus, blood, etc.
Note any odour that may be present	e.g. acetone, ammonia

Specific gravity. Measure specific gravity. If there is insufficient urine to float hydrometer, either (a) use a narrow container, or (b) after chemical testing dilute the urine with an equal quantity of water and double the last two figures of the hydrometer reading.

For further information regarding colour reactions and precautions see *Aids to Diagnosis—A Short Technical Manual*, published by Ames. BCL will also have similar information. Both organizations supply multiple test systems as well as individual test strips. Ames, however, produce a Multistix SG strip which measures the sp. gr. of the urine based on the pK_a change of certain preheated polyelectrolytes in relation to ionic concentrations.

In the presence of an indicator, colours range from deep blue-green in urine of low ionic concentration, through green and yellow-green in urines of increasing ionic concentration. N-Multistix SG strips (Ames) test for sp. gr., pH, protein, glucose, ketone, bilirubin, blood, nitrite and urobilinogen in urine. The Combur 8 Test (BCL) tests for pH, protein, glucose, ketone, urobilinogen, bilirubin, blood and nitrite in urine.

All these combined test strips give reactions which are identical to the single test strips, some of which are included in this chapter and in Chapter 9.

Ketones

In diabetes mellitus, if there is a depression of carbohydrate metabolism, or in starvation, there is an increased oxidation of fat to provide energy. Under these conditions the liver yields acetoacetic acid, some of which is decarboxylated to give acetone and some reduced to β-hydroxybutyric acid. This results in the accumulation of ketone bodies in the blood (ketonaemia), some of which are excreted in the urine (ketonuria).

Ketone bodies

1. $CH_3CO.CH_2COOH$
   acetoacetic acid
2. $CH_3CHOH.CH_2COOH$
   β-hydroxybutyric acid formed from the reduction of acetoacetic acid
3. $CH_3CO.CH_3$
   acetone formed in the body from acetoacetic acid by the loss of carbon dioxide.

It is important to test for these substances as part of the routine urine examination of diabetic patients.

Acetoacetic acid

Gerhardt's test

Principle

Ferric chloride reacts with many substances to give characteristic colours, one of which is acetoacetic acid.

Reagents

10% ferric chloride.

Method

1. Add the ferric chloride solution drop by drop to 5 ml of urine in a test-tube.
2. A red or purplish colour is given by acetoacetic acid.
3. When the urine contains a large amount of phosphate, a precipitate of ferric phosphate is produced.

4. Filter or centrifuge the urine and add a few more drops of ferric chloride to the clear sample.

Salicylates

A similar colour is given by salicylates and they can be differentiated from acetoacetic acid by their behaviour on heating. If the urine is boiled, acetoacetic acid loses carbon dioxide and is converted into acetone. Acetone will not give a positive reaction with ferric chloride. Salicylates, on the other hand, are unaffected by boiling:

$$CH_3CO.CH_2COOH \rightarrow CH_3.CO.CH_3 + CO_2 \uparrow$$

If the heating is carried out after adding the ferric chloride, the acetoacetic acid colour will disappear, while the salicylate colour persists.

Rothera's nitroprusside test

Principle

Nitroprusside in alkaline solution reacts with a ketone group to form a purple colour.

Reagents

Ammonium sulphate, sodium nitroprusside and concentrated ammonia.

Method

1. Saturate about 5 ml of urine with ammonium sulphate and add a small crystal of sodium nitroprusside.
2. Mix well and then add 0.5 ml of concentrated ammonia.
3. A purple colour indicates the presence of acetoacetic acid, acetone, or both, and is maximal in 15 min.
4. The rate of colour development is a better quantitative guide than the intensity of colour. The reaction is more sensitive than Gerhardt's test for acetoacetic acid and is less sensitive with acetone than it is with acetoacetic acid.

Modifications

Several workers have modified the test by using a powdered reagent:

1. Mix 100 parts of ammonium sulphate and 1 part of sodium nitroprusside and use this for saturating the urine. Mix well and then add the concentrated ammonia.
2. Prepare a powdered mixture of 1 g fine sodium nitroprusside, 20 g ammonium sulphate and 20 g anhydrous sodium carbonate. The powder is mixed completely and if kept dry will keep for at least 1 year. A small pinch of powder is placed on a white tile; add one drop of urine and note colour development. Acetone and acetoacetic acid will give a violet colour.

Acetest

This is Rothera's test in a tablet form.

Composition

The tablet contains sodium nitroprusside, aminoacetic acid (glycine), lactose and disodium phosphate.

Principle

The ketone group of acetone and acetoacetic acid react with sodium nitroprusside at the optimum alkaline pH provided by the buffer system to give a lavender or purple colour. Lactose enhances the colour.

Directions

1. Place the reagent tablet on a clean white surface, preferably a piece of filter paper.
2. Put one drop of urine on tablet.
3. Compare colour of tablet with colour chart exactly 30 s later.

Interpretation of colour reaction

1. Tablet turns lavender or purple within 30 s— ketones present.
2. Tablet remains white at 30 s (or turns cream)— ketones absent.

Precautions

1. Make sure that container for urine is absolutely clean and free from contaminants, for example acids, disinfectants and detergents.
2. Test only fresh specimens if possible; refrigeration is required if the specimen has to be kept.
3. Recap the bottle tightly as soon as a tablet has been removed, to avoid uptake of moisture.

Sensitivity

In ketosis, the urine contains a considerable preponderance of the acetoacetic acid over acetone. The sensitivity to acetoacetic acid is 1.0 mmol/l and acetone 4 mmol/l. As the tablets are supposed to have a greater sensitivity for the acetoacetic acid, the colour produced is almost entirely due to that acid.

Specificity

The only substance besides acetone and acetoacetic acid likely to be present in the urine which is known to give colours with these tablets is phenolsulphonphthalein (used occasionally in renal function tests). The colour is not the same as those shown on the colour chart, but it can be mistaken for it.

Commercial test strips

The two commercial test strips for ketones are made by Ames (Ketostix) and BCL (Ketur Test). They are both plastic strips, one end of which is impregnated with a buffered mixture of sodium nitroprusside and glycine.

Ketostix

Principle

As for the Acetest, except there is no lactose in this strip.

Directions

1. Dip test end of the reagent strip in fresh specimen and remove immediately, or pass briefly through urine stream.
2. Briefly touch tip of strip on container to remove excess liquid.
3. Compare colour of test end with colour chart exactly 15 s later.

Interpretation of colour reaction

1. Test end turns lavender or purple within 15 s— ketones present.
2. Test end remains off-white at 15 s—ketones absent.

Ketur Test

This is used in the same way as Ketostix, except that comparison with the colour chart is made 30–60 s later.

Precautions

1. Make sure that container for specimen is absolutely clean and free from contaminants, for example acids, disinfectants and detergents.
2. Test only fresh specimens if possible; refrigeration is required if specimen has to be kept.
3. Do not touch test end of strip.
4. Recap the bottle tightly immediately after removing a strip to avoid uptake of moisture. Do not remove desiccant.
5. Do not leave strip in specimen to avoid risk of dissolving out reagents.

Sensitivity

The Ketostix and Ketur Test are sensitive to 1.0 mmol/l of acetoacetic acid and 13 mmol/l and 7 mmol/l of acetone, respectively.

Specificity

Besides acetoacetic acid and acetone, phenylketones, bromosulphthalein, phenolsulphonphthalein and phenolphthalein will also turn the strip shades of red or purple which, while not matching the chart, could cause confusion.

Phenylpyruvic acid (phenylketonuria)

On the addition of ferric chloride solution to the urine in phenylketonuria, a green or blue colour is obtained, which fades in a few minutes to a yellowish colour. This is a rare condition and must be reported immediately. Phenylketonuria is an inborn error of metabolism, whereby the body is unable to convert phenylalanine to tyrosine by its usual enzymatic pathways.

Phenylalanine accumulates in the blood, urine and CSF; transamination converts the phenylalanine into phenylpyruvic acid, which is excreted in the urine as early as two to three weeks after birth. Early recognition of phenylpyruvic acid is important, as dietary control is necessary to prevent the infant from becoming mentally retarded.

Phenistix

Phenistix are used for detecting the presence of phenylpyruvic acid and *p*-aminosalicylic acid (PAS).

Composition

The test area of the strip is impregnated with ferric ammonium sulphate, magnesium sulphate, and cyclohexylsulphamic acid.

Principle

Ferric ions at a suitable pH react with phenylketones (notably phenylpyruvic acid) to give a greyish-green colour, and with PAS and its metabolites to give a brownish-red colour. The desired acidity (pH 2.3) is provided by cyclohexylsulphamic acid, and the magnesium salt minimizes interference by phosphates.

Directions

1. Press test end of strip against freshly wet napkin (not merely damp), or dip in urine and remove immediately, so as to avoid dissolving out test reagents.
2. Compare colour of test end with colour chart

exactly 30 s later, read in good light and ignore any colour developing after 30 s.

Interpretation of colour reactions

1. Test end turns greyish-green within 30 s—phenylpyruvic acid positive.
2. Test end turns off-white or cream within 30 s—phenylpyruvic acid negative.
3. When the test end turns brownish-red at once, this indicates the presence of ingested PAS.

Precautions

1. Do not leave strip in contact with wet napkin or urine to avoid risk of dissolving out reagents. For same reason also do not place strip in dry napkin and read it when this has been used.
2. Phenylpyruvic acid decomposes on standing, especially in a warm atmosphere, therefore:
   (a) Always test *fresh* urine.
   (b) Use only a really wet napkin; a partially dried one or one that has been rewetted with water gives unreliable results.
   (c) Do not use a napkin contaminated with faeces; certain faecal bacteria specifically and rapidly destroy phenylpyruvic acid.
   (d) Do not leave the strip to be read some time later; a positive result will fade.
3. Do not touch test end of strip. Recap bottle tightly as soon as strip has been removed.

Sensitivity

0.5–0.6 mmol/l.

Specificity

The test may be unreliable, particularly if carried out on napkins. Cases are also occasionally missed because of the instability of phenylpyruvic acid when using alkaline urines. The test is not specific for phenylpyruvic acid, as the following substances also give a positive reaction: PAS, *p*-hydroxyphenylpyruvic acid, imidazolepyruvic acid, tetracycline and a few phenothiazine tranquillizers or their metabolites.

A further disadvantage is that since phenylpyruvic acid only appears in the urine from about 2–3 weeks after birth, the test is usually done at 4–6 weeks. Since treatment should begin as soon as possible to prevent brain damage, the methods for detecting the presence of an increased level of plasma phenylalanine, i.e. the ferric chloride and Phenistix tests, should no longer be used. Chromatographic methods or the Guthrie Bacterial Inhibition Assay technique are far better. The chromatographic methods will also detect the presence of other amino-acid abnormalities and these procedures are now favoured by an increasing number of scientific workers.

β-Hydroxybutyric acid

There is no test in everyday use for this ketone. Although it occurs together with the other ketones, it can be tested for by boiling the urine at an acid pH to remove the acetone and acetoacetic acid. The β-hydroxybutyric acid is oxidized to acetoacetic acid with hydrogen peroxide and then tested with Rothera's reagent. A positive reaction indicates the presence of β-hydroxybutyric acid in the urine.

Multiple test strips

These are reagent test strips combining rapid convenient tests for pH, blood, glucose, ketones, bilirubin and urobilinogen produced by Ames (Multistix) or BCL (BM-Test 7). Other combinations are also available, such as the Labstix (Ames) and BM-Test 5L (BCL); further information can be obtained from the manufacturers.

Quantitative blood and urine analysis

In certain diseases it may be essential to estimate quantitatively constituents in blood and urine to help with a diagnostic problem or treatment.

Urine glucose

In the majority of cases sufficient information is obtainable from qualitative tests for glucose, but if an estimate of the amount of glucose lost daily is required then a 24-h sample of urine is collected and the glucose content estimated accurately, using any of the blood glucose methods described in Chapter 8. If these methods are used, the urine needs diluting in order to bring the concentration of glucose to within the range of the method to be adopted. Benedict's quantitative reagent was formerly used to estimate the total amount of reducing substance in urine, but this method has now been superseded. The best value to aim for is about 20 mmol/l glucose, the dilution of which can be gauged from the qualitative tests. Semi-quantitative results can be obtained with the Clinistix or BM-Test glucose test strips. When using glucose oxidase methods, it is necessary to remove interfering substances by using 0.5 g activated charcoal per 10 ml of urine or appropriate dilution. Mix for 1–2 min, stand for 15 min, centrifuge or filter and then use an appropriate aliquot for glucose estimations.

Urine proteins

In renal disease or other diseases affecting renal

function, the estimation of urinary proteins may be of considerable importance. The increased excretion of proteins in the urine may be the result of changes in the glomeruli, thereby allowing increased passage of proteins, which is called glomerular proteinuria, or of impaired reabsorption of protein in the tubules, when it is called tubular proteinuria.

Turbidimetric method

This method is similar to that given for cerebrospinal fluid protein (Chapter 11). It may be necessary to centrifuge or filter the urine before analysis. A blank consisting of 1 ml urine plus 4 ml 0.9% sodium chloride must be put through the assay each time. Subtract the blank absorbance from the test absorbance before working out the concentration.

Colorimetric method (Biuret reaction)

Principle

Alkaline copper solution reacts with the peptide bonds in the protein molecule, producing a violet colour which is directly proportional to the amount of protein present.

Reagents

1. 20% trichloracetic acid.
2. 1M sodium hydroxide, 40 g per litre of water.
3. Standard protein solution: 5.0 g/l in 0.90% NaCl. Store distributed into small volumes below −18°C. The standard can be prepared from diluted pooled serum, or by making suitable dilutions of commercial control serum. The protein content of the standard should be checked beforehand against a standard solution of accurately known protein nitrogen content (Armour's standard protein solution).
4. Stock Biuret reagent. Dissolve 45 g of sodium potassium tartrate in approximately 400 ml of 0.2M NaOH. Add with constant stirring 15 g copper sulphate ($CuSO_4.5H_2O$); when in solution add 5 g of KI and dilute to 1 litre with 0.2M NaOH.
5. Working Biuret solution. Dilute 200 ml of stock solution to 1 litre with 0.2M NaOH containing 5 g KI per litre.

Method

Test:
1. To 1 or 2 ml of urine add an equal volume of trichloracetic acid.
2. Mix well and allow to stand for a few minutes.
3. Centrifuge.
4. Decant the supernatant fluid without disturbing the deposit.

5. Dissolve the precipitated protein in 1 ml of 1M NaOH.
6. Add 2 ml of distilled water.

Blank: 3 ml of distilled water.
Standard: 3.0 ml of standard protein solution.

To all three tubes add 5 ml of working Biuret reagent, mix thoroughly and place them in the 37°C water bath for 10 min. After colour development allow the tubes to cool and compare the absorbances in the photoelectric absorptiometer, using a green filter or absorbance at 540–560 nm. Use the blank to zero the instrument.

Calculation

Grams protein per litre of urine are found by the following system:

$$\frac{\text{Absorbance of test}}{\text{Absorbance of standard}} \times \text{Strength of standard} \times \frac{100}{\text{Amount of urine taken}}$$

Let absorbance of test = 0.25 and absorbance of standard = 0.50. The standard protein solution contained 5.0 g/litre, so 3 ml of protein solution will contain 0.015 g protein. If 2.0 ml of urine was used in the precipitation stage, then:

$$\text{g protein/litre} = \frac{0.25}{0.50} \times \frac{0.015 \times 1000}{2} = 3.75$$

24 h excretion of protein may be required when following the treatment of nephrotic patients.

Urine chlorides

The measurement of chloride in urine is not often requested, but when required the most convenient method is the coulometric procedure described in Chapter 6, p. 81. As the chloride excretion can vary, depending upon dietary conditions, the volume of urine taken for the estimation may have to be adjusted accordingly; the appropriate factor must then be incorporated into the calculation.

The average adult excretes about 200 mmol of sodium chloride per day, but this value is greatly influenced by the salt content of the diet. Urinary chloride determinations do not always reflect the true chloride balance of the body. After surgical operations a reduced chloride excretion may be found in cases of hyperchloraemia, while patients with hypochloraemia may excrete a lot of chloride (see also Sweat Tests in Chapter 8).

Urea

Urea is one of the end products of protein

metabolism. It is formed in the liver from deaminated amino acids, most probably by way of the ornithine–arginine cycle. The enzyme arginase is found in large quantities in the liver:

Any excess urea in the circulation is eliminated from the blood stream by the kidneys and passes out into the urine.

In health, blood always contains some urea; the level varies, but ranges from 2.5 to 8.3 mmol/l for a normal person on a full ordinary diet. In the elderly, values slightly higher than these are found, even without significant renal dysfunction. In general, a blood urea of over 8.3 mmol/l is suggestive of impaired renal function.

As urea is one of the principal end products of protein metabolism, it follows that the urea content of the blood and urea is influenced over a period of time by the amount of protein in the diet. People on low-protein diets tend to have lower blood ureas.

Urea diffuses very readily through body fluids. For this reason, similar results are obtained if the estimation is carried out on whatever samples are most readily available; for example, cerebrospinal fluid, oedema fluid, plasma, serum or whole blood.

The estimation of blood urea is valuable not only in cases of renal failure, but in a wide variety of conditions which are not primarily renal. Less frequent causes of raised blood urea are diarrhoea and vomiting, and circulatory failure. In childhood and pregnancy, low values are often found.

Blood urea estimation

Collection of samples

The estimation can be carried out on whole blood, plasma or serum. Any of the routine anticoagulants may be used, except the following:

1. Sodium fluoride, generally not used as an anticoagulant, but as an enzyme inhibitor, and therefore unsuitable for urease methods.
2. Ammonium oxalate, which must never be used, as most of the routine methods depend upon the measurement of ammonia.

Principles of blood urea determination

1. One of the methods of estimating urea is based on the action of the enzyme urease, which decomposes urea to form ammonium carbonate:

$$H_2N \!\!\diagdown \!\! C=O \xrightarrow[+\,enzyme]{+H_2O} 2NH_3 + CO_2$$

urea

$$\xrightarrow{+H_2O} (NH_4)_2CO_3 \quad \text{ammonium carbonate}$$

The ammonia produced may be measured either by using Nessler's reagent or by the phenol–hypochlorite reaction.

2. When urea is heated with diacetyl monoxime a coloured compound is formed which is used as the basis of its estimation. This is a direct method which does not depend upon the enzyme urease, and there is no interference from ammonia or acetone.
3. The phenol–hypochlorite reaction is better known as the Berthelot reaction, a more sensitive technique than Nessler's reaction, giving a more stable colour and obeying Beer's law.

Estimation of blood urea using the Berthelot reaction

Principle

The ammonia formed from the enzyme reaction as described above reacts with phenol in the presence of hypochloride to form indophenol which in an alkaline medium gives a blue-coloured compound. Nitroprusside in the phenol reagent acts as a catalyst, thereby increasing the speed of the reaction, the intensity of the colour obtained and its reproducibility.

Reagents

1. Urea solution, 20 mmol/l (1.2 g/l).
2. Phenol–sodium nitroprusside solution, 50 g phenol analytical reagent (AR) and 0.25 g sodium nitroprusside per litre. Dilute 1 to 5 for use.
3. Sodium hydroxide–sodium hypochlorite solution. Sodium hypochlorite solution is available commercially containing 10–14% w/v available chlorine. If the solution contained 10% w/v available chlorine, then 210 ml would be diluted to 1 litre. Taking the mid-part of its concentration to be 12%, then 175 ml of hypochlorite is diluted in 1 litre. This will give approximately 2.1 g of available chlorine per litre. The method can withstand a ± 20% variation in concentration without affecting the result.
   25 g of sodium hydroxide and 2.1 g hypochlorite per litre. Dilute 1 to 5 for use.
   Solutions 2 and 3 keep at least 2 months in the refrigerator in amber bottles.
4. Buffered urease solution. Dissolve 100 mg urease Type III powder (Sigma Chemical Co.) in about

90 ml of a solution containing 1 g sodium EDTA, adjust the pH to 6.5 and dilute to 100 ml with distilled water. Store in the refrigerator for up to 4 weeks.

Method

Test: 20 µl serum or plasma.
Blank: 20 µl 0.9% NaCl.
Standard: 20 µl urea standard.

To each tube add 200 µl urease buffer and incubate at 37°C for 15 min. To all tubes add 5 ml phenol–nitroprusside solution. Mix well, then add 5 ml hypochloride reagent. Mix again and place in 37°C water bath for 15 min. After 15 min, measure the absorbance of the test and standard against the blank at 630 nm.

Calculation

Serum, plasma urea

$$= \frac{\text{Absorbance of test}}{\text{Absorbance of standard}} \times 20 = \text{mmol/l}$$

Preparation of calibration curve

Serum urea (mmol/l)	0	5	10	15	20	25	30
ml standard urea (20 mmol/l)	0	1	2	3	4	5	6
ml water			10	9	8	7	6	5	4

Mix thoroughly and estimate 200 µl of each solution in the same way as described above.

Estimation of blood urea using diacetyl monoxime

Reagents

1. Trichloracetic acid (TCA)—dissolve 100 g in distilled water and dilute to 1 litre.
2. Stock diacetyl monoxime—dissolve 25 g in distilled water and dilute to 1 litre.
3. Stock thiosemicarbazide, 2.5 g/l distilled water.
4. Acid ferric chloride solution. To a 50 g/litre aqueous ferric chloride solution add very carefully 1 ml concentrated sulphuric acid.
5. Acid reagent. Add 10 ml orthophosphoric acid (sp. gr. 1.75), 80 ml concentrated sulphuric acid and 10 ml acid ferric chloride to 1 litre of distilled water. Allow to cool and mix well.

6. Colour reagent. To 300 ml acid reagent add 200 ml distilled water, 10 ml solution 2 and 2.5 ml solution 3. Mix well and allow to cool.
7. Urea standards, 10 mmol/l.

Method

Test: 0.2 ml blood, serum or plasma.
Blank: 0.2 ml water.
Standard: 0.2 ml standard.

To all tubes add 1 ml water and 1 ml TCA. Mix well and centrifuge. Remove 0.2 ml from each tube and add to 3 ml colour reagent. Mix well and place in the boiling water bath for 20 min. Cool to room temperature. Read absorbance of test and standard against the blank at 520 nm within 15 min. If Beer's law is obeyed, the following calculation can be used.

Calculation

Urea concentration

$$= \frac{\text{Absorbance of test}}{\text{Absorbance of standard}} \times 10 = \text{mmol/l}$$

To confirm that Beer's law is obeyed, prepare the following calibration curve, using the method described above, and the following urea standards:

0, 5, 10, 15, 20, 30, 40 and 50 mmol/l

Urine urea

It is often necessary to know the urea concentration in urine, either on a single specimen or as part of a timed collection. This can be an important estimation in cases of renal failure. As urine urea is greatly in excess of the blood level, the estimation can be performed by a similar method as those for blood analysis after first diluting the urine about 1 in 20 with water or isotonic saline.

Urine excretion in a normal adult is about 500 mmol per day or approximately 330 mmol/l. The excretion, however, depends upon the protein content of the diet. A low-protein diet results in low urea excretion, while a high-protein diet is accompanied by a high urea excretion. Urine urea estimations were most commonly carried out as part of urea clearance and concentration tests, but these tests have now been replaced by a far better parameter, the creatinine clearance test. This estimation measures very closely the glomerular filtration rate of the kidney.

11

Chemical analysis of cerebrospinal fluid

Examination of the cerebrospinal fluid (CSF) is used in the clinical investigation of the central nervous system, which consists of the brain, spinal cord and peripheral nerves.

The brain is about one-fiftieth of the body weight and lies within the cranial cavity. It is divided structurally into the cerebrum (greater brain), the brain stem consisting of the midbrain, pons varolii and medulla oblongata, and lastly the cerebellum or lesser brain (*Figure 11.1*). The four irregularly shaped ventricles, namely the right and left lateral, and third and fourth ventricle, play an important part in the formation of CSF (*Figure 11.2*). Completely surrounding the brain and spinal cord are three membranes known as dura mater (outer membrane), the arachnoid mater (middle membrane) and pia mater (the inner membrane). The pia mater and arachnoid mater are separated from each other by the subarachnoid space. Between the tough

outer coat (dura mater) and arachnoid mater is the subdural space containing a small amount of tissue fluid (*Figure 11.3*).

Formation of CSF

Within the lateral ventricles are the choroid plexuses, where the CSF is formed. They are a network of complex capillaries projecting into the ventricular cavities, covered only by the pia mater and a single layer of cells lining the ventricular system of the brain. The CSF formed by the choroid plexuses passes into the third ventricle via the interventricular foramen (foramen of Monro), then by the aqueduct of the midbrain into the fourth ventricle. From the roof of the fourth ventricle the CSF flows through the foramina into the subarachnoid space to completely surround the brain and spinal cord. At the same time, CSF also flows from

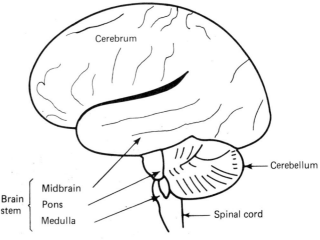

Figure 11.1. The major divisions of the brain

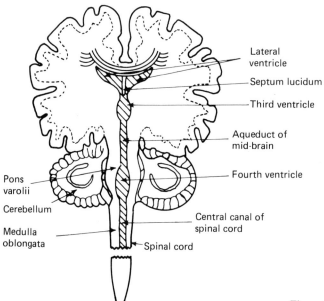

Lateral ventricle

Septum lucidum

Third ventricle

Aqueduct of mid-brain

Fourth ventricle

Pons varolii

Cerebellum

Central canal of spinal cord

Medulla oblongata

Spinal cord

Figure 11.2. Ventricles of the brain, anterior view

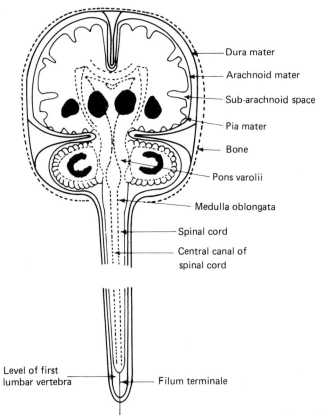

Dura mater

Arachnoid mater

Sub-arachnoid space

Pia mater

Bone

Pons varolii

Medulla oblongata

Spinal cord

Central canal of spinal cord

Level of first lumbar vertebra

Filum terminale

Figure 11.3. The meninges of the brain and spinal cord

the floor of the fourth ventricle downwards through the central canal of the spinal cord. The production of CSF is balanced by an equal absorption of fluid, the reabsorption probably taking place in the blood capillaries of the arachnoid mater. By this process the total volume of CSF will be completely returned to the circulating blood every 6–8 h.

Function of CSF

1. Supports and protects the delicate structures of the brain and spinal cord.
2. Acts as a cushion and shock absorber.
3. Used as a reservoir to regulate the contents of the cranium, i.e. if the volume of the brain or blood increases, CSF drains away; if the brain shrinks, more fluid is retained.
4. Keeps the brain and spinal cord moist.
5. May act as a medium for the interchange of metabolic substances between nerve cells and CSF.

Obtaining CSF

Specimens of CSF are obtained by introducing a long needle between the third and fourth lumbar vertebrae into the spinal subarachnoid space, with the patient's back flexed to separate the vertebrae. The cord comes to an end at the level of the first lumbar vertebra and cannot be damaged by the needle entering the subarachnoid space an inch or so lower.

A lumbar puncture is far safer than a cisternal puncture, which involves passing the needle between the occipital bone and the atlas into the cisterna magna at the base of the brain.

Composition of CSF

The volume of CSF averages between 120 and 150 ml, and is produced at the rate of about 0.3 ml per min (430 ml/day). It consists of water, dissolved oxygen and a number of solids. The sp. gr. is about 1.005, pH 7.4–7.6, and it contains up to 5 lymphocytes per mm^3. It is a clear colourless fluid and should show no coagulum or sediment on standing. The composition is very similar to that of plasma, except in protein concentration (*Table 11.1*). CSF can therefore be considered an ultra-filtrate of blood.

A sample of CSF sent to the laboratory for routine examination requires the following investigations: appearance, cell count, total protein, globulin, chloride and glucose. In place of the Lange colloidal gold curve and electrophoresis, which is required in certain hospitals, the estimation of the specific globulin IgG to that of albumin is a far better parameter to determine.

The diagnostic importance of CSF examination lies in the cytological and chemical changes produced by certain diseases. Normal ranges and values obtained in various conditions can be seen in *Table 11.2*.

All examinations should be carried out as soon as possible after the specimen is taken. If delay is unavoidable the specimen should be placed in a refrigerator at between 2 and 10°C and dealt with at the earliest opportunity. Place a small amount of the CSF in a sodium fluoride tube to prevent glycolysis.

Pathological variations and methods of estimation

Appearance

The presence of blood is the main cause of an abnormal colour.

1. Blood

(a) Trauma—while collecting the CSF, some blood may be introduced as a result of trauma; in this

Table 11.1 Composition of CSF

	Plasma	CSF
Total protein	6–8 g/l	0.15–0.45 g/l
Glucose	3.0–5.3 mmol/l	2.8–4.4 mmol/l
Chlorides (as NaCl)	96–106 mmol/l	120–130 mmol/l

Table 11.2 Changes in CSF in various conditions

Condition	Appearance	No./type of leucocytes per mm^3	Protein (g/l)	Globulin	Chlorides (mmol/l)	Glucose (mmol/l)
Normal	Clear and colourless	Up to 5 lymphocytes	0.15–0.45	No increase	120–130	2.8–4.4
Tubercular meningitis	Clear or slightly turbid	Increased lymphocytes and polymorphs	Markedly increased	Increased	85–120	Less than 2.8
Subarachnoid haemorrhage	May be bloodstained and/or yellow	Normal or increased lymphocytes	Increased	Increased	120–130	2.8–4.4
Xanthochromia	Yellow	Normal or increased lymphocytes	Normal or increased	No increase or increased	120–130	2.8–4.4

case the first few ml should be collected separately, and the subsequent fluid should be almost, if not completely, clear. Centrifuging will reveal the presence of a small number of red cells.

(b) Subarachnoid haemorrhage—the CSF will be heavily bloodstained. Furthermore, haemolysis of red cells occurs, liberating haemoglobin, which will eventually be converted into bilirubin. If the CSF is taken a few days after the haemorrhage, the supernatant fluid will be coloured yellow and xanthochromia is present.

2. Turbidity

Turbidity is usually due to an increase in leucocytes or leucocytes plus organisms. Leucocytes may reach about 400 per mm^3 before the fluid appears turbid. In TB meningitis, the fluid, as a rule, is not turbid. For the types of organisms present in CSF see Chapter 27.

3. Coagulum

A fibrin clot may form on standing in pathological specimens containing enough fibrinogen. This usually indicates that the protein concentration is greater than 1.0 g/l, but a coagulum can form with a lower protein concentration. Sometimes in TB meningitis a fine web-like clot will form; this usually contains the tubercle bacilli, revealed on microscopic examination.

4. Cell count

The cells in CSF are counted by using a Fuchs–Rosenthal counting chamber (see Chapter 31, p. 322).

Protein

Turbidimetric methods are the most commonly used techniques for the estimation of total protein, although a colorimetric method is available. In the colorimetric technique, CSF is treated with alkaline copper tartrate to form cupric–amino acid complexes. On the addition of phosphomolybdotungstic acid (Folin and Ciocalteau's phenol reagent), the complexes form an intense blue colour due to the reduction of molybdate to molybdenum oxides. The coloured complex is then compared against standard protein solution similarly treated.

Turbidimetric procedures

Principle

Proteins in CSF are precipitated by either dilute trichloracetic acid or dilute sulphosalicylic acid in

sodium sulphate solution, and the turbidity of the resultant uniform suspension is measured spectrophotometrically against a standard solution similarly treated.

Methods

A. Trichloracetic acid method

Reagents
1. 3% aqueous w/v trichloracetic acid solution.
2. Stock standard protein solution, 5.0 g/l, as prepared on p. 158.
3. Working standard protein solution, 0.5 g/l. Dilute stock standard 1 in 10 with 0.9% NaCl (saline). Prepare fresh each week and store in about 1.5 ml quantities at about −18°C. Thaw a sample for use each day.

Technique
1. *Test:* Add 1.0 ml of CSF dropwise with constant mixing to exactly 4.0 ml trichloracetic acid.
2. *Standard:* Mix 1.0 ml of standard protein solution in the same manner with exactly 4.0 ml trichloracetic acid.
3. *Blank:* Mix 1.0 ml distilled water with 4.0 ml trichloracetic acid.
4. After standing at room temperature for 10 min, remix the turbid solutions.
5. Read the absorbance of the standard and test against the blank at 450 nm or by using a blue filter.

Calculation
T = test reading, S = standard reading, and since the test and standard are treated in the same manner:

$$\frac{T}{S} \times 0.5 = \text{g CSF protein per litre}$$

e.g.

$$T = 0.20 \qquad S = 0.25$$

$$\frac{0.20}{0.25} \times 0.5 = 0.4\,\text{g protein per litre}$$

■ Notes

1. If the value of the unknown exceeds the upper limit of the method as established by a calibration curve, repeat the determination by using an appropriate saline dilution of the CSF.
2. A calibration curve will show whether a linear relationship holds for increasing protein concentration and should be constructed for each photometric instrument.
3. A standard method of mixing the tubes (5 times) should be used as in turbidimetric methods; the size and shape of the particles depend on this and thus the absorbance reading.
4. Standard diameter tubes *must* be used, as the method is temperature dependent and the calibration curve would vary accordingly.

Preparation of standard calibration curve

Dilute the stock standard protein (5 g/l) 1 in 5 with saline and prepare a series of tubes as follows:

g protein per litre CSF	0	10	20	30	40	50	60	70	80	90	100
ml of standard protein solution (1 g/l)	0	1.0	2.0	3.0	4.0	5.0	6.0	7.0	8.0	9.0	10.0
ml of saline	10	9.0	8.0	7.0	6.0	5.0	4.0	3.0	2.0	1.0	0.0

Mix well, and treat 1.0 ml of each standard protein solution with 4.0 ml trichloracetic acid as before. If the absorbances are linear, in other words a straight-line relationship is obtained, further standards can be prepared up to 2.5 g/l by diluting the stock standard 1 in 2 and setting up the following series of tubes:

g protein per litre CSF	150	175	200	225	250
ml of standard protein solution (2.5 g/l)	3.0	3.5	4.0	4.5	5.0
ml of saline	2.0	1.5	1.0	0.5	0.0

Mix well and treat as above.

B. Micromethod

This method can be used when the volume of CSF available is less than 0.5 ml.

Reagents

The same as for method A.

Method

Using automatic micropipettes add to 75 mm × 12 mm tubes as follows:

Blank: 0.2 ml of 0.9% NaCl
Standard: 0.2 ml of protein standard
Test: 0.2 ml of CSF

To all tubes add 0.8 ml of 3.0% trichloracetic acid. Stopper and mix by inverting × 5. Leave for 10 min. Mix once by inverting. Read the absorbance of the standard and test against the blank at 450 nm using glass microcuvettes having a 1 cm light path.

Calculation

$$\frac{\text{Test reading}}{\text{Standard reading}} \times 0.5 = \text{g CSF protein per litre}$$

Notes

1. This method is linear up to 1.7 g/l. Any results above this should be repeated by using 0.1 ml of CSF plus 0.1 ml of saline in place of 0.2 ml of CSF. Multiply the result by 2.
2. Standard tubes and adequate mixing are very important in this method.

C. Method using permanent standards

This method is less accurate than the methods given above, but since it is a rapid technique, many laboratories find it of acceptable accuracy.

Reagents

1. 3% sulphosalicylic acid.
2. Permanent protein standards supplied by Gallenkamp Ltd.

Technique

1. Add 1.0 ml CSF to a standard tube containing 3.0 ml of sulphosalicylic acid.
2. Mix contents and allow to stand for 5 min.
3. Compare the tube with the turbidity standards, which are usually marked in mg protein per 100 ml of fluid. To convert to g/l, divide the mg amount by 100.

Results

The protein content of normal CSF lies between 0.15 and 0.45 g/l and is almost entirely albumin in nature. An increase in protein content is the commonest abnormality found, when the protein is a mixture of albumin and globulin, with albumin predominating.

Globulin

Two tests for showing an increase in globulin content are given. Pandy's method is the more sensitive, but is unreliable.

1. Pandy's method

Principle

If globulin is added to a saturated aqueous solution of phenol, water is absorbed onto the globulin molecules and the phenol is displaced from the solution, causing a fine and persistent turbidity.

Reagent—Pandy's reagent

Saturated aqueous solution of phenol (8–10 g/100 ml). This solution should be clear and colourless.

Technique

1. Using a Pasteur pipette, carefully add 1 drop of CSF to 0.5 ml Pandy's reagent in a small test-tube.
2. The tube is held against the light to detect any turbidity.
3. Normal CSF remains quite clear.
4. A turbidity or precipitate indicates an increase in globulin content.

2. Nonne–Apelt's method

Principle

Globulin is precipitated out of solution by half-saturation with ammonium sulphate.

Reagent

Saturated ammonium sulphate. Dissolve 85 g of ammonium sulphate in 100 ml hot distilled water. Allow to stand overnight, filter and store in well-stoppered bottle.

Technique

1. Pipette 1 ml of saturated ammonium sulphate into a small test-tube.
2. Add 1 ml of CSF and mix.
3. Smaller volumes of sample and reagent can be used providing equal volumes are adhered to.
4. Stand for 3 min and note whether there is any opalescence or turbidity.
5. Normal CSF will remain clear or only show the faintest degree of opalescence.
6. It has been suggested that 1 ml of CSF should be layered on top of 1 ml of ammonium sulphate solution when a white ring at the junction of the two liquids will be obtained, in increased globulin concentration.
7. This is not recommended as the junction of the two liquids may be greater than 50% saturation.

Results

A small amount of globulin is always present in normal CSF, but this cannot be detected by the above techniques. For a given rise in total protein there is a corresponding rise in globulin content.

In tabes and disseminated sclerosis, an increased globulin content can be obtained with CSF showing a normal total protein content.

Quantitative globulins

In inflammatory conditions of the cerebral tissues, such as found in tuberculous meningitis, syphilitic meningitis and multiple sclerosis, CSF globulins are raised, especially the immunoglobulin IgG. Various methods have been used to detect this increase as it is a valuable test if multiple sclerosis is suspected. Electrophoresis may be used, but it needs a lot of experience to interpret the bands.

The electrophoresis of normal ventricular CSF shows a pattern similar to that of a plasma ultrafiltrate. When this is compared with normal lumbar fluid there will be a difference in electrophoretic pattern both in concentration and type because of the alteration in composition during passage down the spinal canal. In multiple sclerosis there is sometimes an increase in the level of gamma globulin (IgG), but its measurement needs to be made in relation to either the total protein or its albumin concentration. The quantitation of albumin and IgG in CSF is preferred, and both these levels are done by immunological methods such as radial immunodiffusion.

Radial immunodiffusion test

Radial immunodiffusion for IgG and albumin concentrations involves the diffusion of an antigen (IgG and albumin) through a semi-solid medium containing an antibody (anti-IgG or anti-albumin), resulting in the formation of a circular zone of precipitation. The diameter of this precipitation zone is then measured, which is then a function of the concentration of the antigen (IgG or albumin).

This procedure allows the determination of the IgG/albumin ratio which is of diagnostic significance in multiple sclerosis and other neurological diseases.

Normal values:

Albumin	0.061–0.713 g/l
IgG	0.011–0.012 g/l
IgG/albumin ratio	0.051–0.433

Chlorides

Chloride levels in CSF can, if necessary, be estimated by any of the methods for plasma chlorides, the most convenient being the coulometric titration procedure, as described in Chapter 6. Mohr's method, described below, has been retained because of its simplicity and also because it helps students to understand the principle of how a simple titration procedure was used. It is now obsolete. The conversion into SI units is shown at the end of the calculation.

1. Mohr's method

Principle

Chlorides are estimated as sodium chloride by titration against silver nitrate using potassium chromate as indicator. Silver nitrate is added until all the chloride ions present in the CSF have combined with the silver ions. Any further silver nitrate added is now free to combine with the potassium chromate indicator to yield a red precipitate of silver chromate. The solution at this point suddenly changes from pale yellow to faint brick-red colour.

$$NaCl + AgNO_3 \rightarrow AgCl + NaNO_3$$

Reagents

1. Standard silver nitrate solution (2.906 g of silver nitrate is dissolved in and made up to 1 litre with distilled water). Keep in an amber bottle and standardize against an accurately prepared sodium chloride solution containing 500 mg NaCl per 100 ml using the method described below. Check at frequent intervals, and determine the factor (see Chapter 5):

    1 ml standard $AgNO_3 \equiv 1$ mg NaCl

2. 5% potassium chromate solution.

Technique

1. Pipette 1.0 ml CSF into a conical flask containing about 10 ml of distilled water and 2–3 drops of potassium chromate.
2. Slowly add the silver nitrate from a 10 ml burette and continuously rotate the flask, to ensure thorough mixing.
3. As the end-point nears, the silver nitrate solution should be added slowly and carefully to avoid adding excess of the reagent.
4. Note the titre and repeat the titration again if sufficient CSF is available.
5. Normal fluid usually requires between 7.0 and 7.6 ml of silver nitrate.

Calculation

$$NaCl + AgNO_3 \rightarrow AgCl + NaNO_3$$
$$58.5 \qquad 170$$

From the above equation it can be seen that 58.5 g of sodium chloride are equivalent to 170 g of silver nitrate. Therefore

58.5 mg NaCl $\equiv$ 170 mg $AgNO_3$

Now the standard solution of $AgNO_3$ contains 2.906 g per litre

$\equiv 2.906$ mg per ml

Hence, 2.906 mg or 1 ml of standard $AgNO_3$ corresponds to

$$2.906 \times \frac{58.5}{170} \text{ mg of NaCl}$$

1 ml $AgNO_3 = 1$ mg NaCl

If the titre was 7.3 ml of $AgNO_3$ (or 7.3 ml × factor), then mg NaCl per 100 ml CSF =

$$\text{Titre} \times 1 \times \frac{100}{\text{Amount taken}}$$

$$= 7.3 \times 1 \times 100 = 730 \text{ mg per 100 ml}$$

Convert the NaCl value in terms of mmol per litre, using the following formula:

$$\text{mmol per litre} = \frac{\text{mg per 100 ml} \times 10}{\text{Molecular weight}}$$

$$= \frac{730 \times 10}{58.5} = 124.8 \ (125) \text{ mmol/l}$$

∎ Note

A solution of $AgNO_3$ containing 5.812 g/l can be used, in which case 1 ml of $AgNO_3 \equiv 2$ mg NaCl.

2. Coulometric titration method

In this type of titration a constant electric current is passed between two silver electrodes which dip into an acid buffer solution to which a known volume of fluid is added. Silver ions are released from the anode and combine with the chloride ions in the sample during titration. The digital display starts registering as the silver and chloride ions combine ion to ion, until all the chloride has been precipitated as silver chloride. This causes a sudden increase in potential between the silver electrodes and stops the digital display which is then a measure of the chloride concentration of the sample.

Equipment

Several different manufacturers produce equipment of this nature, but the Corning 925 Chloride Meter is the most popular.

Principle

A constant electric current is passed between two silver electrodes which dip into an acid buffer solution to which the CSF is added. The insoluble silver chloride formed by electrochemistry is usually held in solution by gelatine added to the acid buffer. At the end of the titration, free Ag ions appear in solution, an increase in potential occurs and the current is switched off, which is then a measure of the chloride content of the CSF.

Reagents and method

Consult the appropriate manufacturer's manual.

Results

Normal CSF contains 120–130 mmol NaCl/l and is higher than the plasma level, 96–106 mmol/l. In meningitis, there is usually a fall in chloride content, while an increase can sometimes be found in hypertension.

Glucose

The method for glucose estimation is the same as for blood glucose (see p. 127). Since the glucose content of CSF is normally lower than that in blood and in, for example, tuberculous meningitis, a further reduction occurs; a large volume of CSF should be used, making sure the diluent is reduced correspondingly and the calculation is amended for this change.

■ Note

It is imperative to carry out the assay as soon as possible after withdrawal of CSF. Glycolytic enzymes present in the CSF will cause a reduction in the glucose content, and therefore the estimation becomes valueless after a few hours.

Results

The normal glucose content is between 2.8 and 4.4 mmol/l, although a range of 2.25–5.6 mmol/l is often allowed. In meningitis, the most important pathological change is a decrease in glucose content and in some cases glucose may be absent. Small increases are found in poliomyelitis and raised values may occur in diabetes mellitus.

Section 3

Cellular pathology

12

Introduction to histology

Histology is the microscopic study of the normal tissues of the body, whereas histopathology is the microscopic study of tissues affected by disease. The procedures adopted for the preparation of material for such studies are known as histological or histopathological techniques, and it is with these techniques that the medical laboratory scientist in the pathology department is primarily concerned. The various ways of preparing and examining smears, preserving and processing tissues, cutting and staining sections and the ability to recognize whether or not the procedures have been performed correctly constitute the skills of the medical laboratory scientist in this subject. For the work to be executed competently a knowledge of the structure of cells and the organs and tissues formed by them is essential.

The basic substance of all living things is *protoplasm*, which is contained within small units, called *cells*, many millions of which go to make up the human body.

Protoplasm is the general name given to the main constituents of a cell (of a colloidal nature), together with water, protein, carbohydrates, lipids and inorganic salts. If the cell is studied by histological methods and light microscopy, it is seen to contain structures, as shown in *Figure 12.1*. Electron microscopy, however, shows complete tubular structures in the cytoplasm, and detail in the nucleus not seen by ordinary microscopy (*Figure 12.2*).

The cell

A cell may be conveniently described as a mass of protoplasm enclosed within a membrane (cell or plasma membrane) containing a subdivision, the

nucleus, which is bounded by the nuclear membrane. The portion of cell lying between the plasma and nuclear membranes is known as the cytoplasm. Within the cytoplasm a variety of fine structures called organelles may be identified. These are specialized structures with individual functions and consist of the living material of the cell.

Cell membrane

This is a semi-permeable membrane which permits the selective passage of substances to and from the cell. The exchange of materials through the cell membrane is due to osmotic pressure exerted by the intercellular fluid and cytoplasmic ground substance, or by an active transport mechanism. Electron microscopical studies have shown that the membrane contains three layers which are thought to be composed of protein and lipid molecules.

Cytoplasmic organelles

Endoplasmic reticulum

Cytoplasm is organized into a network of fine branching tubules known as the endoplasmic reticulum (ER). These tubules are lined by a membrane which in places is coated with granules of ribonucleoprotein (ribosomes), and is known as 'rough' or granular ER. It is associated with protein synthesis. Parts of the membrane of the reticulum which are not coated with ribosomes are called 'smooth' or agranular ER and are thought to be associated in some cells with synthesis of fats and similar substances. Although the endoplasmic reticulum cannot be resolved by light microscopy, the amount

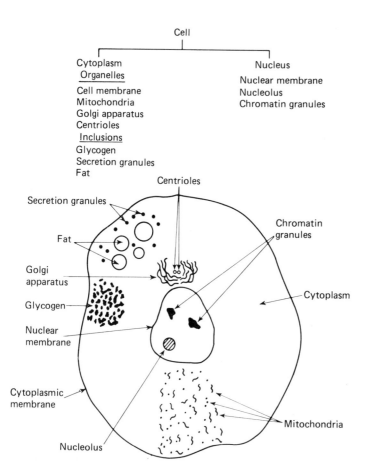

Figure 12.1. Diagram of living cell with its components and inclusions which can be demonstrated by methods using light microscopy. It is unlikely that more than one type of inclusion would be present but fat, glycogen, pigments and secretory granules are all included

present in a cell appears to have some effect on the staining reaction of the cytoplasm.

Golgi apparatus

This is a specialized area of smooth ER comprising membranous canals and vacuoles. It may be distinguished by its selective reaction with silver salts and osmium tetroxide. Secretory products are concentrated around this area where they may possibly combine with a synthesized carbohydrate component.

Mitochondria

These small filamentous or granular bodies may be distributed evenly throughout the cytoplasm or accumulated in selected sites according to cell type. The number of mitochondria may be very large; as many as 2500 have been found in liver cells. Mitochondria vary in length up to 7 μm and are between 0.5 and 1.0 μm in diameter. They can be demonstrated in fresh unfixed tissue by special microscopic techniques, or in fixed and stained

preparations. Electron microscopy shows these organelles are bound by double membranes. The innermost membrane is reflected to run across the inside of the mitochondria at several points to form shelf-like cristae, and the aggregation and shape of the cristae varies in cells of different functions. Mitochondria have been described as the power houses of the cell and appear to be concerned with cell respiration and enzymatic activity. They are rapidly affected by autolysis and are some of the first structures to disappear after the death of the cell. Acetic acid causes destruction and distortion of mitochondria and should be avoided in fixing solutions.

Lysosome

This is a minute spherical organelle with a diameter of about 0.25 μm. Lysosomes are bounded by a single membrane and contain hydrolytic enzymes, i.e. enzymes which break down large complex molecules into smaller molecules. Rupture of the lysosome membrane releases the enzymes and causes eventual destruction of the cell. This process

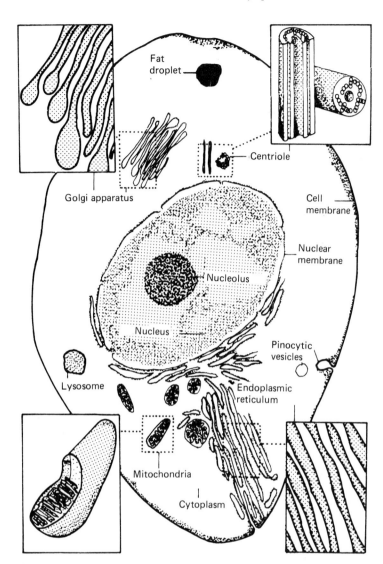

Figure 12.2. Diagram of a normal cell as shown by electron microscopy

is known as autolysis. Lysosomes are abundant in leucocytes and macrophages in which they are thought to play an important part in phagocytosis (intracellular digestion) of bacteria and nutrient particles.

Centrosome

The cell centre or centrosome is present in all cells, although it is not readily visible except during cell division. It is seen in sections as a clear area of cytoplasm less than 1.0 μm in diameter, often lying in a concavity of the nucleus, and containing two dark dots, the centrioles. Electron microscopy reveals the centrioles to be short cylindrical bodies whose walls are composed of fine fibres arranged

longitudinally like a bundle of twigs. The centrioles are thought to be associated with the formation of fibrillary material, e.g. cilia, the hair-like processes which extend from certain cells, and with the spindle of fibrils which extend from the parted centrioles upon which the chromosomes arrange themselves during cell division.

Cytoplasmic inclusions

Non-living substances that may be seen in the cytoplasm of cells are referred to as inclusions. They usually consist of stored nutrients, materials produced by the cell, or ingested particles. The following are those most commonly seen.

Glycogen

Accumulations of glycogen are stored in the cytoplasm of liver cells and skeletal muscle. In stained sections it is seen either as fine granules or as larger amorphous masses.

Fat

Fat is generally stored in fat cells, but it may also occur normally or pathologically in other cells. It accumulates in the form of minute globules which tend to fuse together to form larger globules, often distending the cytoplasm and displacing the nucleus to the periphery of the cell. It is dissolved out when tissues are prepared by the paraffin wax or celloidin techniques unless special fixatives are used, but it is easily demonstrated in frozen sections.

Secretion granules

These are products of cell synthesis and are found in the cytoplasm of specialized cells which have a secretory function. They are dispersed throughout the cytoplasm as small globules which on fixation usually become coagulated to form granules.

Pigments

These are frequently present in the cytoplasm of cells and may be either *endogenous* or *exogenous* in nature. Endogenous pigments such as melanin and haemosiderin are produced within the body; exogenous pigments are particles of foreign matter such as coal dust, which are ingested by phagocytosis and absorbed.

Artificial pigments produced as a result of fixation or precipitation of the staining solutions may be present. Such pigments can be easily identified and removed.

The nucleus

Nuclear membrane

The nucleus contains most of the genetic material of the cell. It is bounded by two membranes each rather similar to the cytoplasmic membrane.

Chromatin

Aggregations of a material with an affinity for basic dyes are scattered throughout the nucleus; these are known as chromatin granules. The intense staining reaction of these granules and of the chromosomes which appear during cell division is due to their nucleoprotein content. Nucleoprotein is composed of basic proteins and nucleic acid and the chief nucleic acid present in chromatin is deoxyribonucleic acid (DNA).

Nucleolus

This is a small spheroidal body present within the nucleus of most cells. It contains a high proportion of ribonucleic acid (RNA) and is thought to be concerned with the synthesis of proteins.

Chromosomes

These are small thread-like bodies which are seen within nuclei during cell division. Each chromosome has a bifid structure formed by two *chromatids* lying side by side and linked at one point, the *centromere*.

Normal somatic (body) cells in man contain 46 chromosomes arranged in pairs, one of each pair derived from the father and the other from the mother. Because of this pairing they are known as the *diploid* set and consist of 1 pair of sex chromosomes and 22 pairs of somatic chromosomes (autosomes). The sex chromosomes in the female are similar to each other and are designated by the symbol 'XX', in the male they are dissimilar and are designated 'XY'.

The mature female and male germ cells, namely the *ovum* and *spermatozoan*, contain only a single set of chromosomes, i.e. 23, and these are referred to as the *haploid* set. The chromosomes of the ovum consist of 22 autosomes and 1 'X' chromosome; the chromosomes of the spermatozoan consist of 22 autosomes and 1 sex chromosome which may be 'X' or 'Y', as half the spermatozoan contain an 'X' chromosome and the other half a 'Y' chromosome. On fusion of the ovum and spermatozoan, the diploid set of chromosomes is formed and the sex of the resulting embryo is determined according to the sex chromosome carried by the spermatozoan.

Cell division

The process by which most human cells divide is called *mitosis* (*Figure 12.3*). Before cell division occurs, the amount of deoxyribonucleic acid in the nucleus is doubled so that one-half is passed to each new cell. Four stages of mitotic division are recognized, although it should be borne in mind that the whole process is continuous with no intervals between stages.

Prophase

The chromatin of the nucleus becomes concentrated into a tangled mass of filaments which resolve themselves into pairs of chromosomes. The centrioles meanwhile have separated and move towards opposite poles of the cell, drawing with them a

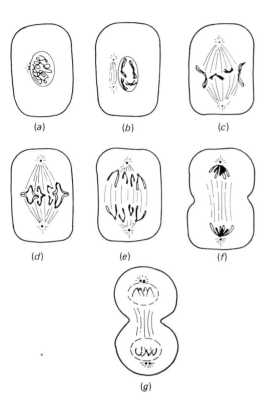

(a)   (b)   (c)

(d)   (e)   (f)

(g)

Figure 12.3. The four phases of cell division. (a) Early prophase: concentration of chromosomes into a tangled mass but constituent chromatids are not apparent. (b) Later prophase: the centrioles have separated and the shortened chromosomes are each seen to be composed of two chromatids. (c) Metaphase: disappearance of the nuclear membrane and the chromosomes are arranged in the equatorial region of the spindle. (d, e, f) Anaphase: longitudinal division of the chromosomes, the two halves move apart towards the poles of the spindle; constriction of the cytoplasmic membrane begins. (g) Telophase: the chromosomes become thread-like and condensed, nuclear membranes form around both groups, and the cell membrane constricts until cleavage into two daughter cells is complete

number of delicate fibres, known as the *achromatic spindle*, along which the paired chromosomes become orientated. The nucleolus and nuclear membrane disappear and are not seen again until division is complete.

Metaphase

The chromosomes arrange themselves in the equatorial region of the achromatic spindle and each divides longitudinally into two chromatids.

Anaphase

The centrioles move further apart and the two chromatids of each chromosome move away from one another along the spindle towards opposite ends of the cell. The cell now contains two sets of identical chromosomes. The cytoplasmic membrane begins to constrict.

Telophase

In this terminal stage of mitosis each of the two groups of chromosomes are invested with a nuclear membrane. The chromosomes become thread-like again and appear to coalesce to form chromatin granules. The cytoplasmic membrane continues to constrict and finally divides; the two daughter cells are separated from each other to form exact replicas of the parent cell.

Intercellular substances

Living cells are bound together with other non-living materials, the *intercellular substances*, to form tissues. Some tissues are composed mainly of one type of cell which carries out the particular function of that tissue, but most tissues contain in addition other, less specialized cells whose function is to support the main cell type.

The intercellular substances include tissue fluid and various fibres, notably collagen, elastic and reticular fibres. The functions of these substances are to support and strengthen the tissue or to maintain and nourish the cells whose environment they constitute.

Collagen

This is a tough, fibrous protein comprised of fine fibrils of 0.3–0.5 μm diameter aggregated to form microscopically visible fibres and ribbons ranging up to 100 μm thick. The fibres are sometimes referred to as *white fibres* and they are the characteristic element of all types of connective tissue.

Elastic fibres

These consist of the fibrous protein elastin. They are long, branching homogeneous threads or ribbons, much thinner than collagen fibres. Known also as *yellow fibres* because of the colour they impart to tissues when present in large numbers, their function is to give such tissues the power of elastic recoil. Elastic fibres are found abundantly in the walls of blood vessels, trachea, lungs and dermis.

Reticular fibres

Structurally similar to collagen fibres to which they are often connected, these fibres differ from collagen in certain methods of demonstration. The delicate networks formed by reticulum fibres offer support for cells, capillaries and nerve fibres, and are also found at the junctions between connective and other types of tissue.

Examination of tissues

Numerous techniques can be used to prepare tissue for microscopical examination, the method selected being governed by a number of factors. These include the structures or inclusions to be studied, the amount and nature of the tissue to be examined, whether the specimen is fresh or preserved and the urgency of the investigation.

Fresh specimens

Fresh specimens may be examined as teased and squash preparations, touch preparations or frozen sections.

Teased preparations

These are prepared by carefully dissecting, with mounted needles, the tissue to be examined. The dissection is carried out while the specimen is immersed in an isotonic solution, such as normal saline or Ringer's solution in a petri dish or watch glass. Selected pieces of the tissue are transferred carefully to a microscope slide and mounted as a wet preparation beneath a coverglass, care being taken to avoid the formation of air bubbles. The preparation is then examined by bright field microscopy, the illumination being reduced either by closing the iris diaphragm or lowering the substage condenser. Many details can be studied in slides prepared by this method, which has the advantage of permitting the cells to be examined in the living state; the preparations, however, are not permanent. The use of the phase contrast microscope greatly increases the structural detail of the cells examined, allowing movement and mitotic division to be observed. The application of certain stains such as methylene blue can also be of great value.

Squash preparations

The cellular contents of small pieces of tissue not exceeding 1 mm in diameter can be examined by placing the tissue in the centre of a microscopic slide and forcibly applying a coverglass. Staining can be carried out if necessary by making use of capillary attraction; a drop of a vital stain placed at the junction of the coverglass and slide is drawn into contact with the tissue which absorbs it.

Smears

The microscopic examination of cellular material spread lightly over a slide in the form of a smear is a technique which has wide application in histopathology. The method of preparing the smear differs according to the nature of the material to be examined, but as a general rule smears are made either by spreading the selected portion of the specimen over the surface of the slide with a platinum loop or, alternatively, by making an apposition smear with the aid of a second slide. Smears may be examined either as fresh preparations in a similar manner to that described for teased preparations, or by using a supravital staining technique in conjunction with a warm stage. Both of these techniques suffer from the same disadvantage, namely, that the preparations are not permanent. Permanent stained preparations can be made from fresh smears by fixing them while still wet, staining to demonstrate specific structures and inclusions and mounting the cleared specimen beneath a coverglass with a suitable mounting medium. Details of these methods are given in Chapter 19.

Impression smears

These are prepared by bringing into contact the surface of a clean glass slide with that of a freshly cut piece of tissue. Cells transferred to the surface of the slide are examined microscopically by phase contrast or after applying vital stains. Alternatively, the impression smear, which is also known as a touch preparation, can be fixed and stained according to the methods described in Chapter 18.

Frozen sections

Sections of 10–15 µm in thickness can be cut from fresh tissue frozen on a microtome with the aid of carbon dioxide or electrothermal coupling units. The sections are transferred from the microtome knife to a dish containing an isotonic solution, from which they may be either attached to slides prior to staining or carried through the staining solutions by means of a glass rod.

The impetus given to histochemistry in recent years has led to the commercial development of the cryostat, a microtome housed in a form of deep freeze cabinet which permits thin sections to be cut at an atmospheric temperature of −10 to −20°C from previously frozen fresh tissue. The sections are cut by using controls positioned outside the cabinet at room temperature. This instrument, which has become standard equipment in a large number of histological laboratories, definitely facilitates the preparation of sections from unfixed tissues (see p. 203).

Many cell products are soluble in aqueous solutions and for this reason cryostat sections, which may be transferred directly from the microtome knife to the microscope slide, are the method of choice for many histochemical investigations. Details of the techniques used for preparing frozen sections are given in Chapter 16.

Fixed tissues

The most effective means of studying normal and diseased tissues of the body microscopically is by the examination of thin sections, previously stained to demonstrate certain structures or inclusions, and mounted on glass slides beneath a thinner glass coverslip. The sections are normally prepared from fixed tissue. Fixation is necessary to prevent the post-mortem changes which occur shortly after death, or on removal from the body.

A number of sectional methods may be used, all of which necessitate that the tissue be supported during the process of cutting the sections. The following factors help to determine the fixative and sectional method to be used:

1. The urgency of the examination.
2. The structure or inclusions to be demonstrated.
3. The material to be sectioned.
4. The staining procedure to be employed.
5. Whether or not serial sections are required.

Frozen sections

The use of frozen sections of fresh tissue has already been mentioned. With tissue fixed in formol–saline, this method is invaluable as a rapid diagnostic technique and also for demonstrating lipids and the supporting elements of the central nervous system.

Paraffin sections

Paraffin wax is the most widely used embedding medium for preparing histological slides. The fixed tissue not being miscible with the wax, selected pieces are passed through baths of alcohol of ever-increasing concentration in order to remove all water. The alcohol-saturated tissue is then transferred to an ante-medium which is miscible with both the alcohol and the paraffin wax. Many ante-media raise the refractive index of the tissue, imparting to it a transparent appearance. For this reason, they are commonly referred to as 'clearing agents', but as this is a property not possessed by all of them, the term is incorrect. The ante-medium is eventually replaced by molten paraffin wax and when sufficiently impregnated, the tissue is embedded in fresh wax which solidifies on cooling.

The paraffin wax technique permits thin individual and serial sections to be cut with ease from the majority of tissues. It also allows a multitude of staining techniques to be employed and facilitates storage of the blocks and unstained mounted sections.

Celloidin and low-viscosity nitrocellulose sections

Celloidin is a purified form of nitrocellulose and is soluble in a number of solvents. In histology, the solvent generally used consists of equal parts of ethyl alcohol and ether. As an embedding medium, celloidin has certain properties which make it a valuable auxiliary technique.

The use of celloidin permits thicker sections to be cut than is possible with the paraffin wax technique, and for this reason the method is used for studying the central nervous system. Its rubbery consistency makes it of great value as an embedding medium when sections are required from blocks of tissue that are either very hard or are composed of a number of tissues of varying consistency. As heat is not required during the process of impregnating the tissue, less shrinkage occurs in celloidin sections than in those prepared by the paraffin wax technique.

The disadvantages of the method are that it is slow (impregnating and embedding taking several weeks), the blocks and sections must be stored in 70% ethyl alcohol, sections of less than 10 μm cannot easily be cut and serial sections are difficult to prepare owing to each one having to be handled individually during cutting and staining.

Low-viscosity nitrocellulose (LVN) is now more widely used as an embedding medium than celloidin. LVN, which is usually dissolved in equal parts of absolute alcohol and diethyl ether to which 5% of tricresyl phosphate has been added, dissolves more readily than celloidin and permits the preparation of more concentrated solutions which form firmer blocks and allows thinner sections to be cut.

Resin sections

Resin embedding is a relatively new technique for use with light microscopy. It is adapted from embedding methods used to support tissue during the preparation of sections for electron microscopy. The principal advantage of resin embedding is that it permits the preparation of much thinner sections for which specially adapted knives and microtomes are required. A number of different resins are now commercially available, but the most popular are those miscible with water.

13

Fixation

Shortly after death or removal from the body, cells and tissue begin to undergo changes, which result in their breakdown and ultimate destruction. These are referred to as post-mortem changes, which may be either putrefactive or autolytic in nature.

Putrefaction is due to the invasion of the tissue by bacteria, which generally disseminate from the alimentary tract and spread quickly into surrounding organs causing decomposition. Autolysis is due to the action of enzymes from the dead cell. This phenomenon occurs chiefly in the central nervous system and the endocrine system.

These changes may be retarded by low temperatures or prevented by the use of chemical fixatives. Fixation is the basis of histological technique, and the results of all subsequent procedures depend on the correct selection and use of the fixative employed. It is therefore essential to understand the action which different fixatives have upon the cell and tissue constituents.

A fixative may be described as a substance which will preserve after death the shape, structure, relationship and chemical constituents of tissues and cells. It is mainly due to the action of fixatives on the protein elements of cells and tissues that the structural stabilization is achieved. The preservation should be such that the fixed tissue resembles as closely as possible the form which it had during life. In addition to preserving the tissue and cells, the fixing fluid or vapour must also render them insensitive to such subsequent treatment which may be necessary for the production of the final slide or specimen.

A good fixative should be capable of fulfilling the following requirements:

1. It must kill the cell quickly without shrinking, or swelling, or other distortion.
2. It must penetrate the tissue and cells rapidly and evenly.
3. It must render insoluble the substance of the cell and give good optical differentiation.
4. It must inhibit bacterial decay and autolysis.
5. It must harden the tissue and render it insensitive to subsequent treatment.
6. It must permit at a later date the application of numerous staining procedures in order to render the constituents of the tissue and cells more readily visible.
7. It should allow tissue to be stored for long periods of time.
8. It should permit the restoration of natural colour for photography and mounting as museum specimens.
9. It should be simple to prepare and economical in use.

No single fixing solution has yet been evolved which will comply with each of the conditions outlined above. As a result, it is necessary for the histologist to have at his command a wide range of fixatives in order that he may draw upon the one most suited to his needs as occasion demands.

Temperature has an important effect upon the action of fixatives. A low temperature will retard fixation but will also reduce the autolytic action of the enzymes released after death; a high temperature will decrease the time required in the fixative but will also increase autolysis. Where time is of no object, fixation at a low temperature for a prolonged period is advocated. In cases where fixation is not possible until some time after death, storage at a low temperature (e.g. 2–5°C) is essential.

Simple and compound fixatives

In order to obtain a fixative which will comply as nearly as possible with the conditions previously outlined, it is necessary to mix together several substances, each of which has its own particular effect upon the cell and tissue constituents, in order to obtain the combined effect of their individual actions. These individual substances are known as simple fixatives, and the solutions resulting from the mixing of two or more of them are referred to as compound fixatives.

Compound fixatives may thus be described as the product of two or more simple fixatives mixed together in order to obtain the combined effect of their individual actions upon the cell and tissue constituents. The formula of some compound fixatives is completely irrational, strong oxidizers being combined with equally strong reducers. Provided that the tissue is only immersed in these irrational solutions for the specified period however, and provided also that it receives the correct treatment subsequent to fixation, excellent results can nevertheless be obtained.

Fixatives are usually grouped under headings according to their action upon the cell and tissue constituents. Those which preserve the tissue in a manner which permits the general microscopical study of the tissue structures and allows the various layers of tissues and cells to retain their former relationship with each other are termed *micro-anatomical fixatives*; those which are employed for their specific action upon a specific part of the cell structures are termed *cytological fixatives*. This last group may be further subdivided into *nuclear* and *cytoplasmic fixatives* depending upon which of the cell inclusions they act. Generally speaking, those cytological fixatives which contain glacial acetic acid or have a reaction of pH 4.6 or less are nuclear fixatives, while those which do not include glacial acetic acid as a constituent and have a reaction above the critical level of pH 4.6 are cytoplasmic fixtures.

Some simple fixatives are used to preserve certain cell products for histochemical demonstration. Chief among these are cold acetone (0–5°C) and formol–saline buffered to a reaction of pH 7. The cold acetone is used when it is required to demonstrate phosphatases; buffered formol–saline permits the majority of histochemical procedures to be performed. Absolute ethyl alcohol may also be used as a histochemical fixative, usually on sections cut from freeze-dried material or which were prepared by the use of a cryostat.

To preserve an accurate picture of the cell, it is necessary to 'fix' the tissue as soon as possible after it is removed from the body. The specimen is immersed in a large volume of fixative. With routine fixatives, the volume of fluid should be about 50–100 times that of the tissue. In the case of the chrome–osmium fixatives, for example Flemming's fluid, the volume need only be ten times that of the tissue.

Simple fixatives

Actions and properties

Many fixatives have been devised, but only about ten formulae are used in routine work. The action of the simple fixatives upon the cell and tissue constituents will now be described.

Formaldehyde

Formaldehyde (HCHO) is a gas produced by the oxidation of methanol, and is soluble in water to the extent of 40% by weight (sold commercially as formalin). Fats and mucin are preserved, but not precipitated, by formaldehyde. It is a powerful reducing agent, but is often used irrationally in conjunction with certain oxidizing agents (for example, Zenker–formol*).

After prolonged storage, formaldehyde often develops a white deposit of paraformaldehyde. The formation of this precipitate is said to be avoided by storage at room temperature, but its presence does not impair the fixing qualities of the formaldehyde. The solution is usually acid in reaction, due to the presence of formic acid. Though not harmful, this acid can be neutralized by the addition of a small quantity of magnesium carbonate, or a few drops of sodium hydroxide. Care should be exercised when neutralizing formaldehyde with magnesium carbonate, as carbon dioxide may be released suddenly. Insufficient gas space can result in a violent explosion and it is therefore recommended that neutralization be performed in a wide-mouth vessel. When the immediate reaction between the formic acid and the magnesium carbonate has ceased, the solution may be stored in a Winchester quart bottle.

Mercuric chloride

Mercuric chloride ($HgCl_2$) is included in many fixatives and is frequently used in saturated aqueous solution. (At room temperature its solubility in water is approximately 7%.) It precipitates all proteins, but does not combine well with them, and penetrates and hardens tissues rapidly. Fixatives containing mercuric chloride leave a black precipitate in the tissue, and this must be removed by one of the methods described in the section on 'pigments' (p. 219).

Mercuric chloride is corrosive and should not be allowed to come into contact with metal surfaces. It is poisonous and must be handled and disposed of with great care.

---

*Although some workers adopt the term 'formal' as the abbreviation of formalin, various reference works use the alternative abbreviation 'formol' which is retained in this sixth edition.

Osmium tetroxide

Osmium tetroxide (OsO_4), commonly known as osmic acid, is a pale yellow powder which dissolves in water (up to about 6% at 20°C), forming a solution which is a strong oxidizing reagent. Osmium tetroxide is extremely volatile and is easily reduced by contact with the smallest particle of organic matter, or by exposure to daylight. It should therefore be kept in a dark, chemically clean bottle. Exposure to the acid vapour must be avoided since the black oxide, OsO_2, can become deposited in the cornea, resulting in blindness.

Although an expensive reagent, osmium tetroxide is widely used in cytological fixatives. It is the only substance that permanently fixes fat, rendering it insoluble during subsequent treatment with alcohol and xylene. (The Golgi element and mitochondria are also preserved.) Osmium tetroxide is seldom used alone as a fixative, but is usually combined with a chromium salt. After fixation in these solutions, tissues should be washed in running water. Osmium tetroxide is a poor penetrating agent, suitable only for small pieces of tissue. The vapour of osmium tetroxide may be used to fix some tissues, such as the adrenal. The vapour penetrates better than the solution, 'washing out' is unnecessary and the production of artefacts is minimized.

Picric acid

Picric acid ($C_6H_2(NO_2)_3OH$) is normally used in saturated aqueous solution, that is approximately 1% solution. It precipitates all proteins and combines with them to form picrates. These picrates are soluble in water, and the tissue must not come in contact with water until the picrates have been rendered insoluble by treatment with alcohol. Picric acid is explosive when dry.

Acetic acid

Acetic acid (CH_3COOH) is a colourless solution with a pungent smell. At approximately 17°C it solidifies, which accounts for its name 'glacial acetic acid'.

Acetic acid is included in a number of histological fixatives. It is not a general protein precipitant but a powerful precipitant of nucleoprotein. When used alone it causes considerable swelling of the tissue, and this property is used in certain compound fixatives to counteract the shrinkage produced by other components. In Heidenhain's 'Susa', for example, the shrinkage produced by mercuric chloride is reduced by the addition of acetic acid. It is often used by cytologists in studying chromosomes, and its chromatin-precipitating properties make it useful in nuclear studies. It destroys mitochondria and the Golgi element, and when used

in conjunction with potassium dichromate destroys the lipid-fixing properties of that reagent.

Ethyl alcohol

Ethyl alcohol (C_2H_5OH) is a colourless liquid that is readily miscible with water. It was used extensively by early histologists, but today its use as a simple fixative is confined to histochemical methods. It is frequently incorporated into compound fixatives. Ethyl alcohol is a reducing agent, and should not be mixed with chromic acid, potassium dichromate or osmium tetroxide. As a simple fixative it is used at concentrations of 70–100% which preserves glycogen, but does not fix it. Ethyl alcohol produces considerable hardening and shrinkage of tissue. It is also a highly flammable solution.

Chromic acid

Chromic acid is prepared by dissolving crystals of the anhydride CrO_3 in distilled water, and is conveniently stored as a 2% stock solution. Chromic acid is a strong oxidizing agent, and should not be combined with reducing agents, such as alcohol and formalin. It is a strong protein precipitant, and preserves carbohydrates. Tissue fixed in chromic acid should be thoroughly washed in running water before dehydration, to avoid the formation of the insoluble sub-oxide.

Potassium dichromate

Potassium dichromate ($K_2Cr_2O_7$) is one of the oldest and most widely used of the simple fixatives. Two entirely different forms of fixation can be produced, depending upon the pH of the solution. At a more acid reaction than pH 4.6, the results are similar to those produced by chromic acid. At a more alkaline reaction than pH 4.6, the cytoplasm is homogeneously preserved and the mitochondria fixed.

One of the most important properties of potassium dichromate is its strong fixative action on certain lipids. This attribute is used particularly in the study of myelinated nerve fibres. If a fixative contains potassium dichromate, tissues preserved in it should be well washed in running water, prior to dehydration.

Trichloracetic acid

Trichloracetic acid (CCl_3COOH) is sometimes incorporated into compound fixatives. It is a general protein precipitant but has a marked swelling effect on many tissues, a property made use of to counter the shrinkage produced by other simple fixatives. It can be used also as a slow decalcifying agent and the softening effect which it has on dense fibrous tissue is found to facilitate the preparation of sections from blocks of this nature.

Compound fixatives

Compound fixatives may conveniently be considered under two headings: (1) micro-anatomical, and (2) cytological. Micro-anatomical fixatives are used for preserving the various layers of tissue and cells in relation to one another, so that general structure may be studied. Cytological fixatives are usually subdivided into two groups: (a) nuclear, and (b) cytoplasmic. They are used for preservation of the constituent elements of the cells, although this often entails loss of the properties of the micro-anatomical fixatives.

Micro-anatomical fixatives

10% Formol–saline

Formol–saline is a micro-anatomical fixative, but not a compound one. It is described here merely for convenience.

This is recommended for the fixation of material from the central nervous system and general post-mortem tissue. The period of fixation required is 24 h or longer, depending on the size of the tissue.

Formula

Formaldehyde, 40%	100 ml
Sodium chloride	8.5 g
Distilled water	900 ml

Advantages

This fixative is excellent for post-mortem material and is consequently very widely used. It causes even fixation and produces very little shrinkage. Large specimens may safely be fixed for an indefinite period provided that the solution is changed every three months. Fixation with formol–saline can be followed by most staining techniques, and it is particularly valuable for work on the central nervous system. Although fat is not fixed, it is preserved and may be demonstrated by suitable staining procedures. This is the only routine fixative which conveniently facilitates the dissection of specimens; 10% formalin is the basis of all museum fixatives, for it is the only fixative that allows the natural colour to be restored to the specimen.

Disadvantages

It is a slow fixative and tissue which has been fixed in formol–saline is liable to shrink during dehydration in alcohol. This shrinkage may be reduced by secondary fixation in formol–saline–sublimate (see p. 185). The metachromatic reaction of amyloid is reduced, and acid dyes stain less brightly than they do after mercuric chloride fixation. Formalin has an irritant vapour which may injure the nasal mucosa and cause sinusitis. Rubber gloves must be worn when handling specimens fixed in formol–saline, for dermatitis may be produced by prolonged contact of formalin with the skin. A pigment is often formed in tissue containing a great deal of blood.

10% Neutral buffered formalin

This is recommended for the preservation and storage of surgical, post-mortem and research specimens. The period of fixation is 24 h or longer.

Formula

Sodium dihydrogen phosphate (anhydrous)	3.5 g
Disodium hydrogen phosphate (anhydrous)	6.5 g
Formaldehyde, 40%	100.0 ml
Distilled water	900.0 ml

Advantages

This fixative has the same advantages as formol–saline, but in addition it prevents the formation of the troublesome post-mortem precipitate (acid formalin pigment)—see p. 219.

Disadvantages

The disadvantages of this fixative are similar to those listed for formol–saline. It does also, however, have the disadvantage of taking longer to prepare and in a busy routine laboratory where large volumes of the fluid are used daily this is an important factor to consider. It is also more expensive for routine use.

Heidenhain's 'Susa'

This is recommended mainly for biopsies. The period of fixation required is from 3 to 12 h.

Formula

Mercuric chloride	45 g
Sodium chloride	5 g
Trichloracetic acid	20 g
Glacial acetic acid	40 ml
Formaldehyde, 40%	200 ml
Distilled water	800 ml

Advantages

This fixative penetrates rapidly, producing good and even fixation, with the minimum of shrinkage and hardening. It allows brilliant subsequent staining results with sharp nuclear detail, and may be followed by most staining procedures, including silver impregnations. Large blocks of fibrous tissue may be sectioned more easily after this fixative than for any other. The tissue is transferred directly from the fixative to 95% or absolute alcohol.

Disadvantages

Slices of tissue should not exceed 1 cm in thickness, as prolonged fixation necessary for thicker material produces shrinkage and hardening. Red blood corpuscles are poorly preserved. Some cytoplasmic granules are dissolved.

Formol–sublimate

This is recommended for routine post-mortem material. The period of fixation required is from 3 to 24 h, depending on the thickness of the tissue.

Formula
Saturated aqueous mercuric chloride	90 ml
Formaldehyde, 40%	10 ml

Advantages

This is an excellent routine fixative, and it produces little or no shrinkage or hardening of the tissue. It can be followed by most staining procedures, including the silver reticulum methods, with excellent results. Cytological details and red blood cells are well preserved. The tissue is transferred directly from the fixative to 70% alcohol.

Disadvantages

Slices of tissue should not exceed 1 cm in thickness.

Formol–saline–sublimate

Good results are obtained if the formol–sublimate solution (see above) is diluted with an equal volume of 10% formol–saline. The results obtained are similar to those following formol–sublimate. The solution is recommended for secondary fixation.

Zenker's solution

This is recommended for the fixation of small pieces of liver and spleen. The period of fixation required is from 12 to 24 h.

Formula
Mercuric chloride	5.0 g
Potassium dichromate	2.5 g
Sodium sulphate (optional)	1.0 g
Distilled water	100.0 ml

Add 5 ml of glacial acetic acid just before use.

Advantages

Tissue fixed in Zenker's solution permits excellent staining of nuclei and of connective tissue fibres. It is recommended particularly for tissues which are to be stained by one of the trichrome techniques.

Disadvantages

Penetration is poor, and pieces of tissue should not exceed 0.5 cm in thickness. Tissue immersed in the fluid for more than 24 h tends to become brittle. After fixation, the tissue must be washed in running water for several hours. Zenker's solution is not recommended for frozen sections. The solution does not keep well after addition of the acetic acid.

Zenker–formol (Helly's)

This is recommended for the fixation of pituitary tissue and bone-marrow. The period of fixation required is from 12 to 24 h.

Formula
Mercuric chloride	5.0 g
Potassium dichromate	2.5 g
Sodium sulphate (optional)	1.0 g
Distilled water	100.0 ml

Add 5 ml of 40% formaldehyde just before use.

Advantages

Although this fixative contains both oxidizing and reducing agents, it produces excellent nuclear fixation. Staining of nuclei is even more intense than after fixation with Zenker's solution. Cytoplasmic granules are well preserved.

Disadvantages

The disadvantages are comparable with those of Zenker's solution. If material is allowed to remain in the fixative for longer than 24 h, a brown scum is produced on the tissue.

Bouin's solution

This is recommended for the fixation of embryos The period of fixation required is from 6 to 24 h.

Formula
Saturated aqueous picric acid	75 ml
Formaldehyde, 40%	25 ml
Glacial acetic acid	5 ml

Advantages

This fixative produces very little micro-anatomica distortion and permits brilliant staining results. The tissue should *not* be washed in running water, bu transferred directly from fixative to 70% alcohol. Bouin's solution preserves glycogen and may be used for fixing tissue in which this carbohydrate is to be demonstrated. The yellow colour which Bouin's fluid imparts to tissue is useful when handling fragmentary biopsies.

Disadvantages

This fixative penetrates poorly, restricting its usefulness to small pieces of tissue.

Gendre's fluid

A general micro-anatomical fixative which is also widely used for the preservation of glycogen.

Formula

Acetic acid, glacial	5 ml
Picric acid, saturated solution in 95% alcohol	80 ml
Concentrated formaldehyde solution (40%)	15 ml

Advantages

The results produced are very similar to Bouin's solution (see above), but the combined action of both the alcohol and high picric acid content make it an excellent fixative for glycogen. When fixation is complete the tissue is washed in several changes of 80% alcohol.

Disadvantages

These are similar to those listed under Bouin's fluid.

Cytological fixatives

As has been previously mentioned, cytological fixatives are usually divided into two groups: (a) nuclear, and (b) cytoplasmic.

Nuclear fixatives	*Cytoplasmic fixatives*
1. Flemming's fluid	1. Flemming's fluid without acetic acid
2. Carnoy's fluid	2. Helly's fluid
	3. Formalin with 'post-chroming'

Nuclear fixatives

Flemming's fluid

This fixative is recommended for the preservation of nuclear structures. The period of fixation is from 24 to 48 h.

Formula

Chromic acid, 1%	15 ml

Aqueous osmium tetroxide, 2%	4 ml
Glacial acetic acid	1 ml

Advantages

This fixative is the most commonly used of the chrome–osmium–acetic fixatives. Excellent fixation of nuclear elements, especially chromosomes, is produced. It is the only fixative which permanently preserves fat. The reagent is costly, but relatively small volumes are required, i.e. the tissue may be fixed in ten times its own volume of Flemming's fluid.

Disadvantages

Owing to the poor penetrative powers of this fixative it should only be used for small pieces of tissue. The solution deteriorates rapidly, and must be prepared immediately before use. Tissue fixed in Flemming's fluid should be washed for 24 h in running tap water prior to dehydration.

Carnoy's fluid

This is recommended for fixing chromosomes, lymph glands, and urgent biopsies. The period of fixation required is from ½ to 3 h.

Formula

Absolute alcohol	60 ml
Chloroform	30 ml
Glacial acetic acid	10 ml

Advantages

This fixative permits good nuclear staining, but is not recommended for detailed nuclear studies. It fixes rapidly and also dehydrates, and is therefore useful for biopsy material. Glycogen is preserved. Following fixation, the tissue is transferred directly to absolute alcohol.

Disadvantages

Excessive shrinkage is caused by this solution and it is only suitable for small pieces of tissue. Red blood corpuscles are haemolysed.

Cytoplasmic fixatives

Flemming's fluid without acetic acid

This is recommended for mitochondria and the period of fixation required is from 24 to 48 h.

Formula

Flemming's fluid, but omitting the acetic acid (see above).

The advantages and disadvantages of this solution are similar to those listed for Flemming's fluid. The omission of acetic acid improves the cytoplasmic detail.

Helly's fluid

This is synonymous with Zenker–formol (see p. 182).

10% Formol–saline

Fixation in 10% formol–saline, followed by the post-chroming of the tissue, in 3% potassium dichromate for 3–7 days, permits good cytoplasmic staining and improves myelin preservation.

The fixation of smears

Smears which are to be examined for the presence of malignant cells may be fixed in the following solutions (see also Chapter 19).

Alcohol–ether

This is a widely used cytological fixative, especially recommended for use with the Papanicolaou staining methods. It is highly flammable.

Formula

Absolute ethyl alcohol	1 volume
Ether	1 volume

1. Fix the smears for 15 min or longer.
2. Rinse in alcohol followed by distilled water and continue to stain by the selected procedure.

Schaudinn's fluid

This is a rapidly penetrating fixative used in diagnostic exfoliative cytology for preserving smears which are to be stained with haematoxylin and eosin.

Formula

Mercuric chloride, saturated aqueous solution	66 ml
Absolute ethyl alcohol	33 ml
Glacial acetic acid	1 ml

1. Fix the smears for upwards of 2 min.
2. Wash in distilled water.
3. Remove the mercuric chloride pigment according to the method given on p. 219.
4. Continue to stain by the selected procedure.

Carbowax fixative

This is useful for the transportation of smears to the laboratory.

Formula

Carbowax	3.0 g
Glacial acetic acid	0.2 ml
Absolute ethyl alcohol	100 ml

Flood the smear and allow the fluid to evaporate (10–15 min). Remove the film of carbowax by immersing in absolute ethyl alcohol for 10 min, or longer, immediately prior to staining.

Aerosol spray fixatives

A number of alcohol-based fixatives in aerosol spray containers are now available commercially. These aerosol spray fixatives are intended for the preservation of cells smeared on glass slides. In addition to being alcohol based, they also contain a water-soluble wax which provides a protective barrier.

The fixation of gross specimens

It is often necessary to fix specimens of entire organs. This may be done with 10% formol–saline, or with one of the museum fixatives consisting of formaldehyde in conjunction with various acetates, such as Wentworth's solution.

Formula

Sodium acetate	40 g
Formaldehyde, 40%	100 ml
Distilled water	900 ml

The technique of fixation varies with the organ to be preserved. A detailed description of the technique is outside the scope of this book, but the following brief notes will act as a guide.

Central nervous system

Tissue from the central nervous system should be fixed as soon after death as possible, to prevent the autolytic changes which rapidly take place. If the whole brain is to be preserved, it should be suspended in 10% neutral formol–saline by means of a cord passed under the basilar artery. If the spinal cord is required whole, it should be laid flat on a narrow strip of wood or cork and the dura mater incised along its entire length. The dura mater should now be reflected and pinned onto the board with plastic pins (metal pins are not recommended for this purpose, as they rust and leave unsightly holes in the tissue). Fixation is accomplished by floating the pinned specimen, board uppermost, in 10% neutral formol–saline.

Lungs

Formol–saline, 10%, is run into each of the major bronchi from an aspirator placed 1.2 m (4 ft) higher than the specimen. The fluid is run in until the contours of the lung appear sharply outlined. The bronchi should be plugged with absorbent cotton wool and the specimen immersed in a large volume of the fixative.

Heart

The heart should be packed with small balls of absorbent cotton wool saturated with 10% formol–saline. The specimen should then be immersed in a large volume of 10% formol–saline.

Liver, kidney and spleen

Such specimens are best fixed by injection. Formol–saline, 10%, is injected into the blood vessel of the organ by means of a Roberts' bronchogram syringe, and the specimen then immersed in a large volume of fixative.

Intestine

The method of fixation depends on the pathology to be demonstrated. If the natural shape is to be preserved, as in Crohn's disease, the specimen should be packed with absorbent cotton wool and soaked in 10% formol–saline. If it is desired to demonstrate such parasites as *Trichuris trichiura*, the gut is opened and pinned out, in a similar manner to that described for the spinal cord.

Secondary fixation

Following fixation with formol–saline it is sometimes advantageous to refix the tissue for a further 4 h in a second fixative. The fixatives usually selected for this purpose are formol–sublimate, Zenker–formol and Heidenhain's 'Susa'. This procedure, which is known as secondary fixation, has the advantage of imparting a firmer texture to the tissue and in many instances improves the subsequent staining results.

Post-chromatization

In order to facilitate certain staining procedures, fixed tissues or sections can be immersed in 3% potassium dichromate for several hours prior to staining. This procedure is known as post-chromatization or post-chroming, and is used mainly with tissue fixed in formol–saline.

The purpose is to mordant the tissue. Post-chroming should not be confused, however, with post-mordanting (see p. 215). This latter procedure is carried out after staining, a classic example being the application of the iodine in Gram's stain.

'Washing out'

Reference has been made to the washing of tissue in running water, after certain fixatives have been used. This may be done in several ways, but whatever the method, it is important to ensure that the specimen is bathed in a constant stream of fresh water. It is important that neither the tissue nor the accompanying label are washed out of the container. It is also important to make sure that the water surrounding the tissue is constantly being changed, preferably by means of a siphon system. Failure to observe this point may result in the fixative being insufficiently removed from the tissue.

The purpose of washing the tissue in running water is to remove oxidizing agents such as potassium dichromate and osmium tetroxide to prevent reduction when coming into contact with the alcohol. It is also important to remove all traces of formaldehyde from tissue to be embedded in gelatin.

14

Decalcification

When heavy deposits of calcium salts are present in tissue, the cutting of sections is facilitated by decalcification. Inadequate decalcification results in poor section-cutting and severe damage to the knife-edge. Calcium is normally present in large amounts in bone and teeth, but pathologically deposits may be found in varying amounts in other tissues, notably those involved in tuberculous or cancerous changes. Calcified deposits are often present also in the heart valves and walls of large blood vessels, particularly the aorta, of elderly people.

An acid is the essential constituent in most decalcifying solutions, and a second substance is often incorporated to prevent distortion of the tissue, although this should be minimal if adequate fixation has been given. Buffer solutions of pH 4.4–4.5 and organic chelating agents, e.g. ethylene-diamine tetra-acetic acid (EDTA), can also be used.

A good decalcifying agent should remove all calcium without damage to cells or tissue fibres and with no impairment of subsequent staining or impregnation.

The four acids most commonly used for removing calcium salts from tissues are formic, nitric, hydrochloric and trichloracetic acid.

The speed at which the calcium salts are dissolved out of the tissue is dependent upon the strength, temperature and volume of the decalcifying solution in relation to the size and consistency of the tissue undergoing decalcification. An increase in either the concentration of the acid acting as the decalcifying agent or the temperature at which decalcification takes place, can markedly decrease the time required, but this is usually attended by partial digestion of the tissue and inferior staining results. These adverse effects, produced by a higher temperature, do not apply to EDTA which may be used successfully at 40–60°C.

Selection of tissue

Bone

Blocks of tissue suitable for sectioning are selected from the gross specimen by means of a sharp, fine-toothed hacksaw after preliminary fixation in neutral 10% formalin. To facilitate fixation and decalcification, the selected block of tissue should not exceed 5 mm in thickness. Damage to the surface of the tissue and impacted bone-dust produced by sawing can be removed by trimming the decalcified tissue with a sharp knife. It is always advisable, however, to discard the first sections cut in order to avoid possible artefacts in the final preparation.

Teeth

Blocks of teeth for sectioning are usually best taken when the specimen is either completely or partially decalcified. They may then be selected with a sharp knife, thereby causing the minimum of damage and distortion to the tissue.

Calcified tissue

Blocks of tissue suitable for processing and sectioning can usually be selected from fixed soft tissues containing calcified areas by means of a sharp knife. If large calcified areas are encountered a hacksaw is gently applied until the deposits are cut through and the surrounding soft tissues are again dealt with by knife. Considerable damage to knife-edge and tissues will occur if the cutting of such areas is attempted by knife alone. The selected tissue block should preferably not exceed 5 mm thickness as immersion in the decalcifying solution for too long a period is to be avoided.

Tissues should be completely fixed before commencing decalcification and neutral 10% formalin is the recommended fixative for this purpose. At least 48 h fixation is required for tissue blocks of 5 mm thickness.

Technique of decalcification

1. The selected tissue slice is suspended in the decalcifying solution by means of a waxed thread. This allows the solution free access to all surfaces of the tissue, while the wax protects the thread from the action of the acid. With few exceptions, the volume of decalcifying fluid should be approximately 50–100 times the volume of the tissue.
2. The progress of decalcification should be tested at regular intervals, usually daily, but in the final stages and with some decalcifying solutions more frequent tests are made. The fluid is renewed following each positive test.
3. When decalcification is complete the tissue is transferred directly to 70% alcohol and given several changes over 8–12 h. This not only effectively washes out the acid, but also establishes the first stage of dehydration for either the paraffin wax, celloidin or LVN infiltration techniques (see Chapter 15).
4. The tissue is then completely dehydrated and processed according to the required embedding technique. If the paraffin wax method is used, it is recommended that at least part of the wax impregnation be carried out in the vacuum oven (see p. 196).

Assessment of decalcification

Tissues should be immersed in the acid decalcifying solutions only for as long as is necessary for complete calcium removal. Prolonged immersion beyond this stage will result in deterioration of cell and tissue morphology and the quality of subsequent staining reactions. The stage to which decalcification has progressed and its eventual end-point can be assessed by (1) X-ray examination, and (2) a chemical test. The simplicity of the chemical test has fortunately led to the abandonment of several crude methods for decalcification assessment. These included probing of the tissue block by needle, knife or finger nail in an effort to detect residual gritty fragments of calcium. Such malpractices were the direct cause of tissue damage, and small spicules of bone often remained undetected.

1. X-ray examination is the most satisfactory method, depending on the availability of facilities and a good relationship between laboratory and radiography department. X-ray is the only means by which tissues treated with EDTA can be adequately controlled, but it cannot be used on material fixed in mercuric chloride because this fixative renders such material radio-opaque. It can also be inconvenient during the final stages of decalcification when frequent examination may be necessary.
2. A chemical test is a simple and reliable expedient when radiography is unavailable. It is a two-stage test which depends on the detection of dissolved calcium in the decalcifying fluid. A positive result at either stage indicates that further decalcification of the tissue in fresh fluid is required and the test should be repeated after a suitable interval.

Method

1. Decant 5 ml of the used decalcifying fluid into a clean test-tube and add a small piece of litmus paper.
2. Add strong ammonia (sp. gr. 0.88) drop by drop while agitating the tube until the litmus paper just turns blue, indicating alkalinity.
3. If the solution becomes turbid at this stage calcium is present in considerable amounts and the tissue should be transferred to fresh decalcifying fluid.
4. If the solution remains clear proceed with the second stage of the test. Add 0.5 ml saturated aqueous ammonium oxalate, mix and allow to stand for 30 min. Any turbidity developing during this period indicates the presence of calcium and re-immersion of the tissue in fresh decalcifying fluid is necessary.

   If the solution remains clear it may be assumed that decalcification is complete.

   It is important that sufficient time is allowed between tests to ensure dissolution of calcium by the fresh decalcifying fluid. Intervals of 3–4 h are considered adequate for most decalcifying solutions.

When using the chemical test to control the degree of decalcification it is essential that the decalcifying fluid is prepared with distilled water. Failure to observe this precaution may result in false positive readings being produced by the presence of calcium ions in tap water.

Decalcifying solutions

Formic acid (HCOOH)

This is recommended for post-mortem and research tissue. The time necessary for decalcification is from 2 to 7 days.

Formula

Formic acid (sp. gr. 1.20)	5 ml
Distilled water	90 ml
Formaldehyde (40%)	5 ml

Advantages

This solution permits excellent staining results and it is regarded by many workers as being the best decalcifying solution for routine purposes.

Disadvantages

At the above strength decalcification is slow, and the solution is therefore unsuitable for urgent work. Decalcification may be speeded up by increasing the formic acid content up to 25 ml (Gooding and Stewart's fluid). A disadvantage of using concentrations of formic acid in excess of 8%, however, is that the opacity of the solution interferes with the chemical test used in controlling the degree of decalcification. While the used fluid can be diluted in order to apply this test, the final result is not always as accurate as when used with a sample of the undiluted decalcifying solution.

Nitric acid–formaldehyde

This is recommended for urgent biopsies. The time required for decalcification is from 1 to 3 days.

Formula

Nitric acid (sp. gr. 1.41)	10 ml
Formaldehyde (40%)	5–10 ml
Distilled water	to 100 ml

Advantages

This is a rapidly acting decalcifying solution which permits good nuclear staining.

Disadvantages

Nuclear staining is not as good as that obtained after more slow-acting solutions. Nitric acid frequently develops a yellow colour when used as a decalcifying agent owing to the formation of nitrous acid. This increases the speed of decalcification but also impairs the subsequent staining reactions. The addition of 0.1% urea to the pure concentrated nitric acid temporarily arrests the discoloration and does not appear to affect the efficiency of the acid.

Aqueous nitric acid

A rapidly acting decalcifying solution which is recommended for routine use.

Formula

Nitric acid (sp. gr. 1.41)	5–10 ml
Distilled water	to 100 ml

Advantages

This is a rapid decalcifying solution which causes very little hydrolysis, provided that the tissue is not allowed to remain immersed beyond the stage when decalcification is completed. The subsequent staining results are good.

Disadvantages

The disadvantages of the solution are similar to those given above under nitric acid–formaldehyde. The remarks relating to the use of urea to stabilize the nitric acid also apply with this solution.

Perenyi's fluid

This solution was introduced originally as a fixative for ova, but it has gained popularity in recent years as a good routine decalcifying fluid. The time required for decalcification is from 2 to 10 days.

Formula

Nitric acid, 10% aqueous solution	40 ml
Absolute ethyl alcohol	30 ml
Chromic acid, 0.5% aqueous solution	30 ml

When freshly mixed the solution is yellow, but it rapidly assumes a clear violet colour.

Advantages

No hardening occurs in tissues treated with Perenyi's fluid; indeed it is often used as a softening agent, prior to dehydration, for dense fibrous tissues. Cellular detail is well preserved and subsequent staining is good. When decalcification is complete, tissues do not require washing in water and may be transferred directly to several changes of 70% alcohol.

Disadvantages

It is rather slow for decalcifying dense bone. The chemical test given on p. 187 cannot be used to determine decalcification end-point because a precipitate is formed when ammonia is added to Perenyi's fluid even in the absence of calcium ions. This difficulty may be overcome, however, by a simple modification:

1. Transfer 5 ml of used decalcifying fluid to a chemically clean test-tube and add a small square of litmus paper.
2. Add ammonium hydroxide solution (sp. gr. 0.88) drop by drop, mixing between drops, until the reaction is alkaline.
3. Add glacial acetic acid drop by drop until the precipitate is dissolved.
4. Add 0.5 ml saturated aqueous solution of ammonium oxalate.

The appearance of a white precipitate within 30 min indicates the presence of calcium, and that the tissue requires further treatment with fresh fluid.

Ebner's fluid

The use of this fluid is recommended for teeth and the time necessary for decalcification is from 3 to 5 days. Various formulae have been given for this method, but the following gives good results:

Formula

Saturated aqueous sodium chloride (36% approx.)	50 ml
Distilled water	50 ml
Hydrochloric acid	8 ml

Advantages

This is a fairly rapid decalcifying solution and subsequent staining results are usually good. It is particularly useful for decalcifying teeth. The excess acid is removed by several changes of 90% alcohol for 24 h. Dehydration is thereby hastened.

Disadvantages

Nuclear staining is not as good as that obtained after formic acid.

Trichloracetic acid

This is recommended for small pieces of delicate tissue which require decalcification. The time necessary for decalcification is from 4 to 5 days.

Formula

Trichloracetic acid	5 g
10% formol–saline	95 ml

Advantages

It permits good nuclear staining. The excess acid is removed by washing in several changes of 90% alcohol.

Disadvantages

It is a slow decalcifying solution, and is not recommended for use with dense bone.

Citrate–citric acid buffer (pH 4.5)

This is recommended when speed is not an important factor. The period required for decalcification is approximately 6 days, during which time the solution should be changed daily.

Formula

Citric acid (monohydrate), 7% aqueous solution	5.0 ml
Ammonium citrate (anhydrous), 7.4% aqueous solution	95.0 ml
Zinc sulphate, 1% aqueous solution	0.2 ml
Chloroform, as preservative	a few drops

Advantages

This solution produces no damage to the cells or tissue constituents and permits excellent staining results.

Disadvantages

This method is too slow for routine work.

Ion exchange resins

The incorporation of an ion exchange resin (an ammonium form of polystyrene resin) into the decalcifying solution has been claimed to speed up the process of decalcification and to improve staining. The principle of the method is that the calcium ions are removed from the solution by the resin, thereby increasing the rate of solubility of the calcium from the tissue. However, subsequent workers have shown that no obvious improvement in decalcification speed, preservation or staining is achieved by the use of these resins. A layer of the resin, approximately 13 mm (½ in) thick, is spread over the bottom of the vessel being used and the specimen is allowed to rest on it. The decalcifying solution is added, the volume of the solution being approximately 20–30 times that of the tissue. The end-point is determined by radiological examination, the chemical test not being applicable.

The use of ion exchange resins is limited to decalcifying solutions which have a non-mineral acid as their active constituent, formic acid being the usual choice. Two baths of 0.1M hydrochloric acid followed by three washes of distilled water will regenerate the used resin for further use.

Chelating agent

This is a very slow decalcifying solution recommended only for detailed microscopical studies where time is not an important factor. It is not suitable for use with urgent surgical specimens. The time required for decalcification is approximately 3 weeks, during which time the solution must be changed at intervals of 3 days, reducing to 1 day in the final stages.

Formula

Ethylene diamine tetra-acetic acid (EDTA) disodium salt	5.5 g
10% neutral formalin	100 ml

Advantages

Histological artefacts are minimized by the use of this solution, there being no carbon dioxide bubbles produced to destroy the pattern of the remaining organic material. The subsequent staining results are also excellent.

Disadvantages

It is slow and unsuitable for urgent work. The chelating agent also tends to harden the tissue slightly.

RDC

RDC (Bethlehem Instruments Ltd) is a proprietary fluid which is more rapid than conventional fluids. The manufacturer's instructions must be followed.

Softening of dense fibrous tissue

Some specimens are composed of dense fibrous tissue which, while not containing calcium salts, is nevertheless too tough for sectioning. Blocks of tissue taken from such specimens may be softened, as described by Lendrum, by the addition of 4–6% phenol to the dehydrating alcohols.

Commercially produced reagents such as Mollifex (BDH plc) are available for softening tissue after embedding in paraffin wax.

15

Dehydration, impregnation and embedding techniques

Many fixatives, including formaldehyde, can produce harmful effects when inhaled or when in contact with the skin. A special area should therefore be set aside for the examination of all specimens. This should take the form of a stainless steel bench provided with running water and a drainage point. Extraction facilities should also be provided to remove harmful vapours. Special benches with extraction hoods specifically designed for this purpose are now available commercially, and are strongly recommended.

Disinfectant should always be used to wash down surfaces on which specimens have been examined. Disposable gloves should always be worn and discarded after use.

Suitable instruments must be kept available and should include a large ham knife, probes, scalpels, plain and toothed forceps of varying sizes. Several pairs of scissors should also be provided, including fine dissecting, blunt-nosed and bowel scissors.

A plastic rule is necessary to measure tumours and cavities and scales to record the weight. Finally, bone forceps and a bone saw or fine hacksaw should be provided to take blocks of tissue from calcified specimens.

Selection of tissue

Following fixation, pieces of tissue for histological examination are selected from the gross specimen. A brief description of the nature of the tissue and site of origin should be recorded, either on a working card, or in a book reserved for the purpose. Small cardboard tickets bearing the general laboratory number and pathology number (this information varies according to the system employed) should be written out in waterproof ink or pencil

and placed in the compartment of the processing basket or specimen bottle, together with the tissue.

The introduction of the Tissue Tek II (Miles Scientific) and similar systems has greatly facilitated the processing of tissue and reduced the risk of possible error. The Tissue Tek II system consists of small plastic cassettes, available in various sizes and colours, with an integral lid and roughened sides which permit the necessary information to be recorded in pencil. The cassettes eventually form part of the final paraffin wax block, which means that the tissue is always identified.

Tissue requiring special attention should have an asterisk marked on the ticket, and details of the special attention to be given to the specimen should be recorded on the working card. Frequently, blocks are to be sectioned from a particular surface. This may be identified by passing a thread through one corner of the opposite surface of the tissue to that which is to be sectioned.

At no time after the pieces of tissue have been selected should their identifying label be removed. Failure to observe this rule could lead to a positive malignancy report being issued for the wrong patient. The use of the cassettes eliminates this risk.

Paraffin wax technique

Dehydration

The original fixative solutions used are not miscible with paraffin wax; therefore preliminary dehydration is necessary. The solution commonly used for this purpose is alcohol; acetone and dioxane have also been used in the past.

Table 15.1 Alcohol method of dehydration (time in hours)

	10% formol–saline	Zenker or Helly	Bouin's fluid	Susa, Carnoy or formol–sublimate	Flemming's fluid
Running water	–	1–12	–	–	1–12
Alcohol, 30%	–	1–6	–	–	½–3
Alcohol, 50%	–	1–6	–	–	½–3
Alcohol, 70%	3–12	1–6	3–12	–	½–3
Alcohol, 90%	3–12	1–6	3–12	1–6	1–3
Absolute alcohol 1	3–12	1–6	3–12	1–6	1–3
Absolute alcohol 2	3–12	1–6	3–12	1–6	1–3
Absolute alcohol 3	3–12	1–6	3–12	1–6	1–3

The alcohol method

This consists in passing the tissue through a series of progressively more concentrated alcohol* baths. Tissues together with their identifying labels are carefully transferred by forceps from one container to another at the appropriate times, allowing them to drain for a few seconds on blotting paper between each change. The containers should be fitted with ground-glass stoppers under which the accompanying labels should be clipped. The more delicate the tissue, the lower is the grade of alcohol suitable for commencing dehydration, and the smaller the intervals there should be between the strengths of the ascending alcohols.

The strength of the initial alcohol and the time required in each grade depend on the size and type of tissue and on the fixative which was used. *Table 15.1* may be followed as an approximate guide.

To ensure that the final bath of alcohol is pure, and free from water, it is advisable to keep a layer of anhydrous copper sulphate 6 mm (¼ in) in depth and covered with filter paper, on the bottom of the

*The purchase and use of absolute ethyl alcohol is subject to many restrictions for customs and excise purposes. 74° OP spirit (Absolute Industrial Methylated Spirit), which is not subject to these restrictions, is normally used in laboratories.

Proof spirit is legally defined as 'That which, at the temperature of 51°F weighs exactly twelve-thirteenth parts of an equal volume of distilled water'. At 60°F it has a sp. gr. of 0.9198 and contains 57.1% v/v, or 49.2% w/w, of ethyl alcohol. Spirits are described as so many degrees over-proof (OP) or under-proof (UP). Proof spirit is the standard and is referred to as 100°. A spirit stated as 70° would therefore be 30° UP (100° − 70°). A spirit stated simply as 160° would be 60° OP (100° + 60°).

Ninety-five per cent alcohol is equivalent to 60° OP, which means that 100 volumes of this would contain as much ethyl alcohol as 166 volumes of proof spirit.

As proof spirit (100°) contains approximately 57% ethyl alcohol, 74 OP (174°) would contain

$$\frac{57 \times 174}{100} \text{ % ethyl alcohol} = \text{approx. } 99\%$$

vessel used. This salt *also* acts as an indicator, turning blue when water is present. The alcohol should be discarded if a blue tinge becomes apparent. Isopropyl alcohol may be used for dehydration purposes.

The period necessary for dehydration may be reduced by processing at 37°C instead of room temperature. This procedure is sometimes of value when sections are required urgently from small fragmentary biopsies. These specimens should be wrapped carefully in filter paper prior to processing.

The acetone method

This is used for the most urgent biopsies. Only small pieces of tissue should be treated, and dehydration takes from ½ to 2 h. Considerable shrinkage is produced during the process, rendering it unsuitable for routine work.

The dioxane method

Dioxane (diethylene dioxide) is a unique reagent which has the unusual property of being miscible with both water and molten paraffin wax. It produces very little shrinkage and is simple to use. It is now known to be toxic and its use is no longer recommended.

Clearing

'Clearing' or 'de-alcoholization' is the term applied to the removal of alcohol from blocks or sections of tissue by immersing them in an ante-medium. Most of the original ante-media raised the refractive index of de-alcoholized tissues, thereby imparting to them a degree of transparency which resulted in this stage of processing being designated the 'clearing stage' and the media used as 'clearing agents'. Not all of the present-day ante-media (e.g. chloroform) cause this transparent effect and the term 'clearing' is therefore strictly incorrect.

Clearing agents must be miscible with both alcohol and paraffin wax. The most common clearing agents are xylene, toluene, chloroform and cedar wood oil.

Xylene

A rapid clearing agent suitable for urgent biopsies. It is cheap and highly flammable. Tissues are rendered transparent by xylene and it volatilizes readily in the paraffin oven. Biopsies, and tissue blocks not exceeding 3 mm in thickness, are cleared in 15–30 min but some material, notably brain and blood-containing tissues, tends to become brittle if immersion is prolonged.

Toluene

This appears to have superseded benzene as an ante-medium for routine work because of its lower toxicity. Like xylene it is highly flammable, has similar 'clearing' properties, but without the same brittle effect on tissues. It is somewhat more expensive than xylene. Clearing time is from 15 to 180 min, depending on tissue type and thickness.

Chloroform

An expensive routine 'clearing agent', being non-flammable and causing minimal shrinkage or hardening of tissues even when the optimum clearing time is exceeded. It is relatively slow in its displacement of alcohol and tissue-blocks are not rendered transparent so that the end-point is difficult to assess. Most tissues of 3–5 mm thickness are de-alcoholized in 6–24 h. It should be pointed out that chloroform vapour is both anaesthetic and toxic and in addition it may have a deleterious effect on the rubber sealing ring of the vacuum impregnating bath.

Cedar wood oil

Rarely used for routine clearing purposes because of its cost and slow action. This reagent causes little or no damage to even the most delicate tissues. It is therefore of particular value in research laboratories and in embryological procedures. Certain tissues, notably skin and dense fibrous material, benefit from treatment with cedar wood oil in that it imparts to such tissues a consistency which facilitates subsequent section cutting. Tissue-blocks become transparent after alcohol displacement, but the oil is difficult to eliminate in the wax oven, several changes of wax being necessary. Alternatively, the cleared tissues may be treated with toluene for 30 min before being transferred to molten paraffin wax. Cedar wood oil for histological purposes is a thin, colourless, slightly yellow fluid distinct from the more viscous type used for oil immersion objectives and which is unsuitable for de-alcoholization.

Other agents

Carbon disulphide, carbon tetrachloride, paraffin oil, cellosolve (2-ethoxyethanol) and methyl benzoate are less commonly used as ante-media. Methyl benzoate, however, dissolves celloidin, and is used in conjunction with it for the double impregnation of tough or fragile objects (see p. 199).

Proprietary reagents

There are a number of commercially produced reagents available. They have the advantage of being more economical in use, but the efficiency of some has been queried. Before using these reagents routinely it is advisable to test them under routine laboratory conditions.

Impregnation with paraffin wax

Tissues are transferred from the clearing agent to a bath of molten paraffin wax in the embedding oven. During this stage, the clearing agent is eliminated from the tissues by diffusion into the surrounding melted wax and the wax in turn diffuses into the tissues to replace it. At least one change of wax should be given in order to remove the clearing agent that has been displaced from the tissue and to ensure its replacement with pure wax. The exact number of changes of wax and the time which the tissue requires in each is dependent upon the density and size of the block of tissue and the clearing agent used. A guide to impregnation times suitable for most tissues is given in *Table 15.2*. The wax used should be of suitable melting point. This varies with the nature of the tissue; hard tissue requires a higher

Table 15.2 Impregnation times in paraffin wax technique

Thickness of tissue (mm)	*Clearing agent employed*	*Molten paraffin wax* (h)	*No of wax changes*
<3	Xylene Toluene	1½	One
<3	Chloroform Cedar wood oil	2–3	Two
3–5	Xylene Toluene	2–3	Two
3–5	Chloroform Cedar wood oil	3–5	Three
5–8	Xylene Toluene	3–5	Two
5–8	Chloroform Cedar wood oil	5–8	Three

melting point wax than soft tissue to give the necessary consistency and support during section-cutting. The waxes commonly used have melting points in the range between 50 and 60°C, the most popular, suitable for both the English climate and most surgical and autopsy material, having a melting point of 58°C.

Complete wax impregnation is necessary for the production of good sections, but if tissues are subjected to the high temperatures of the wax oven beyond this point, over-hardening may result, which is thought by some to be detrimental to sectioning. On the other hand, inadequate impregnation leads to ultimate drying and shrinking of the embedded tissue block which, being inadequately supported by wax, cracks or crumbles when section-cutting is attempted.

The wax infiltration oven is an electrically heated cabinet which may be water-jacketed or anhydric, with or without a circulating fan. A reliable thermostat should maintain the internal temperature at 2–3°C above the melting point of the wax. The interior of the oven should be large enough to accommodate an enamel jug and funnel, fitted with Whatman No. 1 filter paper for the filtration of new or reclaimed wax, and a number of glass containers of suitable size for the wax infiltration of tissues. Some purpose-built ovens are fitted with a separate upper compartment enclosed with a hinged lid. This houses several plated metal containers for wax infiltration purposes, thus allowing the entire oven space to be utilized for wax filtration and storage.

The storage and dispensing of molten paraffin wax has been facilitated by the recent introduction of the wax dispenser. This is essentially an electrically heated, temperature-controlled, insulated tank of one imperial gallon (4.5 litre) capacity, with an integral outlet filter, heated tap, and loose-fitting lid. Temperature is adjustable up to 70°C and a safety cut-out device operating at 90°C prevents accidental overheating of the wax with its attendant fire risk. Only new wax should be stored in the dispenser unless an additional filter, suitable for the reclamation of used wax, has been installed.

Tissue density

Dense tissues require longer immersion in molten paraffin wax to ensure complete impregnation, and therefore structures such as bone, fibromas and brain require approximately twice as long as soft tissues such as kidney or liver. The excessive hardness of dense tissues caused by this increased exposure to hot wax is (with the exception of brain and other CNS material) undesirable because of possible difficulties during section-cutting. Complete wax infiltration of such tissues can be obtained without undue hardening by means of the vacuum impregnation techniques (see p. 196).

Size of the block of tissue

The amount of clearing agent carried over into the wax depends on the surface area of the tissue-block. When treating large pieces, the effects of this contamination may be minimized by frequent changes of wax. The time required for thorough impregnation depends on the thickness of the tissue; a piece 5 mm thick, for example, takes an average time of 3 h, whereas a piece 10 mm thick may take up to 10 h.

Automatic tissue processors

The automatic tissue processors (*Figure 15.1*) are an excellent example of the practical application of automation in the medical laboratory. These machines decrease both the time and labour necessary for processing tissue, thereby allowing a more rapid diagnosis to be made while freeing the laboratory staff for work of a more technical nature. The decrease in the processing time is due to the constant agitation which the tissue undergoes, a procedure which also improves the penetration and produces more consistent results.

A variety of these machines is manufactured for use on the laboratory bench. Most machines incorporate a 12-stage cycle with the last two baths being thermostatically controlled to contain paraffin wax. They are designed with a 24-hour clock, but a 1-hour clock is available for rapid processing. A 7-day clock is also available. Modern machines are equipped with an electronic timer which permits greater programming flexibility.

Safety devices

When the processing cycle is completed and the tissue has reached the second wax bath, a cut-out device operates. The tissue then remains in the wax until removed by hand. A second safety device comes into operation should the first wax bath have solidified. Failure of the transfer mechanism to return to its normal position results in the tissue containers being carried over to the second wax bath, thereby avoiding damage to the tissues. In addition to the above automatic safety devices, an alarm bell powered by two dry cell batteries can be installed in a convenient position in the laboratory. This is intended to provide warning in the event of a power failure or a fuse being blown.

Tissue containers

Special containers made of either stainless steel or plastic are provided. The stainless steel containers are designed with one, two, four or six divisions and are supplied with close-fitting lids and with a choice

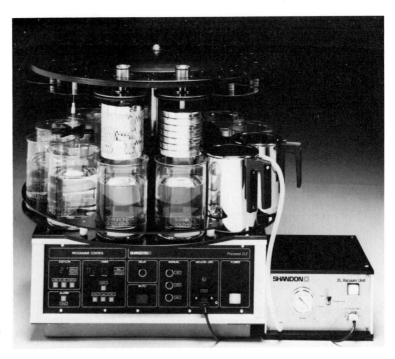

Figure 15.1. An automatic tissue processor (reproduced by courtesy of Shandon Southern Products Ltd)

of mesh sizes. Special baskets for curettings and fragmentary tissue are available.

Plastic containers with up to six compartments are also available. These are of value when processing tissues fixed in corrosive sublimate. The plastic containers are loaded onto a central spindle and are designed to interlock. This dispenses with lids, with the exception of the top basket.

Processing schedule for automatic tissue processor

The processing schedule used with the automatic tissue processor will vary according to the type of tissue, the nature of the work, the clearing reagent used and personal preference. Two examples are given in *Table 15.3*, both of which provide good results.

Vacuum-impregnation technique

The vacuum-impregnation technique depends on the production of negative pressure inside the embedding oven. This pressure reduction hastens the extrusion of air-bubbles and of the clearing agent from the tissue-block, facilitating rapid penetration by the wax.

Table 15.3   Examples of schedules for tissue processor

Schedule I		*Schedule II*	
Reagent	*Processing time* (h)	*Reagent*	*Processing time* (h)
70% alcohol	2	70% alcohol	2
90% alcohol	3	90% alcohol	2
Absolute alcohol 1	3	96% alcohol	2
Absolute alcohol 2	3	Absolute alcohol 1	2
Absolute alcohol 3	3	Absolute alcohol 2	2
Toluene 1	0.5	Absolute alcohol 3	2
Toluene 2	1	Chloroform 1	2
Wax 1	3	Chloroform 2	2
Wax 2	3	Chloroform 3	2
Wax 3 (vacuum bath)	0.5	Wax 1	2
		Wax 2	2
		Wax 3 (vacuum bath)	0.5

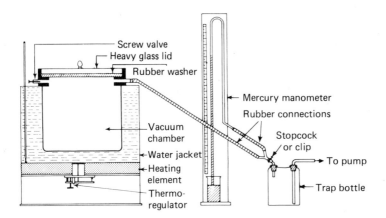

Figure 15.2. Diagram illustrating the assembly of the vacuum-impregnation apparatus

It is useful for the following tissues: (a) urgent biopsies; (b) dense tissue; (c) lung tissue; and (d) tissue which contains a large amount of fat.

Vacuum-impregnation oven

There are several types of vacuum-impregnation bath (or vacuum-impregnation oven). A type in common use has a vacuum compartment which is a flat-bottomed brass chamber, with a heavy glass lid resting on a thick rubber washer, which creates an airtight junction. The vacuum chamber is immersed in a thermostatically controlled water-jacket. A valve is fitted on one side of the chamber by means of which air may be admitted when the bath is under negative pressure. On the opposite side of the chamber is a small tube by which the interior is connected to the vacuum pump (*Figure 15.2*).

Some automatic tissue processors are now manufactured with a vacuum-impregnation facility.

Assembly of apparatus

1. Fit a Venturi water pump to a cold water tap on the mains supply.
2. Connect the pump to a trap bottle with pressure tubing.
3. Connect the bottle to a glass Y-piece with pressure tubing.
4. Attach one end of the Y-piece to a manometer and the other end to a vacuum bath. A glass stopcock should be inserted in the 'pressure' tubing between the Y-piece and the trap bottle.

Method of using the vacuum-impregnation oven

1. Transfer the cleared tissue to a container of molten paraffin wax, and place it in the vacuum bath.
2. Place the heavy glass lid in position and press it firmly down.

3. Close the valve and exhaust the chamber with the Venturi pump, until a negative pressure of 400–500 mm is shown on the manometer.
4. Close the stopcock between the Y-piece and the trap bottle, and turn off the pump.
5. When the tissue has been immersed in the wax for the requisite period, unscrew the valve gradually, allowing the pressure inside the bath to rise to that of the atmosphere.
6. Remove and change the wax, or embed the tissue, as necessary.

■ Note

Never turn off the water pump while the stopcock between the Y-piece and the trap bottle is still open. If this precaution is not observed, water may be sucked back into the trap bottle and the vacuum chamber. An electric pump may be used in place of the water pump.

When the oven is not in use, the rubber washer should be removed. Prolonged exposure to high temperatures causes the rubber to perish.

Moulds for embedding

A variety of moulds is available for 'blocking out' or embedding the tissue in paraffin wax.

Leuckhart embedding boxes

These are convenient moulds for routine work and are widely used. They consist of two L-shaped pieces of metal, usually brass, and may be purchased in a variety of sizes. They are arranged on a glass or metal plate to form a mould of the desired size. When the embedding wax has solidified, the moulds and the encased blocks are removed from the base plate and tapped on the bench. The two L-pieces immediately come away from the wax block and are ready to be re-used.

Plastic ice-trays

These form convenient moulds for the busy routine

laboratory, one block being embedded in each compartment. When set, the wax blocks are easily removed by flexing the plastic tray. This may be facilitated by smearing the inside of the mould with a little glycerol or liquid paraffin. Aerosol sprays are also available.

Watch glasses

These are ideal for embedding fragmentary biopsies. While it is not essential to smear them with glycerol before use, it is a sensible precaution as the blocks are sometimes difficult to remove.

Technique for embedding

1. Fill the mould with molten paraffin wax.
2. Warm a pair of blunt-nosed forceps (electrically heated forceps may also be used), and use them to transfer the tissue from the paraffin bath to the mould.
3. Warm the forceps again, and orientate the tissue until it is lying in the desired plane. Run the warm forceps round the tissue to ensure that any wax which may have solidified during the transferrence from the paraffin bath to the mould is melted.
4. Remove the corresponding label from the paraffin bath, and place it against the side of the mould adjacent to the tissue.
5. Blow on the surface until a thin film of wax has solidified.
6. Transfer the mould to a container of cold water, and immerse it gently. The mould should remain submerged until the wax hardens. This may take 10–30 min, but solidification may be hastened by transferring the mould to running water.

Plastic embedding cassettes

These are disposable products available in a number of sizes and intended to speed up the paraffin wax embedding technique. The plastic cassettes are used in conjunction with special stainless steel base moulds. The tissue to be embedded is positioned in a base mould which has been previously sprayed with an aerosol provided for the purpose. The plastic cassette is placed in position and the paraffin wax poured in until it reaches the top.

After cooling, the base mould is easily detached, leaving the embedded tissue ready for cutting. No trimming is necessary and the wax-filled plastic cassette serves as a block holder. Following sectioning, the blocks are stored in the plastic cassettes. This method undoubtedly saves a great deal of time and is of value when blocks have to be re-cut, but it has the disadvantage of requiring a much greater storage space, and the plastic cassettes are relatively expensive.

Glass tubing

Glass tubing which has one end sealed with a cork is useful for embedding cytological specimens which are to be sectioned. The processing and embedding can be carried out in the tubing, the specimen being centrifuged between each stage. The small particle of tissue will collect at the bottom of the tubing and make the sectioning easier. After the paraffin wax has solidified, the cork may be removed and the block pushed out of the tubing.

Gelatin embedding

As a general rule, tissue from which frozen sections are to be prepared is not embedded, the freezing of the tissue providing sufficient support for sectioning. When frozen sections are required from tough or friable tissue, however, it is advantageous to embed the tissue in a supporting medium, in order to prevent the tissue from fragmenting.

The usual embedding medium for this purpose is gelatin, and when embedded the blocks of tissue are transferred to formalin in order to harden them. The formalin changes the structure of the gelatin from the hydrosol to the hydrogel condition.

Aschoff's gelatin embedding method

Solution 1:

Gelatin	12.5 g
Distilled water	87.5 ml
Phenol crystals, as preservative	1 g

Solution 2:

Gelatin	25 g
Distilled water	75 ml
Phenol crystals, as preservative	1 g

Solution 3:

Concentrated formaldehyde solution (40%)	5 ml
Distilled water	95 ml

Mode of preparation

Solutions 1 and 2. Heat the distilled water to 37°C and dissolve the phenol. Add the gelatin and incubate at 37°C until solution is effected. Filter through surgical gauze, bottle and label.

Solution 3. Add the concentrated formaldehyde solution to the distilled water. Mix well and label.

Preparation for use

Melt the gelatin by heating in a water bath or by incubation.

Procedure

1. Place thoroughly washed formalin fixed tissue not exceeding 3 mm in thickness in solution 1 and incubate at 37°C for 12–24 h.
2. Transfer to solution 2 for 12–24 h at 37°C.
3. Embed in solution 2 using a Leuckhart embedding box, cool and trim. Excess gelatin inhibits the freezing.
4. Place the trimmed block in solution 3 for 24 h and then cut frozen sections, according to the technique described on p. 210.

■ **Notes**

1. Following embedding the gelatin block may be cooled in a refrigerator but must not be allowed to freeze.
2. Excess gelatin may be removed by floating the sections onto paper and trimming with scissors.
3. Tissues permeated with gelatin take far longer to freeze than unimpregnated tissues of an equivalent size.
4. By using the above method, sections of 5 μm upwards may be obtained.

Celloidin

Celloidin is the trade name given to a purified form of nitrocellulose. It is of particular value as a histological embedding medium for sectioning hard tissues of a mixed consistency, for cutting very thick sections or when the minimum of shrinkage is required and the frozen section technique is not practicable.

Celloidin is usually supplied in the form of wool dampened with alcohol. The working strengths are 2, 4 and 8%, the solvent being equal parts of ether and alcohol.

Necoloidine, a similar compound available from B.D.H. plc, is used in many laboratories in place of celloidin. It is supplied as a solution of about 8% of pyroxylin in ether–alcohol, but for use should be thickened to a 16% solution. Thickening is a simple matter, the solvent being allowed to evaporate in a fume-cupboard until the volume has become reduced by approximately half.

Evaporation is a constant problem when using celloidin and the working solutions should always be stored in bottles fitted with ground-glass stoppers. An ideal bottle for this purpose is a wide-mouthed oil bottle, fitted with a ground-glass stopper and a ground-glass covering cap. It must be remembered that ether vapour is highly dangerous and celloidin should never be used in the vicinity of an open flame.

Celloidin impregnation and embedding technique

Impregnation

1. Dehydrate the tissue through ascending grades of alcohol, completing the dehydration by using a bath of absolute alcohol containing copper sulphate.
2. Transfer the tissue to a mixture of equal parts of alcohol and ether for 24 h. The purpose of this step is to speed up the subsequent impregnation.
3. Transfer the tissue to a thin (2%) solution of celloidin for 5–7 days.
4. Transfer the tissue to a medium (4%) solution of celloidin for 5–7 days.
5. Transfer the tissue to a thick (8%) solution of celloidin for 2–3 days.

Embedding

1. Half-fill a suitable embedding mould with thick (8%) celloidin and place the tissue in position, with the surface to be cut uppermost. Top up the mould with more of the embedding solution. The mould should be considerably deeper than the thickness of the tissue, in order to prevent the tissue from becoming exposed, as the celloidin shrinks on hardening.
2. Place the mould in a desiccator containing ether vapour, in order to remove all air-bubbles. Immediately all air-bubbles are removed from the embedding medium, invert the tissue so that the surface to be cut is face downwards in the mould. This prevents any air-bubbles from being trapped beneath the tissue.
3. Transfer the mould to a second desiccator containing chloroform vapour, until the celloidin is hardened to the required consistency. This can be tested by pressing the ball of the thumb (not the nail) against the surface of the block, the celloidin being hard enough when no impression is left on the surface.
4. Remove the block from the mould and place it in pure chloroform. The block floats at first but eventually sinks to the bottom of the solution. When the block has sunk, transfer it to a solution of 70% alcohol until required for cutting. The block may now be trimmed with the exception of the cutting surface.

Attaching the block to the holder

Celloidin blocks are attached to wooden or vulcanite holders which have deep serrations cut into them. The block holder is coated with medium (4%) celloidin and the trimmed block pressed firmly into position. Pressure is maintained by means of a lead weight or by winding a piece of thread around the holder and the block. After about 1 h, during which time the block and holder can be returned to the chloroform desiccator, the celloidin is set firm and the block and holder should be reimmersed in 70% alcohol for 30 min. The cutting surface of the block may now be trimmed with a sharp hand razor.

It is a common practice to store both the blocks and holders in 70% alcohol until all work on the sections is finished. Wooden blocks should therefore be made from a hard wood and should be soaked before use in order to ensure that discoloration of the alcohol and block does not occur.

In many laboratories, chloroform is not used to harden the block. Hardening is then done very slowly by placing the mould beneath a bell jar and raising one side slightly, allowing the vapour to escape and the solution to thicken. When using this method the edge of the bell jar that is raised must be changed periodically to ensure that even evaporation takes place and should be lowered overnight and at weekends.

Necoloidine is used in a similar manner to celloidin, but the impregnating solutions are twice as thick, being 4%, 8% and 16%. The tissue is embedded in the stock solution, thickened as described earlier.

Low viscosity nitrocellulose (LVN)

Low viscosity nitrocellulose is used by some workers as an embedding medium in preference to celloidin. This preference is based upon a harder block being formed with LVN than with celloidin, thinner sections thus being made possible. The sections have a tendency to crack, but plasticizers can be incorporated into the medium to overcome this problem. The addition of 0.5% oleum ricini (castor oil) is recommended for embedding chrome mordanted tissues, and this method is described here.

Solution 1:
Low viscosity nitrocellulose	7 g
Ethyl alcohol, absolute	42 ml
Ether	50 ml
Oleum ricini	0.5 ml

Solution 2:
Low viscosity nitrocellulose	14 g
Ethyl alcohol, absolute	42 ml
Ether	50 ml
Oleum ricini	0.5 ml

Solution 3:
Low viscosity nitrocellulose	28 g
Ethyl alcohol, absolute	42 ml
Ether	50 ml
Oleum ricini	0.5 ml

Mode of preparation

Solutions 1, 2 and 3. Dissolve the LVN in the alcohol and ether. Add the oleum ricini, mix well and label.

Procedure

1. Dehydrate tissue according to the celloidin technique.
2. Place in solution 1 for 4–7 days.
3. Place in solution 2 for 4–7 days.
4. Embed in solution 3 and continue according to the celloidin technique.

■ Notes

1. Sections should be cut dry and collected into 70% alcohol.
2. LVN is highly explosive and should be handled with respect. Exposure to direct sunlight should be avoided.

Peterfi's double-impregnation method

This method is a valuable aid for preparing sections from blocks of tissue of varying consistency (e.g. eyes).

Celloidin, dry	1 g
Methyl benzoate	100 ml

Weigh out the dry celloidin and transfer it to a 250 ml flask. Add the methyl benzoate and stopper the flask firmly. Shake several times each day, occasionally inverting the flask, until solution of the celloidin is effected.

Procedure

1. Dehydrate according to the normal schedule.
2. Transfer to the methyl benzoate–celloidin from absolute alcohol and impregnate for 24–72 h.
3. Pass through three changes of toluene over a period of 24 h.
4. Impregnate and embed in paraffin wax according to the normal schedule.

■ Note

Many modifications of the above method have been suggested. Some workers prefer to clear in pure methyl benzoate before impregnating with the celloidin solution; others impregnate for a further 24 h in a second solution containing 2% celloidin in methyl benzoate; the period in toluene is also reduced by many workers.

16

Section cutting

The microtome

The microscope is designed to facilitate the study of animal tissue by transmitted light and for this purpose the tissue must be sliced into thin lamellae or 'sections'. These are cut at a predetermined thickness which depends on the character of the tissue. Uniform thickness can only be assured by using a microtome.

Microtomes of various designs are made for use with different tissue-supporting media. For preparing paraffin sections, the rocker, rotary and sledge patterns are normally used.

Cambridge rocking microtome

Although no longer manufactured, the Cambridge rocking microtome (*Figure 16.1*) remains a firm favourite with many microtomists because of its simplicity of operation and maintenance and its ability to produce sections of high quality. It consists of a heavy base and two arms; the lower arm rests on a column and supports the upper, both being pivoted on knife edges which act as a fulcrum. The lower arm is located by a spring behind the supporting column and is also attached by means of a trapped nut directly to the micrometer screw, at the base of which is mounted the ratchet wheel of the feed mechanism. The upper arm, which carries the block-holder, is located in front of the supporting column by a second spring and is retained at the opposite end by means of an adjustable cord. The cord passes via a pulley to the operating handle. Preliminary movement of the handle lowers the rear of the upper arm and raises the block to clear the knife prior to producing movement of the feed mechanism. Continued movement of the operating handle causes a pawl to engage in the ratchet wheel of the feed mechanism, turning it according to the predetermined thickness. The turning of the ratchet

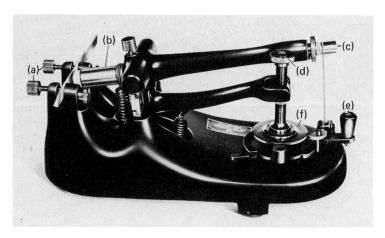

Figure 16.1. The Cambridge rocking microtome: (a) knife clamps; (b) block-holder; (c) tension adjustment; (d) micrometer screw; (e) operating handle; (f) feed mechanism (photograph by courtesy of Raymond A. Lamb)

wheel rotates the micrometer screw and elevates the lower arm to a more obtuse angle, producing a forward movement at the fulcrum. This movement is relayed to the upper arm, thereby moving the block-holder forward. By slowly releasing the pressure on the operating handle, the tension on the locating spring causes the upper arm to return through an arc to its former position, a section being cut as the tissue passes the knife edge. Sections prepared on the Cambridge rocking microtome are thus cut in a slightly curved plane; its feed mechanism is graduated in units of 1 or 2 µm.

The Cambridge rocking microtome was one of the first instruments to be incorporated into a cryostat (see p. 203) by British manufacturers for the preparation of sections from unfixed tissue at a temperature of approximately −20°C. The simplicity of its mechanism and the small number of moving parts made it an ideal microtome for low-temperature work.

Rotary microtome

The rotary microtome (*Figure 16.2*) is an excellent machine for research work and is particularly valuable for the preparation of serial sections.

Section cutting is effected by the vertical rise and fall of the object against the knife edge, together with the co-ordinated advancement of the object controlled by a micrometer screw and set of slides. Both the vertical and advance movements are actuated by rotation of the operating handle. The block-holder is equipped with adjusting screws to ensure that the block is parallel to the microtome knife in all planes. The knife-holder is movable and the knife clamps may be adjusted to vary the angle of tilt.

Base sledge microtome

The base sledge microtome (*Figure 16.3*) is a rigidly constructed machine readily adaptable for sectioning specimens embedded in all forms of media. It is excellent for cutting sections from blocks of tough tissue, especially if the blocks are large and offer marked resistance to the knife. The sections may be cut with the knife at an angle to the face of the block or parallel to it. Larger sections can more easily be cut with the knife set at an angle, less resistance being offered by the block.

The microtome consists essentially of a heavy base and two movable pillars which hold the adjustable knife clamps. Two accurately machined metal guides traverse the length of the base and carry the movable carriage. The hand-propelled movement of this carriage is checked by a buffer stop.

Movement of the operating handle on the carriage causes a pawl to become engaged in the upper of three ratchet gear wheels, turning it and actuating the two companion wheels and the micrometer screw. The movement of the micrometer screw raises the block-holder which is connected to it by means of a split nut clasp, the use of which adjusts the height of the block in relation to the knife.

The thrust exerted by the feed mechanism is determined by the setting on the thickness gauge,

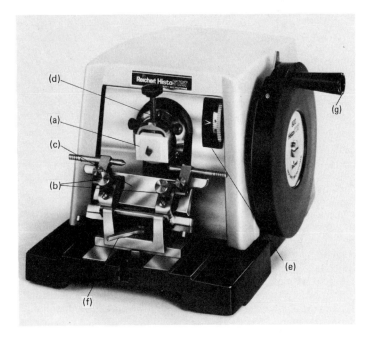

Figure 16.2. Rotary type microtome: (a) block-holder; (b) knife clamp screws; (c) knife clamps; (d) block adjustment clamp; (e) thickness gauge; (f) angle of tilt adjustment; (g) operating handle (reproduced by courtesy of Reichert-Jung Ltd)

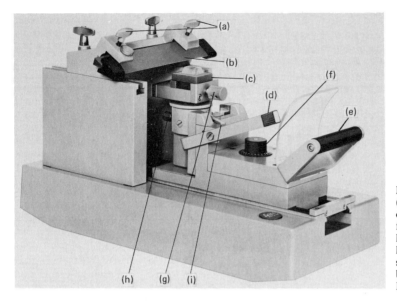

Figure 16.3. Base sledge microtome: (a) angle of tilt adjustment; (b) knife clamps; (c) block-holder; (d) coarse feed adjustment; (e) operating handle; (f) thickness gauge; (g) adjustment locking nut; (h) block adjustment screw; (i) split nut clasp (reproduced by courtesy of E. Leitz (Instruments) Ltd)

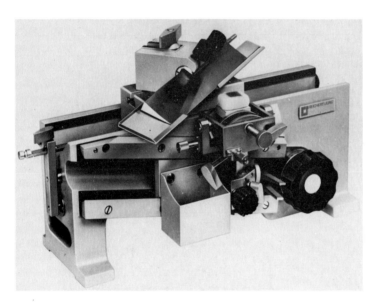

Figure 16.4. The Reichert Universal sliding microtome. This instrument is equipped with an automatic feed mechanism, which can be adjusted in steps of 1 μm, to allow sections to be cut up to 30 μm in thickness. Facilities for adjusting the slant of the knife and the clearance angle are provided and the object clamp can be orientated in two directions to adjust the block to the knife edge (reproduced by courtesy of Reichert-Jung)

which is graduated in divisions of 1 μm up to 20 μm. This gauge limits the movement of the operating handle which must be fully turned while the carriage is in the position shown to ensure that the sections are cut at the correct thickness. For obvious reasons the operating handle must not be turned while the block is on the opposite side of the knife to that illustrated in *Figure 16.3*.

This microtome may be adapted for frozen section cutting by replacement of the paraffin wax object holder with either a CO_2 freezing stage or a thermomodule (see p. 203).

Sliding microtome

The fundamental difference between the sliding microtome and those models described earlier is that with this instrument the block remains stationary while the microtome knife moves during the process of sectioning. The main value of the sliding microtome is the ease with which it cuts sections from tissue embedded in celloidin. A number of instruments of varying design are produced commercially, one of the most popular being that illustrated in *Figure 16.4*.

Freezing microtome

The freezing microtome is primarily used for cutting sections of fixed tissue (a) when speed is of the utmost importance, (b) when a cryostat is not available. It is required to demonstrate fat histologically, and when certain neurological structures are to be studied.

Several types of freezing microtomes are available, but those most widely used take the form of the one illustrated in *Figure 16.5*. The freezing microtome differs markedly from those machines used for the preparation of paraffin wax sections. The stage of the freezing microtome, to which the CO_2 cylinder is connected by means of a reinforced flexible lead, is hollow and perforated around the perimeter. These perforations are an essential part of the cooling, allowing the gas to flow and freely escape, thereby producing even freezing of the tissue. A second cooling device for lowering the knife temperature to facilitate sectioning is also incorporated in most modern machines.

As the operating handle is moved back the knife edge clears the tissue. Continuation of the movement causes a pawl to engage with a ratchet wheel and turn it according to the predetermined thickness. Rotation of this wheel turns the micrometer screw which raises the block-holder. By pulling the operating handle forwards a section is cut as the knife edge slices through the raised tissue. The thickness at which the sections are cut is variable in units of 5 µm. The number of units by which the feed mechanism is turned is determined by the position of the knife stop on the graduated runner. To ensure that the section thickness is correct the operating handle must be pushed back along the runner until checked by the knife stop.

Thermoelectric cooling units may be used in place of CO_2 gas to freeze the tissue and cool the knife. These units, referred to as thermomodules, have a considerable refrigeration capacity and function by a phenomenon known as the 'Peltier' effect. When a direct current is passed across the junction of two dissimilar metals, heat is emitted or absorbed, according to the direction of the current. A flow of cold water maintained through the cooling unit ensures that the heat from the hot face is absorbed. The cooling produced by the thermoelectric unit is dependent upon the flow of the direct current and this may be regulated by means of power packs. The stage temperature can be reduced from ambient to −36°C in 60 s, but the optimum cutting temperature for the tissue is usually about −20°C.

These units are produced commercially and are designed to fit a large number of microtomes. Their popularity has decreased following the ever-growing use of the cryostat.

Cryostat

The best method of preparing sections from unfixed tissue is by use of a cryostat. This consists essentially

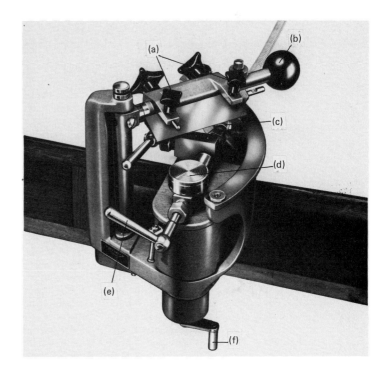

Figure 16.5. A type of freezing microtome: (a) knife clamps; (b) operating handle; (c) thickness gauge; (d) stage; (e) stage valve; (f) coarse adjustment (reproduced by courtesy of Reichert-Jung)

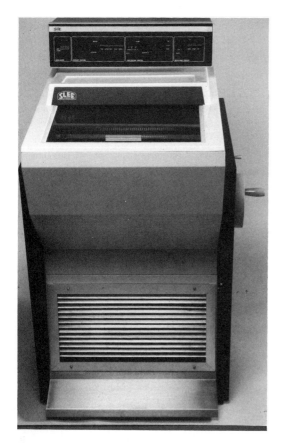

Figure 16.6. Photograph of the SLEE cryostat (reproduced by courtesy of Slee Medical Equipment Ltd)

of a microtome housed in a deep freeze cabinet, maintained at a temperature of approximately −15°C to −30°C. Sections from fresh tissue can be cut on standard freezing microtomes, but they cannot be handled satisfactorily. This applies particularly when fluorescent antibody staining techniques or certain histochemical enzyme methods are to be applied. To obtain satisfactory sections which can be transferred directly from the microtome knife to a slide or coverglass, the tissue, microtome knife and surrounding atmosphere must all be at a low temperature. The conditions are achieved by the use of a cryostat (*Figure 16.6*).

There is a variety of cryostats manufactured, the major fundamental difference between them being the type of microtome employed. The earliest models manufactured in the UK incorporated the Cambridge rocking microtome (no longer manufactured). Cryostats equipped with purpose-built microtomes are now widely used, and models fitted with sledge microtomes, suitable for cutting larger and tougher tissue blocks, are also available. Some models are equipped with a motor drive, while a

microprocessor control is also becoming a standard fitting.

In order to avoid the formation of large disruptive ice crystals when freezing fresh tissue, rapid freezing (quenching) is necessary. Cryostats are usually provided with a rapid freezing attachment, such as a Freon quick-freeze stage, for this purpose and for attaching blocks of tissue to the block-holder. This latter refinement is extremely valuable when the instrument is to be used for preparing urgent sections from biopsies. Blocks of fresh tissue not to be sectioned immediately should be quenched and stored at a temperature of −20°C in airtight containers or aluminium foil.

Microtome knives

These are classified according to their cross-section (profile) as follows: (a) planoconcave—hollow ground on one side; (b) wedge-shaped—plane on both sides; (c) biconcave—hollow ground on both sides; (d) tool-edge—plane on both sides with a steep cutting edge.

Each of the profiles was originally introduced on knives designed for a specific purpose. In practice, however, there is considerable latitude in the utilization of each type and, provided that a knife is sharp and will fit the microtome, it may well be used effectively for cutting most types of tissue and embedding materials. Planoconcave knives are obtainable with profiles of greater or lesser degrees of concavity and are usually recommended for celloidin or wax-embedded tissues. The sturdy wedge-shaped knife is used for cutting frozen and paraffin sections and hard objects embedded in celloidin. Biconcave knives are used mainly for wax-embedded tissues. The popular Heiffor knife has a biconcave profile. This knife with its distinctive integral handle was designed for use with the Cambridge rocking microtome. The tool-edge knife is used in conjunction with a heavy, robust microtome for cutting extra hard materials such as undecalcified bone. With the exception of the Heiffor knife most knives have detachable handles fitted at one end.

The cutting facet (bevel)

In cross-section all microtome knives are basically wedge-shaped, but the cutting edge is not the extension of the two converging sides of a wedge to form a point. Such an edge emanating from a relatively narrow base would be fragile, and subject to considerable vibration during section cutting. A more obtuse angle is therefore ground onto the tapering sides of the knife to form the actual cutting edge. This angle is referred to as the facet angle and

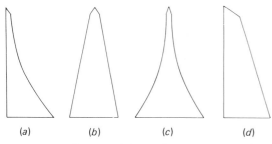

Figure 16.7. Microtome knives: (a) planoconcave; (b) wedge; (c) biconcave; (d) tool edge

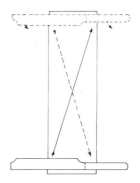

Figure 16.8. Diagram to illustrate the honing of a microtome knife

the sides that enclose it as the cutting facets or bevel (*Figure 16.7*). In order to manually sharpen microtome knives with one or more plane surfaces, it is necessary for them to be fitted with a special device to produce and maintain the cutting facets. This is a spring-loaded semicircular metal sheath which is slipped onto the back of the knife and is known as a tubular knife back, or stropping device. Each knife should have its own back which should be marked to ensure that it is always fitted to the knife in the same way.

Sharpening of microtome knives

A microtome knife requires to be sharpened whenever its cutting edge becomes blunt or damaged. The process of sharpening is divided into two stages, honing and stropping, and each of these operations may be performed either by hand or by means of automatic knife-sharpening machines. Honing entails the grinding of metal from the knife edge with an abrasive substance until all nicks have been removed and the edge is sharp and straight; stropping is cleaning or polishing the knife edge on a softer material, usually leather.

Manual honing

The hone is a rectangular block of natural or synthetic stone, graded coarse, medium or fine according to the degree of its abrasiveness. A widely used natural stone of medium grade is the Belgian yellow stone, which gives good results at reasonable speed.

The size of the hone used is dependent upon that of the knife; the length should always be sufficient to permit the whole of the knife edge to be sharpened in a single stroke, while the width should provide sufficient support to prevent any rocking of the knife. Before honing, the knife should be cleaned with xylene, and where necessary, fitted with its handle and tubular back.

The hone is positioned on a bench of suitable height in front of the operator, who should be

comfortably seated. A damp cloth placed beneath the stone will prevent its movement during use. The surface of the stone should be cleaned to remove any grit or dust and then lubricated with either a fine oil or soapy water.

The knife is placed at one end of the hone (*Figure 16.8*) and is pushed diagonally forward with the cutting edge leading, so that the whole edge is equally ground. Just before it reaches the end of the stone the knife is turned over *on its back*, and with the cutting edge leading again, it is steadily pulled back along the hone towards the operator. Pressure on the knife needs to be just sufficient to maintain its edge in contact with the surface of the hone. The number of strokes required depends on the condition of the knife, but honing is complete when all large nicks have been removed and the edge is straight and sharp. When viewed under a low-power microscope the edge will be seen to be finely but regularly serrated. These serrations are due to the abrasiveness of the stone and are removed by the polishing action of subsequent stropping.

Other stones in common use include:

1. *Arkansas*. A natural stone of clear white to pale yellow colour. It is less abrasive than the Belgian stone and is consequently slower in action.
2. *Aloxite*. A series of composite stones ranging in abrasiveness from coarse to superfine. Only the fine and superfine grades are suitable for microtome knife sharpening.

Plate glass may be used as a hone (lapping plate) in conjunction with an abrasive such as aluminium oxide. This abrasive, available in a range of particle sizes, is suspended in oil or water and applied to the surface of the glass plate, which is then used in the same way as an ordinary hone. The advantage of this method is that by varying the grade of abrasives, all types of honing can be carried out. When a satisfactory edge has been obtained by either the stone or plate glass methods, the knife should be thoroughly cleaned and dried before stropping is attempted.

Stropping

This is performed in a manner similar to honing except that the knife is reversed and lightly stroked back and forth over a leather surface with its cutting edge *trailing* (*Figure 16.9*). Strops may be either flexible (hanging) or rigid. A good quality leather

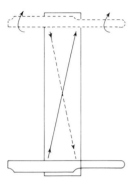

Figure 16.9. Diagram to illustrate the stropping of a microtome knife

such as horsehide, noted for its durability and effectiveness, is recommended. It should be kept supple by the occasional application of a little vegetable oil to its undersurface. Strop-dressings containing mild abrasives or polishing agents such as jeweller's rouge may be used. These are sparingly applied to the leather surface.

It is essential that hanging type strops are pulled as taut as possible during use to prevent rounding **the cutting edge of the knife, which will occur if**

sufficient tension is not maintained. The prepared canvas back fitted to most of these strops serves not only for support but also as a preliminary stropping surface before using the leather. Some hanging strops are available with two leather sides, one side impregnated with a fine abrasive paste, the other with a polishing agent.

The rigid type is essentially a leather strop stretched over a solid wooden block. This type is preferred by many workers because it gives firm support to the knife during stropping, thereby reducing the possibility of producing a rounded cutting edge.

Some authorities regard the practice of knife-stropping to be completely unnecessary, especially if a knife has been honed correctly, using a superfine abrasive or stone. It cannot be denied, however, that very sharp edges are obtained, and maintained for a long time, on microtome knives which are stropped not only after honing, but also after each section-cutting session.

Knife-sharpening machines

These machines offer tremendous saving in time and relatively inexperienced personnel can produce well-sharpened knives with a uniform bevel.

Some automatic machines are available which require hand feeding of the knife against revolving glass or metal wheels. Sharpening is undertaken with the aid of lapping compounds composed of

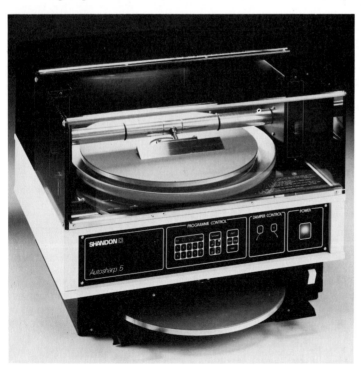

Figure 16.10. A fully automatic knife-sharpening device (reproduced by courtesy of Shandon Southern Products Ltd)

suspensions of alumina or diamond grit which are continuously recirculated by means of a built-in pump. The grade of lapping compound selected is dependent upon the condition of the knife edge.

The great drawback to using machines of this nature is that the knife is fed across the revolving wheel by hand. Uneven pressure and variation in the speed with which the knife is sharpened can result in an irregular knife edge. To hesitate too long with the knife in contact with the revolving wheels can cause considerable damage. A semi-automatic machine with facilities for both honing and stropping, and which is completely dry in operation, is also marketed.

Fully automatic knife sharpeners at economic prices are now manufactured. An example of a type which is widely used is shown in *Figure 16.10*. The knife is held in a holder attached to the main spindle, in such a way that the cutting edge is in contact with a glass or metal plate. A mechanism is provided for adjusting the height of the glass plate to agree with the bevel of the knife. To ensure that the abrasive is spread evenly over the surface of the plate and that no uneven wear occurs, a combined oscillatory and rotary motion is incorporated. A mechanism incorporating a damping device automatically turns the knife over at suitable intervals to ensure that each facet is sharpened equally and a choice of speeds is provided, a slower speed being used for knives in poor condition.

Disposable blades

Disposable blades which eliminate the necessity of sharpening are now in common use. These blades can be adapted to fit most types of microtome. They are expensive to purchase but are excellent labour-saving devices.

The blade is supported in a special holder which permits easy loading and replacement when loaded. The holder is clamped into the microtome in the usual way.

Technique of section cutting

Preparation of paraffin sections

Trimming the block

If several pieces of tissue are embedded in the same mould, it must be divided into individual blocks. This may be done by cutting a V-shaped groove in the intervening wax, and breaking it along this line. If the pieces of tissue are embedded too closely to permit this, the mould should be divided with a fine fret-saw.

The individual paraffin blocks should then be trimmed with a hand razor to within 3 mm (⅛ in) of the tissue, taking care that the sides of the block are parallel. Excess wax on the face of the block should also be pared off. The shavings produced may be returned to the wax oven and used again. The trimmed blocks should be stored in cardboard boxes, each with its accompanying ticket.

Attaching the block to the holder

Heat a wooden-handled spatula over a bunsen burner, and hold it on the surface of the block-holder. Place the paraffin block on the spatula. The hot spatula melts the wax on the block-holder and the base of the block. After a few seconds the spatula is withdrawn and the paraffin block pressed down firmly on the holder. The junction between the two is now sealed by reheating the spatula and running it round the base of the paraffin block.

Orientation of the block on the microtome

1. Fix the block-holder in position on the microtome.
2. Turn back the feed mechanism. On the rotary and base sledge microtomes a special 'split nut clasp' is provided for this purpose.
3. Insert a suitable knife in the microtome, and secure it with the tightening screws.
4. Move the block-holder forward until the paraffin block is almost touching the knife edge.
5. If the microtome has no centring screws, such as in the case of the rocker type microtome, the block must be accurately trimmed before it is attached to the block-holder. When adjusting screws are present they are used to orientate the block-holder so that the surface to be cut and the lower edge of the block are parallel to the knife edge at the moment of impact. In the case of the base sledge microtome it is often advantageous for the leading edge of the block to be set at an angle to the knife.
6. Check all tightening screws on the microtome.
7. The gauge controlling section thickness is set to 15 μm, and the extreme end of the knife is used to trim the block until the whole surface is being cut. The block is now ready for sectioning.

Cutting the sections

Set the gauge to the required thickness and position the knife so that the centre of the blade is positioned for cutting. Screw back the feed mechanisms slightly.

■ Note

This precaution should be taken whenever the knife is moved, for the slightest discrepancy in the knife may cause the cutting edge to dig into the paraffin block when the next section is cut.

After trimming, the block should be cooled with ice. Operate the microtome until complete sections are again being cut and then maintain a regular cutting rhythm. The cutting rate varies with the nature of the tissue, the size of the block and the pattern of the microtome. The optimum cutting speed is determined empirically for each individual block. If the block face and upper and lower edges are parallel to the knife, the sections will form a ribbon. This ribboning is due to the slight heat generated between the block and the knife edge. Continue cutting until the ribbon produced is about 15 cm (6 in) long, supporting its free end all the while with a moistened camel-hair brush. Moisten a second camel-hair brush and gently raise the last section cut, thereby freeing the ribbon which is placed, matt surface uppermost, onto a section board or sheet of black paper. When serial sections are being prepared, the section board is essential, for the glass cover protects the sections from draught and dust.

If the knife of the base sledge microtome is set at an angle, the sections should be removed individually, for ribboning does not usually occur.

If instructions for trimming the block and orientating it on the microtome have been correctly observed, poor results are usually due to one of the following causes (see also *Table 16.1*).

Inadequate impregnation

If dehydration, clearing or wax impregnation are inadequate, crumbling of sections may occur. This fault is easily detected, as the block usually smells of the clearing agent. The block should be trimmed down as near to the tissue as possible, returned to the embedding oven to melt the remaining wax, and then transferred to the cleaning agent. If dehydration is suspected as being at fault, the tissue should be taken back to absolute alcohol (74° OP spirit).

Imperfect knife edge

More failures can be attributed to badly prepared knives than to any other single factor. Nicks in the knife edge frequently result in scoring of the sections with vertical lines. To overcome this, resharpen the knife or move it along in the holder. If the knife is

Table 16.1 Some faults encountered in cutting paraffin sections

Fault	Probable cause	Remedy
Sections scored or split vertically	(a) Knife edge is damaged	(a) Sharpen the knife
	(b) Embedding medium contains dirt	(b) Re-embed the tissue in filtered wax
	(c) Knife edge is dirty	(c) Clean the knife edge with xylene
Sections and block have parallel lines across them (chatters)	(a) Tissue is too hard	(a) Treat the tissue with Mollifex or take a fresh block and treat with phenol during processing
	(b) Tilt of knife is too great	(b) Decrease the tilt of the knife
	(c) Knife or block-holder is loose	(c) Tighten all locking/adjusting screws
Sections cut alternately thick and thin	(a) Knife is blunt	(a) Sharpen the knife
	(b) Tilt of knife is too great	(b) Decrease the tilt of the knife
	(c) Knife or block-holder is loose	(c) Tighten all locking and adjusting screws
Sections roll up on cutting	(a) Knife is blunt	(a) Sharpen the knife
	(b) Tilt of knife is too great	(b) Decrease the tilt of the knife
Sections are squashed, the width of each section being less than that of the block	(a) The bevel on the knife has been lost due to incorrect sharpening	(a) Resharpen the knife using the correct knife back or setting on the automatic knife sharpener, until the bevel is restored.
Sections crumble on cutting	(a) Ante-medium or alcohol is not properly removed	(a) Return to ante-medium or alcohol, as described above.
	(b) Wax is too soft	(b) Apply ice to the cutting surface or re-embed in harder wax
	(c) Knife is blunt	(c) Sharpen the knife
Sections form a curved ribbon	(a) Knife is sharp and blunt in patches	(a) Sharpen the knife
	(b) Horizontal edges of block are not parallel	(b) Retrim block
	(c) Horizontal edges of block are not parallel to the knife edge	(c) Adjust block until it is parallel to knife edge
Sections fail to ribbon	(a) Horizontal edges of blocks are not parallel to each other	(a) Retrim block
	(b) Wax is too hard	(b) Coat horizontal edges of block with wax of lower melting point

blunt, the sections may cut alternately thick and thin. This may be remedied by resharpening the knife.

Incorrect setting of the knife

The knife is set at a tilt on the microtome to allow a clearance angle between the cutting facet and the block of tissue (*Figure 16.11*). Clearance angles between 1 and 6 degrees have proved to be most

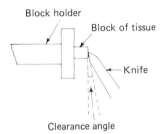

Figure 16.11. Diagram illustrating the angle of clearance of a microtome knife

satisfactory. Biconcave knives require a smaller clearance angle than wedge-type knives. The tilt of the knife may be adjusted by special attachments on the knife-holder of the microtome.

Faults due to an incorrect tilt are as follows.

Chattering

This term is used to describe horizontal lines or furrows across the section. The knife makes a hard metallic scraping sound as the sections are cut. This may be remedied by reducing the tilt of the knife.

Intermittent cutting

If the angle of tilt of the knife is too small, the block is compressed by the cutting facet and a section is not cut. The degree of compression increases until the tissue expands suddenly, and results in the cutting of a thick section. This may be remedied by increasing the angle of tilt of the knife.

Brittle and tough tissue

When possible the block should be cut on the base sledge microtome with the knife positioned to form an angle to the leading edge of the block, to decrease the resistance. The angle so formed is known as the angle of slant. The block should be carefully orientated so that the sections are cut along the line of least resistance.

Dirt

When dirt is present in the paraffin wax, re-embedding of the tissue in freshly filtered wax is necessary.

Minute particles of calcium in the tissue

Once the tissue has been embedded in paraffin wax, decalcification is difficult but the base sledge microtome, using a wedge knife set at an angle, will often allow the cutting of good sections.

Attaching sections to slides

As sections tend to crease slightly on cutting they must be flattened by gentle heat before being attached to slides. Two methods in common use are described below.

The water bath method

A cut section or short ribbon of sections is gently lowered, by means of a camel-hair brush or fine forceps, onto the surface of warm water in a water bath. The temperature of the water should be approximately 10°C below the melting point of the wax. When the section is flat and fully expanded, a prepared clean, grease-free slide is dipped obliquely into the water as close to the section as possible. Slowly withdraw the slide, allowing its surface to touch the edge of the section. Completely remove slide with attached section from the water. Adjust the section to a suitable position on the slide with a mounted needle. Drain off the excess water, identify with the appropriate number by means of a diamond pencil and transfer the slide to an incubator or hot plate (45–50°C) for at least 1 h to ensure that the section is thoroughly dried before being stained.

The hot plate method

A clean grease-free slide is placed on a warm hot plate and flooded with distilled water. A section or short ribbon is laid on the surface of the water and any major creases removed by stretching the surrounding wax carefully with mounted needles. As the water warms up the section will flatten out, and when it is fully extended remove the slide from the hot plate and drain off any excess fluid. Orientate and dry the section as in the previous method.

Use of section adhesives

The attachment of sections to slides by either of the foregoing methods usually results in a firm bond, so that the sections are capable of withstanding the several washings and manipulations of most of the common staining techniques. The two most important conditions governing their attachment are that the sections must be of good quality and the slides must be completely grease-free. Under certain circumstances, however, and in spite of the correct attachment technique, sections will become partly or completely detached from slides during staining. Some of the causes of section detachment are: prolonged immersion of sections in alkaline solutions, the fixation of tissues in powerful protein-coagulant fluids, e.g. Bouin's fixative; tissues containing blood clot or bone. The use of a section adhesive is advised in such cases and may be used routinely for all sections to ensure their attachment to slides. A well-established adhesive is Mayer's glycerol–albumin mixture*:

Combine equal parts of glycerol and white of egg. Mix well, filter through muslin and add a small crystal of thymol as a preservative.

This mixture is lightly smeared over the surface of a clean slide before attachment of the section by the water bath or hot plate methods. Fresh serum may be used as an alternative to glycerol–albumin.

Starch paste* is an adhesive of exceptional quality but because of its carbohydrate nature cannot be used for sections to be stained by the PAS technique. It is prepared as follows:

| Powdered starch | 3 g |
| Cold distilled water | 30 ml |

Mix to a paste and add to

| Boiling distilled water | 60 ml |
| Concentrated hydrochloric acid | 0.5 ml |

Boil for 5 min. Cool and add 0.1 g thymol. Use in the same way as Mayer's albumin mixture.

The addition of an adhesive to the warm water used for flattening sections is both simple and effective. The following combination is recommended:

| Potassium dichromate | 1% in distilled water |
| Gelatin | 1% in distilled water |

These are kept as separate stock solutions, and are added to the water bath to give a concentration of 0.002% of each.

Preparation of frozen sections

Method of cutting frozen sections

1. Clamp the microtome to the bench and connect the CO_2 cylinder by means of the flexible lead provided. If an ordinary CO_2 cylinder is used it must be positioned in such a way that the cylinder valve is the lowest point of the cylinder. Special

cylinders containing a central tube may be supported in a floor stand with the valve uppermost.
2. Close the release valve on the microtome and open the valve on the cylinder. Watch carefully to see that the connection between the lead and the cylinder does not leak and then open the release valve on the microtome. Allow a short burst of CO_2 gas to escape, 1–2 s, to ensure that the connection to the microtome does not leak and that there is gas in the cylinder.
3. Slip the blade of the microtome knife into the knife clamps and secure it by tightening the locking screws.
4. Place a piece of filter paper soaked in gum syrup on the stage of the microtome, lift the stage release valve and allow a short burst of CO_2 gas to escape, freezing the filter paper to the stage.
5. With the microtome knife well clear, position the selected block of tissue on the stage and apply a few drops of gum syrup from a Pasteur pipette. The tissue should be approximately 3–5 mm in thickness. Open the stage release valve and give several short bursts of gas, each of 1–2 s duration, at intervals of 5 s. When the gum is frozen apply more and again freeze with short bursts of CO_2 gas. Continue to build up the gum in this way until the tissue is supported to a height of about 3 mm.
6. Rack up the stage by means of the coarse feed adjustment at the bottom of the microtome until the surface of the tissue is just about level with the edge of the knife.
7. Rub the top surface of the tissue with the ball of the finger until the tissue and supporting gum has a rubbery consistency. Take great care to see that the microtome knife is well clear while doing this. Trim down the block either by setting the feed mechanism to 20 μm or, if more experienced, by turning the coarse feed adjustment. Trim the block until complete sections are being cut.
8. Set the thickness gauge to the required thickness (usually 10 μm) and quickly cut the sections, maintaining a steady rhythm on the microtome. The sections usually collapse on the microtome knife and require removing with a camel-hair brush, from which they are transferred to a dish of water. Some workers use a jerking movement to cut the sections, projecting them forward and catching them in a dish of water, but the technique demands that the cutting temperature of the tissue is correct, an assessment which requires considerable practice. Intermittent cooling of the knife while cutting the sections often helps to produce better results.

If the tissue is frozen too much, the sections will splinter and crumble and the knife edge may be damaged. Soften the surface of the block with the ball of the finger or thumb. If the tissue is not frozen enough, any attempt at section cutting will produce only a streak of useless slush on the edge of the knife. To remedy this give more bursts of CO_2 gas.

A thermomodule (p. 203), operated in conjunction with a suitable power control unit, may be used to freeze the tissue instead of the conventional freezing stage and CO_2 gas. The apparatus is quiet in operation and allows more accurate control of section cutting temperatures.

The thermomodule, suitably connected to a supply of cold running water and power unit, replaces the freezing stage of the microtome. A block of tissue is placed on the platform of the thermomodule together with a drop of water or gum syrup. The current is switched to maximum and the tissue commences to freeze. When the block is completely frozen the current supply is reduced until the required degree of freezing is obtained. This temperature can be maintained for several hours. The knife is inserted in the microtome, the tissue is trimmed, and section cutting and collection is performed as in the CO_2 method.

Handling frozen sections

Frozen sections may be handled loose by the careful use of a brush, mounted needle, seeker or glass hockey stick. They can also be attached to a slide and stained in a similar manner to paraffin wax sections. The latter is usually the method of choice when preparing sections in the theatre from biopsies on which an urgent diagnosis is required. Sections which are to be stained for fat or structural elements of the nervous system are usually 'floated through' the various stains and reagents and mounted when finished. Slides prepared for the demonstration of fat must be mounted in an aqueous mounting medium.

Floating out frozen sections

Orientate the section in a deep, glass dish of distilled water. The dish should preferably be placed on a sheet of black paper in order to give a dark background. Insert a slide beneath the section and slowly withdraw the slide and attached section from the water. Drain the excess water from the slide and remove any creases which may be present in the section by returning the slide to the water in such a way that only half of the section is submerged or floating. The creases will be removed easily by a little careful manipulation. Remove the slide from the water, drain and if necessary insert the opposite half of the section into the water. Drain the slide carefully again and continue according to the method being used for attaching the section permanently to the slide.

Attaching frozen sections to slides

Frozen sections may be attached to slides by celloidinization, albumin or starch adhesive or by being floated onto gelatinized slides.

Celloidinization

Float the section onto a clean, grease-free slide, drain off excess water and blot gently but firmly with a Whatman No. 1 filter paper. The blotting should be done with a rolling action using the fleshy part of the hand. Blot the section a second time with fresh filter paper which has been soaked with absolute alcohol and then coat the slide with 1% celloidin in ether–alcohol. The slide is coated by standing it in a Coplin jar of the celloidin for 1 min or longer, the back is then wiped and the slide transferred to a dish of 70% alcohol for a few minutes to harden the celloidin. When the celloidin has hardened the section can be stained in the normal manner. Following staining the celloidin should be remove by immersion in equal parts of alcohol and ether. Once the celloidin is removed the slides must be handled carefully to prevent the sections from becoming detached.

Albuminized or starched slides

Float the section onto a slide smeared with albumin or starch paste (see p. 210) and drain off the excess water. Blot the section carefully with a Whatman No. 1 filter paper and cover with a few drops of a mixture of equal parts of clove and aniline oil. Allow the mixture to coagulate the adhesive for 3 min and then remove it from the slide with xylene followed by absolute alcohol. The section can now be stained in the normal manner. As an additional safeguard the sections may also be coated with celloidin following immersion in absolute alcohol.

Gelatinized slides

Float the section onto a slide which has been coated with 0.2% gelatin and allowed to dry. Drain off the excess water and transfer the slide to a dish of formalin vapour, the action of which converts the gelatin to an irreversible gel and holds the section in place. Remove the slide after several minutes' exposure and wash in running tap water. The section can now be stained in the normal manner.

Preparation of cryostat sections

Mounting tissues

The tissue to be sectioned is placed in a drop of water in the centre of a previously cooled block-holder. The holders are usually stored in the cryostat and are ready for use when required. Rapid freezing by conduction through the metal block-holder is then carried out. This is effected either by standing the block-holder in a bath of alcohol or acetone containing dry ice, or by placing the block-holder in the special freezing attachment and exposing the tissue to carbon dioxide gas. When the tissue is frozen, the holder is positioned in the microtome. O.C.T. (Miles Scientific) may be used in place of water. The use of a cork disc in the chuck-holder is useful as it facilitates handling, storage and future orientation of the block of tissue.

Section cutting

The tissue should be adjusted to the microtome knife and trimmed in the normal manner, using the remote controls situated outside the freezing chamber. The microtome knife should be placed in position at least 15–30 min before sectioning commences in order to ensure that it is cooled to the correct temperature. The cutting temperature is determined empirically for each piece of tissue, but as a general rule a chamber temperature of $-20°C$ is satisfactory. To obtain the best results the quenched tissue should be left in the cryostat for 15–30 min prior to trimming and sectioning. This does not apply when sections are required urgently for diagnostic purposes.

Sectioning at the predetermined thickness, usually between 5 and $10\,\mu m$, is performed at a slow rate, care being taken to ensure that a steady stroke is maintained during the period that the tissue is in contact with the knife edge. To produce flat sections an anti-roll plate is used. This device consists of either a piece of plastic sheet or, more usually, a piece of glass microscope slide with two narrow strips of Sellotape attached to its vertical edges. The plate is carried in a holder which is fitted to the microtome so that the strips of Sellotape, resting on the knife face, act as spacers between plate and knife. The gap between the plate and knife is approximately $70\,\mu m$, which is sufficient to prevent the sections from curling as they are cut. After each section is cut, the anti-roll plate is slowly moved back and the section removed from the knife.

Section handling

These sections may be attached directly to slides or coverglasses kept at room temperature, merely by touching the glass surface against the section. This is facilitated by using a special holder fitted with a suction cup. When mounted, the sections may be air-dried, fixed in an appropriate fixative (this step may be omitted) and stained by the chosen technique.

Preparation of celloidin sections

The microtome most suited for sectioning celloidin embedded tissue is the sliding type (see *Figure 16.4*).

The base sledge microtome may also be used for this purpose and special attachments designed to hold the knife at an oblique angle are manufactured for some rotary microtomes to allow celloidin sections to be cut. To avoid dehydration and shrinkage, the sections are usually cut by the 'wet method', the sections and block being kept wet at all times with 70% alcohol. While actually cutting, the knife, sections and block are kept wet by applying 70% alcohol to the knife by means of a large camel-hair brush. When cut, the sections and block are stored in a similar solution in jars with tightly fitting lids.

Technique of section cutting

Clamp the vulcanite block securely into the object holder and turn back the feed mechanism. Secure a planoconcave knife in the knife-holders, adjust the angle of slant to about 40° and reduce the tilt to a minimum. Raise the block with the feed mechanism until it is almost touching the knife edge and, with the adjustment screws provided, orientate until the surface to be cut and the edge of the knife are parallel. Set the automatic thickness gauge to about $15\,\mu m$, flood the knife and block with 70% alcohol and trim until complete sections are being cut. Reset the automatic feed mechanism to the required thickness, reflood with 70% alcohol and continue to cut the sections.

The method of cutting varies according to personal preference. Some workers favour a smooth cutting action, the section being kept flat on the knife by means of the camel-hair brush; others prefer to cut by using a jerking action, the section again being kept flat with the camel-hair brush; a third method used is to cut the section quickly, thereby causing it to roll up and necessitating flattening out when transferred to a dish of 70% alcohol. With this method the sections frequently leave the knife.

When using either of the first two methods, the sections are removed from the knife with forceps. The rate of cutting can be increased if the sections are slid along the knife as they are cut, five or six sections being accumulated before being removed. A small piece of wire twisted around the handle of the brush serves as a mounted needle and may be used to move the section along the knife.

When serial sections are required, a small piece of paper is placed over each section. The section and paper are then removed and stored in piles in suitable containers, being kept saturated in alcohol. Each piece of paper should preferably be numbered, but for speed, many workers only number every tenth piece.

The sliding microtome is the most dangerous type of microtome to use owing to the exposed knife-blade being movable. Great care should be taken when using this instrument.

17

Biological staining

Cellular elements often have different refractive indices which can be utilized to permit identification by means of various forms of microscopy. For detailed study, however, and to prepare permanent preparations, staining procedures are invariably employed.

Biological stains are prepared from dyes which have been manufactured to rigid specifications for this purpose or have been subject to rigid quality assurance procedures to ensure that they are suitable for the specialized purposes for which they are to be used. These dyes are classified into two groups—synthetic, which are by far the larger group, and natural. Some of the more important biological stains such as haematoxylin and carmine do, however, belong to the natural group. Dyes can be further subdivided into acid and basic groups, a combination of which can produce a neutral stain (p. 215).

One of the problems confronting biologists is the precise identification of dyes used in staining procedures owing to the enormous number of synonyms employed. The standard reference work used for the identification of dyes is the Colour Index, which first appeared in 1923. The Colour Index is published jointly by the Society of Dyers and Colourists and the American Association of Textile Chemists and Colorists.

The 3rd edition published in 1971 consists of five volumes which have subsequently been updated (see Bibliography). Dyes are grouped under generic names according to colour and usage. A constitution number (CI No.)* is allocated when the chemical constitution of a dye is known, and dyes of similar constitution but different trade names receive the same CI No.

*CI = Colour Index.

The quality assurance procedure used by reputable manufacturers and suppliers of biological stains to test the efficiency of the products they sell are based upon the procedures advocated by the Biological Stain Commission of the USA. These tests comprise spectrophotometry, titanous chloride precipitations and biological staining procedures. Minimum standards and dye content have been defined for 57 of the dyes more widely used in biological staining procedures.

In the UK, the Association of Medical Microtomists (AMM) have conducted performance tests on dyes on behalf of commercial organizations since the 1950s. More recently, the Institute of Medical Laboratory Sciences (IMLS) have introduced a Dye Approval Scheme based on the methods used by the Biological Stain Commission.

Natural dyes

Haematoxylin

Haematoxylin is a dye derived by ether extraction from the wood of the Mexican tree *Haematoxylon campechianum*. Haematoxylin has poor staining properties and is normally used in conjunction with a mordant (see p. 215). Prior to use it must be ripened.

Haematoxylin can be 'ripened' by exposure to air and sunlight, which oxidize the haematoxylin to form the essential staining element haematein. This is a slow process, but it can be hastened by the addition of a little neutral solution of hydrogen peroxide or other powerful oxidizing agent.

Mordants have been described as substances which combine with the tissue and the stain, linking the two, and causing a staining reaction between them. Those commonly used in histology are compounds of aluminium and iron, but chromium and copper are also used. Aluminium compounds are suitable for the progressive staining (see p. 215) of tissues in bulk, but iron compounds may be used only for sections which permit differentiation. Mordants need not necessarily be included in the staining solution; some fixatives are used partly for their mordanting qualities. When myelinated fibres of the central nervous system are to be demonstrated the tissue is usually fixed in 10% formol saline and, prior to embedding, is mordanted in Weigert's primary mordant, which is a mixture of potassium dichromate and fluorchrome.

Cochineal and its derivatives

Cochineal is one of the oldest histological dyes. It is extracted from the bodies of female cochineal insects. The dye obtained is treated with alum, yielding a product relatively free of extraneous matter, and known as *carmine*. It is extensively used for staining zoological specimens and when combined with picric acid (picrocarmine) it is extremely useful in neuropathology. It is a powerful nuclear stain and it is used for the demonstration of glycogen (Best's carmine) or mucin (Southgate's mucicarmine) in permanent preparations.

Orcein

Orcein is a vegetable dye extracted from certain lichens by the action of ammonia and air. It has a violet colour, and is a weak acid, soluble in alkalis. A synthetic version is now available. Its main use in histology is the demonstration of elastic fibres (Taenzer–Unna orcein stain).

Litmus

Litmus is also obtained from lichens, but they are treated with lime and potash or soda, in addition to exposure to ammonia and air. Litmus is a poor dye and is not used as a histological stain. It was widely used as an indicator, but has been largely superseded by synthetic dyes.

Saffron

Saffron, a natural pigment extracted from the stigmata of *Crocus sativus*, is not widely used in histology, but has been incorporated by Masson into a connective tissue stain.

Synthetic dyes

Synthetic dyes are sometimes referred to as 'coal tar dyes', since they are manufactured from substances

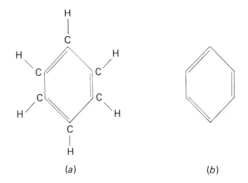

Figure 17.1. Hydrocarbon benzene: (a) showing hydrogen atom attached to each free valency; (b) as usually illustrated

which, until recently, were only obtained from coal tar. All these compounds are derivatives of the hydrocarbon benzene (C_6H_6), which consists of 6 carbon atoms at the corners of an equal-sided hexagon, with a hydrogen atom attached to each carbon atom (*Figure 17.1a*). For simplicity, benzene may be drawn with the C and H atoms omitted (*Figure 17.1b*).

Simple benzene compounds have absorption bands in the ultraviolet range of the spectrum. Certain substances ('chromophores') are capable of moving this absorption band into the visible portion of the spectrum, thereby producing visible colour. Benzene compounds containing chromophores are known as 'chromogens'.

The nitro group (NO_2) is a chromophore. If three of these groups displace three hydrogen atoms of benzene, the compound trinitrobenzene is formed (*Figure 17.2a*).

The chromogen trinitrobenzene is coloured but it is not a dye. Chromogens differ from dyes in that any colouring they impart to tissue is easily removable. Before a substance can be called a dye, it must be capable of retention by tissue. A chromogen becomes a dye after the addition of another radical, known as an 'auxochrome'. If a further hydrogen atom is replaced by a hydroxyl

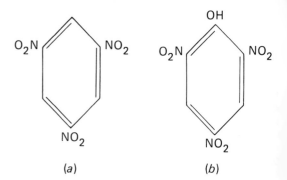

Figure 17.2. (a) Trinitrobenzene; (b) picric acid

group, which is an auxochrome, the compound results as shown in *Figure 17.2b*.

This compound, picric acid, is a dye by virtue of its capacity to form salts with alkalis. Picric acid is unique in that it is the only substance which may be used as a fixative, a differentiator and a stain. A synthetic dye may be described as a benzene derivative, to which a chromophore and an auxochrome have been added.

Care must be taken when handling dyes, both in powder and solution form, especially in cases of prolonged exposure. Inhalation of the powder should be avoided and dyes coming in contact with the skin should be cleaned off immediately to prevent absorption.

Basic, acid and neutral dyes

The nature of the auxochrome ordinarily determines whether the resulting dye is acid or basic in character.

Basic dyes

In basic dyes, such as methylene blue, the colouring substance is contained in the basic part of the compound. The colourless acid radical is usually derived from hydrochloric, sulphuric or acetic acid.

Acid dyes

In these dyes, for example eosin, the colouring substance is contained in the acid component, and the base is usually sodium.

Neutral dyes

These are obtained by combining aqueous solutions of basic and acid dyes. The resultant precipitates are usually insoluble in water, but soluble in alcohol, for example Leishman's stain.

Nuclei are usually stained by basic dyes, and cytoplasm by acid dyes. Neutral dyes stain both nuclei and cytoplasm.

Solubility

Solubilities, expressed as g per 100 ml of solvent, of the more common histological stains in water and ethanol at room temperature, are given in *Table 17.1*.

The staining properties of dyes

Dyes may be considered as having micro-anatomical or cytological staining properties, as already mentioned in Chapter 13.

Micro-anatomical stains are used for demonstrating the general relationship of tissues to each other. Nuclei and cytoplasm are differentiated but their included structures are not necessarily emphasized.

Cytological stains demonstrate the minute structures in the nucleus and cytoplasm of cells without necessarily aiding in the general differentiation of the various tissue types.

Staining brought about by the aid of a mordant is called *indirect staining*, for example haematoxylin. Conversely, where a mordant is unnecessary, as in the majority of the aqueous or alcoholic aniline stains, the term *direct staining* is used. *Mordants* are metallic substances which act as a link between the stain and the tissue to be stained. They may be used in three ways:

1. Before application of the stain (pre-mordanting), e.g. Heidenhain's iron haematoxylin.
2. In conjunction with the stain (metachrome staining), e.g. Ehrlich's acid alum haematoxylin.
3. After the application of the stain (post-mordanting), e.g. Gram's stain.

Substances which, when incorporated into a staining solution, increase the staining power of that solution without acting as a mordant, are termed *accelerators*.

Stains which colour the tissue elements in a definite order are termed *progressive stains*. Those which colour all the tissue elements at the same time, and necessitate 'washing out' (differentiating), before the individual elements can be studied are termed *regressive stains*.

The staining of inclusions in live cells is referred to as *vital staining*. Living cells may be stained after removal from the organism (supravital staining), or while still part of the body (intravital staining). *Specific* stains act only on certain constituents of cells and tissues, and have little or no effect upon the remaining elements. The specificity, however, is usually dependent upon the use of a definite procedure. Most dyes stain the tissue in various shades of their own fundamental colour. Some tissues, however, assume a different colour from that of the solution in which they are immersed. This is known as *metachromatic* staining, a phenomenon seen only with the basic aniline dyes, such as methyl violet, which is frequently used in pathology to demonstrate amyloid infiltration.

Negative staining is used for the examination of bacterial morphology. The organisms and substance of choice are mixed on a slide. When the slide is examined microscopically, the unstained organisms are sharply contrasted against a blue background.

Certain tissue constituents and some organisms are demonstrated by a procedure known as *impregnation*. The solutions used in the impregnation

Table 17.1 CI number and solubility table of some common histological stains

Stain	CI No.	Water	Alcohol
Acid fuchsin	42685	18.0	0.3
Alcian blue	74240	9.5	6.0
Alizarin	58000	nil	0.125
Alizarin red S	58005	5.3	0.15
Auramine O	41000	0.35	7.0
Aurantia	10360	1.3	0.3
Basic fuchsin	42510	0.4	7.6
Bismarck brown Y	21000	1.2	1.1
Brilliant crystal scarlet	16250	1.75	0.8
Brilliant green	42040	3.0	3.3
Carminic acid	75470	8.3	0.2
Celestine blue	51050	2.0	1.5
Chlorantine Fast Red 5B	28160	1.0	0.45
Congo red	22120	4.5	0.8
Crystal violet	42555	1.5	7.0
Eosin	45380	40.5	3.5
Eosin—alcohol soluble	45386	nil	0.45
Haematoxylin	75290	1.75	60.0
Janus Green B	11045	5.3	1.1
Light green	42095	18.5	0.85
Martius yellow	10315	4.7	0.16
Methyl blue (Aniline blue)	42755	10.4	nil
Methyl green	42585	9.2	3.0
Methyl violet 6B	42555	4.2	6.2
Methylene blue	52015	2.5	1.5
Neutral red	50040	3.2	2.0
Nile blue	51180	1.0	1.0
Oil Red O*	26125	nil	0.5
Orange G	16230	7.1	0.3
Phloxine	45410	36.4	8.0
Picric acid		1.1	8.5
Purpurin	58205	nil	0.76
Pyronin B	45010	10.0	0.5
Pyronin Y	45005	11.0	0.5
Safranin O	50240	6.0	2.5
Scarlet R	26105	nil	0.2
Soluble blue	42755	40.0	nil
Sudan II	12140	nil	0.3
Sudan III	26100	nil	0.15
Sudan IV	26105	nil	0.08
Sudan black B	26150	nil	0.23
Tartrazine†		11.0	0.13
Thionin	52000	0.22	0.23
Toluidine blue	52040	3.1	0.5
Trypan blue	23850	10.4	0.02
Victoria blue 4R	42563	2.0	18.4

*Oil red O: 0.1% in isopropyl alcohol.
†Tartrazine: 2.3% in Cellosolve.

The above figures can only be a guide since batches of stain vary slightly in solubility; room temperature, which varies between 19°C and 25°C, also affects the solubility.

techniques are not stains, but are solutions of metallic salts. They differ from stains in being colourless. Opaque chemicals are precipitated on the surface of the tissue or bacteria. A stain is absorbed by the tissue, but an impregnating agent is deposited on its surface. This makes certain organisms (such as Spirochaetes) appear larger than they actually are.

Theory of staining

A great deal of research has been undertaken in an attempt to solve the complex problem of why certain stains have an affinity for certain tissue structures and inclusions. A number of theories have been advanced to explain this phenomenon but at the present time no single explanation has been accepted as being entirely satisfactory. The practice of supporting either a purely physical or chemical theory has been decreasing in recent years and modern workers tend to base their observations upon all of the individual factors, both physical and chemical, which, separately or jointly, are thought to play a part.

The physical factors which are considered as significant are (a) osmosis and capillarity, (b) absorption, and (c) selective adsorption. Osmosis and capillarity are simple physical forces which are considered by some workers as being at least partly responsible for the penetration of stains into porous tissues. The absorption factor is also very simple and is demonstrated in the presence of certain mineral salts, by the action of certain stains on certain tissues. The third physical factor, adsorption, is thought by many authorities to provide an acceptable explanation of a great many staining reactions. Selective adsorption, which is a principle well known to physical chemists, is the property possessed by certain substances to adsorb certain ions from a solution more readily than others. It is also known that the presence of other ions in the solution can have a marked effect upon the ratio of adsorption, and it would appear, therefore, that the action is controlled in part by the concentration of the hydroxyl and hydrogen ions present in the solution.

The main factor in the chemical theory is the assumption that certain parts of biological tissue are acid in character, for example the nuclei of cells, while others such as the cytoplasm have a basic reaction. As has been shown earlier, the colouring substance in basic dyes is contained in the basic part of the compound, the acid radical being colourless; conversely, with acid dyes, the colouring substance is contained in the acid component while the basic is colourless. It has been suggested that differential staining reactions could well be due to chemical combinations being formed between the tissue and stain, the actual reaction depending upon the character of the tissue and stains involved. Thus, acid tissue elements such as nuclei will have an affinity for a basic stain, while cytoplasm, which is basic in character, will have an affinity for acid stains.

Bacteria which are rich in ribonucleic acid, therefore, have an affinity for basic stains and tend to be unaffected by acid stains. In bacteriology, the latter are used mainly in negative staining techniques in which the bacteria are seen unstained against a stained background.

18

Staining procedures

Staining equipment

There are three methods of staining slides in common use: (a) using staining dishes; (b) using a staining rack; and (c) using a staining machine.

Staining dishes

A variety of these dishes is available. Small jars are used for staining single slides; Coplin jars hold 5–10 slides. Large staining troughs with separate baskets enable up to 20 slides to be stained at the same time.

Staining racks

Staining racks are often used in medical laboratories. Two glass rods, 50 mm (2 in) apart, are fixed across the sink. The slides are laid across these rods and the solutions poured onto the slides, using drop bottles. This method is not recommended for prolonged staining procedures.

Staining machines

These are used for staining large numbers of slides by a routine staining procedure. They have a greater usage in cytology and haematology for staining smears than for staining sections. Machines are designed with up to 23 stations to accommodate various staining procedures.

Other apparatus

Other apparatus required for staining includes the following:

1. A bunsen burner for heating stains.

2. A hot plate (thermostatically controlled) for hardening mounting media.
3. A microscope and lamp for controlling the degree of staining.

Procedure for staining paraffin wax sections

Before sections prepared by the paraffin wax technique can be stained, the surrounding wax must be removed and the section transferred, through graded alcohols, to distilled water. To avoid undue repetition in the following staining procedures, the phrase 'de-wax and hydrate' will be used to indicate that the following procedure should be adopted:

1. Free the section from paraffin wax by immersing the slide in xylene for 2 or 3 min. This process may be speeded up by first warming the section in a 60°C oven until the paraffin wax just begins to melt.
2. Transfer the slide to absolute alcohol for 30 s to remove the xylene. Blunt-nosed forceps should be used for transferring the slides from one reagent to another.
3. Transfer the slide to a second dish of absolute alcohol for a further 30 s to ensure that all the xylene is removed and not carried over into the lower grade alcohols.
4. Transfer the slide to 90% alcohol for 30 s.
5. Transfer the slide to 70% alcohol for 30 s.
6. Wash the slide thoroughly in distilled water.

The section is now ready for staining by the appropriate technique.

218

After staining, the section is passed back through the graded alcohols (that is, 70%, 90% and two changes of absolute alcohol), washing very thoroughly in the absolute alcohol.

The section is next cleared in two changes of xylene. The object of this is two-fold. First, the section, after having been immersed in xylene, is miscible with the xylene–balsam (or DPX). Secondly, the refractive index of the tissue is raised so that it is approximately the same as that of the glass slide to which it is attached. This is an important factor, as the refraction of the light is reduced to a minimum when the section is examined under the microscope.

Staining frozen sections

Frozen sections may be attached to slides before staining (see p. 211) or may be stained separately. Some sections in which fat is to be demonstrated are normally stained by being passed through small quantities of staining solutions by means of a tapered glass rod, the end of which is bent to form an angle of 60° (hockey stick). After staining, the sections are floated out in a dish of water, picked up on a slide and mounted in an aqueous mounting medium.

Control and test slides

Known positive slides should be used as controls with all specialized staining procedures. New batches of stain should also be tested with control slides before being used for routine staining purposes.

Pigments

When stained sections are examined microscopically, a deposit or pigment is frequently observed. This may be either artificial or natural in origin.

Artificial pigments

There are two artificial pigments commonly encountered, both being formed by the action of certain fixatives. They are: (a) mercuric chloride deposit; and (b) formaldehyde (post-mortem) precipitate.

Mercuric chloride deposit

The exact nature of this deposit is not known. It is found in all tissue which has been preserved in a fixative containing mercuric chloride, and appears in the form of black clumps, differing from the fine brown deposit of the formaldehyde precipitate. It may be removed from sections by treatment with iodine, as described on p. 221.

An alternative method is to add a few drops of a saturated solution of alcoholic iodine to each of the dehydrating alcohols, when dehydrating the bulk tissue. The disadvantage with this method is that the iodine tends to make the tissue rather brittle for sectioning.

Formaldehyde post-mortem precipitate

This pigment frequently occurs in post-mortem tissue if removed 24 h or more after death has occurred. It is believed to be a breakdown product of haemoglobin, and occurs chiefly in blood-forming organs, such as the liver and spleen. It does not occur when the formaldehyde solution has been neutralized or buffered to a reaction of pH 7 and for this reason is referred to also as the acid formalin pigment. It is readily soluble in saturated alcoholic picric acid or in alkaline solutions, and is easily removed by one of the methods described on p. 222.

Natural pigments

Natural pigments are divided into two classes, exogenous and endogenous.

Exogenous pigments

These pigments consist of foreign matter absorbed by the body during life. The most commonly encountered is carbon, which occurs as a jet-black pigment in sections of the lung and bronchial glands. It is impossible to remove the carbon pigment from sections. Another example of an exogenous pigment is tattooing ink.

Endogenous pigments

These are produced within the organism. There is a variety of pigments in this class which may be encountered when studying sections. Haemosiderin (free iron) is the one which occurs most commonly, and this can readily be demonstrated histochemically by the Prussian blue reaction (see p. 233) or, if required to be removed, it is soluble in acid. Other true pigments which fall into this class are melanin and calcium. Endogenous pigments can be identified easily by means of chemical tests.

Mounting of sections

After the section has been stained it must be prepared as a permanent preparation for microscopic examination. This is accomplished by mounting the section in a suitable medium under a glass coverslip.

The mountants most commonly used for mounting stained sections are Canada balsam, which may be either acid or neutral, and DPX. The choice of medium depends entirely upon the staining procedure used.

Method of mounting sections

1. Clean a coverslip of the appropriate size, and place it on the bench on a sheet of Whatman No. 1 filter paper.
2. Wipe off the excess xylene from the slide with a dust-free cloth.
3. Lay the slide on the filter paper in front of the coverslip.
4. Gently blot the section with a folded sheet of Whatman No. 1 filter paper.
5. Place the necessary amount of mounting medium on the section.
6. Quickly invert the slide and lower it onto the coverslip, applying gentle pressure until the mounting medium flows evenly to the edge of the coverslip.
7. Turn the slide over and, if necessary, square up the coverslip by means of a mounted needle.
8. After the sections have been mounted, the slides should be transferred to the 37°C incubator for 12–24 h in order to harden the mounting medium. Slides which are examined before the mounting medium has hardened frequently have their coverslip moved, resulting in damage to the section. If the slides are required for examination quickly, they can be placed on a hot plate to dry.

■ Notes

1. The object of blotting the section is to remove all *excess* xylene. If this is not done, the xylene will mix with the mounting medium and form air-bubbles which become trapped beneath the coverslip. On no account should the section be blotted so hard that it becomes dry, as shrinkage and cracking will result.
2. Excess balsam may be removed by wiping with a clean duster, dipped in xylene.
3. If DPX is used as the mounting medium, an excess amount should be placed on the slide, the surplus being stripped off 24 h later when it has hardened. This is necessary in order to counteract the shrinkage which it undergoes on drying.

Coverslips for mounting stained preparations should be kept stored in absolute alcohol on the staining bench. The coverslips most commonly used are approximately 0.17 mm in thickness. For use with 3 in by 1 in (76 mm × 25 mm) slides, the sizes range from 22 mm square to 50 mm by 22 mm.

Mounting media

Media for the mounting of microscopical preparations may be divided into two main groups: (a)

aqueous media; (b) resinous media. The media in group (a) are designed to make either temporary or permanent mounts of water-miscible preparations, e.g. frozen sections stained for fat. Their formulae consist of a solidifying agent such as gelatin or gum arabic to which is added glycerol to prevent drying and cracking, various sugars to bring about an increase in the refractive index and a preservative.

Group (b) may be divided into the natural and synthetic media. The most important of the natural resins is Canada balsam; a large number of synthetic resins are available commercially.

Aqueous mountants

Karo corn syrup (refractive index 1.47)

Formula

Karo corn syrup	1 vol
Distilled water	2 vol
Thymol, as preservative	1 crystal

Mode of preparation

Dilute the corn syrup with the distilled water and add the thymol. Mix well, label and store in a refrigerator at 4°C.

Laevulose (fructose) syrup (refractive index 1.47)

Formula

Laevulose (fructose)	70 g
Distilled water	20 ml

Mode of preparation

Dissolve the laevulose in the distilled water by heating at 37°C for 24 h. Mix well and label.

Farrant's medium (refractive index 1.43)

Formula

Gum arabic	50 g
Distilled water	50 ml
Glycerol	50 ml
Arsenic trioxide, as preservative	1 g

Mode of preparation

Dissolve the gum arabic in the distilled water with the aid of gentle heat, add the glycerol and arsenic trioxide. Mix well and label.

■ Notes

1. The addition of 50 g of potassium acetate to the above solution will give a neutral medium (pH 7.2) instead of an acid one (pH 4.4) and raises the refractive index to 1.44.
2. Sodium merthiolate (0.025%) may be substituted with advantage for the arsenic trioxide as a preservative.

Glycerine jelly (refractive index 1.47)

Formula

Gelatin	10 g
Glycerol	70 ml
Distilled water	60 ml
Phenol crystals, as preservative	0.25 g

Mode of preparation

Weigh the gelatin into the distilled water and incubate in a water bath at 60°C until solution is effected. Add the glycerol and then the phenol crystals. Mix well, label and store in a refrigerator at 4°C.

Preparation for use

Melt the glycerine jelly by heating in a water bath or incubator at 60°C.

■ **Note**

To avoid the formation of air-bubbles in the mounted specimen do not shake or stir the melted medium prior to use.

Resinous mountants

Neutral balsam (refractive index 1.52)

Mode of preparation

Dissolve Canada balsam in xylene to form a fairly thin solution (approximately 40–50%). Add calcium carbonate to excess and stir thoroughly. Allow the mixture to settle, decant the supernatant fluid into a stock bottle and discard the residue. Record date and label.

■ **Notes**

1. The Canada balsam dissolves more readily in the xylene when placed in an incubator at 37°C or a paraffin wax oven at 58°C.
2. Toluene may be used as a solvent in place of xylene.
3. Canada balsam is a natural resin obtained from *Abies balsamea*. Mountants prepared from this resin can only be neutralized temporarily, becoming acid and brown on storage.

Acid balsam (refractive index 1.52)

Mode of preparation

Dissolve Canada balsam in xylene to form a fairly thin solution (approximately 40–50%). Add salicylic acid to excess and stir thoroughly. Allow the mixture to settle, decant the supernatant fluid into a stock bottle and discard the residue. Record date and label.

■ **Note**

See Notes under Neutral balsam above.

Xylene damar (refractive index 1.53)

Mode of preparation

Prepare a thin solution of the gum damar by dissolving in chloroform. Filter through paper in a Buchner funnel, using negative pressure, and evaporate the filtrate until all traces of the chloroform are removed. Dissolve the purified gum in xylene until a suitable solution results (approximately 60%). Record date and label.

■ **Notes**

1. Gum damar is a natural resin obtained from the East Indian tree *Sherea wiesneri*. The commercial product invariably contains solid impurities and should always be purified before use.
2. Unlike Canada balsam, gum damar does not become brown on keeping.

Synthetic resins

A wide range of mountants prepared from synthetic resins is available commercially. The formula of most commercial synthetic mountants is kept secret, but in general they are prepared by dissolving a polystyrene in an aromatic hydrocarbon solvent, and adding a plasticizer such as dibutylphthalate or tricresyl phosphate to prevent the formation of air spaces on drying.

DPX mountant (refractive index 1.52)

Polystyrene (lubricant-free)	10 g
Dibutylphthalate	5 ml
Xylene	35 ml

Mode of preparation

Combine the dibutylphthalate with the xylene, mix and dissolve the polystyrene. Record date and label.

■ **Notes**

1. To remove the coverglasses from preparations mounted with DPX immerse in trichlorethylene.
2. Preparations mounted in DPX should be cleared in xylene free from paraffin wax.

Procedures for the removal of pigments

Mercuric chloride precipitate

The removal of the mercuric chloride precipitate.

Lugol's iodine

Solution 1:

Potassium iodide	2 g
Iodine	1 g
Distilled water	100 ml

Solution 2:

Sodium thiosulphate	5 g
Distilled water	100 ml

Mode of preparation

Solution 1. Dissolve the potassium iodide in the distilled water and then add the iodine. Record date and label.

Solution 2. Dissolve the sodium thiosulphate in the distilled water, mix and label.

Procedure

1. Bring sections to water.
2. Immerse in solution 1 for 10 min.
3. Rinse in water.
4. Bleach in solution 2 for 3–5 min.
5. Wash thoroughly in water.
6. Continue with required staining procedure.

Schridde's method

The removal of the formalin post-mortem pigment.

Formula

Ammonia (sp. gr. 0.880)	1 ml
Ethyl alcohol, 75%	200 ml

Procedure

1. Bring sections to 70% alcohol.
2. Treat with ammoniacal alcohol for 30 min.
3. Wash thoroughly in tap water.
4. Continue with required staining procedure.

■ **Note**

Sections may become detached from the slide when using this method.

Verocay's method

The removal of the formalin post-mortem pigment.

Formula

Potassium hydroxide, 1% aqueous solution	1 ml
Ethyl alcohol, 80%	100 ml

Procedure

1. Bring sections to 80% alcohol.

2. Treat with alcoholic hydroxide solution for 10 min.
3. Wash with two changes of water.
4. Transfer to 80% alcohol for 5 min.
5. Wash in water.
6. Continue with required staining procedure.

Barrett's alcoholic picric acid

The removal of the formalin post-mortem pigment:

1. Deparaffinize with xylene and wash thoroughly in absolute alcohol.
2. Immerse in saturated alcoholic picric acid (approximately 8.5%) for 30 min or more.
3. Wash in absolute alcohol to remove the picric acid.
4. Bring the section to water and continue staining in the normal way.

Haematoxylin staining solutions for cell nuclei

The mordants used in conjunction with haematoxylin for demonstrating the nucleus and the cytoplasmic contents are alum and iron. Of these, the solutions containing alum stain the nucleus a dark transparent blue which rapidly turns red in the presence of acid. The solutions containing iron as a mordant stain the nucleus a more intense grey-black colour and are less susceptible to acid. Iron–haematoxylin is of particular value when the counterstain to be employed is of a strongly acidic nature. It is also used when fine structural details of the nucleus and cytoplasm are required.

Alum–haematoxylin solutions

A large number of haematoxylin solutions which contain alum as their mordant have been devised, but only three are commonly employed. Alum–haematoxylin is used as a routine stain in conjunction with eosin, for demonstrating the general structure of tissue.

Iron–haematoxylin solutions

There are two main iron–haematoxylin solutions employed for routine work in the laboratory: Heidenhain's and Weigert's. Of these two solutions, that of Weigert has the advantage of being a much more rapid stain and is of particular value in pathological work where time is an important factor. It is commonly used to stain the nuclei of sections which are to be counterstained with Van Gieson stain, to demonstrate collagen fibres. The Heidenhain's solution, on the other hand, has the advantage of giving very precise staining of both nuclei and cytoplasmic inclusions. It is also used as a routine stain for demonstrating the striations in muscle fibres.

Techniques and results

Mayer's acid–alum–haematoxylin and eosin

A general-purpose staining procedure.

Mayer's acid–alum–haematoxylin

Solution 1:

Ammonium alum	50 g
Chloral hydrate	50 g
Haematoxylin (CI No. 75290)	1 g
Citric acid	1 g
Sodium iodate	0.2 g
Distilled water	1000 ml

Dissolve the haematoxylin in the water with the aid of gentle heat and add the sodium iodate and alum, shaking at intervals to effect solution of the alum. Dissolve the citric acid and chloral hydrate, record date and label. The haematoxylin solution, which turns reddish-violet in colour, is ready for immediate use, no further ripening being necessary owing to the inclusion of the sodium iodate. The solution remains stable for several months.

Acid–alcohol

Solution 2:

Hydrochloric acid (sp. gr. 1.19)	1 ml
Ethyl alcohol, 70%	99 ml

Scott's tap water substitute—see Note 3 below

Solution 3:

Sodium bicarbonate	3.5 g
Magnesium sulphate	20 g
Tap water	1000 ml
Thymol, as preservative	1 crystal

Solution 4:

Eosin, w/s yellowish (CI No. 45380)	1 g
Distilled water	100 ml
Thymol, as preservative	1 crystal

Procedure

1. De-wax and hydrate.
2. Stain in solution 1 for 10–30 min.
3. Wash thoroughly in running tap water.
4. Differentiate in solution 2 until only the cell nuclei retain the stain.
5. Blue in running tap water for 5–10 min, or solution 3 for 1–2 min followed by running tap water.
6. Counterstain in solution 4 for 1–2 min.
7. Wash with running water until the excess eosin is removed.
8. Dehydrate, clear and mount in neutral balsam or DPX.

Results

Cell nuclei, blue; red blood corpuscles, red; muscle, connective tissue and cell cytoplasm, varying shades of pink.

■ Notes

1. Alum–haematoxylin can be used progressively, the optimum staining period being determined for each new batch of stain by staining a control section. For routine work, the common practice is to use it as a regressive stain, owing to factors such as fixation and the type of tissue which influence the staining time.
2. When alum–haematoxylins which are ripened spontaneously are used for routine work, the laboratory requirements should be calculated some months ahead.
3. Sections require thorough washing in tap water after staining with acid–alum–haematoxylin in order to remove all traces of the acid and to bring out the required colour. In districts where the tap water is alkaline in reaction, satisfactory blueing will be obtained without recourse to the use of solution 3.
4. 20 ml of glacial acetic acid may be substituted for the citric acid in the preparation of solution 1.
5. The addition of up to 1% acetic acid to solution 4 is preferred by some workers.
6. The use of 4–5 drops of concentrated formaldehyde solution (40%) may be used as a preservative in place of thymol in solution 4.

Ehrlich's haematoxylin

A general-purpose nuclear stain.

Formula

Ammonium or potassium alum	3 g
Haematoxylin (CI No. 75290)	2 g
Ethyl alcohol, 95%	100 ml
Glycerol	100 ml
Distilled water	100 ml
Acetic acid, glacial	10 ml

Mode of preparation

Dissolve the haematoxylin in the alcohol, in a 1 litre flask, and then add the water. Add the alum and shake until solution is effected. Incorporate the remaining ingredients. Plug the flask lightly with cotton wool and oxidize by exposing to the air and sunlight for 2 weeks or more, shaking daily. Transfer to a suitable storage bottle, record date, label and store in a warm place for 3 or 4 weeks. Repeat the shaking at intervals. The solution remains stable for several years.

Procedure

Proceed as for Mayer's acid–alum–haematoxylin (see p. 223), using the above solution in place of solution 1.

Results

Cell nuclei, blue; other constituents according to counterstain.

■ **Notes**

1. The addition of 0.4 g of sodium iodate will produce instant oxidation, but the stability of the solution will be affected and the period of optimal activity will be reduced. When iodate is employed, it must be added prior to the addition of the acetic acid.
2. The inclusion of the glycerol reduces evaporation and retards the staining rate of the solution.

Harris alum–haematoxylin

A general-purpose nuclear stain of exceptional value in exfoliative cytology.

Formula

Ammonium or potassium alum	20 g
Haematoxylin (CI No. 75290)	1 g
Mercuric oxide	0.5 g
Distilled water	200 ml
Ethyl alcohol, absolute	10 ml

Dissolve the haematoxylin in the alcohol and the alum in the distilled water with the aid of gentle heat. Combine the two solutions in a 500 ml boiling flask and bring rapidly to the boil. Add the mercuric oxide and then cool immediately by immersing the flask in cold water. The solution should assume a dark purple colour on the addition of the mercuric oxide. Transfer to a suitable storage bottle, record date and label. The solution remains stable for several months.

Procedure

Proceed as for Mayer's acid–alum–haematoxylin (see p. 223), using the above solution in place of solution 1. See also Note 2 below.

Results

Cell nuclei, blue; other constituents according to counterstain.

■ **Notes**

1. The addition of 4% acetic acid gives more precise nuclear staining and should be used for cytology.
2. The usual staining time for smears is 4 min.

Cole's haematoxylin

A general-purpose nuclear stain.

Formula

Saturated aqueous aluminium sulphate	750 ml
Haematoxylin (CI No. 75290)	1.0 g
1% iodine in 70% alcohol	50 ml
Distilled water	250 ml

Using a 2 litre flask, dissolve the haematoxylin in the distilled water with the aid of gentle heat.

Add the iodine solution and the aluminium ammonium sulphate solution and mix well. Bring rapidly to the boil and then cool.

Transfer to a suitable dark storage bottle, record date, label and store in a cool place. The solution remains stable for several months.

Procedure

Proceed as for Mayer's acid–alum–haematoxylin (see p. 223), using the above solution in place of solution 1.

Results

Cell nuclei, blue; other constituents according to counterstain.

Gill's haematoxylin

A general-purpose nuclear stain.

Formula

Haematoxylin	2.0 g
Sodium iodate	0.2 g
Aluminium sulphate	17.6 g
Glacial acetic acid	20 ml
Ethylene glycol	250 ml
Distilled water	730 ml

Using a 2 litre flask, mix the distilled water and ethylene glycol. Add the haematoxylin, sodium iodate, aluminium sulphate and glacial acetic acid in that order. Stir for 1 h at room temperature and filter.

Transfer to a suitable dark storage bottle, record date and label. The solution is ready for immediate use.

Results

Cell nuclei, blue; other constituents according to counterstain.

Celestin blue

A stain which, when used in conjunction with Mayer's acid–alum–haematoxylin (see p. 223), is resistant to strong acid dyes and gives good nuclear definition.

Solution 1:

Iron alum	25 g

Celestin blue R (CI No. 900)	1.25 g
Glycerol	35 ml
Distilled water	250 ml

Dissolve the alum in the distilled water. Solution is generally effected by allowing the flask to remain at room temperature overnight. Add the celestin blue and boil for 3 min. Cool, filter and add the glycerol. Record date and label. The solution remains stable for 6–12 months.

Solution 2. Mayer's acid–alum–haematoxylin (see p. 223) or Cole's haematoxylin (see p. 223).

Procedure

1. De-wax and hydrate.
2. Stain in solution 1 for 10–20 min.
3. Rinse in tap water.
4. Stain in solution 2 for 5–10 min.
5. Rinse in water.
6. Blue in running tap water.
7. Counterstain as required.
8. Dehydrate, clear and mount.

Results

Cell nuclei, blue; other constituents according to counterstain.

◀ **Note**

Celestin blue is frequently used in conjunction with Mayer's acid–alum–haematoxylin in place of the older iron–haematoxylin solutions, the combined result being resistant to acid dyes.

Weigert's iron–haematoxylin and Van Gieson's stain

A widely used stain for differentiating muscle fibres and connective tissue.

Haematoxylin solution A:
| Haematoxylin (CI No. 75290) | 1 g |
| Ethyl alcohol, 95% | 100 ml |

Iron chloride solution B:
Iron chloride (ferric) 29%	
aqueous solution	4 ml
Hydrochloric acid (sp. gr. 1.19)	1 ml
Distilled water	95 ml

The working solution

Solution 1:
| Haematoxylin solution (see above) | 1 vol |
| Iron chloride solution (see above) | 1 vol |

Combine the solutions and mix well. The mixture, which is deep purple in colour, is best prepared for use as required. The working solution will remain active for 1–2 days.

Solution 2: Acid–alcohol 1% (see p. 223).

Van Gieson's stain

Solution 3:
Picric acid, saturated aqueous	
solution (approx. 1%)	100 ml
Acid fuchsin (CI No. 42685), 1%	
aqueous solution	5–10 ml

Procedure

1. De-wax and hydrate.
2. Stain in solution 1 for 20 min.
3. Wash in tap water.
4. Differentiate in solution 2, controlling the degree of differentiation microscopically, until the nuclei are just overstained.
5. Wash in tap water.
6. Counterstain in solution 3 for 3–5 min.
7. Blot lightly; do not wash in water.
8. Dehydrate rapidly with 90% and absolute alcohol, clear and mount in acid balsam or DPX.

Results

Cell nuclei, black; collagen, red; muscle fibres, cell cytoplasm and red blood corpuscles, yellow.

■ **Note**

The addition of a few drops of saturated alcoholic picric acid to the dehydrating alcohols is to be recommended. Alcohols used to dehydrate sections stained with Van Gieson's stain should not be used with haematoxylin and eosin.

Heidenhain's iron–haematoxylin

A precise cytological stain which may be used for demonstrating both nuclear and cytoplasmic inclusions. Striations in voluntary muscle are also well stained.

Solution 1:
| Iron alum | 2.5 g |
| Distilled water | 100 ml |

Solution 2:
Haematoxylin (CI No. 75290)	0.5 g
Ethyl alcohol, 95%	10 ml
Distilled water	90 ml

Dissolve the haematoxylin in the alcohol and add the water. Bottle, stopper with a cotton-wool plug and allow the solution to ripen for 4–5 weeks. Record date and label. The solution remains stable indefinitely.

Procedure

1. De-wax and hydrate.

2. Mordant in solution 1 for 3 h or longer.
3. Rinse in water.
4. Stain in solution 2 for a period equal to that for which the sections were mordanted in solution 1.
5. Rinse in distilled water.
6. Differentiate in solution 1, controlling the degree of differentiation microscopically.
7. Wash thoroughly in running tap water for 5–10 min to remove all traces of the iron alum.
8. Counterstain as required.
9. Dehydrate, clear and mount.

Results

Cell nuclei, cytoplasmic inclusions and muscle striations, black; other constituents according to counterstain.

■ Notes

1. The addition of 0.1 g of sodium iodate will render the haematoxylin solution ready for use immediately.
2. Solution 2 may be diluted 1:1 with distilled water to give greater control during differentiation.
3. By heating solutions 1 and 2 to 45°C, the period of staining may be reduced to 45 min.

Verhoeff's elastic fibre stain

For the demonstration of elastic fibres:

Alcoholic haematoxylin
Haematoxylin (CI No. 75290)	5 g
Ethyl alcohol, absolute	100 ml

Ferric chloride solution
Ferric chloride	10 g
Distilled water	100 ml

Lugol's iodine solution (see p. 222)

Solution 1:
Alcoholic haematoxylin	20 ml
Ferric chloride solution	8 ml
Lugol's iodine solution	8 ml

Add the ferric chloride and Lugol's iodine to the alcoholic haematoxylin.

Solution 2:
Ferric chloride solution	20 ml
Distilled water	80 ml

Solution 3: Van Gieson's stain (see p. 225).

Procedure

1. De-wax and hydrate.
2. Stain in solution 1 for 15–60 min.
3. Rinse in water.
4. Differentiate in solution 2, controlling the degree of differentiation microscopically.
5. Transfer to 95% alcohol.

6. Wash in water.
7. Counterstain with solution 3.
8. Dehydrate, clear and mount.

Results

Elastic fibres, black; nuclei, blue to black; collagen, red; muscle fibres, yellow; red blood cells, yellow.

■ Notes

1. Solution 1 will only remain active for 24–48 h.
2. To decrease nuclei staining double the quantity of Lugol's iodine solution.
3. Sections which have been over-differentiated may be returned to solution 1 and restained, provided that they have not been in contact with 95% ethyl alcohol.

Resorcin fuchsin

The demonstration of elastic fibres.

Solution 1:
Basic fuchsin (CI No. 42510)	2 g
Resorcinol	4 g
Ferric chloride, 29% aqueous solution	25 ml
Distilled water	200 ml
Ethyl alcohol, 95%	(approx.) 205 ml
Hydrochloric acid (sp. gr. 1.18)	1 ml

Measure the distilled water into an enamel dish and dissolve the basic fuchsin and resorcinol. Bring to the boil and add the ferric chloride solution. Boil for 3–5 min, stirring constantly, when a thick precipitate should form. Cool and filter. Discard the filtrate and allow the filter paper and enamel dish to dry. Place the filter paper in the enamel dish and dissolve the precipitate in 200 ml of alcohol by heating carefully with constant stirring. Remove the filter paper, cool and filter. Make up the volume to 200 ml with the alcohol and add the hydrochloric acid. Record date and label. The solution remains stable for 3–4 months.

Solution 2: Acid–alcohol 1% (see p. 223).

Procedure

1. De-wax and bring sections to 95% alcohol.
2. Stain in solution 1 for 20 min or longer.
3. Rinse in 95% alcohol.
4. Differentiate in solution 2.
5. Wash thoroughly in water.
6. Counterstain as desired.
7. Dehydrate, clear and mount.

Results

Elastic fibres, dark blue to black; other tissues according to counterstain used.

Martius scarlet blue (MSB) (Lendrum *et al.*) for the demonstration of fibrin

Solution 1: Celestin blue (see p. 224).
Solution 2: Mayer's haemalum (see p. 223).
Solution 3: 0.25% Hydrochloric acid in 70% ethyl alcohol.
Solution 4: 0.5% Martius yellow (CI No. 10315) in 95% ethyl alcohol containing 2% phosphotungstic acid.
Solution 5: 1% Brilliant crystal scarlet (CI No. 16250) in 2.5% aqueous acetic acid.
Solution 6: 1% Phosphotungstic acid.
Solution 7: 0.5% Soluble blue (CI No. 42755) in 1% aqueous acetic acid.

Procedure

1. De-wax and hydrate.
2. Stain in solution 1 for 5 min.
3. Rinse in tap water.
4. Stain in solution 2 for 5 min.
5. Rinse in tap water.
6. Differentiate in solution 3.
7. Wash thoroughly in tap water.
8. Rinse in 95% ethanol.
9. Stain in solution 4 for 2 min.
10. Rinse in water.
11. Stain in solution 5 for 10 min.
12. Rinse in water.
13. Transfer to solution 6 for 5 min.
14. Rinse in water.
15. Stain in solution 7 for 10 min.
16. Dehydrate, clear and mount.

Results

Cell nuclei, blue; fibrin, red; collagen, blue; red blood cells, yellow.

Note

The procedure may be shortened and differentiation eliminated by staining in a single solution of the following for 8 min in place of steps 9–15. Solution 4, 3 vol, solution 5, 2 vol, solution 7, 3 vol. Rinse in water before dehydration.

Gordon and Sweet's reticulin stain

A routine method which demonstrates reticulin fibres but does not stain the cells.

Solution 1:

| Potassium permanganate, 0.5% aqueous solution | 95 ml |
| Sulphuric acid, 3% aqueous solution | 5 ml |

Solution 2:

| Oxalic water | 1 g |
| Distilled water | 100 ml |

Solution 3:

| Iron alum | 2.5 g |
| Distilled water | 100 ml |

Solution 4:

Silver nitrate, 10.2% aqueous solution	5 ml
Sodium hydroxide, 3.1% aqueous solution	5 ml
Ammonia (sp. gr. 0.880)	as required
Glass-distilled water	as required

Measure the silver nitrate solution into a chemically clean 100 ml graduated cylinder and add ammonia water, drop by drop, with constant shaking, until the precipitate formed is redissolved. Add the sodium hydroxide solution and again dissolve the precipitate by adding ammonia water drop by drop. The precipitate should be only just dissolved and the final solution should be slightly turbid. Make up the volume to 50 ml with glass-distilled water. The solution must be prepared at the time of use.

Solution 5: Formalin, 10% aqueous solution in distilled water.

Solution 6: Gold chloride, 0.2% aqueous solution.

Solution 7: Sodium thiosulphate, 5% aqueous solution.

Solution 8: Saffranine O, 5% aqueous solution.

Procedure

1. Bring sections to water.
2. Oxidize in solution 1 for 1–5 min.
3. Wash in water.
4. Bleach in solution 2 for 3–5 min.
5. Wash thoroughly in tap water and several changes of distilled water.
6. Mordant in solution 3 for between 10 min and 2 h (10 min will usually suffice).
7. Wash in several changes of distilled water.
8. Impregnate with solution 4 for 30 s.
9. Wash in several changes of distilled water.
10. Reduce in solution 5 for 1 min.
11. Wash in tap water and then distilled water.
12. Tone in solution 6 for 10–15 min.
13. Rinse in distilled water.
14. Fix in solution 7 for 5 min.
15. Wash in water for 1–2 min.
16. Counterstain nuclei with solution 8.
17. Dehydrate, clear and mount.

Note

It is dangerous to store the ammoniacal silver solution as gas is produced and this may result in an explosion.

Gomori's trichrome stain

A simple connective tissue stain for general use.

Solution 1: Harris alum–haematoxylin (see p. 224).

Solution 2: Acid–alcohol (see p. 223).

Solution 3:

Phosphotungstic acid	0.6 g
Chromotrope 2R (CI No. 16570)	0.6 g
Fast green, FCF (CI No. 42053)	0.3 g
Distilled water	100 ml
Acetic acid, glacial	1 ml

Dissolve the phosphotungstic acid in the distilled water. Incorporate the chromotrope 2R and fast green, add the acetic acid and label.

Solution 4:

Distilled water	100 ml
Acetic acid, glacial	0.2 ml

Procedure

1. Bring sections to water.
2. Stain and differentiate according to the procedure given on page 223.
3. Stain in solution 3 for 5–20 min.
4. Rinse in solution 4 for 1 min.
5. Dehydrate, clear and mount.

Results

Cell nuclei, blue; cytoplasm, red; collagen, green; muscle, red.

Mallory's phosphotungstic acid–haematoxylin

A differential stain designed to demonstrate collagen, neuroglia cells and fibres, myofibrils and striations in muscle tumours.

Solution 1: Mercuric chloride, saturated aqueous solution (approx. 7%).

Solution 2: Lugol's iodine (see p. 222).

Solution 3: Sodium thiosulphate, 5% aqueous solution.

Solution 4:

Potassium permanganate	0.25 g
Distilled water	100 ml

Solution 5:

Oxalic acid	5 g
Distilled water	100 ml

Solution 6:

Haematoxylin	1 g
Phosphotungstic acid	20 g
Distilled water	1000 ml
Potassium permanganate	0.177 g

Dissolve the haematoxylin in 500 ml of the distilled water with the aid of gentle heat. Dissolve the phosphotungstic acid in the remaining 500 ml of distilled water. Combine the two solutions when cool and add the potassium permanganate. Record date and label.

Procedure

1. Bring sections to water.
2. Mordant in solution 1 for 3 h.
3. Rinse in water.
4. Transfer to solution 2 for 10 min.
5. Rinse in water.
6. Bleach in solution 3 for 5 min.
7. Rinse in distilled water.
8. Oxidize in solution 4 for 5 min.
9. Rinse in distilled water.
10. Bleach in solution 5 for 5 min.
11. Wash well in tap water.
12. Stain in solution 6 overnight at room temperature.
13. Rinse in tap water.
14. Dehydrate, clear and mount.

Results

Cell nuclei, deep blue; neuroglia, deep blue; fibroglia and myoglia fibrils, deep blue; red blood corpuscles, deep blue; fibrin, deep blue; collagen, brownish red.

Southgate's mucicarmine

For the demonstration of mucin secreted by epithelial cells.

Solution 1: Mayer's acid–alum–haematoxylin (see p. 223).

Solution 2:

Carmine (CI No. 75470)	1 g
Aluminium hydroxide	1 g
Aluminium chloride, anhydrous	0.5 g
Ethyl alcohol, 50%	100 ml

Weigh the carmine and aluminium hydroxide into a 500 ml flask and then add the alcohol. Shake well and while still shaking add the aluminium chloride. Place in a boiling water bath for 2.5 min exactly. Cool, filter, record date and label.

Procedure

1. De-wax and hydrate.
2. Stain with solution 1.
3. Stain with solution 2 diluted 1:5 with distilled water for 30–45 min.
4. Rinse in distilled water.
5. Dehydrate, clear and mount.

Results

Cell nuclei, blue; mucin, red.

■ **Note**

More precise staining may be achieved by diluting solution 2 1:10 with distilled water and prolonging the staining period.

Periodic acid Schiff method

The periodic acid Schiff reaction (PAS) is widely used in histopathology. The reaction is due to certain carbohydrates that contain 1,2-glycol groups being converted to aldehydes by oxidation with periodic acid. The aldehydes become coloured when treated with Schiff's reagent. It is particularly valuable for demonstrating glycogen, fungi and mucin.

Solution 1:

Periodic acid	1 g
Distilled water	100 ml

Solution 2: Schiff's reagent:*

Basic fuchsin (CI No. 42510)	1 g
Distilled water	200 ml
1.0M hydrochloric acid (98.3 ml HCl, sp. gr. 1.16 made up to 1 litre with distilled water)	20 ml
Sodium bisulphite (anhydrous)	1 g
Activated charcoal	0.5 g

Measure the distilled water into a 500 ml flask, bring to the boil and dissolve the basic fuchsin. Cool to 50°C, filter and add the hydrochloric acid. Cool to 25°C and add the sodium bisulphite. Store in the dark for 24–48 h, during which time the solution becomes straw-coloured. Shake up with the charcoal, filter immediately, transfer to a brown bottle and label. Store in a refrigerator.

Solution 3: Sulphurous acid rinse:

Sodium metabisulphite, 10%	6 ml
1.0M hydrochloric acid	5 ml
Distilled water	100 ml

Solution 4: Harris alum–haematoxylin (see p. 224).

Procedure

1. De-wax and hydrate.
2. Place in solution 1 for 5 min.
3. Rinse in tap water.
4. Rinse in distilled water.
5. Place in Schiff's reagent (solution 2) for 5 min.
6. Place in 3 baths of solution 3 for 2 min in each bath.
7. Rinse in tap water.
8. Stain with solution 4 for 30 s.
9. Blue in tap water.
10. Dehydrate, clear and mount.

*Available commercially from several reputable sources.

■ **Note**

Step 6 can be omitted and the section washed in running tap water for 10 min.

Results

Cell nuclei, blue; mucin and glycogen, purple; basement membrane of kidney and skin, reddish-purple.

Control tests

A control test slide containing known positive material should always be stained to test the efficiency of the solutions.

The Fuelgen reaction

For the demonstration of nucleoproteins.

Solution 1: Hydrochloric acid, 1.0M solution (see Appendix II).

Solution 2: Schiff's reagent (see above).

Solution 3: Sulphite rinse:

Potassium metabisulphite, 10% aqueous solution	5 ml
Hydrochloric acid, 1.0M solution	5 ml
Distilled water	90 ml

Add the potassium metabisulphite solution and hydrochloric acid to the distilled water. Prepare immediately before use.

Procedure

1. De-wax and hydrate.
2. Rinse briefly in cold solution 1.
3. Transfer to solution 1, preheated to 60°C. The optimum period of hydrolysis varies according to the fixative used, but is usually 5–25 min.
4. Rinse briefly in cold solution 1.
5. Rinse in distilled water.
6. Transfer to solution 2 (Schiff's reagent) for 30–90 min.
7. Drain and transfer to 3 baths of solution 3 for 1, 2 and 2 min in each, respectively.
8. Rinse well in distilled water.
9. Counterstain as desired.
10. Dehydrate, clear and mount.

Results

Deoxyribonucleic acid (DNA), reddish-purple; other tissues according to counterstain.

■ **Note**

It is advisable to stain several slides, varying the period of hydrolysis.

Methyl green–pyronin

For the identification of deoxyribonucleic acid and ribonucleic acid.

Trevan and Sharrock's methyl green–pyronin

Solution 1:		Final concentration of stain (%)
Pyronin Y, 5% aqueous solution	17.5 ml	0.16
Methyl green, 2% aqueous solution	10 ml	0.036
Distilled water	250 ml	
Acetate buffer, pH 4.8	277.5 ml	

Add the pyronin Y and methyl green solutions to the distilled water. Dilute with an equal quantity of the acetate buffer (see Appendix II). Record date and label. The solution is best prepared just before use, but it should remain stable for 2–3 months.

Jordan and Baker's methyl green–pyronin

Solution 2:		Final concentration of stain (%)
Pyronin Y, 0.5% aqueous solution	37 ml	0.185
Methyl green, 0.5% aqueous solution	13 ml	0.065
Acetate buffer, pH 4.8	50 ml	

Add the pyronin Y and methyl green solution to the acetate buffer. Record date and label. The solution is best prepared just before use, but it should remain stable for 2–3 months.

Solution 3:	
Acetone	1 vol
Xylene	1 vol

Procedure

1. Bring sections to water.
2. Stain in either solution 1 or 2 for 15–60 min (see Note 2 below).
3. Rinse quickly in distilled water.
4. Blot with non-fluffy filter paper.
5. Flood with 2 changes of acetone.
6. Flood with solution 3.
7. Clear in xylene and mount in neutral balsam or DPX.

Results

Deoxyribonucleic acid (DNA), green; ribonucleic acid (RNA), red.

■ **Notes**

1. The methyl green should be dissolved in the distilled

water, transferred to a separating funnel and washed with successive changes of chloroform until no more violet colour is extracted.
2. Solution 1 is preferred for staining sections from formalin fixed tissue and solution 2 for sections from tissue fixed in Zenker's fluid (see p. 182).

Gomori's aldehyde fuchsin

The demonstration of cells of the islets of Langerhans and elastic fibres.

Solution 1: Lugol's iodine (see p. 222).

Solution 2:
Sodium thiosulphate, 5% aqueous solution.

Solution 3: Aldehyde–fuchsin:	
Basic fuchsin (CI No. 42510)	1 g
Ethyl alcohol, 70%	200 ml
Hydrochloric acid (sp. gr. 1.18)	2 ml
Paraldehyde	2 ml

Solution 4. Light green (CI No. 42095) 0.2%.

Dissolve the basic fuchsin in the alcohol and then add the hydrochloric acid and paraldehyde. Shake the mixture well and stand at room temperature until deep purple in colour (24–48 h). Record date and label.

Procedure

1. De-wax and hydrate.
2. Mordant in solution 1 for 10–60 min.
3. Rinse in water.
4. Bleach in solution 2 for 5 min.
5. Wash in running tap water for 3 min.
6. Rinse in 90% alcohol.
7. Stain in solution 3 for 5–10 min.
8. Rinse in 90% alcohol.
9. Counterstain as desired.
10. Dehydrate, clear and mount.

Results

Elastic fibres, purple; other tissues according to counterstain used.

Trichrome–PAS method (Pearse)

A useful staining procedure for demonstrating the alpha and beta cells in the anterior lobe of the pituitary gland, following fixation in formol saline or Helly's fluid.

Solution 1: 1% aqueous periodic acid (see p. 229).

Solution 2: Schiff's reagent (see p. 229).

Solution 3: 0.5% sodium metabisulphite (see p. 229).

Solution 4: Celestin blue (see p. 224).

Solution 5: Mayer's haemalum (see p. 223).

Solution 6: 1% HCl in 70% ethyl alcohol.

Solution 7: 2% Orange G in 5% phosphotungstic acid.

Procedure

1. De-wax and hydrate.
2. Oxidize in solution 1.
3. Wash in distilled water.
4. Transfer to Schiff's reagent (solution 2) for 20 min.
5. Rinse quickly in 3 changes of reducing bath (solution 3).
6. Wash in water for 10 min.
7. Stain in celestin blue (solution 4) for 1–3 min and rinse in water.
8. Stain in Mayer's haemalum (solution 5) for 1–3 min and wash in tap water.
9. Differentiate rapidly in solution 6.
10. Wash in running tap water for 5 min.
11. Stain in solution 7 for 10–20 s.
12. Differentiate in water until a yellow tinge is just visible, usually 1 min.
13. Dehydrate, clear and mount in DPX.

Results

Cell nuclei, blue-black; beta cell granules, red; alpha cell granules and other acidophilic substances, varying shades of yellow.

Alcian blue–periodic acid Schiff method

For the demonstration of acidic groups and 1,2-glycols of carbohydrates.

Solution 1: Alcian blue 8GX (CI No. 74240), 1% in 3% acetic acid.

Solution 2: Periodic acid, 1% aqueous solution.

Solution 3: Schiff's reagent (see p. 229).

Procedure

1. De-wax and hydrate
2. Stain with solution 1 for 5 min.
3. Wash in running tap water for 2 min.
4. Rinse in distilled water.
5. Oxidize in solution 2 for 2 min.
6. Wash in running tap water for 5 min.
7. Rinse in distilled water.
8. Treat with solution 3 for 8 min.
9. Wash in running tap water for 10 min.
10. Dehydrate, clear and mount.

Results

Acid mucins, blue; neutral mucins, magenta; mixtures of acid and neutral mucins, purple.

■ Note

Cell nuclei may be stained with Cole's haematoxylin (see p. 224) after step 9 if desired.

Alcian blue–chlorantine fast red

For the demonstration of mucin and connective tissue.

Solution 1: Ehrlich's haematoxylin (see p. 223).

Solution 2:

Alcian blue 8GX (CI No. 74240)	0.5 g
Distilled water	100 ml
Acetic acid, glacial	0.5 ml
Thymol, as preservative	10–20 mg

Dissolve the alcian blue in 50 ml of the distilled water and add the acetic acid to the remainder. Combine the two solutions, filter and add the thymol. Record date and label.

Solution 3:
Phosphomolybdic acid, 1% aqueous solution.

Solution 4:

Chlorantine fast red 5B (CI No. 28160)	0.5 g
Distilled water	100 ml

Procedure

1. De-wax and hydrate.
2. Stain with solution 1 for 10–15 min.
3. Blue in tap water.
4. Stain with solution 2 for 10 min.
5. Rinse in distilled water.
6. Mordant in solution 3 for 10 min.
7. Rinse in distilled water.
8. Stain with solution 4 for 10–15 min.
9. Rinse in distilled water.
10. Dehydrate, clear and mount.

Results

Cell nuclei, purplish-blue; mucin, ground substance of cartilage, certain connective tissue fibres and mast cell granules, bluish-green; cell cytoplasm and muscle fibres, pale yellow; collagen fibres, red.

Gram's stain (after Hucker and Conn) for bacteria

Ammonium oxalate–crystal violet solution

Solution 1:

Crystal violet (CI No. 42555), 10% alcoholic solution	2 ml

Distilled water	18 ml
Ammonium oxalate, 1% aqueous solution	80 ml

Dissolve the potassium iodide in the distilled water and then add the iodine. Record date and label.

Gram's iodine

Solution 2:

Potassium iodide	2 g
Iodine	1 g
Distilled water	100 ml

Decolorizer

Solution 3: Ethyl alcohol, 95%

Counterstain

Solution 4:

1% neutral red (CI No. 50040)	15 parts
Carbol fuchsin (see below)	1 part

Procedure

1. De-wax and hydrate.
2. Apply solution 1 for 1 min.
3. Rinse with water.
4. Apply solution 2 for 1 min.
5. Rinse with water.
6. Apply several changes of solution 3 until no more colour appears to flow from the preparation.
7. Wash with water.
8. Apply solution 4 for 10 s.
9. Dehydrate, clear and mount.

Results

Gram-positive organisms, blue-black; Gram-negative organisms, red.

Ziehl–Neelsen's stain for the staining of acid-fast bacteria

Solution 1: Ziehl–Neelsen carbol fuchsin:

Basic fuchsin (CI No. 42510)	1 g
Absolute ethyl alcohol	10 ml
5% phenol in distilled water	100 ml

Dissolve the basic fuchsin in the ethyl alcohol. Combine with the phenol solution, record date and label.

Solution 2: Acid–alcohol, 1% (see p. 223).

Solution 3: Methylene blue, 0.2% aqueous solution.

Procedure

1. De-wax and hydrate.
2. Flood the slide with solution 1. Heat by flaming until stain rises and reheat at intervals. Stain for 10–15 min.
3. Wash with running tap water.
4. Differentiate with solution 2 until only the red blood corpuscles retain the stain when examined under the staining microscope with the 10× objective.
5. Wash with running tap water for a minimum of 10 min.
6. Counterstain with solution 3 for 2 min.
7. Wash with running tap water.
8. Dehydrate rapidly, clear and mount in neutral balsam or DPX.

■ Note

Although the classical method, the practice of flaming slides is no longer approved under the Health and Safety at Work regulations.

Results

Acid-fast bacilli, red; cell nuclei, blue; red blood corpuscles, pink.

Carbol–fuchsin–tergitol method

Solution 1: Kinyoun's carbol fuchsin:

Basic fuchsin (CI No. 42510)	40 g
Phenol, cryst.	80 g
Ethyl alcohol, absolute	200 ml
Distilled water	1000 ml

Dissolve the basic fuchsin in the alcohol and the phenol in the distilled water. Combine the two solutions, mix and allow to remain at room temperature overnight. Filter through wet paper and label.

Solution 2: Tergitol 7.

Solution 3: Acid–alcohol (see p. 223).

Solution 4: Methylene blue (CI No. 52015), 3% aqueous solution.

Procedure

1. De-wax and hydrate.
2. Flood the slide with solution 1.
3. Add one drop of solution 2 to the slide and stain for 1 min at room temperature.
4. Wash in water.
5. Differentiate in solution 3 for 10–15 s until the tissue appears clear.
6. Counterstain with solution 4 for 1 min.
7. Wash in water.
8. Dehydrate in 95% alcohol and acetone.
9. Clear in xylene and mount in balsam.

Results

Acid-fast organisms, bright red; background, blue.

■ Notes

1. Tergitol, wetting agent 7, is a 25% aqueous solution of the sodium sulphate derivative of 3,9-diethyltridecanol-6 obtainable from B.D.H. plc.
2. Solution 4 is a saturated solution and should be filtered before use. Any methylene blue solution will suffice, provided it does not contain potassium hydroxide, as this gives a blurred counterstain.

Methenamine–silver nitrate method for fungi

For the demonstration of fungi in sections.

Stock methenamine–silver nitrate solution

Stock solution:

Silver nitrate, 5% aqueous solution	5 ml
Hexamethylene-tetramine (Hexamine), 3% aqueous solution	100 ml

Add the silver nitrate to the methenamine solution. A white precipitate forms which dissolves on shaking. Record date and label. The solution remains stable for several months if stored at 4°C.

Solution 1: Chromic acid, CrO_3, 5% aqueous solution.

Solution 2: Sodium bisulphite, 1% aqueous solution.

Solution 3:

Borax, 5% aqueous solution	2 ml
Distilled water	25 ml
Stock solution (see above)	25 ml

Dissolve the borax in the distilled water and add the methenamine–silver nitrate stock solution. The solution should be prepared as required.

Solution 4: Gold chloride, yellow, 0.1% aqueous solution.

Solution 5: Sodium thiosulphate, 2% aqueous solution.

Solution 6:

Light green, 0.2% aqueous solution	10 ml
Distilled water	50 ml
Acetic acid, glacial	0.1 ml

Procedure

1. Bring sections and a control slide to water.
2. Oxidize in solution 1 for 60 min.
3. Wash in running tap water.
4. Transfer to solution 2 for 1 min to remove residual chromic acid.
5. Wash in tap water for 5–10 min.
6. Rinse in several changes of distilled water.
7. Impregnate with solution 3 for 30–60 min at 58°C. Examine the control slide under the microscope to check for adequate impregnation.
8. Rinse in several changes of distilled water.
9. Tone in solution 4 for 2–5 min.
10. Rinse in distilled water.
11. Fix in solution 5 for 2–5 min.
12. Wash thoroughly in tap water.
13. Stain with solution 6 for 30–45 s.
14. Dehydrate, clear and mount.

Results

Fungi, sharply outlined in black; inner parts of hyphae and mycelia, reddish; background, pale green.

Perls' method for ferric iron

For the demonstration of ferric salts in tissue.

Solution 1:

Potassium ferrocyanide, 2% aqueous solution	1 vol
Hydrochloric acid, 2% aqueous solution	1 vol

Solution 2: Neutral red (CI No. 50040), 1% aqueous solution.

Procedure

1. De-wax and hydrate.
2. Transfer to freshly prepared solution 1 for 30–60 min.
3. Wash in distilled water.
4. Stain with solution 2 for 3 min.
5. Wash in distilled water.
6. Dehydrate, clear and mount.

Results

Cell nuclei, red; ferric iron, blue.

Von Kóssa's method for calcium

For the demonstration of calcium.

Solution 1:

Silver nitrate	5 g
Glass distilled water	100 ml

Dissolve the silver nitrate in the distilled water. Store in a brown reagent bottle and label.

Solution 2: Sodium thiosulphate, 5% aqueous solution.

Solution 3: Kirkpatrick's carmalum.

■ Notes

1. Solution 1 should be colourless. If tinged with blue it must be discarded. The distilled water must be iron free.

2. Fixatives containing an acid or potassium dichromate should be avoided.

Procedure

1. De-wax and hydrate.
2. Immerse in solution 1 for 5 min or longer, exposing to bright daylight.
3. Wash in distilled water.
4. Fix in solution 2 for 5 min.
5. Wash in distilled water.
6. Stain with solution 3 for 3–5 min.
7. Dehydrate, clear and mount.

Results

Calcium phosphate and carbonate, black; cell nuclei, red.

Oil red O in isopropanol (Lillie and Ashburn)

For the demonstration of neutral fats.

Stock solution:
Oil red O (CI No. 26125)	0.5 g
Isopropyl alcohol, 99% (isopropanol)	100 ml

Solution 1:
Stock solution	6 vol
Distilled water	4 vol

Dilute the stock solution with the distilled water. Allow the diluted stain to stand for 10 min and filter through a Whatman's No. 2 filter paper. The filtrate will remain stable for several hours.

Solution 2: Mayer's acid–alum–haematoxylin (see p. 223).

Procedure

1. Stain formalin-fixed frozen sections in solution 1 for 10 min.
2. Wash in distilled water.
3. Stain lightly in solution 2 for 1–2 min.
4. Blue in tap water.
5. Float out onto a slide.
6. Mount in glycerine jelly.

Results

Lipids, red; cell nuclei, blue.

■ Note

Sudan black B (CI No. 26150) may be substituted for oil red O.

Propylene glycol sudan method (Chiffelle and Putt)

For the demonstration of neutral fats

Solution 1:
Sudan IV (CI No. 26105)	0.7 g
Propylene glycol	100 ml

Dissolve the sudan IV in the propylene glycol by heating to 100°C for a few minutes. Filter the solution while still hot through a Whatman's No. 2 filter paper. Cool the filtrate and refilter through glass wool or a coarse sintered glass funnel using negative pressure. Record date and label.

Solution 2: Propylene glycol, 85%.

Solution 3: Mayer's acid–alum–haematoxylin (see p. 223).

Procedure

1. Wash formalin-fixed frozen sections in several changes of distilled water.
2. Dehydrate in pure propylene glycol for 3–5 min.
3. Stain with solution 1 for 5–7 min, periodically agitating the sections.
4. Differentiate in solution 2 for 2–3 min.
5. Wash in distilled water.
6. Counterstain lightly in solution 3 for 1–2 min.
7. Wash in distilled water.
8. Blue in tap water.
9. Float onto a slide.
10. Mount in glycerine jelly.

Results

Neutral fats, myelin, mitochondria and other lipids, orange-red; cell nuclei, blue.

19

Cytological techniques

Exfoliative cytology entails the microscopical examination and interpretation of cells which are shed (exfoliated) spontaneously from epithelial surfaces of the body, or which may be removed from such surfaces or membranes by physical means.

Spontaneous exfoliation is a characteristic of normal epithelial surfaces which, because of constant growth, continue to shed cells from their superficial layers as they become replaced by new cells, but cells of malignant tumours exfoliate more readily than those from normal tissue even though the lesion may be so small as to escape clinical detection.

The diagnosis of cancer from smear preparations has been carried out in pathology laboratories for many years, but considerable impetus was given to diagnostic cytology by the work of Papanicolaou and the introduction of his colourful staining procedures, which led to a greater knowledge of cell morphology and its alteration in disease. Papanicolaou employed alcoholic fixing and staining solutions, thus giving increased transparency to stained preparations and allowing overlapping cells to be more readily seen and identified.

Exfoliated cells can be found in smears taken directly from epithelial membranes or certain accessible cavities of the body where they may accumulate, for example vagina, buccal mucosa; or from a variety of body fluids and effusions including sputum, urine, pleural fluid and gastric juice.

All fluids, urines, washings and sputa should be regarded as potentially hazardous and, for this reason, the employment of safety cabinets is essential. Smears and pulps should be stored in the safety cabinet until fixed. Staff should wear protective clothing, and disposable tubes, containers and similar vessels should be placed in a sterilizing solution prior to being discarded.

Cytology has become an established aid for the diagnosis of malignancy in various organs, particularly those of the respiratory, urinary and female genital tracts. The collection of material for vaginal cytology for example is readily available with minimal discomfort to the patient; this offers a relatively simple means of 'screening' for the detection of asymptomatic cancer in women.

Assessment of hormone activity in the female, which is of value in some cases of sterility and certain endocrine disorders, also can be established from vaginal smear study.

It has been found that the majority of nuclei belonging to the female sex show a conglomeration of chromatin which is thought to represent the X–X chromosome; this observation is used to determine genetic sex. Scrapings from the oral (buccal) mucosa provide suitable material for this purpose.

Unlike histopathology, in which diagnosis of malignancy is formed often on the general behaviour and arrangement of cell aggregates, cytological diagnosis is based on the appearances of individual cells or small groups of cells. Most of the information in this respect is obtained from study of the nuclei, whereas the cytoplasm may assist to identify cell type. Nuclear abnormalities associated with cancer include the following:

1. Nuclear enlargement without an increase in the overall size of cell, giving a decreased cytoplasm/nucleus ratio.
2. Irregularity of nuclear outline, and variation in size and shape.
3. Hyperchromasia. Due to increased amounts of deoxyribonucleic acid (DNA), the nuclei of malignant cells often stain more deeply with basic dyes.

4. Multinucleation, resulting from abnormal cell division.
5. Uneven distribution and variation in size of chromatin particles.
6. Increase in size and number of nucleoli.

Fixation

To prevent cellular distortion it is essential that all smear preparations for cytological study be fixed immediately before drying of the material occurs.

The fixative should be capable of penetrating rapidly, with good preservation of cell morphology. The fixing fluid advocated by Papanicolaou, consisting of equal volumes of ether and 95% ethyl alcohol, is commonly used, but a mixture containing tertiary butyl alcohol, 3 vol; 95% ethyl alcohol, 1 vol, is equally effective and does not evaporate so readily. Smears should remain in fixative for a minimum of 15 min prior to staining, although prolonged fixation of several days or weeks is not harmful. The fixative supplied by the Department of Health and Social Security, free of charge, has been used successfully for the fixation of all types of cytological smears. It requires dilution with 95% alcohol before use.

A useful container and carrier for smear fixatives is the polythene screw-capped Coplin jar grooved to take up to 10 slides. It is suitable for the transportation of smears from wards and clinics to the laboratory, but it should not be used for postal transmission because of the inflammable nature of the contained fixing fluids.

Smears which require to be sent by post to a cytology laboratory may be air-dried after fixation is complete and placed in suitable wooden, cardboard or plastic slide mailers. Alternatively, aerosol sprays are obtainable which offer an effective and convenient form of fixation and, with certain exceptions, are relatively cheap. They consist usually of polyethylene glycols, isopropyl alcohol and propellants. The alcohol fixes the smear and the wax sets to form a water-soluble protective coating. Some workers advise coating prefixed smears with glycerin or water-soluble wax before mailing; alternatively, they may be fixed and despatched in jars containing a non-combustible glycol fixing mixture.

On collection, each slide should be clearly marked with the patient's name or number; this is a simple matter if the smears are made on slides having a frosted patch at one end. The relevant information is written on the patch with a graphite pencil and this will survive normal handling of the slide throughout fixation and subsequent staining.

Preparation of smears

The successful evaluation of cytological material depends, to a great extent, on the technical quality of the preparations. The material often contains only scanty diagnostic evidence, and this may be unrecognizable at screening unless care is taken during the preparation of smears. The smears must be spread evenly, and be free from lumps. Areas containing unresolved lumps cannot be stained accurately and are usually too thick for critical microscopical study.

It is desirable that smears are made and fixed by a member of the cytology laboratory staff in order to obtain some uniformity of spread, and specimens such as sputum, bronchial aspirations, urine, pleural and abdominal fluids should be dealt with invariably by laboratory personnel.

Smears from the vagina, cervix, breast, etc., are prepared at the side of the patient and sent to the laboratory in containers of fixative, a supply of which should be maintained regularly in participating clinics and wards. Alternatively, they should be fixed with a wax base fixative (see p. 184) and sent to the laboratory in a slide box.

Vaginal smears

Material is usually obtained by aspiration of the posterior vaginal fornix with a stout-walled, slightly curved, glass pipette fitted with a rubber bulb (*Figure 19.1*). The aspirate should be spread rapidly and evenly onto prelabelled clean glass slides which are put without delay into a jar of fixative before drying occurs. Smears prepared by this method may contain not only vaginal cells but also cells exfoliated from other parts of the genital tract, for example endometrium and cervix. Another method, whereby material is gently scraped from the lateral

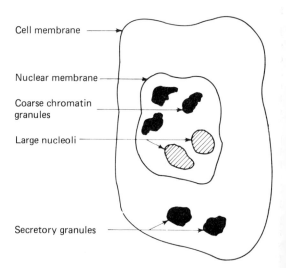

Figure 19.1. Diagrammatic representation of a malignant cell. Compare with *Figure 12.1*. Note the enlarged nucleus with consequent alteration of nucleus/cytoplasm ratio

wall of the vagina with a wooden spatula, is reliable only for hormonal studies.

Cervical smears

To assist in the collection of material for this type of smear the clinician employs an instrument known as a speculum. The appliance is inserted into the vagina and allows the uterine cervix to be directly observed. A spatula or cotton-wool tipped applicator is introduced via the speculum and the cervical surfaces are gently swabbed or scraped. The Ayre spatula (*Figure 19.2*), made of wood or plastic

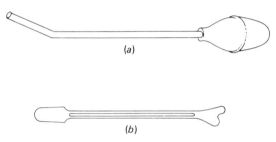

(a)

(b)

Figure 19.2. (a) Bulb and pipette for aspiration of posterior fornix; (b) Ayre spatula

material, is specially designed for this purpose, one end being shaped to fit the contours of the cervix. On withdrawal, the material contained on the swab or spatula is spread onto clean slides and fixed immediately.

Sputum smears

Early morning specimens are recommended and should be produced by a deep cough. Several consecutive daily samples are advised ranging from 3 to 9 days. Suitable materials on subsequent microscopical examination should contain histiocytes and if these are not present the specimen may be discarded.

The sputum is poured from its container into a petri dish and examined microscopically against a black and white background for the presence of blood-flecked or white solid particles. If present, portions of these areas are removed and spread on a slide with a wire loop or spatula, the solid particles being crushed by means of a second slide. If no particles are found, smears should be made so as to include several representative portions of the specimen. The ideal smear should be somewhat thicker than one prepared for tubercle bacilli examination and should show a variation of thickness along its length. The prepared slides are transferred directly to fixative for 15 min.

Smears from urine, pleural and ascitic fluids and gastric washings

It is of the utmost importance that smears from fluid specimens are prepared and fixed as soon as possible after collection, otherwise much cellular detail will be lost. Cells of gastric fluids in particular undergo rapid degeneration and digestion at room temperature. Refrigeration will arrest these destructive processes for a short time only.

On receipt, the specimens are placed in 50 ml tubes, carefully balanced, and centrifuged at 2000 rpm for 20 min. The supernatant fluid is decanted and the sediment spread evenly onto slides with a wire loop. The prepared slides are placed immediately in fixative in the same manner as other smears.

Sediments of fluids containing little or no protein, for example urine and gastric washings, tend to wash off the slides during fixation and staining. Adhesion of these sediments is improved if the slides are lightly coated with Mayer's albumin before spreading.

It must be remembered that many of the specimens sent for cytological investigation may be infected. Aseptic precautions should be observed during the handling of *all* specimens received for cytology, and specimens, glassware and other materials used in the preparation of smears must be autoclaved or placed in antiseptic solution before cleaning or discarding.

Membrane filters

Cellulose acetate membrane filters of graded pore size are useful for the concentration of cells from most body fluids. They are particularly useful where only a few cells are present because the total cellular content of a fluid may be collected onto a single membrane. A variety of pore sizes are available, the most useful being one with a mean flow pore size of 5 µm.

The specimen is filtered through a membrane attached to a special funnel-type holder using controlled negative pressure. Immediately following filtration the cells are fixed by placing the membrane in 96% alcohol. It is then clipped to a slide, stained by the Papanicolaou method, dehydrated and cleared. After clearing, the membrane filter pad may be cut into several strips and mounted onto microscope slides for examination. Special mounting media may be required for certain types of membrane filters.

Fixation of cells in fluid specimens may be carried out by adding an equal volume of formol saline prior to filtration, but generally the cells adhere to the membrane more readily and securely if fixation follows filtration.

Cytological staining techniques

Papanicolaou method

The Papanicolaou method is designed to give sharp nuclear staining, transparency of cytoplasm and good differential colouring of acidophilic and basophilic cells.

Where large numbers of slides are stained by the Papanicolaou method, the use of an automatic staining machine is recommended for convenience and uniformity. Schedules will vary according to individual requirements, but that given below provides satisfactory results.

The solutions required are Harris's alum–haematoxylin, Orange G (OG 6), and a triple-dye mixture designated EA 36 or EA 50. All these solutions may be purchased commercially and give consistently good results. The formulae are as follows:

Harris alum–haematoxylin (see p. 224)

Orange G solution (OG 6)

0.5% Orange G (CI No. 16230) in 95% alcohol	100 ml
dodeca-Tungstophosphoric acid	0.015 g

EA 36 or EA 50

0.5% light green SF (yellowish) (CI No. 42095) in 95% alcohol	45 ml
0.5% Bismarck brown Y (CI No. 21000) in 95% alcohol	10 ml
0.5% Eosin (CI No. 45380) in 95% alcohol	45 ml
Phosphotungstic acid	0.2 g
Saturated aqueous lithium carbonate	1 drop

Mix well and store in tightly capped, brown bottles. A variation known as EA 65, requiring 0.25% light green, is recommended for sputum staining.

Procedure for manual staining

1. Remove smears from fixative and rinse in descending grades of alcohol (80, 70, 50%), for 8–10 s each.
2. Stain in Harris alum–haematoxylin for 4 min.
3. Wash in tap water for 1–2 min.
4. Differentiate in 0.5% hydrochloric acid until only the nuclei are stained.
5. Wash and 'blue' in tap water for 3–5 min.
6. Transfer to 70% alcohol followed by two changes of 90% alcohol for a few seconds each.
7. Stain in OG 6 for 2 min.
8. Rinse in three changes of 95% alcohol.
9. Stain in EA solution for 2–4 min.
10. Rinse in three changes of 95% alcohol.
11. Complete dehydration in absolute alcohol and clear in xylene.
12. Mount in DPX.

Results

Nuclei	Blue
Acidophilic cells	Red
Basophilic cells	Blue-green
Erythrocytes	Orange-red

Procedure for automatic staining

Prepare and fix smears.

Trough	Reagent	Timing
1	70% alcohol	1 min
2	50% alcohol	1 min
3	Distilled water	2 min
4	Harris alum–haematoxylin	4 min
5	Distilled water	1 min
6	Tap water	1 min
7	0.5% HCl in 70% ethanol	30 sec
8	Tap water	1 min
9	Tap water	1 min
10	70% alcohol	1 min
11	70% alcohol	1 min
12	95% alcohol	1 min
13	95% alcohol	1 min
14	OG 6	2 min
15	95% alcohol	30 sec
16	95% alcohol	30 sec
17	EA 36 or EA 65	3 min
18	95% alcohol	1 min
19	95% alcohol	1 min
20	Absolute alcohol	1 min
21	Absolute alcohol	2 min
22	Xylene	1 min
23	Xylene	2 min

Remove from machine and mount in DPX

Results

Nuclei	Blue
Acidophilic cells	Red
Basophilic cells	Blue-green
Erythrocytes	Orange-red

Hormone assessment

Vaginal smears stained by the Papanicolaou technique may be used for the evaluation of hormonal (oestrogen) activity. Two of the methods commonly employed are the karyopyknotic index (KPI) and the more accurate maturation index (MI). The KPI is calculated by the counting of at least 200 squamous cells and expressing as a percentage those that exhibit condensed, deeply stained, structureless (pyknotic) nuclei, with pink- or red-stained cytoplasmas. These are the superficial cornified squamous epithelial cells. Smears should be taken regularly, e.g. every 3 days, throughout the menstrual cycle, thereby obtaining a simple but useful assessment of oestrogenic influence. The maturation index is an extension of the above method and requires a differential count of at least 200 squamous cells. The degree of cell maturation is determined by means of their morphology and staining reactions and classified as being of superficial intermediate or parabasal type. The result is expressed as a percentage. High or low oestrogenic activity is indicated by the preponderance of superficial or parabasal cells, respectively.

Additional methods

Following fixation in ether–alcohol, smears may be treated as blood-films and stained by any of the Romanowsky stains (see p. 317), or they may be brought to water via descending grades of alcohol and stained with haematoxylin and eosin as for sections (see p. 218). Good results are obtained by these methods, although they lack the transparency of cytoplasm that can be seen in Papanicolaou preparations.

Schaudinn's fluid (see p. 184) is often used as the fixative for smears prior to staining with haematoxylin and eosin.

Shorr staining method

Suitable for hormonal studies in vaginal smears. The method requires a single differential staining mixture.

Staining solution

50% ethyl alcohol	100 ml
Biebrich scarlet (CI No. 26905), water-soluble	0.5 g
Orange G (CI No. 16230)	0.25 g
Fast green FCF (CI No. 42053)	0.075 g
dodeca-Tungstophosphoric acid	0.5 g
dodeca-Molybdophosphoric acid	0.5 g
Glacial acetic acid	1 ml

Procedure

1. Fix smears while moist in equal parts of ether and alcohol. 1–2 min is adequate.
2. Stain for 1–2 min in Shorr's stain.
3. Rinse in 70% alcohol to remove excess stain.

4. Transfer to 95% alcohol, followed by absolute alcohol for a few seconds each.
5. Clear in xylene and mount in DPX.

Results

Nuclei	Red
Superficial cornified cells	Brilliant orange-red
Non-cornified cells	Green-blue

Methylene blue

A single-stain rapid method may be employed in the cytological examination of fresh sputum for malignant cells.

Staining solution

Methylene blue	1 g
Distilled water	100 ml

Procedure

Purulent or blood-flecked particles are selected from the sputum with a wire loop. These are transferred to a clean slide and mixed thoroughly with one drop of the stain. The stained mixture is then covered with a large coverslip and spread by gentle pressure. The prepared slide can be examined immediately.

The preparations are not permanent and any suspicious areas detected on microscopical examination should be recorded photographically. Alternatively, the coverslip may be removed and the smear placed in ether–alcohol to fix. It can then be stained with haemotoxylin and eosin for confirmation.

Fluorescence methods have been applied to the differentiation of malignant cells from benign cells. These are based on the principle that certain substances emit visible light when excited by ultraviolet or blue light, usually of 350–400 nm wavelength.

The fluorescent dye acridine orange is capable of combination with both deoxyribonucleic acid (DNA) and ribonucleic acid (RNA). When excited by ultraviolet light, the DNA emits a green or greenish-yellow fluorescence and the RNA an orange-red fluorescence. Malignant cells have an increased RNA content in their cytoplasm and will appear brilliant red.

Techniques based on this knowledge, and which permit the rapid scanning of smear preparations, have been devised. One such technique is as follows:

Acridine orange technique (Bertalanffy)

Solutions required:

1. *0.067M Potassium dihydrogen orthophosphate.* Dissolve 9.072 g potassium dihydrogen

orthophosphate (KH$_2$PO$_4$) in 1000 ml distilled water.

2. *0.067M Disodium hydrogen orthophosphate.* Dissolve 9.465 g disodium hydrogen orthophosphate anhydrous (Na$_2$HPO$_4$) in 1000 ml distilled water).

Phosphate buffer (pH 6): 87.8 ml of solution 1 are mixed with 12.2 ml of solution 2.

Acridine orange stock solution

Acridine orange (CI No. 46005)	0.1 g
Distilled water	100 ml

Dissolve and store in a dark bottle in a refrigerator.

Acridine orange staining solution

Acridine orange stock solution	10 ml
Phosphate buffer (pH 6)	90 ml

0.1M Calcium chloride differentiator

Calcium chloride (CaCl$_2$)	11.099 g
Distilled water	1000 ml

Procedure

1. Fix smears in ether/alcohol (1:1) mixture for 15 min.
2. Hydrate in descending grades of alcohol (80, 70 and 50%) and distilled water.
3. Rinse rapidly in 1% acetic acid and wash in distilled water.
4. Stain with acridine orange staining solution for 3 min.
5. Wash with phosphate buffer for 1 min.
6. Differentiate with 0.1M calcium chloride solution until nuclei are clearly defined.
7. Wash thoroughly with phosphate buffer.
8. Mount with a coverslip using phosphate buffer as the mountant and examine by fluorescent microscopy.

It should be noted that orange-red fluorescence is not specific for malignant cells. Certain normal cells, micro-organisms and trichomonads also exhibit varying degrees of red or orange-red fluorescence. The examiner must be experienced, therefore, in the identification of cells and cell structures.

Sex chromatin (Barr bodies)

Twenty to thirty per cent of cells from the female show a mass of chromatin beneath the nuclear membrane which is not evident in the male. Material for examination is most conveniently obtained from scrapings of the buccal mucosa where Barr bodies are usually seen attached to the membrane of the interphase nuclei of epithelial cells. The 'drumstick' form attached to the lobed nuclei of polymorphs in blood films has the same significance.

A method for the demonstration of sex chromatin in buccal smears and which requires no differentiation is both simple and effective.

Staining solution

Cresyl fast violet acetate	1.0 g
Distilled water	100 ml

Procedure

1. Fix smears before drying occurs in 95% alcohol for 30 min.
2. Transfer to 50% alcohol for a few seconds and then to distilled water.
3. Stain with Cresyl fast violet acetate solution for 5 min.
4. Rinse quickly in tap water.
5. Dehydrate with 95% alcohol followed by absolute alcohol.
6. Clear in two changes of xylene and mount in DPX.

Section 4

Microbiology

20

Introduction to microbiology

Historical survey

In 1675 Antony van Leeuwenhoek (1632–1723), a draper living in Delft, Holland, described 'little animals' he found when examining stagnant rainwater under his home-made microscope. The making of lenses was a hobby, yet the scrupulous way in which he recorded and illustrated his experiments would have done credit to any present-day scientist. Many of the first 'animalcules', as he called them, were protozoa, but later experiments yielded the first recorded account of micro-organisms.

After his death, very little progress was made in determining the relation between bacteria and disease, until towards the end of the eighteenth century. It was then that Dr Edward Jenner (1749–1825) substantiated the belief that cowpox gave protection to people against smallpox. He introduced the term vaccine (from the Latin *vacca*—cow) and established the idea of immunity.

The quality of microscopes was rapidly improving and many more micro-organisms were being discovered, but it was still not generally accepted that they were the cause of disease.

Barri in 1836 helped to establish that micro-organisms could cause disease when, using a heat-sterilized pin, he transmitted a disease from a silkworm infected with a fungus to a healthy silkworm.

Even after evidence such as this, the real science of bacteriology did not begin until the middle of the nineteenth century.

Much credit must be given to Louis Pasteur (1822–1895), a French chemist. It was through his work on the sterilization of liquids that today we have the autoclave. His work on fermentation proved that the breakdown of sugar to alcohol was the result of the activity of micro-organisms. He learned how to isolate and cultivate bacteria and how to study their effect on animals. In 1878 he read a paper on the germ theory of disease which helped to establish that specific organisms can give rise to specific diseases.

During Pasteur's imaginative studies, Robert Koch (1843–1910) was making enormous contributions to bacteriology in a practical way.

He developed methods of fixing and staining bacteria using aniline dyes, he discovered the tubercle bacillus, he isolated the anthrax bacillus in pure culture, he discovered the cause of cholera, and in 1881 he published a method of producing pure cultures of bacteria by growing them on the surface of a solid medium. The medium he devised was a meat infusion broth solidified with gelatin, and poured onto a glass plate. This was the beginning of our present-day culture media. Agar soon superseded gelatin and later Petri introduced his masterpiece—the petri dish.

Many others, such as Lister, with his introduction of antiseptic and aseptic techniques, contributed to the vast amount of knowledge which has developed into the science of bacteriology. Today, with our ever-increasing knowledge of bacteria, fungi and yeasts, rickettsia, viruses and protozoa, the more appropriate term microbiology (from the Greek *micros*—small, *bios*—life) has come into general use.

A classification of micro-organisms

Although we are mainly concerned with bacteria, described on p. 244, a brief description of other micro-organisms will be helpful. The size of bacteria is measured by the use of a graduated eyepiece calibrated by a micrometre slide, and the unit of measurement is the *micro*metre, written μm. The micrometre is 1/1000 of a millimetre (0.001 mm). Viruses, being smaller than bacteria, are generally measured in millimicrometres (1/1000 of a micrometre, or 0.001 μm or 1.0 mμm), now correctly called *nano*metres (nm).

Protozoa

These are small, single-cell animals belonging to the lowest division of the animal kingdom. They consist of protoplasm, which is differentiated into nucleus and cytoplasm, and they are non-photosynthetic. There are four classes of protozoa:

1. Class I, RHIZOPODA, move by means of protoplasmic projections called pseudopodia. *Entamoeba histolytica*, which causes amoebic dysentery, is an example.
2. Class II, MASTIGOPHORA, move by means of undulating membranes or flagella. *Trichomonas vaginalis*, which causes a vaginal discharge, is a member of this class.
3. Class III, CILIATA, move by the beating of numbers of cilia; one member is *Balantidium coli*, which causes balantidial dysentery, a condition similar to amoebic dysentery.
4. Class IV, SPOROZOA, are non-motile organisms that live parasitically within the cells of the host animals; *Plasmodium vivax*, the causal organism of malaria, belongs to this class.

Many protozoa when placed under unfavourable conditions pass into a resting phase, often with the formation of a distinctive cyst which can be used in identification.

Fungi

Like protozoa, fungi are non-photosynthetic organisms. They grow either as single cells, e.g. yeasts, or as colonies of multicellular filaments (hyphae), i.e. moulds. They reproduce by means of spores and the recognition of these spores is often an aid to identification. Some species cause disease in man and animals. For example, *Candida albicans*, a type of yeast, causes thrush, and *Microsporum canis*, a mould, causes ringworm.

Viruses, rickettsiae and chlamydia

These are minute organisms ranging in size from 20 to 300 nm. They are obligate intracellular parasites which can only multiply with the aid of living cells.

Viruses consist in their simplest form of an outer coat of protein and an inner core of nucleic acid which may be either ribonucleic acid (RNA) or deoxyribonucleic acid (DNA) (no virus has been shown to contain both).

Rickettsiae are small micro-organisms which are in some ways intermediate between viruses and bacteria. They are similar to bacteria in that they contain both RNA and DNA, possess metabolic enzymes and reproduce by binary fission; they resemble viruses by being able to multiply only within living cells.

Chlamydia are related to bacteria in the fact that they have both DNA and RNA and possess muramic acid in their cell walls. They are, however, intracellular parasites, about twice the size of rickettsiae, and unlike rickettsiae are sensitive to interferon.

Bacterial morphology

Bacteria are microscopic unicellular organisms which can be classified into the following types of cell: the ovoid or spheroid, called *coccus*; the rod or cylindrical *bacillus*; the curved *vibrio*, the spiral-shaped *spirillum* and coil-shaped *spirochaetes*.

The *coccus* (plural cocci): size 0.5–1.0 μm in diameter. Cocci generally have one axis approximately equal to any other axis. Sometimes the cell is flattened (giving rise to a kidney-shaped cell) or distorted in some way as to depart from the spherical shape, e.g. in streptococci (see below).

If, after binary fission, the daughter cell remains attached to the parent cell, but separates before fission occurs again, these pairs of cocci are called *diplococci*. If fission continues while they remain attached, forming chains, they are termed *streptococci*, but if the division is not in one plane and random clumps of cocci occur, they are called *staphylococci*. Sometimes the cocci remain in pairs for one further division and a regular aggregate of four cocci is formed—these are called *tetracocci*, and if remaining for one further division at right angles to the former, thereby giving rise to a cubical packet of eight cocci, they are called *sarcinae* (Latin = packets).

The terms *Staphylococcus*, *Streptococcus* and *Sarcina* are used as generic names (note the capital initials).

The *bacillus* (plural bacilli): size 1–10 μm in length, 0.3–1.0 μm in width. The bacilli or rods do not form as many groupings as the cocci, only forming *diplobacilli* or *streptobacilli* (pairs and chains). After fission, some rods form certain positions—the daughter cell, for example, remains attached to the parent cell, but swings away at varying angles, giving the appearance of Chinese lettering: a formation characteristic of the genus *Corynebacterium*. Sometimes a cuneiform bundle is the characteristic form, e.g. *Mycobacterium*.

Some bacteria, under unfavourable conditions, undergo changes resulting in the formation of intracellular spores. There is a localized concentration of nuclear material in the cell, with the subsequent development of a membrane around it. This is the resting stage of the bacillus, and germination does not take place until more favourable conditions arise. The mature membrane has a high resistance to ordinary staining, sunlight and heat. The spore often retains its capacity to germinate (generally the enlargement of the spore into the bacillary form with subsequent shedding of the spore membrane) for many years.

The situation of the spore is an aid in the morphological diagnosis of the organism. Some occur at one end of the bacillus, with or without distension of the cell, others in the centre or towards one end.

The *spirillum* (plural spirilla): size variable— approximately $4 \times 0.2\,\mu m$. Spirilla are rigid rods with helical (corkscrew) shape. They are motile by means of a tuft of flagella and are generally Gram-negative.

The *vibrio* (plural vibrios): size $4 \times 0.5\,\mu m$. Vibrios are short, curved, rigid rods shaped rather like a comma. They are motile usually by means of a single flagellum and are generally Gram-negative.

Spirochaetes are also motile, and possess an axial fibre around which the body is twisted in a helical manner. Their length is usually $10-20\,\mu m$ and thickness $0.2-0.4\,\mu m$. The number of spirals varies with the species. They are not easily stained with aniline dyes, and for the best results the silver impregnation methods (e.g. Levaditi) are used.

Bacterial structure

Figure 20.1 shows a diagrammatic representation of a bacterial cell, with some of the essential constituents. The cell wall is a complicated lattice structure of lipoprotein, lipopolysaccharide and peptidoglycan, which gives the bacterial cell its shape and also protects the cytoplasmic membrane.

The cell wall of certain bacteria is covered with a capsule, which is usually a loosely attached slime layer consisting of polymerized sugars and amino sugars that are secreted by the organism. In some bacteria, notably *Bacillus* spp., the capsular material is polypeptide, e.g. polyglutamic acid in *B. anthracis*. In many cases, possession of a capsule correlates with virulence.

The cytoplasmic membrane consists of a layer of lipoprotein and is $5-10\,nm$ thick. It encloses the cytoplasm, which contains soluble metabolites and precursors of macromolecules together with organelles such as ribosomes in a proteinaceous gel. Lying within the cytoplasm is the bacterial *chromosome*—usually a single closed ring of double-stranded DNA. The information for making all of the cell's proteins is encoded in the DNA, and the assembly of these proteins is carried out on the ribosomes—which are made of RNA and protein. At binary fission a duplicate copy of the chromosome passes to the new cell, thereby ensuring uniformity among the descendants of a single cell (clone).

Recently, it has been found that many bacteria contain smaller circles of DNA, called plasmids, which often carry genes that confer antibiotic resistance on the cells carrying them. Of greater current interest is the fact that these plasmids may be transferred between cells of different type (e.g. non-pathogen to pathogen) by a sort of mating process (*conjugation*) that involves the *sex pili* (see *Figure 20.1*).

Smaller pili (common pili or *fimbriae*) are often found on bacterial cells. They may be important in the attachment of pathogens to host tissue cells. The occurrence of antigenically similar pili on different species of bacteria can be a problem for the diagnostic bacteriologist.

Motile organisms possess flagella, which are thread-like appendages composed of protein called flagellin, and are about $20\,nm$ thick. Their rotation

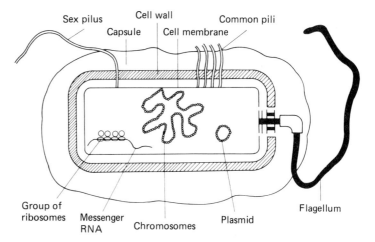

Figure 20.1. Diagram of a bacillus showing essential constituents

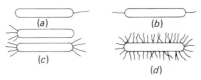

Figure 20.2. The flagella, which enable bacilli to move, may be arranged in one of four ways: (a) monotrichate—one flagellum at one pole; (b) amphitrichate—one flagellum at each pole; (c) lophotrichate—tuft of flagella at one or both poles; (d) peritrichate—flagella completely surrounding the bacterial body

enables bacteria to travel at speeds of up to 50 μm per s. Some organisms possess one flagellum, others more than one. The arrangement of the flagella may be as in *Figure 20.2*.

Bacterial metabolism

Basically, the properties and processes of life are essentially the same in all living things—whatever their size and whether they are plants or animals.

If an individual organism is to survive, it must be able to react to changes in its environment—it must be able to feed and respire and it must be able to reproduce.

To obtain optimum bacterial growth in laboratory-prepared media it is necessary to understand the metabolic role of nutrients. Metabolism can be considered as an interacting set of chemical reactions of which very few occur spontaneously and most have to be catalysed by specific proteins: *the enzymes*. There are two main types of reaction: those resulting in the breakdown of molecules (catabolic reaction) and those resulting in the synthesis of molecules (anabolic reaction). The energy needed to drive the synthetic reactions comes from the breakdown reactions, and the enzymes, which may number about 1000 in a single cell, are involved in its transfer.

The action of enzymes on their specific substrates is often used in the identification of bacteria. For example, the enzyme *urease* breaks down urea, $(NH_2)_2CO$ into ammonia (NH_3) and carbon dioxide (CO_2). The ammonium carbonate so formed can easily be detected in the growth medium by virtue of its alkalinity (pH indicator). The most obvious effect of oxygen on the growth of bacterial cells depends on whether it is used as the final hydrogen acceptor in its respiratory process, i.e. *aerobic respiration*. Bacteria which can grow only in the absence of free oxygen are termed *anaerobes*, and bacteria which can switch to alternative respiratory or energy-yielding pathways and therefore grow with or without oxygen are termed *facultative anaerobes*. Yet another group of bacteria grow best at reduced oxygen levels and these are called *microaerophilic*. All bacteria seem to need some CO_2 in the

atmosphere and most grow more readily when a relatively high concentration (5–10%) is supplied, irrespective of their requirement for oxygen.

Bacteria can be divided into groups based on their nutritional requirements in two different ways; namely, (a) on how they obtain their energy, and (b) on how they obtain the carbon needed for synthesis of all organic molecules.

Energy sources

Some bacteria, found in water and soils, obtain energy from sunlight through the agency of pigments. These are called *phototrophs*. Other bacteria obtain energy for growth from the oxidation of the inorganic compounds (*chemolithotrophs*) or from the oxidation, or fermentation, of organic compounds (*chemorganotrophs*). All bacteria of medical importance fall into this last category or, possibly, into the even more extreme one, the *paratrophs*. Paratrophs obtain their energy from the metabolism of the host cell and include viruses, probably rickettsiae, and possibly some bacteria.

Carbon sources

Some bacteria, notably the phototrophs and chemolithotrophs, are able to grow with CO_2 as the sole carbon source. These are known as *autotrophs*. Most bacteria, however, require to be supplied with organic carbon molecules (e.g. sugars) and these are called *heterotrophs*. The range of possible carbon compounds that can be used for energy production or as carbon sources by different bacteria forms the basis of the 'sugar' fermentation reactions commonly employed in diagnostic bacteriology. Again, the most extreme group are the *hypotrophs*; these organisms rely on the enzymatic apparatus of the host cell for replication, e.g. viruses.

All bacteria must be supplied with water, inorganic salts—notably phosphates—a source of sulphur, and a supply of nitrogen (necessary for both proteins and nucleic acids). Most, but not all, bacteria of medical importance will accept nitrogen only in organic form (e.g. peptones).

The range of temperatures over which different bacteria show optimal growth rises to three main groups:

1. The *thermophiles*, which have an optimal temperature of 55–75°C.
2. The *mesophiles*, optimal temperature 30–45°C.
3. The *psychrophiles*, optimum between 15 and 18°C.

Most medically important bacteria are mesophiles.

Bacterial variation

Most of the genetic information of the bacterial cell

is contained in the chromosomal DNA. This information is encoded in permutations of the four nucleotide bases: *thymine, adenine, cytosine* and *guanine*. The code is triplet, non-overlapping, and read sequentially, each set of three bases (Codon) coding for one amino acid, e.g. *adenine–guanine–adenine* codes for *arginine*. The DNA nucleotide sequence is transcribed into a complementary sequence in messenger ribonucleic acid (mRNA). The mRNA is read on the ribosomes in conjunction with transfer RNA (tRNA) to link together amino acids to form polypeptides of the 'correct' sequences needed by the cell for its structural and functional (enzyme) proteins. It follows that if the bacterial cell is to continue to produce progeny identical to itself, the information contained in the DNA must be capable of accurate duplication and transmission during cell division. Genetic changes may result from alterations that affect the sequence of bases. Therefore, while the maintenance of identity through many generations depends on accuracy of nucleic acid replication, transcription and translation, bacterial variability and adaptability depend on 'inaccuracies' occurring in one or other of the processes.

Several factors operate on bacteria which permit the exploitation of the inherent potential for variation to the advantage of the survival of the line of bacteria. Such factors include the rapid division times of bacteria growing optimally (e.g. 20 min for *Escherichia coli*), thereby presenting many opportunities for genetic changes to occur; the essentially haploid nature of the bacterial genome, thereby allowing rapid expression of the results of genetic alterations; and the extremely important selection pressure exerted by the environment (outside or inside the laboratory). Most genetic alterations (mutations) are lethal to the cells receiving them but, because of the vast number of cells produced by optimally dividing bacteria, even low mutation rates (e.g. 10^{-6}) may produce at least one cell better able to cope should the environment itself alter.

This combination of events permits, in the short term, survival of the line during adverse conditions, e.g. during antibiotic treatment of a patient or an antibiotic-containing media in the laboratory. The long-term implication of the same processes is evolutionary exploitation of the many diverse environments in which we find bacteria today.

Bacterial associations

An organism living and multiplying within the living human body is termed a *parasite*, the body in this instance being a host. When harmless to the host, the parasite is termed a *commensal*, when harmful, a *pathogen*. Under certain conditions, commensals may become pathogens, and pathogens may assume a commensal role. Organisms living on dead matter are termed *saprophytes*. When both host and parasite mutually benefit the association is often called *symbiosis*. This same term is used by some authorities irrespective of whether benefit occurs to either partner, but *satellitism* is the more correct term in these instances.

Bacterial pathogenicity

If a microbe penetrates the body surface, enters body tissue and multiplies, *infection* is said to have occurred. An infection which causes noticeable impairment of the body function is called an infectious disease. A disease is a process, not a thing, and is a result of the interaction between host and pathogen. The outcome of this relationship depends not only on the *pathogenicity* or virulence (the ability to cause damage to the host from small numbers of pathogens) of the parasite, but also on the resistance or susceptibility of the host.

A pathogen must first gain access to the host tissues and multiply before producing disease. To do this, the organism must penetrate the surface, such as the skin, mucous membranes or intestinal epithelium, which normally act as barriers. Many pathogens are helped at this early stage by attaching onto specific receptors on the cell surface and indeed many remain at the surface where they multiply, producing a spreading infection in the epithelium before being shed directly to the exterior. This simplest form of microbial pathogenicity is a feature of diphtheria and streptococal infections. Some organisms can penetrate further, breaking through the front-line surface defences and invading the sub-epithelial tissue. Here they have to evade, resist or inhibit the battery of host defence mechanisms, notably the phagocytic cell systems and the antibody-producing systems.

The phagocytic cells are very important because they engulf the bacteria and, once inside, the bacteria are broken down. Some bacteria have therefore evolved elaborate means of evading this system, such as possession of capsules, which prevent engulfment by phagocytes, or the production of substances called *leucocidins* that kill the phagocyte. Others will live quite happily inside these phagocytic cells, having gained the ability, through substances in their cell wall, to resist the killing action of the phagocyte.

Many bacteria have also developed elaborate strategies for dealing with the immune response. These include the suppression of antibody production or varying their cell surface so that the antibody does not recognize them.

Once established, the manner in which pathogens bring about damage to the host are diverse. In many cases specific factors are involved such as toxins. Those produced and secreted into the environment while the organism is living are termed *exotoxins*; those that are liberated into the environment only on lysis of the organism are termed *endotoxins*. Exotoxins are produced mainly by Gram-positive bacteria and are often relatively heat labile (destroyed at 60°C). Endotoxins are often cell wall components of Gram-negative bacteria and are often relatively heat stable (withstanding 100°C).

Exotoxins may be rendered non-toxic by the addition of chemicals such as formalin, or by heat treatment. When this conversion does not significantly impair the immunological properties, they can be used to produce active immunity in man and animals against the toxin and are called *toxoids*.

21

Microscopic examination of bacteria

Both shape and motility of bacteria can be studied by the microscopic examination of unstained preparations suspended in a fluid (the 'hanging drop' method), but to render the structures of cells visible, staining techniques must be used. These will only differentiate relatively gross individual structures, however, and to reveal those not shown by staining, more complex techniques, such as electron microscopy, are needed.

Apart from differentiating and rendering visible the constituents of a cell, staining will help to identify organisms and place them in their own particular group by their individual reactions to certain stains. An example is the Gram-positive or Gram-negative reaction to Gram's stain.

Making of loops

Wire loops or straight wire are necessary for making smears. They may be made of platinum or nicrome wire. Platinum by itself is too soft for making loops, and platinum wire is generally a mixture of platinum (90%) and iridium (10%). Nicrome wire is cheaper,

more elastic and cools faster than platinum. It has to be renewed more frequently, however, as it burns. Disposable plastic loops, obtainable commercially, are now widely used. They are available in a variety of sizes and are particularly valuable when plating-out faeces—when working with Mycobacteria and when using an anaerobic cabinet. They eliminate the need for flaming which could cause spluttering, shedding bacteria-containing particles into the atmosphere.

Loops are usually circles of approximately 1.5 mm and 3 mm in diameter. The thickness of the wire is SWG (Standard Wire Gauge) 26 or 27.

1. Wind the wire once round a metal rod of appropriate diameter (*Figure 21.1a* and *21.1b*).
2. With a pair of old scissors, cut one arm of the wire at junction (*Figure 21.1c* and *21.1d*).
3. Bend back the loop to centre it (*Figure 21.1e*).
4. Insert into a metal wire-holder.

Sterilization of wire loops

Hold the loop in the bunsen flame in a near vertical position. Allow to cool before using. Use a hooded bunsen burner if spluttering is likely to occur.

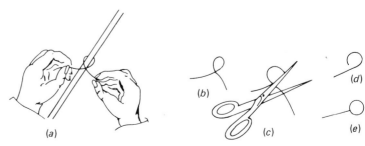

Figure 21.1. The construction of wire loops necessary for making smears; for explanation see text

Making of smears

General notes

1. Use clean slides free from grease.
2. Mark the slide with a glass writing diamond—grease pencil is easily rubbed away.
3. From liquid cultures make fairly heavy smears.
4. From cultures on solid media make thin smears.
5. *Do not* use water taken from rubber tubing attached to taps for making smears, as organisms may be transferred from the rubber.
6. When making films to demonstrate acid-fast organisms, use only one smear per slide and keep the slides apart when staining on a staining rack. This prevents any possibility of transference of acid-fast organisms onto another slide. Throw the slides away after use.
7. *Never* use Coplin or other staining jars for acid-fast material for the same reason as above.
8. When blotting slides, use a fresh portion of paper for each slide, to prevent transference of material.

From liquid media

1. Sterilize loop in bunsen flame.
2. Using aseptic precautions, withdraw 1 loopful of culture.
3. Transfer this to a clean slide and spread it with the loop, to form a thick film of liquid. Sterilize the loop.
4. Allow the film to dry without heating and then rapidly pass the slide 3 times through the bunsen flame. This kills the bacteria and fixes them to the slide.
5. Allow the slide to cool, and then stain the film by the requisite method.

From solid media

Aseptic precautions must be observed during the manipulation of culture tubes or plates.

1. Sterilize loop in bunsen flame.
2. Place 1 drop of distilled water on a clean slide, and resterilize loop.
3. With the loop or preferably a straight wire, transfer to the slide a small portion of the growth to be examined and emulsify it in the drop of water until a thin homogeneous film is produced. Sterilize the loop.
4. Allow to dry, fix and stain.

Making of hanging drop preparations

When suspended in a fluid and examined microscopically many bacteria are seen to be motile, that is,

they move from one position to another. True motility must not be confused with Brownian movement (vibration caused by molecular bombardment) or convection currents. A motile organism is one which *actively* changes its position relative to other organisms present.

1. Clean a slide and a 22 mm square coverslip.
2. On the slide make a ring of plasticine or Vaseline 2 cm in diameter. Alternatively a 'well slide' with a depression in the centre can be used.
3. Transfer a loopful of culture to the centre of the coverslip.
4. Gently press the ring of Vaseline or plasticine on to the coverslip, ensuring that the 'drop' of culture is in the centre of the circle, and does not come in contact with the slide. It is important that the slide and coverslip be completely sealed, otherwise 'draughts' can cause pseudo-motility. If a 'well slide' is used, seal the coverslip with Vaseline or nail varnish.
5. With a quick movement, invert the slide, so that the coverslip is uppermost (*Figure 21.2*).

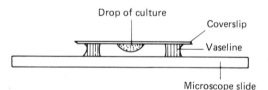

Figure 21.2. Hanging drop preparation

6. Examine under the microscope, focusing first onto the edge of the 'drop', with the 16 mm objective (using a small cone of light), and when in focus swing round to the 4 mm objective to investigate motility.
7. Discard the whole hanging drop preparation into a jar containing a disinfectant, taking care that the disinfectant penetrates into the 'ring' and kills the culture.

Making of wet preparations

1. On a microscope slide, emulsify the specimen (such as faeces) in a small drop of saline, iodine or the required stain.
2. Carefully place a coverslip onto the suspension taking care that no fluid extrudes beyond the edges of the coverslip.
3. Paint the edges of the coverslip with nail varnish, paraffin wax or Vaseline. This effectively seals the preparations and prevents evaporation. Examine microscopically as for 'hanging drop'.

Staining of smears

Gram's stain

In 1884 Gram described this method, which is the most important stain in routine bacteriology. It divides bacteria into two categories, depending on whether they can be decolorized with acetone, alcohol or aniline oil after staining with one of the rosaniline dyes such as crystal violet, methyl violet or gentian violet, and treating with iodine. Those that resist decolorization remain blue or violet in colour, and are designated Gram-positive, those that are decolorized and take up the red counterstain, such as neutral red, safranin or dilute carbol–fuchsin, are termed Gram-negative (see *Table 21.1*).

Table 21.1 Reaction of some organisms to Gram's stain

Gram-positive	*Gram-negative*
Staphylococci	Coliforms
Streptococci	Neisseriae
Pneumococci	Vibrios
Corynebacteria	Spirochaetes
Clostridia	Salmonellae
Mycobacteria	Shigellae
Bacillus group	Haemophilus group

Although many investigators have tried to uncover the mechanism of the Gram reaction, no universal answer has yet been found and it is possible that more than one mechanism exists. It is known, however, that there is a basic chemical difference between Gram-negative and Gram-positive organisms, as well as differences in cell wall composition.

Solution 1:

Methyl violet 6 B (CI No. 42555)	0.5 g
Distilled water	100 ml

Dissolve the methyl violet in the distilled water and filter. Record date and label.

Lugol's iodine

Solution 2:

Iodine	10 g
Potassium iodide	20 g
Distilled water	1000 ml

Dissolve the potassium iodide in about 50 ml of the water, add the iodine, dissolve by shaking and make up to the final volume. Record date, label and store in a tightly stoppered bottle.

Decolorizer

Solution 3:
Absolute ethyl alcohol or acetone or acetone–iodine solution.

Acetone–iodine solution

Iodine	10 g
Potassium iodide	6 g
Distilled water	10 ml
Alcohol 74° OP	90 ml

Dissolve the potassium iodide in the distilled water and then add the iodine. Dissolve by shaking and add the 74° OP spirit. Add 35 ml of this solution to 965 ml of acetone. The presence of iodine in the decolorizer helps to prevent over-decolorization.

Counterstain

Solution 4:
Neutral red, safranin or dilute carbol–fuchsin.

Procedure

1. Prepare a smear, allow to dry and fix with gentle heat.
2. Apply solution 1 for 30 s.
3. Replace solution 1 with solution 2 and allow to act for 30 s to 1 min.
4. Rinse with solution 3 and continue application until no more colour appears to flow from the preparation.
5. Wash with water.
6. Apply solution 4 for 3 min. (If dilute fuchsin is used, stain for 30 s.)
7. Rinse with water, blot carefully and dry with gentle heat.

Safranin

A counterstain for use with Gram's stain:

Safranin O (CI No. 50240)	5 g
Distilled water	1000 ml

Dissolve the dye in the distilled water and filter. Record date and label.

Procedure

Apply the stain for 3 min, wash with water, blot carefully and dry with gentle heat.

■ **Note**

Some workers prefer to dissolve the safranin in ethyl alcohol and to dilute 10 ml of a saturated solution to 100 ml with distilled water.

Neutral red

A counterstain for use with Gram's stain:

Neutral red (CI No. 50040)	1 g
Acetic acid, 1%	2 ml
Distilled water	1000 ml

Dissolve the neutral red in the distilled water and add the acetic acid. Filter, record date and label.

Procedure

Apply the stain for 3–5 min, wash with water, blot carefully and dry with gentle heat.

Dilute carbol–fuchsin

A counterstain for use with Gram's stain:

Ziehl–Neelsen carbol–fuchsin	50–100 ml
Distilled water to	1000 ml

Add the carbol–fuchsin to distilled water and make up the volume to 1000 ml. Filter, record date and label.

Procedure

Apply the stain for 10–20 s, wash with water, blot carefully and dry with gentle heat.

■ Note

While this stain may be of value as a counterstain for routine work, it is not the stain of choice for the demonstration of *Neisseria gonorrhoeae* or other intracellular Gram-negative bacteria. Instead use neutral red.

Stains for acid-fast bacilli

Ziehl–Neelsen stain

The staining of *M. tuberculosis* and other acid-fast organisms.

Carbol–fuchsin

Solution 1:

Basic fuchsin (CI No. 42510)	10 g
Phenol crystals	45 g
Ethyl alcohol, absolute	100 ml
Distilled water	900 ml

(a) Dissolve the phenol in the distilled water. Dissolve the fuchsin in the alcohol with the aid of gentle heat. Combine the two solutions, mix and allow to remain at room temperature overnight. Filter through wet paper and label. Or

(b) Weigh the fuchsin and phenol into a 2 litre flask and dissolve by heating over a boiling water bath. Shake the contents occasionally until solution is effected. Add the alcohol, mix thoroughly and add the distilled water. Allow to remain at room temperature overnight and filter through wet paper. Label.

Acid–alcohol

Solution 2:

Hydrochloric acid (sp. gr. 1.19)	30 ml
Ethyl alcohol, absolute	970 ml

Counterstain

Solution 3: Methylene blue (CI No. 52015) or malachite green (CI No. 42000).

Procedure

1. Prepare a smear, allow to dry and fix with gentle heat.
2. Apply solution 1 and heat until steam rises. Keep the stain hot for 5 min. (Do not allow the stain to boil or to dry on the slide.)
3. Wash with water.
4. Apply several changes of solution 2 until the preparation is colourless or a faint pink.
5. Wash with water.
6. Apply solution 3 for 20–30 s.
7. Wash with water, blot carefully and dry with gentle heat.

Auramine stain

The detection of acid-fast bacilli in sputum by fluorescence microscopy.

Staining solution

Solution 1:

Auramine O (CI No. 41000)	0.3 g
Phenol crystals	3.0 g
Distilled water	97.0 ml

Dissolve the phenol in the water with the aid of gentle heat. Add the auramine gradually and shake vigorously to effect solution. Filter, label and store in a dark stoppered bottle, when the solution will keep for about 3 weeks.

Decolorizer

Solution 2:

Sodium chloride	0.5 g
Hydrochloric acid (sp. gr. 1.19)	0.5 ml
Ethyl alcohol, 75%	100.0 ml

Combine the alcohol with the acid and dissolve the sodium chloride. Label.

Counterstain

Solution 3: Potassium permanganate, 0.1% solution.

Procedure

1. Prepare a thin smear of sputum, allow to dry and fix with gentle heat.
2. Apply solution 1 for 10 min.
3. Rinse in tap water.
4. Apply solution 2 for 5 min.

5. Wash well in tap water.
6. Apply solution 3 for 30 s.
7. Wash well in tap water and drain dry. Do not blot.
8. Examine by fluorescence microscopy.

Result

Acid-fast bacilli appear as bright, luminous yellow rods against a dark background.

Simple stains and counterstains

Methylene blue

A simple stain for routine use and as a counterstain with Ziehl–Neelsen stain.

Methylene blue (CI No. 52015) saturated alcoholic solution (approx. 1.5%)	50 ml
Distilled water	950 ml

Combine the ingredients and filter. Record date and label.

Procedure

Apply the stain for 30 s, wash with water, blot carefully and dry with gentle heat.

Malachite green

A counterstain for use with Ziehl–Neelsen stain.

Malachite green (CI No. 42000)	1 g
Distilled water	1000 ml

Dissolve the dye in the distilled water and filter. Record date and label.

Procedure

Apply the stain for 20–30 s, wash with water, blot carefully and dry with gentle heat.

Stains for corynebacteria

Albert's stain

The routine staining of *Corynebacterium diphtheriae*.

Solution 1:

Toluidine blue (CI No. 52040)	1.5 g
Malachite green (CI No. 42000)	2.0 g
Acetic acid, glacial	10.0 ml
Ethyl alcohol, 95%	20.0 ml
Distilled water	1000.0 ml

Dissolve the dyes in the alcohol and add the water and acetic acid. Allow the solution to stand at room temperature for 24 h and filter. Label.

Solution 2:

Iodine	6 g
Potassium iodide	9 g
Distilled water	900 ml

Dissolve the potassium iodide in about 50 ml of the water, add the iodine, dissolve by shaking and make up to the final volume.

Procedure

1. Prepare a smear from an 18–24 h Loeffler serum culture of the test organism, allow to dry and fix with gentle heat.
2. Apply solution 1 for 3–5 min.
3. Wash with water and blot carefully.
4. Apply solution 2 for 1 min.
5. Wash with water, blot carefully and dry with gentle heat.

Results

Granules bluish-black, remainder of organism green, other organisms usually pale green.

Pugh's stain

The routine staining of *Corynebacterium diphtheriae*.

Toluidine blue (CI No. 52040)	1 g
Ethyl alcohol, absolute	20 ml
Acetic acid, glacial	50 ml
Distilled water	950 ml

Combine the acetic acid with the distilled water and add the dye dissolved in the alcohol. Filter, record date and label.

Procedure

1. Prepare a smear from an 18–24 h Loeffler serum culture of the test organism, allow to dry and fix with gentle heat.
2. Apply the stain for 2–3 min.
3. Wash with water, blot carefully and dry with gentle heat.

Results

Granules reddish-purple, remainder of organism light blue.

Spore stains

The spore wall is relatively impermeable to stains,

but spores can be stained by heating the preparations. The spore wall resists decolorization by such alcohol treatments as would be sufficient to decolorize vegetative organisms.

Fuchsin–methylene blue spore stain

Solution 1: Ziehl–Neelsen carbol–fuchsin.

Solution 2: Ferric chloride, 30% aqueous solution.

Solution 3: Sodium sulphite, 5% aqueous solution.

Solution 4: Methylene blue (CI No. 52015), 1% aqueous solution.

Procedure

1. Prepare a thin smear, allow to dry and fix with the minimum amount of heat.
2. Apply solution 1 for 3–5 min, heating the preparation until steam rises.
3. Wash in water.
4. Apply solution 2 for 1–2 min.
5. Replace solution 2 with solution 3 and allow to act for 30 s.
6. Wash in water.
7. Apply solution 4 for 1 min.
8. Wash in water, blot carefully and dry with the minimum amount of heat.

Results

Spores bright red, remainder of organism blue.

Fuchsin–nigrosin spore stain (Fleming)

Solution 1: Ziehl–Neelsen carbol–fuchsin.

Decolorizer

Solution 2: (A) Nigrosin, 1% solution (CI No. 50420)
    or
    (B) Sodium sulphite, 5% solution.
Solution 3: Nigrosin 10% solution.

Procedure

1. Prepare a thin smear, allow to dry and fix with the minimum amount of heat.
2. Apply solution 1 for 5 min, heating the preparation until steam rises.
3. Wash with water.
4. Apply solution 2 (A) for 5–10 min or (B) for 5–30 s.
5. Wash in water, blot carefully and dry with the minimum amount of heat.
6. Place a small drop of solution 3 at one end of the slide and spread in an even layer over the stained preparation with the edge of another slide.
7. Allow to dry and examine.

Results

Spore bright red, remainder of organism unstained against a dark grey background of nigrosin.

Capsule staining

By ordinary staining methods, carbohydrate capsules are unstained, but are often seen as a clear zone around a stained organism. To demonstrate capsule either a direct staining or a negative staining technique is used.

Crystal violet capsule stain

Solution 1: Crystal violet (CI No. 42555), 1% aqueous solution.
Solution 2: Copper sulphate, 20% aqueous solution.

Procedure

1. Prepare a thin smear, dry in air without fixation.
2. Apply solution 1 for 2 min without heating.
3. Wash with solution 2.
4. Blot carefully, dry in air and examine.

Results

Capsule pale violet, bacterial cell deep violet.

Nigrosin–methylene blue capsule stain

Solution 1:

Nigrosin (CI No. 50420)	5–10 g
Distilled water	100 ml
Formalin, as preservative	0.5 ml

Dissolve the nigrosin in warm distilled water, add the formalin and filter. Label.

Solution 2: Loeffler's alkaline methylene blue (see p. 255).

Procedure

1. To one loopful of culture on a clean slide add one loopful of freshly filtered solution 1. Mix, allow to dry in air and fix with gentle heat.
2. Apply solution 2 for 30 s.
3. Rinse rapidly in water, blot carefully and dry with gentle heat.

Results

Bacterial cell blue, capsule unstained against a dark grey background of nigrosin.

Note

Safranin may be employed in place of the methylene blue in solution 2.

India ink preparation

The demonstration of bacterial capsules in wet films. (Negative staining.)

Procedure

1. Place one loopful of India ink on a perfectly clean glass slide.
2. Emulsify a small portion of solid bacterial culture in the drop of ink, or mix in a loopful of liquid culture.
3. Cover the mixture with a clean coverglass and press the latter down firmly, to form a very thin ink film. Seal the edges of the cover glass with paraffin wax or other suitable medium, and examine using oil-immersion objective.

Results

Bacteria highly refractile, surrounded by a clear zone against a dark grey background of ink particles. Non-capsulated bacteria do not show this clear zone.

Simple stains

Most of the counterstains used in Gram's and Ziehl–Neelsen's method can be used as simple stains to show the morphology of organisms. In addition to these, the following stain can be used.

Loeffler's alkaline methylene blue

A basic dye for routine use in studying the morphology of micro-organisms in smears from cultures. The stain is more intense than neutral solution of methylene blue and may show some degree of polychromatic staining.

Methylene blue (CI No. 52015), saturated alcoholic solution (approx. 1.5 g per 100 ml of 95% alcohol)	300 ml
Potassium hydroxide, 1% aqueous solution	10 ml
Distilled water	990 ml

Measure the potassium hydroxide solution into the water and combine with the methylene blue solution. Mix thoroughly and filter. Record date and label.

Procedure

Apply the stain for 30 s, wash with water, blot carefully and dry with gentle heat.

Polychrome methylene blue

This stain has a similar application to that of Loeffler's alkaline methylene blue and is of special value in McFadyean's reaction for demonstrating anthrax bacilli in blood.

Preparation for use

Proceed as for the preparation of Loeffler's alkaline methylene blue and distribute the stain into bottles. Half-fill the bottles and shake at intervals to thoroughly aerate the contents. Record date and label. The process of ripening may take several months but may be accelerated by chemical treatment.

Procedure

See Loeffler's alkaline methylene blue, above.

22

Sterilization

The term *sterilization* strictly means the killing of all forms of life that may be present in a specimen or an environment. In bacteriology it is used to describe a variety of procedures directed to achieving this objective; examples are the destruction of bacteria in a contaminated sample and the active exclusion of unwanted bacteria from culture media by means of filtration techniques. The methods of sterilization that are used in laboratories may be conveniently divided into physical, chemical and mechanical methods.

Physical methods

Radiation

The commonest forms of electromagnetic radiation used in microbiology are ultraviolet (u.v.) light and the much more energetic gamma (γ) rays. It has long been known that exposure to direct sunlight slowly kills bacteria and that this is due to the u.v. rays which occur at the extreme limit of the visible spectrum. In the laboratory, u.v. light is generated by means of a hot-cathode/low-pressure mercury vapour lamp and its bactericidal effect is maximal at wavelengths between 250 and 260 nm. Ultraviolet light is absorbed by certain types of molecule found in living cells, notably nucleotides, and their electrons thereby gain extra energy. This is often sufficient to disrupt weak intramolecular bonds—such as the hydrogen bonds binding together the double helix of DNA. This, in turn, can cause intramolecular changes that are lethal to the cell. Some genes are more sensitive than others to this damage; for example, those of which a cell has multiple copies will require a higher dosage to achieve the same effect as that observed when a single vital gene is inactivated.

Laboratory use of ultraviolet light is limited by its very poor penetrating power. Even a thin glass coverslip is sufficient to protect bacteria on its undersurface completely, and drops of moisture in aerosols may protect bacteria borne within them. The chief application of u.v. light is sterilization of the (still) air in inoculating cabinets and 'sterile rooms', where the light may be left on for long periods between operations.

Gamma rays are an example of ionizing radiation i.e. their energy is sufficient to knock peripheral electrons out of their orbits around the atomic nucleus and produce ion pairs. These highly reactive ions (H^+, OH^-) may be produced in the extracellular or intracellular water and interact with vital molecules in the cell. Additionally, such ionization may be produced in the DNA itself and cause irreparable damage.

The very high penetrating power of γ-rays make them ideally suited to the sterilization of prepacked disposable plastics, e.g. syringes. They are, however, useless for the sterilization of foods and pharmaceuticals because of chemical alteration produced in the products themselves. Special equipment is necessary for carrying out this procedure, in order to guard against irradiation of the operators (which could be fatal). This equipment is both heavy and costly to install and is therefore more likely to be used by manufacturers than by pathology laboratories.

Dry heat

Dry heat at high temperatures causes destruction of living cells and tissues by oxidation of their components. Its extreme form is simply the incineration of (inflammable and disposable) articles and their contaminating micro-organisms, e.g. the carcasses of infected animals. Less extreme applications are the raising of inoculating loops to red heat and the burning of alcohol on forceps, thereby incinerating the micro-organisms on their surfaces.

The commonest application of dry heat at moderate temperatures is in the use of the *hot-air oven*. This is used for materials that are unaffected by temperatures of 160–180°C and for which autoclaving is unsuitable, e.g. dry glassware and unwettable materials such as powders, oils and waxes.

Air is a poor conductor of heat and the oven must not be packed so tightly as to impede circulation or to trap air pockets; a fan should always be fitted to aid convection. The poor heat conduction must be borne in mind when calculating exposure times. Powder contained in a 125 ml jar may take 45 min to reach the operating temperature of 160°C and the sterilization time must therefore be increased by this period.

The sterilization periods commonly used are 160°C for 1 h or 180°C for 30 min. It is important to allow the oven to cool before removing the contents lest, owing to rapid contraction of the air within petri dishes, unsterile air be sucked in. Occasionally, even modern glassware may be damaged by too rapid cooling.

Moist heat

When heat is applied to water at sea level, the temperature rises until it reaches 100°C. An additional amount of heat energy (heat of vaporization) is then taken up by the water without a change in temperature, whereupon it boils. It is important to remember that the temperature does not go above 100°C, and at high altitudes water even boils several degrees lower than this because of the reduced atmospheric pressure. At high altitudes it will therefore be less effective. If, on the other hand, the atmospheric pressure is increased, the water will boil at a higher temperature and therefore is more effective in killing organisms. This is the principle used in autoclaving (see below).

Boiling water

A temperature of 100°C will kill all non-sporing organisms within 10 min. Most spores will be killed in 30 min at this temperature, but some spores will resist boiling for several hours. The addition of 2% sodium carbonate increases the bactericidal effect of boiling water, and spores that resist boiling water for 10 h have been killed in 30 min by this addition. This method is suitable for infected instruments (such as at animal autopsy) if they are to be used immediately, particularly as the sodium carbonate prevents rusting of the instruments. It is unsuitable if instruments are to be stored in a sterile condition.

Steam at 100°C

Steam at 100°C is used mainly to sterilize certain complex media, where the constituents might be 'broken down' (hydrolysed) at temperatures above 100°C, e.g. sugars, gelatin, etc. Such media are sterilized by a form of intermittent steaming called 'Tyndallization'. This is steaming on three consecutive days. The medium is steamed for 30 min on the first day, incubated at room temperature overnight, steamed for a further 30 min on the second day, reincubated, and steamed again for 30 min on the third day. The first day's exposure kills non-sporing and vegetative organisms; the incubation period, provided the medium is favourable, allows germination of most spores, and the second steaming kills these. The repeated process usually ensures germination and subsequent killing of any spores remaining after the first and second exposures. It will be seen, therefore, that Tyndallization is only effective when the medium to be sterilized is favourable for the germination of spores: it is useless for non-nutrient fluids and may not kill anaerobic spore-bearers, unless the incubation is carried out anaerobically, and it will not kill thermoduric organisms.

Steam under pressure

The sterilizing efficiency of steam under pressure is due to its temperature (>100°C), and its ability to condense on cooler, wettable objects, thereby rapidly transferring its *latent heat of vaporization* and raising their temperature. The change of volume caused by the condensation aids penetration of the steam and the moist environment allows rapid heat coagulation of proteins—a feature that accounts for the ability of the process to achieve sterilization at temperatures much lower than those required by dry (oxidation) methods.

It should be noted that the part played by the *pressure* of the steam is solely the production of moist heat at temperatures above 100°C.

The simplest laboratory autoclaves are merely versions of the domestic pressure cooker. Steam is generated by applying heat (gas or electricity) to a small volume of water contained within the sealed body of the apparatus. All air *must* be displaced from the autoclave before bringing it up to sterilization pressure because it is the pressure, read from a gauge or preset by means of special valves, that is used as a guide to the steam temperature in those simple models. This relation (5 psi = 110°C; 10 psi = 115°C, 15 psi = 121°C, 20 psi = 126°C) is true only if the atmosphere within the autoclave is pure steam. If, for instance, the autoclave contains half air, half steam 15 psi produces a temperature of 112°C. Under these conditions, sterilization might take as long as 12 h in contrast to the 15 psi (121°C) for 20–30 min routinely employed.

Another reason for ensuring that all air is displaced is that air pockets trapped between articles can behave only as 'hot air' at relatively low temperature and so fail to sterilize. This is true also if the steam becomes too dry (as may happen in steam-jacketed autoclaves when there is a higher pressure in the jacket than in the vessel); such steam is called *superheated* and behaves like 'hot air'.

Larger laboratory autoclaves are usually fed with steam from an external supply. The steam is usually admitted to the pressure vessel through a valve and baffle plate. The steam outlet valve is at the bottom and a thermocouple is inserted at this point to allow direct measurement of the temperature during various stages of the process. At the top of the vessel are mounted a pressure gauge and safety valve. Comparison of the pressure and temperature readings gives valuable information on the functioning of the apparatus.

Testing of autoclaves

Whether material is adequately sterilized may be determined by several methods. A method that is of particular value when the time factor for using the material is important is the use of Browne's sterilizer control tubes. These are tubes containing an indicator liquid, which can be purchased for steamer, hot-air oven or autoclave. The liquid will change from red to green if the correct temperature–time combination has been employed; if not, they turn a reddish-brown colour.

Another method is by impregnating filter paper strips with a sporing organism, such as *Bacillus stearothermophilus*. The strip is enclosed in an envelope, and placed in a convenient part of the material undergoing sterilization. It must be remembered that the strip or Browne's tube must be placed in a position where steam is least likely to penetrate. On removal, the spore strip is cultured in a suitable medium and incubated for 7 days at 55°C. This method is excellent when time is not too important. Commercially prepared strips of dried *B. stearothermophilus* are available and are used as described.

It is, however, recommended that whenever possible the working of an autoclave should be monitored by means of a series of thermocouples placed within the contents and calibrated to indicate the temperatures actually attained.

Low-temperature sterilization

Biological fluids may be sterilized by heating them in a water bath at 56°C for periods of 1 h daily as long as may be necessary. The principle is the same as Tyndallization, but the lower temperature may necessitate more than three exposures to heat. If the temperature of 56°C is exceeded, the fluids may be coagulated. This method of sterilization can be used only when the fluid does not contain resistant spores, or very thermoduric organisms.

Vaccines may be sterilized by placing them in a water bath at a temperature of 60°C for 1 h. This is usually adequate, as vaccines are prepared under aseptic conditions and spores are not normally present. Temperatures higher than 60°C may diminish the immunizing power of the vaccine.

Chemical agents

Many chemical agents are referred to as *disinfectants*, a term that is applied to substances which destroy micro-organisms on inanimate objects. Other terms with a similar meaning are *germicide* and *bactericide*. A disinfectant, which is non-injurious to human tissue, is called an *antiseptic* and chemicals which are used to prevent organisms growing in a sterile medium, but do not kill them, are called *bacteriostats*. The action of a disinfectant is modified by several factors. Some disinfectants are very efficient in the absence of organic matter, but are less effective in its presence.

Chemical agents function as sterilizing agents by the following lethal mechanisms:

1. Interfering with the enzymatic system of the organism (enzyme poisons).
2. Disruption of the cell membrane.
3. Coagulation of protein.
4. Oxidation.

Very many different compounds have been used as disinfectants and only a few commonly used examples are given below.

Alcohol (ethanol)

Absolute alcohol is not a very effective sterilizing agent, as at this concentration its power of penetration is very poor. When diluted with distilled water to a concentration of 70%, however, it becomes effective as a skin sterilizer and is used prior to inoculations or venepunctures.

Chloroform

Chloroform is sometimes used to maintain the sterility of serum. When the serum is required for use it is placed in a 56°C water bath for a short while in order to evaporate the chloroform. To be effective, chloroform must be present in a concentration of 0.25%.

Chlorine

Chlorine and its derivatives are used extensively in microbiological laboratories, especially in virology departments, where it is the disinfectant of choice. However, its activity is poor in the presence of organic matter and can be completely lost by combination with thiosulphate, sulphides and ferrous salts. It is necessary to guard against accidental mixture with such inhibitors.

Glycerol

Glycerol in 50% solution will kill contaminating organisms. It is used for the preservation of certain viruses which are not affected by the glycerol.

Phenol and cresols

Phenol and cresols are powerful antiseptics. They are used mainly for discarded cultures, infected pipettes, and other infected material. A 5% solution is generally used: stronger solutions may be less effective owing to protection of organisms in the middle of a cluster of which the outer members have been coagulated into a shield.

Quaternary ammonium compounds

These are cationic detergents which are used mainly for skin disinfection and in the food industry. They are ineffective against *Mycobacterium tuberculosis*, bacterial spores and *Pseudomonas aeruginosa*. A form that is much used in hospitals is cetyl-trimethyl-ammonium bromide ('Cetrimide').

Aldehydes

Two types of aldehydes are commonly used, formaldehyde (supplied as a 40% solution—formalin) and activated glutaraldehyde.

For general purposes, formaldehyde gas and formalin are too irritant, but they have application in the laboratory for disinfecting exhaust protective cabinets.

Activated glutaraldehyde is less irritant than formaldehyde, but it should only be used where there is minimal organic matter present because of its low penetrating power.

Sterilization by filtration

Several types of material have found use as microbial filters, such as diatomaceous earth (in Berkefeld and Mandler filters); porcelain (in Chamberland filters); sintered glass; asbestos (in Seitz filters); and cellulose esters (in membrane filters). The last two types are the only ones in common use.

Seitz-type filters

The asbestos-disc or Seitz filter is a satisfactory one for general purposes (*Figure 22.1*), and consists of an asbestos disc supported, rough side uppermost, in a metal mount.

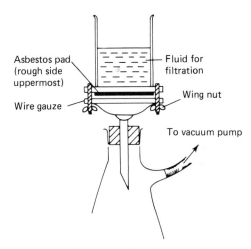

Figure 22.1. Filtration, using a Seitz-type filter

The Seitz filter is attached to a vacuum flask through a silicone rubber bung. Red rubber bungs tend to vulcanize after heating, but the silicone rubber withstands repeated autoclaving.

The side arm of the flask is plugged with non-absorbent wool and the filter unit wrapped in Kraft paper and sterilized at 121°C for 20 min.

After use, sterilize if necessary, then discard the asbestos disc, clean the metal mount, insert a fresh disc, and sterilize by autoclaving. The asbestos discs are supplied in varying grades, the more important being those shown in *Table 22.1*. For small amounts a 'Hemming's filter' can be used. This consists of a filter pad fitted between two bijou bottles. The bottles are centrifuged, and the liquid to be filtered is thereby forced through the pad from one bijou to the other.

Table 22.1 Carlson–Ford filter sheets for sterilization

HP/PYR	For the removal of pyrogens
HP/EKS2	For removal of minute organisms from heavily infected liquids.
HP/EKS	For absolute sterility using controlled standard conditions.
HP/EK	For sterility down to *Serratia marcescens*/*C. prodigiosum*.

■ Notes

1. Never filter material containing solid matter if the latter can be removed by other methods, e.g. by centrifugation.
2. Test sterilizing filter candles periodically by filtering a culture of *Serratia marcescens* (*C. prodigiosum*) and testing the filtrate for sterility. Filtration should not be effected too rapidly; 5–10 drops per min is a suitable rate. When negative pressure is used this should not exceed 200 mmHg.

Membrane filters

In recent years, membrane filters have replaced other types for many applications. These are now made of cellulose esters (cellulose nitrate or cellulose acetate) supported in a matrix of regenerated cellulose. Their advantages include:

1. Ease of handling—they are relatively tough.
2. They are sufficiently inexpensive to be used once only.
3. Electrical neutrality—charged molecules are not taken out of solution as readily as with other types.
4. Minimal retention of solute.
5. Accurate grading of pore sizes over a wide range.

Such membranes can also be used for bacterial counts in, for example, the examination of water supplies. A known volume of water is passed through a membrane filter: commercially available apparatus may pump many gallons through a single membrane. The membrane is then removed and placed on a pad moistened with an appropriate liquid culture medium (which may be selective, e.g. for pathogenic bacteria) and incubated. The colonies which develop can be counted to allow estimation of the numbers of viable cells in the original specimen. If these membranes are treated with microscopic immersion oil, they become transparent so that they can be examined by direct microscopy after staining the bacteria trapped on their surface.

23

The principles and use of culture media

To isolate, identify and study the characteristics of micro-organisms, it is essential to grow them on artificial media, and in routine bacteriology the most important requirement of a culture medium is its ability to allow detectable growth from a minute inoculum within the shortest period of incubation.

Essential requirements of culture media

As the basic requirements for bacterial nutrition are moisture, carbon and nitrogen, it is necessary for an artificial medium to provide these three essentials and, for many pathogenic bacteria, other components as well.

Moisture plays an important part in the nutrition of bacteria; in the absence of water bacteria cannot grow. (This fact is used in preservation of foodstuffs by drying, which although preventing bacteria from growing, will not necessarily kill them.)

Organisms cannot always obtain their nitrogenous and carbon requirements from complex proteins and these substances must be broken down into simpler compounds. This breaking down is performed by the organism's enzyme system. For their carbon requirements some bacteria can utilize the CO_2 in the atmosphere, while others have to decompose certain organic substances. The form in which nitrogen is added to the medium depends on the enzyme-reducing abilities of the organism. The simplest way of ensuring a supply of nitrogen is by the addition of peptone, which is a hydrolysed product of protein and consists of a mixture of proteases, polypeptides and amino acids. It is soluble and easily incorporated in most media. Carbon requirements are provided by amino acids,

provided by the breakdown of peptone, but the addition of carbohydrates often produces a more luxuriant growth.

In addition to the basic requirements of water, carbon and nitrogen, other chemical substances are necessary, such as sulphur, phosphorus, and very small traces of metal salts (referred to as *trace elements*) and in some cases certain vitamins and vitamin-like substances called '*essential metabolites*'.

With the addition of blood or serum, most common pathogenic bacteria can be cultivated.

Environmental factors

Apart from these nutritional requirements, bacteria require certain other conditions before they will grow satisfactorily in or on artificial culture media.

Gaseous requirements

Oxygen is required for the growth of many, but not all, micro-organisms. Those that will grow only in the presence of free oxygen are called *obligatory* or *strict aerobes*, those that can grow only in the absence of free oxygen are called *obligate* or *strict anaerobes*, and those organisms that can grow in either state are termed *facultative anaerobes*. Most organisms of medical importance fall into this last group and generally grow more luxuriously under aerobic conditions. Those organisms which grow best in an atmosphere containing a reduced level of oxygen are termed *microaerophilic*.

Growth of the obligatory anaerobe depends on the state of oxidation or reduction in its environment. This oxidation–reduction (or redox) potential is a measure of the state of oxidation in a solution. It is determined by immersing an electrode in the solution and measuring the electrical potential set up between electrode and solution. This electrode potential, called Eh and measured in millivolts, is higher the more oxidized the system. Strict anaerobes are unable to grow in culture media unless the Eh is below a certain value. One explanation as to why anaerobic organisms do not grow in the presence of oxygen is that many organisms form hydrogen peroxide (H_2O_2) when incubated in the presence of oxygen. Most aerobic organisms produce an enzyme, called catalase, which catalyses $H_2O_2 \rightarrow H_2O + O$. Anaerobes do not have this enzyme, and are therefore destroyed by the peroxide. When grown in the absence of oxygen, however, H_2O_2 is not produced.

Hydrogen-ion concentration (pH)

In culture media the pH refers to its acidity or alkalinity (see p. 74). The optimum growth of most pathogenic bacteria occurs over a very narrow pH range—around the neutral region of pH 6.5–7.4. Some organisms, like lactobacilli, prefer an acid medium of around pH 4.0, while others (e.g. *Vibrio cholerae*) prefer a more alkaline range around pH 8.0–9.0.

Temperature requirements

For all micro-organisms there is a range of temperatures within which growth will take place. The *optimal temperature* is that at which growth is most luxurious. The *minimum temperature* is that below which growth ceases, but death does not necessarily occur, and the *maximum temperature* is that above which death occurs.

Types of media

Liquid media

After introduction into a liquid medium, the organism takes a little time to adjust itself to its new environment—this is called the *lag phase*, but after this initial phase the organism commences to multiply by binary fission (*Figure 23.1*). This is called the *logarithmic phase*, as multiplication is by geometric progression. After a time, due to the exhaustion of the nutritional factors of the medium and the accumulation of waste products, some bacteria die, and there is a balance of dead and living bacteria. That is, the number of bacteria multiplying is equivalent to the number of dying. This is referred to as the *stationary phase*. After this short period of equilibrium the number dying is greater than the number multiplying and the *phase of decline* sets in.

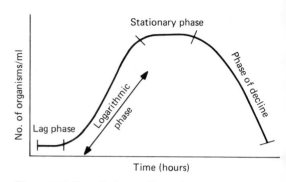

Figure 23.1. Growth phases of bacteria

As the organism grows in liquid media, it utilizes the components of the medium, and excretes by-products of bacterial metabolism into the medium. Provided the medium is originally free of these by-products, use can be made of their production to help identify the organism. For example, certain organisms produce a by-product called indole. By growing these organisms in a medium rich in the amino acid tryptophan and free from indole (e.g. peptone water) tests can be made on the culture to show whether the organism has, or has not, produced indole. Another use for liquid media is to demonstrate whether an organism has the power to ferment specific carbohydrates (sugars). To a sugar-free medium is added the specific carbohydrate, and the organism is then grown in the medium. An indicator included in the medium shows whether acid has been formed due to the fermentation of the sugar, by the organism (see p. 268).

Solid media

In liquid media the bacteria are free to move about but when grown in solid media they multiply at the site of inoculation and form colonies. The appearance of these colonies is often typical of the species. This makes possible the isolation of a single species of bacteria from a mixture. Liquid media are solidified by the addition of solidifying substances referred to as gelling agents, such as agar and gelatin.

Agar is a carbohydrate derived from seaweed. The main supply comes in powder form as distinct from the earlier Japanese shred agar. A satisfactory gel is achieved at approximately 1% concentration in nutrient broth. The *melting point* is 98°C and is cooled to 50°C before adding coagulable body fluid in the form of blood or serum. The *setting point* is 42°C.

Gelatin is a protein derived from the collagen of skin, hide, sinew and bone. It forms a satisfactory gel at a concentration of 12–15% in nutrient broth. Prolonged exposure at temperatures above 100°C destroy its setting properties. The *melting point* is 24°C. Many bacteria produce gelatinase, and their ability to liquefy gelatin is used as a means of classifying them either by their remaining liquid after growth at 37°C or by showing liquefaction after growth at room temperature.

Enriched media

If blood, serum or other enriching factors are added to a basal medium to enable organisms to grow that would not do so on the basal medium alone, that medium is termed 'enriched'. Examples are blood, serum or chocolated blood agar.

Differential media

These are media containing substances or indicators which will differentiate one organism from another. MacConkey agar will distinguish lactose-fermenting organisms from non-lactose fermenters. Blood agar will differentiate organisms by their ability to produce different types of haemolysis. These media are sometimes referred to as indicator media.

Selective media

These are *solid* media containing substances which inhibit the growth of most organisms other than those for which the media are devised; for example, tellurite media for the diphtheria bacillus and deoxycholate–citrate–agar for the *Salmonella* and *Shigella* groups.

Enrichment media

These are *fluid* selective media which incorporate substances that inhibit the growth of organisms other than those for which the medium was devised; for example, Selenite F inhibits coliform bacilli, while allowing the typhoid–paratyphoid organisms to grow freely as an enriched culture.

Auxanographic media

These are defined media lacking in certain nutritional factors. The organism is plated onto the medium and various nutritional factors are spotted onto the medium. Growth in and around these areas indicates the need of the organism for that particular factor. Identification of certain organisms can be carried out by this method.

Transport or carrier media

These are generally semi-solid media that are designed to preserve the viability of organisms for several hours or days. Swabs, containing delicate organisms, taken on a ward or at a clinic, are placed in the transport media and sent to the laboratory. As the organisms remain viable for some considerable time, delay does not prevent their isolation in the laboratory.

Storage of culture media

Media may be dispensed in bottles with rubber-lined metal screw caps, polypropylene caps or tubes plugged with non-absorbent cotton wool. Small bottles may be sterilized with their caps screwed down firmly, but not packed tightly in the baskets. The larger bottles should have their caps loosened before heating and subsequently tightened for storage.

A useful method of distinguishing between types of media is the use of coloured non-absorbent cotton wool plugs in tubes or, in the case of bottles, coloured caps or beads may be used.

Cotton wool plugs must not be so tight that air is excluded. On the other hand, they should be firm enough to allow one to raise each tube by its plug.

Media for current use should always be stored in a dust-free cupboard or in a cool, moist atmosphere. For longer periods store at 4–6°C. Each batch should be tested before use and labelled with a batch number. The shelf-life of media varies considerably. Poured plates will be used within a few days of preparation, but agar slopes should be checked to ensure that moisture is still present. Supplies of the basal media should be such that each batch is renewed within 3 months of manufacture.

Plate cultural methods

If colonial characteristics of an organism are to be examined, the petri dish is an excellent container for the medium. The shallowness of the dish and the large surface area render macroscopic examination of colonies easy, and, if necessary, microscopic examination is possible. The dish should be flat-bottomed, and either of heat-resistant soda-free glass or plastic. The most commonly used petri dishes are 90 mm diameter disposable plastic.

Glass petri dishes may be sterilized in copper tins which have a deep lid to prevent air penetration on cooling. They should be sterilized in a hot-air oven for 1 h at 160°C and allowed to cool slowly in the oven.

Plate inoculation methods

To isolate single colonies, the medium in the petri dish should be inoculated as follows.

Using a sterile loop, smear a loopful of the specimen over area A (*Figure 23.2*). Sterilize the loop in the bunsen flame, and when cool streak over

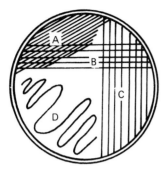

Figure 23.2. Plate inoculation method (see text for explanation)

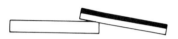

Figure 23.3. Diagram illustrating a method of drying plates

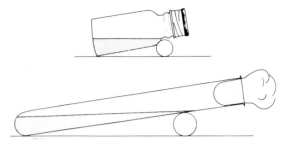

Figure 23.4. Slope cultures. A tube or a bottle containing a quantity of the medium to be solidified is slightly raised at one end

area B. Repeat over areas C and D. Incubate the plates at 37°C. The maximum available area should be used, but care must be taken not to cross a previously inoculated area.

An alternative method is to use a sterile spreader. This is a glass rod, 3 mm in diameter, bent at right angles and sterilized either by boiling, or by wrapping it in Kraft paper and placing in the hot-air oven at 160°C for 1 h. A small amount of the specimen is placed on the medium, and smeared over the whole surface, using a sterile spreader. With the same spreader, another petri dish is inoculated. Any of the specimen remaining from the first inoculation will be transferred to the second petri dish, and single colonies should be obtained. In both methods, it is essential that the medium surface is dry so that discrete colonies are obtained.

The drying of plates is performed by placing the flat surface of the lid onto an incubator shelf (at 37°C) and angling the media-containing dish (media downward) either within or on the edge of the lid (*Figure 23.3*).

Tube cultural methods

Slope cultures

Many tests devised to differentiate organisms require solid cultures. It is not always necessary to grow an organism on a whole petri dish of medium, and slope cultures often suffice. 'Slopes' or 'slants' are tubes or bottles containing a small quantity of medium that has been allowed to solidify with the bottles slightly raised at one end (*Figure 23.4*). Such

slopes are used only for maintenance or biochemical tests *once the organism has been isolated in pure culture.*

Deep cultures

'Anaerobic' organisms (see p. 261) require an oxygen-free atmosphere. For cultivation of these organisms 'shake' or 'deep' cultures are sometimes made. The medium is distributed in 150 mm × 20 mm tubes to a depth of 6–7 cm and allowed to solidify. For use, the medium is melted, cooled to about 45°C, inoculated with the organism, and mixed by rotation between the palms of the hands. When it has solidified, the culture is incubated and the anerobic organisms grow at the bottom of the tube. These shake, or deep, tubes can also be used for counts of viable organisms. In similar fashion, the medium is melted, cooled, inoculated with a known dilution of the organism and mixed. It is then poured into a sterile petri dish, and after incubation a count is made of colonies growing in and on the medium.

Roll tubes

The 'roll tube' method is also useful for counting viable organisms. The medium is distributed into 150 × 15 mm tubes, 1–2 ml per tube, and stored. For use, the medium is melted, cooled to approximately 50°C, and a known quantity of a known dilution of the test sample is added. The tube is then tilted and rolled between finger and thumb, allowing the medium to run all round the sides of the tube just below the half-way mark. This rolling is carried out under cold tap water. A thin film of agar solidifies around the sides of the tube, which is inverted for incubation. Colonies are counted on the following day. By varying the dilution of the bacterial inoculum and taking the mean of several readings, a fairly accurate count of viable organisms in a specimen can be obtained. Commercially made equipment is available for the rolling operation.

24

Preparation of culture media

In most laboratories the preparation of culture media from raw materials—such as ox-hearts—is fast disappearing, and the majority of laboratories either prepare their media from dried or dehydrated products or use ready-prepared media. Excellent as these media are, it is still advisable to check the pH of the finished product and also to perform sterility tests and quality control. Many firms produce manuals giving the composition of the media and their uses, and as these are freely available this chapter will not include precise formulae of all these media.

However, it is important to know why certain ingredients are included, to know the different types of media and to know how to estimate the pH of the medium.

The adjustment of pH

It is essential that all media are adjusted to the correct pH and great care must be taken to ensure that this is performed accurately. Usually the adjustment of pH is performed using a pH meter (see p. 75) and this is the method of choice. However, under certain conditions it may be necessary to use manual methods, and two such methods are included here—the colorimetric and the Lovibond comparator methods.

Colorimetric method

An indicator is added to the medium and to a standard buffer solution. The medium is adjusted until the colours are matched.

Apparatus required

1. Comparator rack.

2. Set of standard pH tubes, that is, tubes containing buffer solution and indicator.
3. Comparator tubes, that is, glass tubes of same bore and wall-thickness as standard tubes.
4. Indicator solution. For media, phenol red is the indicator of choice.
5. Pipettes.
6. 10M, 1.0M and 0.1M NaOH; 10M and 0.1M HCl.
7. Micro-burettes.

Method

1. Measure 5 ml of medium into each of 3 comparator tubes and 5 ml of distilled water into another comparator tube.
2. To one of the comparator tubes of medium add the same amount of indicator as is present in the standard pH tube.
3. Place tubes in comparator rack as shown in *Figure 24.1*. The standard pH tubes used should be those above and below the required pH; for example, if pH 7.5 is the desired reaction of the medium, the two standard tubes to be used should be pH 7.4 and 7.6.
4. If the medium is too alkaline, add sufficient 0.1M HCl from a burette to alter the colour of the tube containing medium and indicator, to a tint midway between those of the two standard tubes. If the medium is too acid add 0.1M NaOH instead of 0.1M HCl.

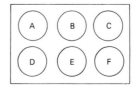

Figure 24.1. The position of tubes in a comparator rack: A and C, 5 ml of medium; B, distilled water; D and F, standard pH tubes; E, 5 ml of medium + indicator

5. Measure the volume of alkali or acid that was necessary to adjust the reaction of 5 ml of the medium.
6. Average two readings and calculate the amount of alkali or acid to add to the bulk of medium. Add the necessary alkali or acid in concentrated form.

Example of calculation

If 0.5 ml of 0.1M HCl is required to adjust the pH of 5 ml of medium, then 5 ml of 0.1M HCl would be required for 50 ml of medium and 100 ml of 0.1M HCl would be required for 1000 ml of medium, or 10 ml of 1.0M HCl, or 1 ml of 10M HCl, which is a suitable small quantity to add.

After the addition of alkali or acid to the bulk of the medium, mix well and check the pH using the same method.

Lovibond comparator

This method is also colorimetric. The sample of medium plus indicator is matched against permanent coloured-glass standards (see Chapter 6).

Method

1. Tubes A and B contain known volume of medium.
2. Add standard volume of indicator to tube B (right-hand tube).
3. Close comparator, and turn indicator disc to required pH reading.
4. Add alkali or acid to tube B, until colours are matched.
5. Calculate amount of acid or alkali to add to bulk of medium, as in the colorimetric method.

Notes on estimating the pH of media

1. Readings must not be made until the medium is cool.
2. If agar is used, the tube containing agar plus indicator, and the tube containing agar alone, must be cooled until the agar has solidified.
3. All tubes must be of the same glass, bore and wall-thickness.
4. Tubes must be thoroughly washed and rinsed with neutral distilled water before they are used again.
5. Never match colours in direct sunlight; use a north light. A special viewing box is used for artificial light.
6. One's perception of the delicate colour tints is soon dulled by prolonged examination. It is advisable to glance at the tubes briefly but frequently, when matching colours.

Preparation of culture media

1. At no stage of the preparation should a medium be overheated, for fear of destroying its nutritive qualities. Sterilization should be effected at the lowest temperature, and for the shortest time that will ensure complete sterility.
2. The adjustment of pH should be carried out accurately.
3. Utensils and glassware should be clean.
4. Fresh batches of peptone should be examined for solubility, colour (which should be pale), reaction (which should be neutral), absence of sugar and suitability for indole production. To test for presence of sugar and suitability for indole production, prepare tubes of peptone water and of peptone water plus indicator. Inoculate them with a culture which is capable of fermenting most sugars (to produce acid) and of liberating indole; the most suitable organisms for this test are those of the *Escherichia coli* group. Alternatively, a chemical test for the presence of sugar may be performed.
5. Follow the manufacturer's instructions faithfully.

Notes on some commonly used media

Nutrient broths

These are basal media used to grow a number of non-fastidious organisms and also as a basis for nutrient, blood, chocolate agar, etc.

Infusion broth

This is prepared by infusing fat-free minced meat in water overnight at 4°C.

Digest broth

Fresh lean fat-free minced meat is treated with sodium carbonate to neutralize any sarcolactic acid present in the meat. The meat is then digested by trypsin.

Meat extract broth

Commercial concentrated meat extract, dissolved in distilled water with peptone added.

Enriched media using nutrient broth

Blood broth

Sterile nutrient broth plus 5% sterile defibrinated or oxalated horse blood added aseptically.

Serum broth

Sterile nutrient broth plus 5% sterile serum added aseptically.

Chocolate broth

Blood broth mixed and heated at 70–80°C until a chocolate colour develops.

Fildes' broth

Sterile nutrient broth plus 5% Fildes' medium added aseptically.

Glucose broth

Sterile nutrient broth plus 0.25% sterile glucose.

Nutrient agar

This is nutrient broth to which agar has been added.

Some media made from nutrient agar

Blood agar slopes, serum agar slopes, chocolate agar slopes and Fildes' agar slopes

These are prepared either from individual agar slopes which are melted down, cooled and the required enrichment added, or from a larger amount of agar, as for blood agar plates, which is distributed aseptically into sterile tubes or bottles which are then sloped.

Nutrient agar plates are used for the cultivation of many easily grown organisms (e.g. staphylococci, *E. coli*). Melt the nutrient agar by steaming, cool to 50°C and pour 15–20 ml aseptically into clean sterile petri dishes.

Blood agar plates are used for the cultivation and differentiation of more delicate organisms (e.g. streptococci, gonococci).

Method 1

Melt the nutrient agar by steaming. Cool to 50°C and add 5–10% sterile defibrinated or oxalated horse blood. Pour 15–20 ml volumes aseptically into clean sterile petri dishes.

Method 2

Pour a thin layer of agar into sterile petri dishes, and when this has set, add the molten blood agar (7–10% blood). It has been stated that this method is preferable to Method 1 in that haemolysis is more easily seen, the blood agar layer is more uniform in thickness and less horse blood is used. In practice, however, now that most petri dishes have flat bottoms, many laboratories use Method 1.

Chocolate agar plates may be used for the cultivation of certain organisms (e.g. *Haemophilus influenzae* and pneumococci). Add blood to nutrient agar, as when making blood agar plates. Heat at 70–80°C for 10 min and pour aseptically into clean sterile petri dishes. *H. influenzae* requires two growth factors, called X and V. Both of these are found in blood. The X factor is haematin, and the V factor nicotinamide adenine dinucleotide (NAD). Blood contains an enzyme NADase which progressively breaks down NAD leaving little available for the bacteria to utilize. The growth of *H. influenzae* is consequently poor on blood agar plates. If, however, the blood is heated as for chocolate agar, the enzyme NADase is inactivated and more NAD is available for the bacteria, with the result that colonies of *H. influenzae* on chocolate plates are greatly increased in size.

Although many laboratories purchase ready-prepared poured plates from the several commercial firms who make them, the pouring of plates is still performed. There are several automatic plate-pouring machines on the market, the more modern of which sterilize, pour and stack the plates without supervision—thus saving valuable time.

Glucose agar

This consists of 10% solution of glucose in distilled water sterilized by Seitz filtration:

1. Taking aseptic precautions, add sufficient glucose solution to melted and cooled agar to give a final concentration of 0.5%.
2. Distribute aseptically into required containers, that is, petri dishes, tubes or bottles.
3. If in tubes or bottles, steam for 20 min, and slope if necessary.

Nutrient gelatin

Nutrient broth	1000 ml
Powdered gelatin	120–150 g

1. Dissolve in the steamer and check that pH is 7.4.
2. Tube or bottle in 10 ml quantities.
3. Sterilize by steaming for 20 min on 3 successive days.

A clear, satisfactory gel is obtained by this method, and clearing and filtering is seldom necessary. Should the medium need clearing, add the white of an egg, and steam for 30 min. Any particles present will adhere to the coagulated egg-white, and be removed by filtration.

The higher concentration of gelatin will be needed to produce firm gel in countries with a warm climate.

Carbohydrate media

Although these media can be bought ready made, many laboratories prefer to make their own and use plugged or capped tubes rather than bottles. For this reason, the preparation of this form of culture media is given in detail.

The ability of different organisms to ferment certain carbohydrates is used in their identification and classification. It is essential that the medium used for this test shall be free from all carbohydrates except those specifically added. Nutrient broth is useless for this purpose, as it contains small amounts of 'muscle' sugar. An aqueous solution of suitable peptone and sodium chloride is prepared. The selected carbohydrate and indicator is added to this solution, and it is dispensed in tubes or bottles containing a small Durham's tube. This must be inverted and completely filled with the medium. The indicator will reveal the production of acid and the inverted Durham's tube will trap any bubbles of gas that may be formed (*Figure 24.2*).

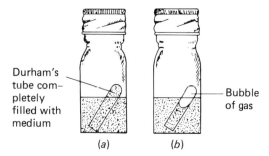

Durham's tube completely filled with medium

Bubble of gas

(a) (b)

Figure 24.2. Production of gas in a Durham's tube

For the fermentation reactions of more delicate organisms such as streptococci, pneumococci and *Corynebacterium diphtheriae*, the medium must be enriched with serum. Other organisms, such as gonococci and meningococci, grow better on a solid medium and for these agar is incorporated in the serum sugar media.

Peptone water

This is used for testing for indole production, for the preparation of sugar media, and, when alkaline, for the cultivation of *Vibrio cholerae*.

Method

Peptone	10 g
Sodium chloride	5 g
Distilled water	1000 ml

1. Dissolve in steamer.
2. Adjust reaction to pH 7.5.
3. Filter through Chardin-type filter paper.

4. Distribute in tubes or bottles.
5. Autoclave at 10 psi for 15 min.

Peptone water sugars

Preparation

1. To sterile peptone water add 1% Andrade's indicator and sufficient of a 10% solution of the required sugar (sterilized by Seitz filtration) to give a final concentration of 0.5%.
2. Distribute aseptically into sterile tubes or bottles containing inverted Durham fermentation tubes.
3. Steam for 30 min. If the medium is of the correct reaction and the indicator is satisfactory, the solution becomes pink during heating but returns to a straw colour on cooling.

Preparation of Andrade's indicator

1. Dissolve 0.5 g of acid fuchsin (CI No. 42685) in 100 ml of distilled water.
2. Add 16 ml of 1.0M NaOH and leave overnight.
3. The colour should change from pink to brownish-red and then to yellow.
4. If it is necessary to add more 1.0M NaOH, small amounts only should be added, and 24 h allowed for any colour change.

Hiss' serum water sugars

These are used for fermentation reactions of *Corynebacterium* and other genera requiring serum for growth.

Ox serum	1 part
Distilled water	3 parts

1. Adjust reaction to pH 7.5 and add Andrade's indicator, 1%, and sugar, 1%.
2. Tube or bottle and steam for 20 min on 3 consecutive days.

Solid sugar medium

This is used for fermentation reactions of *Neisseria*, and other genera requiring serum for growth.

1. Melt nutrient agar and cool to 55°C. Using aseptic precautions, add to each 100 ml the following:

0.04% phenol red solution	5 ml
Sterile rabbit serum	5 ml
10% sterile sugar solution	10 ml

2. Distribute aseptically into tubes or bottles and allow to solidify in a sloping position.
3. Test for sterility by incubation.

■ **Notes**

1. It is essential to use rabbit serum (or human serum) in

this medium, as horse, sheep or ox serum contains maltase, which may lead to a false reaction.

2. The muscle sugar content, that may be present in the nutrient broth, is so diluted that erroneous results are not obtained.

Litmus milk

Constituents

Cream-free milk (skimmed milk)
Litmus

Litmus milk is used for the fermentation of its sugar, lactose and for the clotting and digestion of milk.

Media for special purposes

Media for the isolation and identification of Gram-negative intestinal bacilli

Organisms isolated from faecal and urinary specimens may be lactose fermenters (generally non-pathogenic organisms) or non-lactose fermenters (generally pathogenic organisms). Special media are used for differentiating these organisms and for inhibiting the non-pathogens while allowing the pathogens to grow more freely.

MacConkey's agar

Constituents

Peptone
Sodium chloride
Sodium taurocholate
Lactose
Neutral red
Agar

Prepare according to manufacturer's instructions.

MacConkey's agar is used for differentiating intestinal organisms into lactose- and non-lactose-fermenting organisms. The peptone constitutes the nutrient base, solidified by the agar. Sodium taurocholate (bile salt) inhibits many Gram-positive organisms, and lactose and the indicator (neutral red) differentiate the lactose- and non-lactose-fermenting organisms. The lactose-fermenting organisms, by the fermentation of lactose, produce acids which act upon the bile salt and absorb the neutral red, giving red colonies. The non-lactose-fermenting organisms give an alkaline reaction, do not absorb the neutral red, and produce colourless colonies.

MacConkey's agar can also be prepared without the addition of sodium chloride. The absence of salt provides a low electrolyte medium which prevents most *Proteus* species from spreading.

Desoxycholate–citrate agar

Constituents

Protease peptone
Meat extract
Sodium citrate
Sodium thiosulphate
Ferric citrate
Sodium desoxycholate
Lactose
Neutral red
Agar

Prepare according to manufacturer's instructions.

A selective medium for the isolation of the *Salmonellae* and the dysentery organisms.

Sodium desoxycholate (bile salt) will inhibit the growth of many Gram-positive organisms, while favouring the growth of the intestinal Gram-negative organisms. The neutral red indicator is, however, toxic in the presence of sodium desoxycholate, and sodium citrate and sodium thiosulphate are also toxic for the coliforms and to a certain extent the *Salmonellae*. To neutralize this toxicity for the *Salmonellae*, ferric citrate is added, which does not interfere too greatly with the toxicity for the coliforms. Thus, while coliform organisms do grow on this medium, they do not grow as well as the non-lactose fermenters. The coliforms appear as pink colonies, with a precipitation of desoxycholate (due to acid production) surrounding the colony. *Proteus* species appear as colourless non-spreading colonies, generally with a black central dot, and with the characteristic fishy odour. Pathogens also appear as colourless, later pale pink, colonies sometimes with a black central dot, but rarely after 24 h incubation. This black dot is due to H_2S production by the organisms, which combines with the ferric citrate, present in the medium, to form iron sulphide.

CLED medium (Mackey and Sandys)

Constituents

Peptone
Meat extract
Tryptone
Lactose
L-cystine
Bromothymol blue
Agar powder

Prepare according to manufacturer's instructions.

The cystine–lactose–electrolyte deficient (CLED) medium is recommended for urinary bacteriology. Its electrolyte deficiency prevents the swarming of *Proteus* species and good colonial differentiation is obtained with most urinary pathogens.

Growth characteristics are as follows:

Escherichia coli	Yellow, opaque colonies with a slightly deeper coloured centre about 1.25 mm diameter. (Non-lactose-fermenting strains—blue colonies.)
Klebsiella spp.	Extremely mucoid colonies varying in colour from yellow to whitish-blue.
Proteus spp.	Translucent blue colonies usually smaller than *E. coli.*
Salmonella spp.	Flat blue colonies.
Pseudomonas pyocyanea	Green colonies with typical matt surface and rough periphery.
Streptococcus faecalis	Yellow colonies about 0.5 mm diameter.
Staphylococcus aureus	Deep yellow colonies about 0.75 mm diameter, uniform in colour.
Coagulase negative staphylococci	Pale yellow or white, more opaque than *Strep. faecalis*, often with paler periphery.
Diphtheroids	Very small grey colonies.
Lactobacilli	Similar to Diphtheroids but with a rougher surface.

Wilson and Blair's medium

Constituents

Nutrient agar
Bismuth ammonium citrate scales
Anhydrous sodium sulphite
Dextrose
Ferric–citrate scales
Sodium phosphate crystals ($Na_2HPO_4.12H_2O$)
Brilliant green

Prepare according to manufacturer's instructions.

Wilson and Blair's bismuth sulphite medium is a selective medium used for the isolation of the typhoid–paratyphoid organisms. The brilliant green, incorporated in the medium, inhibits the growth of *E. coli*. As the typhoid organism grows it reduces the sodium sulphite to sulphide which, together with the bismuth, forms bismuth sulphide. The organism in the presence of bismuth sulphide and glucose forms a black colony provided the medium is not too acid. To prevent excess acidity, sodium phosphate is present as a buffer, and ferric citrate is added to neutralize the toxicity of the bismuth.

Salmonella typhi appears as black colonies, usually within 24 h. *S. paratyphi B* appears as black colonies, usually within 48 h.

Coliform organisms are inhibited by the brilliant green and bismuth sulphite in the presence of an excess of sodium sulphite.

Selenite F medium (modified)

Constituents

Sodium acid selenite (sodium hydrogen selenite)
Peptone
Mannitol
Disodium hydrogen orthophosphate (Na_2HPO_4)

Prepare according to manufacturer's instructions.

Sodium acid selenite has, at near neutral pH, a high toxicity for *E. coli*, but not for the salmonella organisms. As the pH increases, this toxicity decreases and the buffer salt is added to help maintain the near neutral pH. A fermentable carbohydrate is included to produce acid, thus neutralizing the alkali produced by the bacterial reduction of the selenite.

It is essential to use sodium acid selenite (sodium hydrogen selenite), as ordinary sodium selenite is very alkaline, but care must be taken when using this chemical as inhalation of the powder may be dangerous.

Phenylalanine agar

Constituents

Yeast extract powder
di-Phenylalanine
Disodium hydrogen orthophosphate
Sodium chloride
Agar

Prepare according to manufacturer's instructions.

Phenylalanine is converted to phenylpyruvic acid by oxidative deamination. This is a specific property of *Proteus* and *Providence* organisms. The phenylpyruvic acid is shown by adding ferric chloride, which results in a green coloration.

Media for isolation of *Corynebacterium* group

Most media used for the isolation of *C. diphtheriae* from mixed cultures contain compounds of tellurium, which inhibit the growth of organisms not of the genus *Corynebacterium*. Once isolated, subcultures of corynebacteria can be maintained on serum media, such as Loeffler's medium.

Hoyle's medium

This is one of many media used for the isolation of corynebacteria.

Constituents

Beef extract
Proteose peptone
Sodium chloride
Agar

Add when melted:

Sterile laked horse blood
Potassium tellurite solution

Laked horse blood

Blood may be laked by freezing and thawing several times and storing in the frozen state, or by adding 0.5 ml of 10% white saponin, sterilized by autoclaving, to 10 ml of blood.

After 24–48 h incubation, colonies of the *gravis* type appear a slate-grey colour with a bluish tinge, the shape approximating to a daisy head. Colour and size of the *mitis*-type colonies are similar to the *gravis* type, but appear more glistening, are convex and have a perfectly circular outline.

Intermediate-type colonies are never larger than 2 mm. They are blacker than the other types and have a poached egg shape. Today, the corynebacteria isolated do not always conform to the above description of the classical types.

Loeffler's serum slopes

These are used for the cultivation of organisms such as *Corynebacterium diphtheriae*.

Ox serum, 3 parts
2% glucose broth, 1 part

1. Sterilize the broth by autoclaving at 115°C for 15 min.
2. Sterilize the serum by Seitz filtration.
3. Mix and distribute aseptically into sterile tubes or bottles.
4. Inspissate at 75°C until set.
5. Next day, inspissate at 75°C for 1 h. It is important not to exceed 75°C.

Egg media

Egg media are generally used for growing the tubercle bacillus, and may be purchased commercially 'ready to use'.

Lowenstein–Jensen medium is one of the most useful for the primary isolation of *Mycobacterium*

tuberculosis, the incorporated malachite green inhibiting the growth of many contaminants.

Glycerol egg

Glycerol egg is used for cultivation of human tubercle bacilli, which grow better in the presence of glycerol.

Egg	78%
Nutrient broth	20%
Glycerol	2%

1. Sterilize the broth and glycerol in the autoclave at 115°C for 15 min.
2. Break the eggs under aseptic conditions into a sterile flask containing glass beads.
3. Shake well and filter through sterile muslin into the sterile glycerol broth.
4. Distribute in sterile tubes or bottles under aseptic conditions and inspissate in a sloping position at 75–80°C. Heat until solidified.

Dorset egg

This is used for cultivation of human and bovine tubercle bacilli.

Egg	80%
Nutrient broth or saline	20%

Proceed as for glycerol egg medium.

Lowenstein–Jensen medium

This is used for the primary isolation of human tubercle bacilli. The addition of 0.5% sodium pyruvate enhances the growth of bovine tubercle bacilli.

Asparagine–mineral salt solution

Potassium dihydrogen orthophosphate (Analar)	0.4%
Magnesium sulphate (Analar)	0.04%
Magnesium citrate	0.1%
Asparagine	0.6%
Glycerol (Analar)	2.0%
In distilled water.	

Steam for 2 h and store in the refrigerator.

1. Add 6 g of potato flour (optional) to 150 ml of this solution, heat over a flame with constant stirring until a smooth mixture is obtained.
2. Sterilize in the autoclave at 115°C for 20 min.
3. Break 5 eggs, under aseptic conditions, into a sterile flask containing glass beads. Shake well and filter through sterile muslin.
4. Mix the eggs with the cool asparagine–potato starch mixture and add 5 ml of 2% malachite green (CI No. 42000) solution.

5. Distribute, under aseptic conditions, in sterile tubes or bottles and sterilize by inspissating at 75–80°C until solidified.

The tubercle bacilli obtain their nitrogen from the asparagin, and their carbon from the glycerol. The malachite green helps to inhibit the growth of other organisms.

The human type of tubercle grows as heaped-up, dry, yellow colonies, and the bovine type, if it grows, as small, discrete, colourless colonies.

Media for isolation of staphylococci

Ludlam's medium

(Selective medium for isolation of *Staphylococcus aureus* from contaminated material.)

Constituents

Beef extract
Peptone
Dipotassium hydrogen orthophosphate
  (anhydrous)
Lithium chloride
Mannitol
Potassium tellurite

Prepare according to manufacturer's instructions.

After 48 hours' incubation: *S. aureus*—dark grey or black shiny colonies; *S. epidermidis*—either no growth or small pale colonies.

Mannitol salt agar

Constituents

Peptone
Mannitol
Sodium chloride
Phenol red
Agar

Prepare according to manufacturer's instructions.

This selective medium is useful when searching for carriers of staphylococci. Presumptive coagulase-positive staphylococci produce colonies surrounded by bright orange-yellow zones. Coagulase-negative staphylococci produce colonies surrounded with a reddish zone. For carrying out the coagulase test, colonies need to be subcultured onto a medium not containing an excess of salt.

Medium for isolation of *Vibrio cholerae*

Thiosulphate citrate bile salt agar (TCBS medium)

Constituents

Peptone
Yeast extract
Sodium citrate (Analar) ($Na_3C_6H_5O_7.2H_2O$)
Sodium thiosulphate (Analar) ($Na_2S_2O_3.5H_2O$)
Sodium taurocholate
Ferric citrate
Thymol blue
Bromothymol blue
Agar

Colonies of *V. cholerae* and the El Tor biotype appear yellow on a bluish-green medium after 10–18 h incubation due to fermentation of sucrose.

Medium for isolation of *Bordetella pertussis*

Bordet-Gengou

Constituents

Potato infusion
Agar
Proteose peptone
Glycerol
Horse blood

Prepare according to manufacturer's instructions.

Two plates should be used per specimen, one containing penicillin.

Media for cultivation of anaerobic organisms

Thioglycollate broth (Brewer's broth modified)

Constituents

Sodium thioglycollate
Glucose
Powdered agar
Methylene blue (CI No. 52015)
Nutrient broth pH 7.4

Prepare according to manufacturer's instructions.

The glucose acts as a primary reducing agent, while the thioglycollate maintains the anaerobic conditions achieved after autoclaving; the sloppy agar prevents convection currents and the methylene blue acts as an indicator, remaining colourless except where oxygen is present at the surface of the medium.

Cooked meat medium

Cooked meat medium prepared in the laboratory is often better than the dehydrated product.

1. Boil 500 g of minced ox heart in 500 ml of 0.05M NaOH, to neutralize its lactic acid content.
2. Drain off fluid and partially dry the meat with a clean cloth.
3. Fill narrow-necked 1 oz bottles, with screw caps and rubber washers, to a depth of 50 mm (2 in).
4. Add nutrient broth to 25 mm (1 in) above the level of the meat.
5. Sterilize at 121°C for 20 min.

The meat particles contain reducing substances which maintain anaerobic conditions at the bottom of the tube, and also prevent convection currents.

Transport media

A transport medium enables delicate pathogens such as *Neisseria gonorrhoeae* and *Bordetella pertussis* to survive on the swab until cultured. The medium is also of value as an aid in the recovery of *Shigella* species from rectal swabs.

Stuart's transport medium

Constituents

Sodium thioglycollate
Sodium glycerophosphate
Calcium chloride
Powdered agar
Methylene blue (CI No. 52015), 1% aqueous solution
Glass-distilled water

Prepare according to manufacturer's instructions.

Amies transport medium

Constituents

Neutral charcoal
Sodium chloride
Sodium hydrogen phosphate
Potassium dihydrogen orthophosphate
Potassium chloride
Sodium thioglycollate
Calcium chloride
Magnesium chloride
Agar

Prepare according to manufacturer's instructions.

The concentration of salt used is optimal for the preservation of *N. gonorrhoeae* and the calcium and magnesium salts control the permeability of the bacterial cells, increasing their survival time. The charcoal increases the survival of *N. gonorrhoeae*.

Instructions sent with transport outfit

'Take the specimen and insert the swab or swabs into the upper third of the medium in the small bottle. Cut off the protruding portion of the swab stick with scissors and screw the lid on the bottle, tightly. This usually forces the swab down slightly and centres it in the transport medium. Label the bottle and return it with swabs enclosed to the laboratory as soon as possible. Keep specimens in a refrigerator at 4°C until ready for shipment.'

Quality control of media

All fresh batches of bulk media should be tested for their quality, by comparison with either a previous batch and/or other media.

Selective media

Viable counts should be performed on plates poured from the bulk. Selected organisms are used. For example, with desoxycholate citrate media, *Escherichia coli*, *Salmonella typhimurium* and *Shigella sonnei* would be the organisms used, and viable counts compared with those performed on MacConkey or nutrient agar plates. The *E. coli* should be suppressed or grow very poorly on the DCA, while the counts and size of the other organisms should be similar on both media.

Enrichment media

These should be tested for their inhibitory and nutritional powers by inoculating with selected organisms.

For example, Selenite F medium would be inoculated with *E. coli* and *Sal. typhimurium*, incubated at 37°C and then plated on to MacConkey agar. The *E. coli* should be inhibited, but the *Sal. typhimurium* should grow.

Fermentation media

These should be tested with selected organisms that will:

1. Ferment the sugar with gas production.
2. Ferment the sugar without gas production.
3. Not ferment the sugar.

Other media should be tested for their ability to support the growth of exacting and other organisms.

Sterility testing

Media prepared from bulk should be tested for sterility by overnight incubation at 37°C.

An exception to this rule may be made in the case of blood agar plates. Selected plates (the last one poured from each flask) are chosen for incubation to check the sterility of the blood, agar and glassware. The rest of the batch are stored at 4°C until they are required for use.

25

Methods for anaerobic cultivation of bacteria

Cultivation of anaerobes (see p. 261) can be performed in several ways.

Growth in special media

Glucose broth

Long thin tubes are half-filled with this medium, boiled for 5 min to remove dissolved oxygen, and the surface of the medium is covered with sterile molten Vaseline. This seals the medium from the air, and inoculation is carried out through the layer of Vaseline by means of a Pasteur pipette.

Thioglycollate broth (see p. 272)

Cooked meat medium (see p. 273)

Iron strips

Heated to redness, cooled, and added to liquid media, iron strips will oxidize in the medium, and produce anaerobic conditions.

The anaerobic jar

Undoubtedly, the best general method of anaerobic cultivation is the use of the anaerobic jar. It is capable of producing conditions sufficiently anaerobic to grow the strictest anaerobes (e.g. *Clostridium tetani*) and allows specimens to be directly streaked out, in the normal way, on solid media.

The jar

A seamless metal or plastic vessel, sufficiently large to contain petri dishes and tubes, is fitted with a gas-tight lid. The lid has inlet and outlet valves and, on its inner surface, a room-temperature catalyst enclosed within a wire gauze envelope. The catalyst consists of alumina pellets coated with 0.5% palladium which catalyses the combination of oxygen in the jar with hydrogen to form water.

Method of use

1. Place cultures in the jar, taking care to loosen the tops of screw-capped bottles. Secure the lid.
2. Close the inlet valve, connect the outlet valve to a vacuum pump, and evacuate to approximately 10 cm Hg. This is monitored on a vacuum gauge. After disconnecting the vacuum pump, the reading on the vacuum gauge should remain constant for 5 min. If it fails to maintain a vacuum, check the lid washer and valve seatings (see below).
3. Connect the inlet valve to a supply of carbon dioxide, nitrogen and hydrogen. A convenient method is to supply the gas from a football bladder or anaesthetic apparatus bag that has been filled from a cylinder.
4. Open the inlet valve. The gas will quickly enter the jar and the residual oxygen will react with the hydrogen to form water on the gauze cover of the catalyst.
5. After 3 min the reaction should be complete' and the inlet valve may be closed. After disconnecting the bag, the formation of a secondary vacuum is checked before placing the jar in the incubator.

One advantage of this type of jar is that the process of evacuation causes oxygen dissolved in liquid media (e.g. sugar fermentation tubes) to be displaced by the reduced pressure, thereby ensuring correct anaerobic conditions *within the tubes*.

'Gas Pak' type of systems

Another version of the anaerobic jar has come into common use, namely the self-contained CO_2–H_2 anaerobic system. The principle employed here is the generation of both hydrogen and carbon dioxide by adding water to prepacked chemicals, thereby eliminating the need for any external apparatus and manipulations. These sachets are available from various commercial sources.

Testing anaerobic jars

In order to test that anaerobic conditions have been achieved, jars are commonly fitted with side arms to which are attached tubes containing chemical redox indicators.

If anaerobic conditions have not been obtained in the anaerobic jar, the reason may be that either the jar leaks, or the capsule is not working.

To test if the jar is leaking, place a piece of cotton wool soaked in ether into the jar. Clamp down the lid and close all taps. Immerse in a bucket of warm water. This will cause the ether to expand in the jar, and force air out of any leak that has occurred, thus producing bubbles at the site of the leak. The capsule may need renovating and heating it will remove the moisture which can interfere with the catalyst activity.

Indicators

Alkaline methylene blue–glucose solution

Solution 1:

0.1M sodium hydroxide	6 ml
Distilled water	94 ml

Solution 2:

0.5% methylene blue (CI No. 52015)	3 ml
Distilled water	97 ml

Solution 3:

Glucose	6 g
Distilled water	100 ml

Add a small crystal of thymol as a preservative.

For use, mix equal volumes of solutions 1, 2 and 3 in a test-tube. Boil until colourless and place in the anaerobic jar. Clamp lid and proceed as previously described.

Alternatively, alkaline glucose broth (pH 8.5) with methylene blue added can be used in the same way.

Semi-solid indicator

Some anaerobic jars have a side arm to which an indicator tube is attached with a short length of rubber tubing. The following indicator is for use with such jars:

Sodium thioglycollate	0.1%
Borax	1.0%
Methylene blue (CI No. 52015)	0.02%
Agar	0.5%

Dissolve by boiling, cool to approximately 50°C and dispense in $6.5 \times 100\,mm$ tubes (as used for freeze drying). Place on manifold of freeze-drying machine, evacuate over P_2O_5 and seal tubes with double-headed burner.

If a freeze-drying unit is not available, the tubes are boiled and sealed immediately the mixture is colourless.

Both these indicators will remain colourless in the absence of free oxygen. If they have turned blue, anaerobic conditions have not been achieved.

Biological indicators

A plate inoculated with a strict anaerobe, e.g. *Clostridium tetani*, can be included in each jar and examined after incubation for growth.

However, the discovery on the following morning that the jar *was* not anaerobic is of little value and no comfort to the bacteriologist. It is therefore of more importance regularly to *check* the jar for air leaks and for catalyst activity.

Use of an anaerobic jar for CO_2 cultivation

It is often necessary to grow organisms in an atmosphere of CO_2. The simplest method is to place the cultures in a jar together with a lighted candle. Screw down the lid of the jar and incubate. The candle utilizes some of the oxygen present, giving an atmosphere of CO_2.

If an exact 10% CO_2 is required the procedure is as follows:

1. Place the cultures in an anaerobic or similar jar, and screw down the lid.
2. Attach one outlet tap on the lid to a manometer and the other to a vacuum pump.
3. Evacuate air, until the manometer reads 100 mmHg.
4. Close the vacuum pump tap, and attach to a source of CO_2 (a rubber football bladder filled from a cylinder).
5. Allow CO_2 to enter the jar until the manometer reads 24 mmHg.
6. Close both taps, take the jar into the incubator, open the taps and allow the warm air to enter the jar.
7. Close the taps and leave to incubate.

■ Notes

1. If a complete vacuum was obtained in the jar the manometer would read 760 mmHg; therefore, 10% of that

atmosphere would be 76 mmHg. By evacuating to 100 mmHg and running in CO_2 until the manometer reads 24 mmHg, 10% of that atmosphere has been replaced with CO_2.

2. The opening of the taps in the incubator warms the cultures and also mixes the CO_2 with the air present in the jar. Using this method, any amount of CO_2 can be introduced into the jar.

Anaerobic cabinets

During the past few years, anaerobic cabinets have been introduced into many laboratories. It is possible to carry out routine bacteriological techniques within these cabinets in an anaerobic atmosphere. Thus, isolation culture techniques and subculture can be performed in the absence of free oxygen.

26

Antigen–antibody reactions

Antigens and antibodies

When certain foreign substances, usually proteins, are introduced into the animal blood stream, they trigger a specific response by certain specialized lymphoid cells resulting in the production of blood proteins called *immunoglobulins*. Each such foreign protein is an *antigen*; a bacterial cell thus contains many different antigens. The specific immunoglobulin produced in response to each different antigen is called *antibody*, and a serum containing antibodies is an *antiserum*.

Antibody molecules combine specifically with their corresponding (homologous) antigens. *In vivo*, this constitutes an important defence mechanism against microbial infection. Motile bacteria are immobilized when their flagellar antigens combine with specific antibodies, and toxic substances—both diffusible toxins, e.g. diphtheria toxin and cell-bound virulence factors, e.g. streptococcal M-substance—can be neutralized by combination with antibodies. The blood also contains a series of proteins known collectively as *complement* (C′). Complement is bound non-specifically by antigen–antibody complexes and can then initiate lysis (if the 'antigen' is a bacterial or other cell) and promote phagocytosis of bacteria in which the antibody has been absorbed.

These same reactions can be exploited by the microbiologist in the routine diagnostic laboratory.

It is important to note that the microbiologist may use a 'known' antiserum to detect specific antigens in an 'unknown' organism and, vice versa, a known antigen preparation to test for specific antibody in an 'unknown' serum. For example, in the diagnoses of typhoid fever, bacteria isolated from faecal specimens may be identified as *Salmonella typhi* by agglutination reactions using a variety of known antisera—some of which have been purified to contain antibodies against a single antigen ('single factor sera'). Conversely, a presumptive diagnosis of typhoid fever may be obtained by agglutination reactions carried out onto patient's serum against known suspensions of *Salmonella typhi* and the closely related bacteria of paratyphoid fever. (This is known as the Widal reaction.) This approach is, in general, less satisfactory, since each bacterial suspension is necessarily a mixture of antigens, many of which are shared by related bacteria. Previous immunization may also confuse the issue.

H and O antigens

In 1903, Smith and Reagh discovered that the motile hog cholera bacillus had a non-motile variant. When agglutination tests were performed using antiserum produced by the motile organism, the non-motile organism gave a different agglutination reaction to the motile type. Whereas the motile organism gave a rapid fluffy type of agglutination, the non-motile organism gave a slower granular agglutination. A year later, Beyer and Reagh heated the motile organisms to 70°C for 15 min and showed that the heated motile organism agglutinated in the same way as the non-heated, non-motile organism did, because the flagellar antigen had been destroyed. These workers proved that a motile organism has two antigens, one flagellar antigen, the other the body antigen, while a non-motile organism only has the body antigen.

In 1917, Weil and Felix were performing agglutination tests with a flagellated motile organism that spread over the surface of an agar plate (*Proteus*). It gave an appearance resembling the mist caused by breathing on glass, and they named it the *Hauch* form—*Hauch* meaning breath. A non-flagellated, and therefore non-motile, variant of the same organism gave discrete colonies on the same media and was named the *Ohne Hauch* form—the non-breath form. The two forms were symbolized as the H and O forms; this designation has been extended, and H is now used as a symbol for all flagellar antigens irrespective of whether the organism spreads on agar, and O as the symbol for the body or somatic antigen. The antibodies against these antigens are called H and O antibodies, respectively.

The main serological methods used by the microbiologist as diagnostic aids and identification are as follows: agglutination, precipitation, complement fixation and labelled antibody tests (fluorescence, etc.).

Agglutination

This is the binding together of antigens and antibodies which results in the formation of *visible* clumps. The antigens are usually particulate (e.g. bacterial cells, as in the case of Salmonella O and H agglutination tests).

Agglutination tests

Tube agglutination

Apparatus required

Pipettes, test-tubes, agglutination tubes, grease pencil, racks for tubes, serum, saline, antigen and 50°C water bath.

1. Place 10 test-tubes in a rack.
2. Add 4 vol of saline to tube 1 and 1 vol to tubes 2–10.
3. Add 1 vol of serum to tube 1 and mix. This dilutes the serum 1 in 5, i.e. 1 vol of serum plus 4 vol of saline, giving 5 vol of solution of which 1 vol is serum.
4. Transfer 1 vol of serum saline solution to tube 2. This dilutes the serum 1 in 10.
5. Repeat the procedure up to and including tube 10. This gives serum dilutions of 1 in 5, 1 in 10, 1 in 20, 1 in 40, 1 in 80, 1 in 160, 1 in 320, 1 in 640, 1 in 1280 and 1 in 2560.
6. Using a fresh pipette and, starting from the highest dilution, transfer 0.5 ml from each test-tube into a corresponding agglutination tube rack.
7. Add 0.5 ml of antigen to each tube. The addition of an equal quantity of antigen dilutes the serum again, the final serum dilution being 1 in 10 in the first tube, 1 in 20 in the second tube, and so on.
8. To another agglutination tube add 0.5 ml of saline and 0.5 ml of antigen. This tube serves as a control and shows if the antigen is salt-agglutinable.
9. Place the agglutination rack in the water bath and adjust the water level until it covers one-third of the tube.

Slide agglutination test

For rapid identification of colonies from an agar medium, slide agglutinations can be performed using the colony suspended in saline as the antigen and mixing with known serum. Only O agglutinations should be performed this way, as solid media are not good for the formation of flagella and false negative slide H agglutinations may occur. Slide agglutinations should be confirmed by the tube technique.

Method

1. Place 1 drop of saline on a slide, and next to it, 1 drop of required serum.
2. Using a straight wire, transfer part of the colony to be tested to the saline and mix, making a smooth suspension.
3. If no auto-agglutination has taken place, mix the serum with the smooth suspension.
4. Look for agglutination, which should occur within 10–15 s.

Notes on agglutination tests

1. Agglutination will take place only in the presence of an electrolyte; therefore, 0.9% sodium chloride should be used as a diluent.
2. Immunoglobulins are thermolabile; therefore, temperatures in excess of 50°C should not be used.
3. Flagellar antigens agglutinate more quickly than the somatic antigens; they can be read after 2 h incubation at 50°C. Somatic antigens are best incubated at 37°C for 2 h followed by refrigeration at +4°C overnight; the results are recorded after warming to 37°C for 10 min.
4. During incubation the water level should be adjusted so that one-third of the tube is immersed. This allows the formation of convection currents which aid mixing and thereby speed the agglutination reaction.

Carrier particle agglutinations

If there is no particulate phase in the system it is possible to bind either the antigen or antibody onto carrier particles such as latex beads, erythrocytes or *Staphylococcus aureus*–protein A complexes (coagglutination).

Latex agglutination

Antibodies to microbial antigens are attracted to the latex particle and the reagent is then used to detect homologous antigens in body fluids. It has been used to detect *Haemophilus, pneumococcus* and meningococcus antigen in CSF, urine and serum or for the serological identification of bacteria such as streptococci.

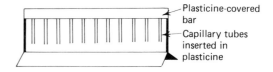

Figure 26.1. Rack for capillary tubes

Haemagglutination

Tannic acid treated erythrocytes will bind *Treponema pallidum* extracts and these can be used in the *Treponema pallidum* haemagglutination (TPHA) test for the detection of syphilis antibodies. In the case of hepatitis B infection, erythrocytes coated with homologous antiserum will detect Australia antigen (HB_sAg) in patient's serum.

Coagglutination

Staphylococcus aureus (Cowan strain) is rich in protein A and this protein binds IgG molecules. The antibody-coated staphylococcus will agglutinate in the presence of homologous antigen and can be used for the rapid detection of antigens in body fluids or for the identification of organisms (e.g. Phadebact test for *Neisseria gonorrhoeae*).

Precipitation

In these tests a *solution* (or a chemical extract) of an antigen combines with specific antibody to form a precipitate. Lancefield's streptococcus grouping is an example of a precipition reaction.

Lancefield grouping (Fuller's formamide method)

1. Centrifuge overnight glucose broth culture or growth from a blood agar plate at 3000 rpm for 5–10 min and discard supernatant.
2. Add 0.1 ml formamide (boiling point 180°C) to the deposit and boil for 1 min.
3. Cool and add 0.25 ml of acid alcohol (95 ml C_2H_5OH + 5 ml 2M HCl) to the clear fluid. This precipitates the protein fraction. Add 0.5 ml of acetone to precipitate the carbohydrate.
4. Dissolve the precipitation in 3–4 drops of normal saline and add 1 drop phenol red. Adjust pH to alkaline using 0.03M NaOH.
5. Centrifuge and remove supernatant which contains the carbohydrate (antigen Ag).

Test

Using capillary tubes inserted in plasticine carry rack, as shown in *Figure 26.1:*

1. Take up a loopful of carbohydrate (Ag)—see *Figure 26.2*—and touch opening of capillary tube (a), allowing a small amount to move up the tube by capillary action (b).
2. Take up a loopful of grouping antiserum (Ab)—see *Figure 26.2*—and touch opening of capillary tube, allowing a small amount to enter (c).

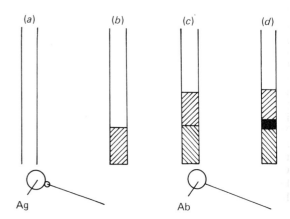

Figure 26.2. Precipitation method

3. Within 1 min a visible line of precipitation should appear if the antigen and antibody are homologous (d).
4. Repeat the test for the other grouping antiserum.

Gel precipitation method

In the above method, precipitation at the interphase of the two reagents results in a visible ring. For other antigen–antibody combinations, the precipitation reaction can be more easily demonstrated in agar gel. There are a number of different gel diffusion methods, such as immunodiffusion and immunoelectrophoresis.

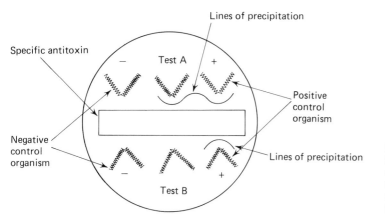

Figure 26.3. Elek plate. Test organism A produces lines of precipitation which identify with the positive control—positive result; test organism A does not produce lines of precipitation—negative result

Immunodiffusion

In this test the antigens and antibodies are allowed to diffuse towards each other and a precipitate occurs when the antigen and antibody meet in optimal proportions. This is the principle employed in the Elek plate for the detection of diphtheria toxin by the demonstration of toxin–antitoxin precipitations. Briefly, a strip of filter paper is dipped in a solution of purified diphtheria antitoxin containing 1000 units/ml and allowed to drain before planing across the surface of a 20% calf serum agar plate. The test organisms, along with a known positive and negative strain, are inoculated as shown in *Figure 26.3* before incubation at 35°C for 24–48 h. When toxin is produced it will diffuse into the agar and lines of precipitation will occur where it meets the antitoxin diffusing from the strip (*Figure 26.3*). Confirmation that the line of precipitation is caused by toxin is obtained by comparing its position with lines formed by the positive control.

Immunoelectrophoresis

These techniques use the same principle as immuno-diffusion except that the antigens are caused to move by the application of an electric current. Where both antigen and antibody are driven towards each other across the gel, the technique is termed counter-current immunoelectrophoresis (CIE). This latter technique has been used for demonstration analysis in body fluids (e.g. meningococci in cerebrospinal fluid) or antibodies in patient serum against fungal agent.

Complement fixation

Complement is a thermolabile group of proteins present in serum (see p. 355). It has the property of binding to antigen–antibody complexes. Free complement is then said to be 'fixed', i.e.

$Ag_1 + Ab_1 \rightarrow Ag{-}Ab$ complex
$Ag{-}Ab$ complex $+ C' \rightarrow Ag{-}Ab{-}C'$ complex

Furthermore, complement has enzymatic activity which breaks down cell membranes and should the antigen be whole bacterial cells or red blood cells, then lysis of these cells will occur, but only in the presence of specific antibody and complement. Thus, using red blood cells (RBC) as antigens and anti-RBC antibody we have a sensitive *inidicator system* for detecting free complement where the cells remain intact (*Figure 26.4*).

Remembering, therefore, that complement only attaches to antigen–antibody complexes, then if antigen or antibody is missing complement will not be fixed; it will be free in the system and thus detectable by the indicator system. Using complement fixation we have a useful technique for detecting both antigen and antibody.

Thus, using a known test antigen (Ag_1), the presence of specific antibody (Ab_1) can be detected in patient's serum. In the example shown in *Figure 26.4*, patient 1 has antibody to the test antigen but patient 2 does not. In a similar way, using a test antibody, antigen can be detected.

Labelled antibody tests

It is possible to bind various 'labels' onto antibodies without altering their ability to attach antigens. Three types of label are commonly used, namely, fluorochromes, enzymes and radioactive substances, giving rise respectively to fluorescent antibody (FAB) tests, enzyme-linked immunosorbent assays (ELISA) and radioimmunoassays (RIA) (see Chapter 6). There are a number of ways in which tests using these labelled antibodies are carried out—direct, indirect or sandwich techniques. *Figure 26.5*

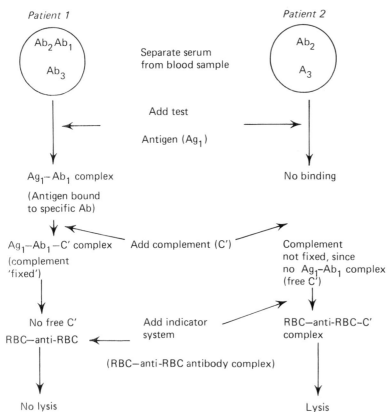

Figure 26.4. Complement fixation tests (A or Ab, antibody; Ag, antigen)

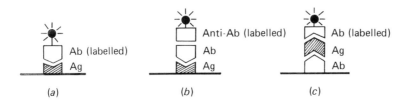

Figure 26.5. The three methods of using labelled antibodies: (a) direct; (b) indirect; (c) sandwich (Ab, antibody; Ag, antigen)

outlines the steps undertaken to detect antibody in patients' serum using the three different labelling methods.

The methods outlined in *Figure 26.6* are examples using a solid phase onto which antigen or antibody is attached. However, it is possible to use a system where the antigen is not bound to a solid phase but is free in solution. The enzyme multiplied immunoassay test (EMIT) is an example of such a system. The EMIT can be used for detecting antibiotics in

patients' serum. Briefly, in this system (*Figure 26.7*) the drug is labelled with an enzyme and when the enzyme-labelled drug becomes bound to an antibody against the drug, the activity of the enzyme is reduced. Drug present in the patient's serum competes with the enzyme-labelled drug for the antibody, thereby decreasing the antibody-induced inactivation of the enzyme. The activity of the enzyme is measured by monitoring the colour change following addition of a suitable substrate.

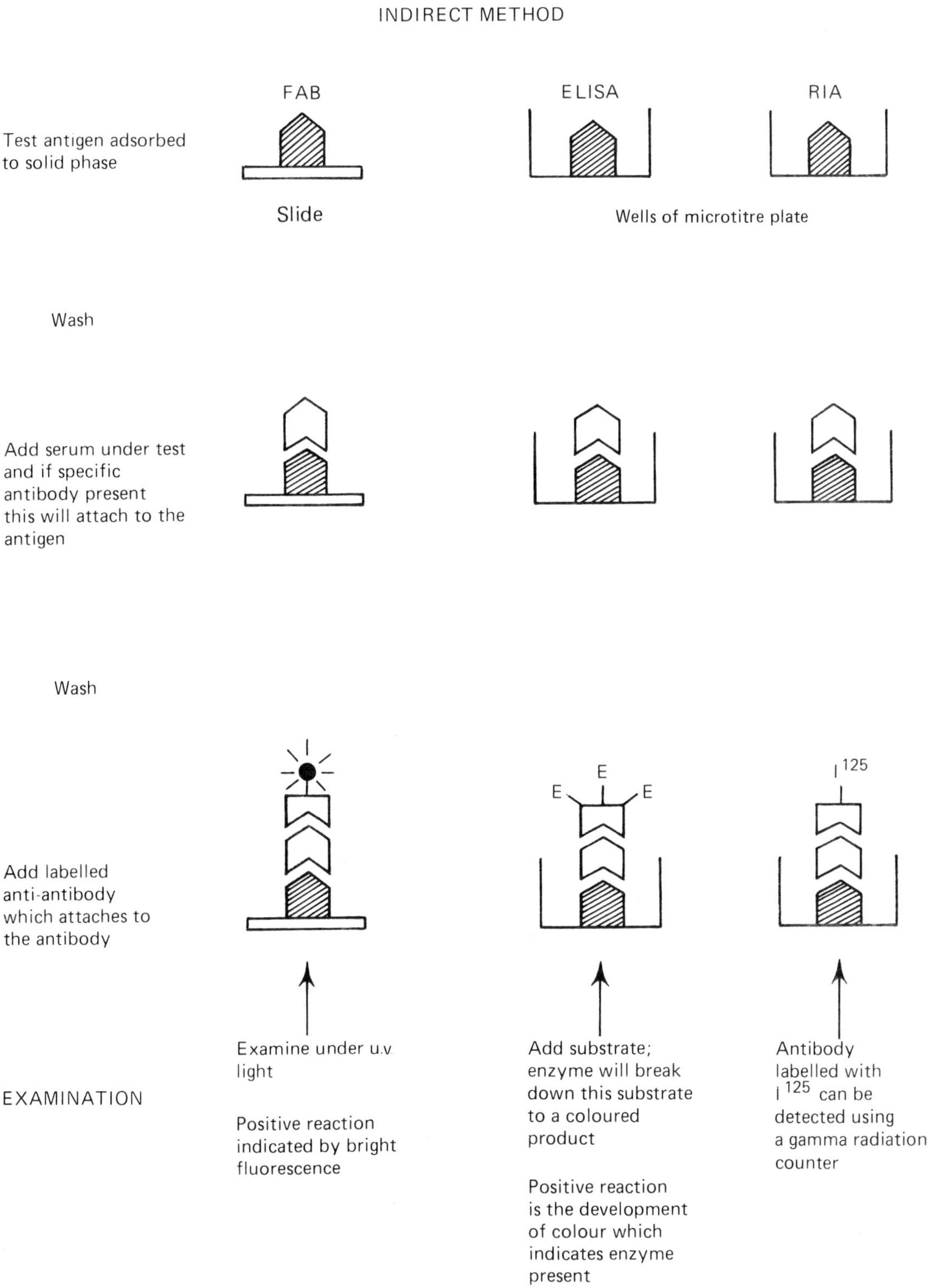

INDIRECT METHOD

Figure 26.6. Labelled antibody tests: fluorescent antibody (FAB) tests; enzyme-linked immunosorbent assays (ELISA); radioimmunoassays (RIA). Shaded, antigen; unshaded, antibody

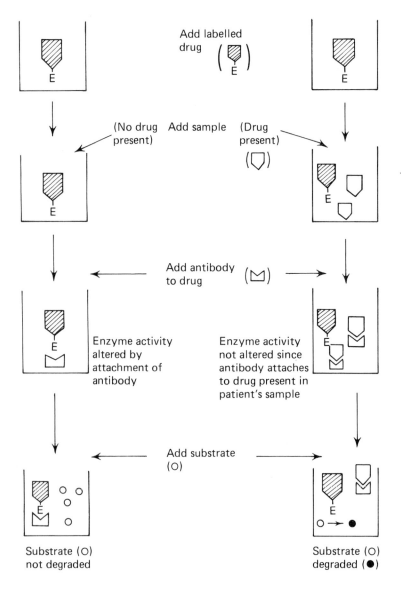

Add labelled drug

(No drug present)   Add sample   (Drug present)

Add antibody to drug

Enzyme activity altered by attachment of antibody

Enzyme activity not altered since antibody attaches to drug present in patient's sample

Add substrate (O)

Substrate (O) not degraded

Substrate (O) degraded (●)

Test sample: NEGATIVE

Test sample: POSITIVE

Figure 26.7. Enzyme multiplied immunoassay test (EMIT)

Dilutions

The preparation of 'dilutions' often causes a certain amount of trouble. The one cardinal rule to remember is that if one volume of a concentrated or neat solution is diluted with an equal volume of diluent (e.g. distilled water), then that solution has been diluted 1 in 2. That is:

1 vol of solution + 1 vol of diluent = 1 in 2

If this 1 in 2 solution is further diluted with an equal volume of diluent then the solution has been diluted 1 in 4. That is:

1 vol of 1 in 2 solution + 1 vol of diluent = 1 in 4

or a ½-solution diluted:

½ = ½ × ½ = ¼ = 1 in 4

If a neat solution is diluted with twice its volume

of diluent, then the resultant dilution is 1 in 3. That is:

1 vol of solution + 2 vol of diluent = 1 in 3

It will be seen, therefore, that if a 1 in 3 solution is diluted 1 in 4, the resultant dilution is 1 in 12. That is:

$\frac{1}{4} \times \frac{1}{3} = \frac{1}{12} = 1$ in 12

If the above approach is taken, any dilution should be readily obtained.

The following equation is useful when the dilution of solutions of known strengths is required: where R is the required concentration, V the total volume of solution required and O the original concentration, then $(R \times V)/O$ gives

Volume of original solution to be diluted with distilled water to the final volume required

Example

The original solution is 70%; 45 ml of 30% solution is required. Using the equation:

$$\frac{30 \times 45}{70} = 19.3$$

Therefore, 19.3 ml of 70% solution must be diluted with 25.7 ml of distilled water to obtain 45 ml of a 30% solution.

27

Routine bacteriological examination of specimens

Strict safety precautions have now been laid down for the handling of specimens suspected of containing pathogens. In the UK, the Advisory Committee on Dangerous Pathogens have issued a report on the categorization of pathogens according to risk and categories of containment. Organisms are classified into four hazard groups:

Group 1. An organism that is most unlikely to cause human disease.

Group 2. An organism that may cause human disease and which might be hazardous to laboratory workers, but is unlikely to spread in the community. Laboratory exposure rarely produces infection and effective prophylaxis or effective treatment are usually available.

Group 3. An organism that may cause human disease and present a serious hazard to laboratory workers. It may present a risk of spread in the community, but there is usually effective prophylaxis or treatment available.

Group 4. An organism that causes severe human disease and is a serious hazard to laboratory workers. It may present a high risk of spread in the community and there is usually no effective prophylaxis or treatment.

For each of these groups there is a defined physical containment level, and it is essential that all laboratory workers are aware of these requirements and adhere to them.

As there are many types of specimens received daily in a routine microbiology laboratory, and laboratories have their own individual methods for treating and examining specimens, only a broad outline will be given here. The student, in addition to being aware of the laboratory's methods, should also refer to the more advanced textbooks on microbiology (see Bibliography).

General procedure

1. The specimen should be properly labelled with the patient's name, hospital number, ward and date of collection. This is essential in order to prevent confusion of specimens from patients of similar name. The date of collection is required so that delays in reaching the laboratory are apparent, and misleading results avoided; for example, pathogens in urine may be overgrown by contaminants if there is a long delay in transit from ward to laboratory.

2. The request form should state the provisional diagnosis and the nature of examination required. This facilitates selection of techniques; for example, if a specimen of sputum is sent for detection of *Mycobacterium tuberculosis* (in a suspected case of pulmonary tuberculosis), detailed examination for other organisms is obviously not required.

3. Any information with regard to the chemotherapy should be noted. Certain precautions may be necessary; for example, specimens from patients receiving sulphonamides should be inoculated on to media containing *p*-aminobenzoic acid, which prevents the bacteriostatic action of sulphonamides on the organisms. Similarly, the use of penicillinase may be required for the isolation of organisms from a patient receiving penicillin.

4. The correct container should be used. Most specimens for bacteriological examination should be received in a sterile container. For sputum, particularly for out-patients who send their specimens by post, urine and blood, wide-mouthed universal bottles are convenient. For specimens that are to be treated by a concentration method for *M. tuberculosis*: plastic cartons are suitable for sputa or faeces; narrow-mouthed

universal bottles, containing 3.8% sodium citrate for pleural fluids; and wide-mouthed universal bottles with 15% trisodium orthophosphate, for specimens of gastric lavage. It is obvious that a specimen received in a gastric lavage bottle would be useless for general investigation of organisms present. By the time it reached the laboratory, many of the bacteria would be destroyed by the trisodium orthophosphate.

Microbiological safety cabinets

All work involving the handling of specimens and cultures containing or suspected of containing Group 3 organisms, or under certain conditions Group 2 organisms, should be performed under cover of a Class I or Class III safety cabinet. The design of a cabinet should be such that it conforms to British Standard (BS) 5726: 1979 'Specification for Microbiological Safety Cabinets' (British Standards Institution, London). This gives a description of the three types of safety cabinet—Classes I, II and III. It also gives methods of testing air speeds, filtration efficiency and for determining the level of protection provided.

Class I cabinets are open-front exhaust protection cabinets that protect the worker against the inhalation of aerosols containing organisms, etc.

Class II cabinets are laminar flow cabinets, primarily designed to control airborne contamination of the material inside the cabinet and offering some protection to the worker.

Class III cabinets are totally enclosed exhaust protective cabinets which are airtight and are fitted with glove ports. This cabinet is the only one that can be used for working with Group 4 organisms.

General precautions

Other precautions when dealing with all specimens or cultures are:

1. Never lay a culture tube on the bench; always place it in a rack or tin.
2. Label clearly *every* tube or plate with the specimen's number.
3. When finished, always discard the cultures into an appropriate discard receptacle for sterilizing. Never remove the cultures once discarded until they have been sterilized.
4. Keep the working space on the bench clear so that if an accident occurs the minimum number of articles will be involved.
5. Handle all apparatus and materials carefully.
6. Do not smoke when working with specimens or cultures. Never lay a pipette mouthpiece on the bench.
7. When pipetting always use a teat or other pipetting device; *never pipette by mouth*.
8. Do not lick gummed labels.
9. Wear rubber gloves when handling all blood specimens.
10. Report any accident, however trivial, to the senior person in the laboratory.
11. Always wash your hands with soap and water after handling cultures and specimens, and before going off duty. It is recommended that disposable paper or continuous roller towels be provided to minimize any possibility of cross-infection.

Postage of pathological specimens

Certain regulations are laid down by the Postmaster-General for the sending of specimens through the post. Universal containers wrapped in absorbent cotton wool and sent in wooden or metal boxes are permissible, provided the label is clearly marked 'Pathological Specimen' and 'Fragile with Care'. These regulations may be obtained from the Post Office, and if the suitability of any box or container is in doubt, it should be submitted to the Secretary of the Post Office, for confirmation of its suitability. Failure to do so may lead to the prosecution of the person sending the specimen.

Examination of specimens

A general plan for examining specimens is as follows.

Macroscopic examination

Note the following:

1. Colour, opacity, consistency.
2. Presence of blood, mucus or pus.
3. Presence of macroscopic bodies, such as parasites.

Microscopic examination

1. Unstained film or negative staining, e.g. when looking for cells or casts in urine deposit.
2. Stained film by (a) Gram; (b) acid-fast bacilli stain; (c) special stains.

Culture

Inoculate the appropriate media according to the specimen being examined.

Examination of cultures

Keep extensive notes on the examination of the cultures set up as follows:

Plate cultures

Note types of colony seen and list as 1, 2, 3, and so on. Note the shape, colour, size, consistency, haemolysis and Gram stain reaction.

Liquid cultures

Note nature of the medium such as colour, type of growth (granular, smooth, surface, etc.) or deposit.

Microscopic appearance of bacteria

Note shape, size, arrangement, motility, staining reaction, spores, capsules, pleomorphism.

For the final report, however, it is only necessary to report the organism or organisms seen in smear and isolated on culture together with the sensitivity pattern.

Blood cultures

In certain diseases, for example, septicaemia and typhoid fever, bacteria may be present in the blood, and the presence of the causative organisms may be detected by cultures. Blood is taken from the patient, and immediately inoculated into tubes or bottles of a suitable medium. These are incubated at 37°C. If possible, a 'pour plate' should be made with the patient's blood and nutrient agar. This is a good guide to the number of organisms present in the blood as well as hastening identification. From normal blood, the cultures are sterile.

The blood must be added to media that inhibit the natural antibactericidal power of the blood and that prevent clotting. Sodium polyethanol sulphonate (Liquoid) not only prevents clotting but also neutralizes the bactericidal power of fresh blood when used at a concentration of 0.03–0.05 g per 100 ml.

The medium is placed in bottles which have perforated caps, thus enabling the syringe needle to be pushed through the rubber liner. Some blood culture bottles have rubber stoppers, which again enable a syringe needle to be used for subculture. The advantage of this type of stopper is that if the pressure inside the blood culture bottle increases (incubator overheats), the stopper gives way to the pressure—allowing the air inside to escape, and the bottle does not burst. This prevents the bottle being opened until required for subculturing. 5 ml of blood is added to 100 ml of glucose broth and, for anaerobic bacteria, 100 ml of thioglycollate broth.

In *Castaneda's method*, a diphasic medium may also be set up. This medium is made up of a slope of nutrient agar to which glucose broth has been added. The exposed surface of the slope is examined daily for growth and by tilting the blood broth over

the agar slope each day, opening the bottle to subculture is avoided. The other bottles should be subcultured daily for 3 days and then after 1 week's incubation. Incubation should be continued for up to 3 weeks, subculturing weekly. Subcultures are usually made into blood agar plates which are then incubated aerobically, anaerobically and in an atmosphere of 10% CO_2.

More modern methods for blood cultures utilize either impedance or radiometry.

Impedance is the resistance to flow of an alternating electrical current through a conducting material. This principle has been used to measure growth rates in blood cultures. Early growth can be detected very rapidly by this method.

Radiometry is based on the detection of radioactive carbon dioxide $^{14}CO_2$ produced metabolically by bacteria from a suitable medium containing a radioactive carbon source. The Bactec is an example of this and is now being used in some laboratories.

There are many modifications to blood culture techniques. In cases such as bacterial endocarditis, a pour plate is of value using the patient's blood, as often identification of any organism present can be performed the next day. A Gram film from a spun deposit often gives an indication of the type of organism present. The use of Thiol broth (Difco) is also recommended for anaerobic cultivation.

The following organisms are associated with septicaemia: *Streptococcus pneumoniae*, *S. pyogenes*, 'viridans streptococci', coliform bacilli, Brucellae, *Salmonella typhi*, *Staphylococcus aureus*, but *any organism* isolated must be investigated carefully and regarded as a pathogen unless it is established as a contaminant. The most common contaminants are *Staphylococcus epidermidis* micrococci, diphtheroids and aerobic sporebearers. These can enter the cultures from the patient's or operator's skin, or from the air. However, some of these 'contaminants' have been incriminated in endocarditis.

Cerebrospinal fluid

It is very important that the clinician should be informed, as soon as possible, of any organisms found in a cerebrospinal fluid specimen (generally sent in a sterile universal bottle). In most cases this can be ascertained by examination of stained direct smears, but cultures should also be set up immediately. Normally cerebrospinal fluid is sterile but contaminants may be introduced by careless technique, both in ward and laboratory.

Method

1. Note the appearance of the fluid—for example whether clear or cloudy—and transfer it to a

clean sterile centrifuge tube, taking a small quantity for cell count.
2. Centrifuge at 3000 rpm for 5 min.
3. Discard the supernatant fluid into a jar of disinfectant (unless required for biochemical or other examination) and make two smears from the deposit.
4. Stain one smear by Gram and the other for acid-fast organisms. If *torulosis* is suspected prepare a 'negative stain' film using Nigrosin or India ink.
5. Inoculate the following media from the deposit: one blood agar plate and incubate aerobically at 35°C; one chocolate agar plate and incubate in 10% CO_2 at 35°C. Direct sensitivity tests may be performed. The following day, any organisms grown should be identified and sensitivity tests performed.
6. If *tuberculous meningitis* is suspected, inoculate two Lowenstein–Jensen slopes (in addition to the plates), and incubate at 37°C for 8 weeks, examining the slopes at weekly intervals.

(In suspected meningococcal meningitis the cerebrospinal fluid may be incubated overnight at 35°C and then cultured as above.)

The following organisms are associated with meningitis: *Neisseria* species, *Streptococcus pneumoniae*, *S. pyogenes*, *Haemophilus influenzae*, *Staphylococcus aureus*, *Listeria*, *Cryptococcus*, *Mycobacterium tuberculosis*. However, any organism isolated should be thoroughly investigated and regarded as a pathogen unless established as a contaminant.

Note

In cases of tuberculous meningitis, a spider-clot is often noted on the fluid. The clot is carefully decanted into a watch glass. If a piece of lens paper is carefully laid on the clot, the clot will adhere to the paper. The clot is then 'blotted' onto a clean glass slide, fixed and stained by the Ziehl–Neelsen method.

Faeces

Faeces are sent to the laboratory in a suitable wide-mouth container with a screw-capped lid or in the form of a rectal swab. Usually the organisms to be isolated are pathogenic Gram-negative bacilli, *Staphylococcus aureus*, Campylobacter, tubercle bacilli, or parasites. The normal flora may include coliform bacilli, *Streptococcus faecalis*, *Bacillus subtilis*, *Clostridium perfringens* and Bacteroides.

Method for Gram-negative bacilli

1. Inoculate a large loopful of the faeces onto a deoxycholate citrate agar plate and into a tube of Selenite F. Incubate at 35°C.

2. Inoculate a Campylobacter plate; incubate in a 5% CO_2/N_2 atmosphere at 43°C.
3. Emulsify a further portion in peptone water; from the peptone water inoculate a MacConkey agar plate and a Wilson and Blair plate if enteric fever is suspected. Incubate at 35°C.
4. The following day examine the plates for colonies.
5. Pick off suspicious colonies and identify by biochemical reactions and agglutination tests.
6. Plate out the Selenite F medium onto a MacConkey agar plate. Incubate at 35°C overnight.
7. Examine and identify any non-lactose-fermenting colonies present.

If *Vibrio cholerae* is suspected, inoculate into alkaline peptone water and thiosulphate–citrate–bile salt–sucrose (TCBS) medium. If *Staphylococcus aureus* is suspected, inoculate into salt cooked meat broth or on Ludam's medium and make a Gram film.

Method for isolation of *Mycobacterium tuberculosis*: ether concentration test

1. Make a thick saline suspension of faeces in a screw-capped bottle.
2. Add an equal volume of ether and shake well.
3. Centrifuge at 3000 rpm for 5 min.
4. Pipette off the supernatant ether into disinfectant and make a smear from the gelatinous layer.
5. Stain smear by Ziehl–Neelsen and examine.
6. If culture is required, remove gelatinous layer, treat as for sputum (see below), and inoculate two Lowenstein–Jensen slopes.
7. Incubate at 35°C for 8 weeks, examining weekly.

Alternatively, treat the faeces by a sputum concentration method.

Fluids

Pleural, peritoneal and other fluids

The fluids are sent to the laboratory in a sterile narrow-mouthed universal bottle containing 3 ml of 3.8% sodium citrate. This prevents any clotting of the fluid. A similar procedure is adopted as for cerebrospinal fluid. These fluids are commonly sterile, but contaminants may occur as in blood cultures.

Method

1. Note the appearance and quantity of fluid.
2. Transfer to a clean sterile centrifuge tube and centrifuge at 3000 rpm for 15 min.

3. Discard the supernatant fluid into disinfectant or keep for protein estimation. From the deposit inoculate two blood agar plates and make two smears.
4. Incubate the blood plates aerobically and anaerobically at 37°C.
5. Stain the smears by Gram, Ziehl–Neelsen, auramine–phenol or Leishman and examine.
6. After incubation identify any organisms isolated.
7. If *M. tuberculosis* is suspected it is inoculated directly on to two Lowenstein–Jensen slopes. Then the deposit is treated as for sputum and two more Lowenstein–Jensen slopes inoculated.

Possible pathogens that might be isolated include *Mycobacterium tuberculosis*, viridans streptococci, haemolytic streptococci, *Staphylococcus aureus, Streptococcus pneumoniae* and anaerobic streptococci.

Pus

The nature of the examination is again governed by the type of pus received, that is, whether from ear, wound or boil. It may be sent in a sterile container or on a swab or gauze. The contaminants found depend on the site of the pus. If from the skin, *Staphylococcus epidermidis* diphtheroids and coliform bacilli may be present as commensals.

Method

1. Note the appearance. If actinomycosis is suspected, examine for sulphur granules.
2. Inoculate two blood agar plates. On one, place a metronidazole disc to detect anaerobes.
3. Make two smears and stain by Gram and for acid-fast bacilli.
4. Incubate the plates aerobically and anaerobically. If gonococci are suspected, incubate a third plate in CO_2.
5. If indicated by smears, a direct sensitivity test should be set up.
6. Next day, identify any organisms isolated. Re-incubate up to 7 days if actinomycosis is suspected.
7. If *Mycobacterium tuberculosis* is suspected, the pus is inoculated onto two Lowenstein–Jensen slopes and then treated as for sputum.

Possible pathogens that might be isolated include *Staphylococcus aureus*, haemolytic streptococci, *M. tuberculosis, Clostridium perfringens, Bacillus subtilis, Proteus vulgaris, Actinomyces israelii*, Bacteroides and Haemophilus species.

Serology

For serological examination, whole blood is sent to the laboratory in a sterile universal bottle. The blood is allowed to clot, then freed from the sides of the bottle with a firm straight wire and incubated at 37°C for a short time to hasten clot retraction. The serum is removed with a sterile Pasteur pipette into a centrifuge tube and spun down to remove any free red cells. For complement-fixation tests it is better to keep the whole blood specimen in the refrigerator overnight before removing the serum.

The serum is pipetted into a clean sterile bottle and clearly labelled with the patient's name, hospital number, ward, date and nature of specimen and kept in the freezing compartment of the refrigerator. The tests to be carried out depend on the provisional diagnosis. These may include: Widal tests in suspected Salmonella or dysentery infections; agglutination tests in suspected Brucella infections; VD serology in suspected syphilis cases; anti-streptolysin titre in cases of rheumatoid arthritis; and virus serology in suspected virus diseases.

Sputum

Sputum examinations can be divided into two main groups. Examination may be for *Mycobacterium tuberculosis* or for other organisms. The normal flora may include viridans and non-haemolytic streptococci, *Neisseria*, diphtheroids, fusiform bacilli and spirochaetes.

Method for organisms other than *M. tuberculosis*

1. Note appearance of sputum, whether salivary, mucoid, purulent or blood-stained.
2. Homogenize the sputum either by shaking with sterile Ringer's (see below) solution and glass beads, or by adding 1% pancreatin (see below) and incubating for 1 h. Culture onto blood agar and any other media routinely used and make smears.
3. Stain the smears by Gram and Ziehl–Neelsen or auramine–phenol.
4. Incubate the blood agar plate aerobically at 35°C.
5. Examine the smears and next day identify any organisms isolated.

Possible pathogens that might be isolated from sputa include *Haemophilus influenzae*, haemolytic streptococci, *Klebsiella pneumoniae, Streptococcus pneumoniae, Staphylococcus aureus* and *Pseudomonas aeruginosa*.

Ringer's solution

Sodium chloride	9.0 g
Potassium chloride	0.42 g
Calcium chloride	0.48 g
Sodium bicarbonate	0.2 g
Glass-distilled water	1000 ml

Table 27.1 Appropriate media for swabs from different sites

Media and incubation conditions	Site				
	Nose/ throat	Ear	Eye	Wound	Genito- urinary
Chocolate agar, CO_2		+	+	+	+
Blood agar, CO_2			+		
Blood agar, O_2	+	+		+	+
Anaerobic blood agar, 24 h AnO_2				+	+
Crystal violet, AnO_2	+	+			
CLED, O_2		+		+	+
MacConkey agar, O_2		+		+	+
Kanamycin–vancomycin agar, AnO_2		+		+	+
Neomycin blood agar, 48 h AnO_2		+		+	+
Tellurite, O_2	+	+			
New York City, CO_2					+

1% pancreatin solution for homogenizing sputum

Add 1 g of pancreatin to the following solution:

Sterile normal saline solution	100 ml
Buffer solution	7 ml

Buffer solution: 0.2M NaOH, 1 vol.
0.2M KH_2PO_4 1.2 vol.

Routine examination for *M. tuberculosis*

A smear from a specimen of sputum will demonstrate the presence or absence of acid-fast bacilli, but will *not* prove they are tubercle bacilli. Culture for *M. tuberculosis* must be performed together with subsequent tests if the culture yields growth. A concentration method is given which will kill most organisms other than mycobacteria.

Petroff's method (modified)

1. Mix the sputum with 3 or 4 times its volume of 4% sodium hydroxide in a sterile, wide-mouth universal bottle.
2. Shake on a mechanical shaker (housed in an exhaust cabinet) for 20 min or shake by hand frequently during a 20-min period, again in an exhaust cabinet.
3. Centrifuge at 3000 rpm for 15 min.
4. Pour the supernatant fluid into disinfectant and resuspend the deposit in 25 ml of sterile glass-distilled water containing 100 iu per ml of penicillin.
5. Spin at 3000 rpm for 15 min. Pour off supernatant fluid and film the deposit.
6. Inoculate two Lowenstein–Jensen slopes.
7. Incubate at 37°C in a flat position for 24 h to allow the fluid to spread evenly over the surface of the medium. Then incubate in an upright position for up to 8 weeks.
8. Examine the cultures weekly.

Swabs

These should be cultured immediately on arrival, as the material soon dries on the swabs. Types of media and incubation conditions are given in *Table 27.1*. If delay in transit is anticipated the swab should be moistened with a little broth before inoculating media, or a suitable transport medium used. Alternatively, utilize the commercially prepared Swab Transport Systems (available from Difco and TCS). All media should be inoculated before films are made, owing to the scantiness of material on the swab. Reliance should not be placed on the film result alone; its main use is to exclude Vincent's infection, that is, the presence of spirochaetes and fusiform bacilli from throat swabs.

The normal flora may include *Neisseria*, viridans and non-haemolytic streptococci and diphtheroids.

Throat swabs

Method

1. Inoculate appropriate agar plates and incubate aerobically and anaerobically at 35°C.
2. In suspected diphtheria cases, a Loeffler's serum slope and blood tellurite plates are also inoculated and incubated aerobically at 35°C.
3. The next day identify any organism grown.

Pharyngeal swabs (post-nasal) and pernasal swabs

These swabs are prepared from 150 mm lengths of SWG 18 copper wire, slightly bent 25 mm from the end. Absorbent wool is wrapped around this end, which has been flattened. The swab is sterilized in a 125 mm × 12 mm tube by hot air. These swabs are received from cases of suspected whooping-cough and meningococcal carriers.

Method

1. In suspected whooping-cough cases inoculate Bordet–Gengou plates with 0.25 units of penicillin per ml and/or Lacey's DPF plates. Incubate at 35°C for 2–4 days.
2. In suspected meningococcal cases inoculate chocolate agar and incubate in 10% CO_2 at 35°C for 1–2 days.

Genito-urinary swabs

These swabs are generally received from cases of suspected puerperal sepsis, gonorrhoea or trichomoniasis. Stuart's or Amies transport medium should be used if delay in sending to the laboratory is likely. Special transport medium is required if isolation of Chlamydia is to be attempted.

The normal flora may include staphylococci, diphtheroids, faecal streptococci, coliform bacilli, fusiform bacilli.

Method

1. Inoculate appropriate plates and incubate anaerobically in 10% CO_2 at 35°C.
2. Make a smear, after inoculation of plates, and stain by Gram's method and a wet preparation for examination for *Trichomonas vaginalis*.
3. The next day, identify any organism grown on the plates and reincubate the plates.

Possible pathogens may include haemolytic streptococci, *Neisseria gonorrhoeae*, *Staphylococcus aureus*, *Clostridium perfringens*, *Candida albicans*, *Gardnerella vaginalis* and other anaerobes.

Eye swabs

Swabs taken from eye infections should be cultured immediately they are taken, to prevent enzymatic action killing any organisms present.

Method

1. Inoculate appropriate plates and incubate aerobically in CO_2 at 35°C.
2. Next day identify any organisms grown on the plates.

Possible pathogens include *Staphylococcus aureus*, pneumococci, *Haemophilus influenzae*, *Neisseria gonorrhoeae*, haemolytic streptococci and diphtheroids.

Laryngeal swabs (for *Mycobacterium tuberculosis*)

Method 1: absorbent wool swabs

1. Immerse the laryngeal swab in a few ml of 6% sulphuric acid for 6 min.

2. Pour off acid and replace with 4% NaOH. Leave for 20 s and inoculate the swab on two Lowenstein–Jensen slopes.
3. Incubate slopes at 35°C for 8 weeks, examining at weekly intervals.

Method 2: alginate wool swabs

1. Immerse the laryngeal swab in 5 ml of 15% trisodium phosphate.
2. Agitate the swab until the wool has dissolved.
3. Centrifuge. Inoculate two Lowenstein–Jensen slopes from deposit.

Films should *not* be made owing to scanty amount of material on the swab.

Gastric lavage

On the wards, the gastric washings are placed in a sterile universal bottle containing 5 ml of 15% trisodium phosphate, and sent to the laboratory. On receipt, the specimen is centrifuged and the deposit treated as for concentration of sputum. By placing the gastric washings direct into trisodium orthophosphate, the acid washed from the stomach (which would be sufficient to kill the tubercle bacilli) is neutralized.

Urine

'Cleaned up' mid-stream specimens of urine should be sent to the laboratory in suitable sterile containers, with the minimum of delay. Catheter specimens should be avoided because of the high incidence of bladder infections after catheterization. A film of the specimen without centrifugation is made and stained. If organisms are seen, this (provided the specimen was freshly voided) indicates that the organisms are present in large enough numbers to cause infection. When culturing, it is suggested that some form of viable count be performed. A standard loop is used which will take up a known amount of urine. Counting of the colonies, next day, on media inoculated this way, will give an approximate number of viable organisms per ml. It has been said that 100000 organisms per ml is indicative of infection. It is imperative that the urine specimen be examined without delay as organisms will reproduce rapidly in urine.

If isolation of *Mycobacterium tuberculosis* is requested, three consecutive early morning specimens should be sent.

Method

1. Note appearance of urine.

2. Using a standard sterile loop*, insert vertically into the urine and inoculate MacConkey or CLED and blood agar plates. Make a film. Incubate at 35°C and next day count and identify any organisms present. A colony count of 400 is indicative of infection.
3. Transfer to centrifuge tube and centrifuge at 3000 rpm for 15 min. Pour off the supernatant fluid into disinfectant.
4. From the deposit make a wet preparation.
5. Examine for cells, casts, crystals, organisms, etc.

Provided the specimen has been taken with adequate aseptic precautions, the following organisms may be considered to be pathogenic: coliform bacilli, *Streptococcus faecalis*, *Staphylococcus aureus*, haemolytic streptococci, *Proteus*, *Shigella* and *Salmonella* species.

Method for *M. tuberculosis*

1. The specimen of urine is allowed to stand overnight in the refrigerator.
2. Discard the supernatant (under cover of inoculating cabinet) and transfer the sediment to universal containers.
3. Centrifuge the bottles at 3000 rpm for 20 min.
4. Discard the supernatant and treat each deposit as for sputum.
5. Inoculate six Lowenstein–Jensen slopes from each deposit.

A generalized scheme for the isolation and identification of bacteria from pathological specimens

On the day that a specimen arrives in the laboratory (i.e. as soon as possible after being taken) it is usually plated out onto a variety of enriched, selective or differential media. The choice of these and of the other conditions of incubation will be guided by the clinical information that should accompany all such specimens. These conditions of incubation include temperature—usually 35–37°C for pathogenic bacteria, and the choice of atmosphere—aerobic, anaerobic, microaerophilic, with or without 5–10% CO_2. With certain specimens it is worthwhile to put up direct drug-sensitivity tests.

After overnight incubation the plates are scanned for growth and individual colonies examined with a ×8 hand lens or a plate microscope. These examinations often yield much information. An experienced bacteriologist can bring together evidence from the colonial morphology, the nature of the media on which the colonies have or *have not* grown, and the effect of the organism's growth on the medium, e.g. haemolysis or pH change. These clues, when taken together with the clinical information, will often point strongly to the identity of the bacteria under examination, *but* they can never be conclusive and confirmatory tests must always be carried out.

One vital procedure is to make films from individual colonies for examination of cellular morphology and arrangement, and staining reaction notably to Gram's method. In some cases it is advantageous to use special techniques, e.g. to demonstrate spores by specialized staining reactions, or motility by the use of a hanging drop preparation.

At this stage it is also possible to carry out certain 'instant' tests, such as the catalase and oxidase reactions and the slide test for cell-bound coagulase.

The bacteriologist is now usually ready to make a provisional report to the physician on the likely identity of the bacteria isolated (and, possibly, their drug sensitivity) so that treatment can be started or modified.

Confirmation usually requires more time-consuming biochemical tests (although rapid methods, such as the API system, have simplified these identifications) and often the determination of the types of antigen on the bacterial surfaces by means of agglutination or precipitation methods (e.g. *Salmonella* and *Streptococcus*). Occasionally, the susceptibility of the bacteria to highly specific bacteriophages may be useful confirmatory evidence (e.g. with *Brucella* spp. and *Bacillus anthracis*).

Toxigenic pathogens, e.g. *Corynebacterium diphtheriae*, may require an animal pathogenicity test for final confirmation.

It is important to realize that the confirmation of an organism as being 'X' may have serious consequences—both medical and legal—for the patient and others. 'Confirmation' based on insecure evidence must therefore be avoided, even when it means a longer wait for the 'Final Report'.

Some of the more common organisms isolated from clinical specimens

Useful pointers to final confirmation are given in parentheses.

*A standard loop containing $\frac{1}{250}$ ml of water can be made by using a metal rod, 3.26 mm diameter (30 Morse Gauge) and nichrome or platinum wire SWG 28. The content of the loop can be checked by weighing a bijou bottle of water, inserting the loop in a vertical position and spreading on a piece of blotting paper. After removal of 500 loopfuls, the bottle and water are reweighed and the loopful content calculated.

Gram-positive cocci

Staphylococcus aureus

Pathogen found in pyogenic infections and often in nose and on skin in health.
(Catalase and coagulase-positive.)

Staphylococcus epidermidis (albus)

Commensal found in the nose and on the skin, but may be pathogenic under certain conditions.
(Catalase-positive and coagulase-negative.)

Streptococcus pyogenes

Pathogen found in tonsillitis, scarlet fever and pyogenic infections.
(Catalase-negative, identified by Lancefield's grouping.)

Streptococcus faecalis

Pathogen found in urinary infections and in normal intestine.
(Catalase-negative and grows on bile salt media and is resistant to penicillin.)

Streptococcus pneumoniae

Pathogen found in respiratory infections and meningitis.
(Catalase-negative, and 'Optochin'-sensitive, unlike 'viridans streptococci'.)

Viridans streptococci

Commensal found in mouth and throat, occasionally pathogenic.
(Catalase-negative, 'Optochin'-resistant.)

Gram-negative cocci

Neisseria gonorrhoeae

Pathogen found in cases of gonorrhoea.
(Oxidase-positive, identified and confirmed by typical sugar reactions.)

Neisseria meningitidis

Pathogen found in cases of meningitis, rarely in healthy persons.
(Oxidase-positive, identified by typical sugar reactions and antigenic structure.)

Neisseria catarrhalis

Commensal found in throat and mouth, in health but especially in catarrhal secretions.
(Oxidase-positive, grows on nutrient agar, fermentation tests negative.)

Neisseria pharyngis

Commensal found in throat and mouth.
(Oxidase-positive, ferments most sugars, grows on nutrient agar.)

Gram-positive bacilli

Clostridium spp.

A group of sporing anaerobic organisms generally pathogenic when isolated from clinical material.

Bacillus anthracis

Pathogen isolated from cases of anthrax.

Bacillus subtilis and B. cereus

Saprophyte found in soil and dust, common laboratory contaminant.

Corynebacterium diphtheriae

Pathogen found in cases of diphtheria.
(Catalase-positive, identified by sugar reactions and toxin production.)

Corynebacterium hofmannii

Commensal found on skin and in the upper respiratory tract.
(No fermentation of sugars used for *C. diphtheriae*.)

Mycobacterium tuberculosis

Pathogen isolated from cases of tuberculosis.
(Acid-fast bacillus identified by special methods.)

Gram-negative bacilli

Escherichia coli

Pathogen or commensal. Found in urinary tract infections and in normal intestine and sewage.
(Identified by indole production, sugar reactions and other tests.)

Klebsiella pneumoniae

Pathogen found in respiratory infections.
(Identified by special biochemical tests.)

Salmonella spp.

Pathogens found in typhoid and paratyphoid fevers and food poisoning.
(Over 1000 species identified by sugar reactions and antigenic structure.)

Shigella spp.

Pathogens found in bacillary dysentery.
(Identified by sugar reactions and antigenic structure.)

Proteus spp.

Pathogens found mainly in urinary tract infections or commensals found in normal intestine and sewage.

Pseudomonas aeruginosa

Pathogen found in wound and urinary infections.
(Special tests.)

Pasteurella multocida

Pathogen found occasionally in respiratory infections and also infections from animal bites.
(Identified by indole production, failure to grow on bile salt media and other tests.)

Haemophilus influenzae

Pathogen found in meningitis and bronchitis, but also in normal nasopharynx.
(Identified by X and V factor requirements.)

Bordetella pertussis

Pathogen found in cases of whooping cough.
(Special tests and antigenic structure.)

Brucella abortus and Brucella melitensis

Pathogens found in undulant fever.
(Identified by special tests and antigenic structure.)

Campylobacter jejuni

Pathogen found in cases of acute diarrhoea. Animals both domestic and wild are the main reservoirs. Outbreaks associated with food, milk, acid water.
(Identified by colonies—oxidase test.)

Legionella pneumophila

Pathogen found in cases of Legionnaires' disease. Widely distributed in nature and commonly found in surface water and soil. May be found in water storage and distribution systems as well as in the recirculating cooling water or air-conditioning plants.
(Identified by biochemical tests, fluorescent antibody technique and gas–liquid chromatography.)

Yersinia enterolitica

Pathogen found in animals, ice cream, mussels, foodstuffs. Associated with outbreaks of diarrhoea. Will grow at 4°C.
(Identified by growth biochemical tests and motility—motile at 25°C, non-motile at 36°C.)

Some tests used for the identification of organisms

Aesculin hydrolysis

To determine the ability of an organism to hydrolyse aesculin to aesculetin and glucose. Used to differentiate Group D streptococci from other streptococci.

Method

Inoculate aesculin agar slope and incubate at 35°C. Hydrolysis is indicated by a brown coloration.

Catalase activity

One use of this test is to differentiate staphylococci (catalase+) from streptococci (catalase−).

Method

To the organism growing on a suitable solid medium add 1 drop of 10 vol hydrogen peroxide. Examine immediately, and after a few minutes, for bubbles of gas which indicates catalase production.

■ Note

Blood-containing media are unsuitable for this test. Alternatively, a small portion of the colony under test is placed in 1 drop of hydrogen peroxide on a microscope slide; catalase-positive strains cause effervescence in the drop. This test should be carried out under an inoculating cabinet.

Coagulase activity

A pathogenic staphylococcus, *S. aureus*, has the power of clotting or coagulating blood plasma. This is due to the production by the pathogenic staphylococci of the enzyme *coagulase*. Coagulase may be bound to the organism, in which case it is demonstrated by the slide test, or 'free', when the tube method is used. The vast majority of pathogenic staphylococci produce both forms. Occasionally, however, some strains only produce one or the other. It is necessary to perform a tube test on all 'slide negative' staphylococci.

Method 1: slide test

1. Emulsify a colony of staphylococci in one drop of distilled water on a clean glass slide. The opacity should be such that the hands of a watch can be seen through the suspension.
2. Add a small loopful of rabbit plasma and mix.
3. A positive coagulase test will show immediate clumping—a negative test will show no clumping.

A known positive staphylococcus should be tested at the same time, to check that the plasma is working properly.

Method 2: tube test

1. Dilute fresh rabbit plasma 1/10 with normal saline.
2. To 0.5 ml of this (in a 75 × 12 mm tube), add 5 drops of an overnight broth culture of the staphylococcus under test.
3. To another 0.5 ml, add 5 drops of sterile broth (this acts as a negative control).
4. To another 0.5 ml, add 5 drops of a known coagulase-positive, staphylococcus culture. This acts as a positive control.
5. Incubate at 35°C for up to 6 h. A positive coagulase test will show clotting usually within 1 h.

Test for indole production

Reagent (Kovak's reagent)

p-Dimethylaminobenzaldehyde	5 g
Amyl alcohol	75 ml
Concentrated HCl	25 ml

Dissolve the aldehyde in the alcohol by gently warming in a water bath (about 50–55°C). Cool and add the acid. Protect from light and store at 4°C.

Method

To a peptone water culture (24–48 h incubation) add 0.5 ml of reagent. Shake well and examine after 1 min.
A red colour indicates the presence of indole.

Optochin sensitivity (ethylhydrocuprein hydrochloride inhibition)

Streptococcus pneumoniae is sensitive to 'Optochin', but 'viridans streptococci' and *S. faecalis* are resistant. This fact is used for the identification of *S. pneumoniae*.

Method

Place a disc impregnated with ethylhydrocuprein on the surface of a blood agar plate inoculated with the organism. Incubate and examine after 18–24 h. Sensitivity to the compound is shown by inhibition of bacterial growth around the disc.

Preparation of discs

To a filter paper disc, 0.5 cm diameter, add 0.02 ml of a 1/5000 solution of ethylhydrocuprein hydrochloride. Dry at 37°C or freeze-dry. Store in a closed container. These discs may be obtained commercially.

Oxidase test

This is used for distinguishing colonies of *Neisseria* from mixed cultures and *Pseudomonas aeruginosa* from enteric bacteria. Both *Neisseria* and *P. aeruginosa* are oxidase-positive; *Neisseria* are *strongly* positive.

Method 1

Flood the colonies with a solution of 1% aqueous tetramethyl-*p*-phenylenediamine hydrochloride solution. A positive oxidase reaction turns the colonies a purple colour; a strong reaction is almost black. It is important to subculture *immediately* after observing the reaction—the reagent is lethal to *Neisseria*.

Method 2

Place 2–3 drops of oxidase reagent on a piece of filter paper. Smear the colony under test across the paper. A positive reaction turns the paper a dark purple within 10 s.

Oxidation–fermentation

To determine the ability of an organism to oxidize or ferment a carbohydrate. Used as an aid in identification of many bacteria.

Method

To the Hugh and Liefson base add 0.5 ml of sterile 10% glucose solution to each tube. Inoculate two tubes with a loopful of growth from an 18 h culture. Add 1.5 ml of sterile paraffin to one tube and incubate both tubes upright for up to 3 days. Alternatively, incubate one tube aerobically and one tube anaerobically.

Results (using bromocresol purple as an indicator)	Aerobic tube	Anaerobic tube
No action on sugar	No change (mauve)	No change (mauve)
Oxidation	Acid (yellow)	No change (mauve)
Fermentation	Acid (yellow)	Acid (yellow)

Phenylalanine deaminase (PDA) test

To determine the ability of an organism to deaminate phenylalanine to phenylpyruvic acid by enzymatic activity. Used to differentiate *Proteus* and *Providencia* spp. from other Enterobacteria.

Method

Inoculate phenylalanine agar slope and incubate for 24 h. Run 0.2 ml of 10% ferric chloride solution rapidly over surface of slope. Positive reaction—green coloration on slope and in fluid at base of slope.

Isolation of organisms from specimens

A guide for the isolation and identification of some common organisms is shown in *Table 27.2*. These methods will, of course, vary from laboratory to laboratory and the student must be familiar with his department's methods and the reasons for their use.

Antimicrobial susceptibility testing

The susceptibility of organisms to antibacterial substances, e.g. antibiotics, is an important factor in the treatment of patients. When antibiotics are given to a patient a certain concentration can be expected to reach the site of infection. If the organism is susceptible to that concentration, then the patient should respond to therapy; if not, then the organism will continue to multiply. Therefore, it is most important to establish the breakpoint between *susceptible* and *resistant* in order to guide the specific therapy of the patient with an infectious disease.

There are two main methods of susceptibility testing, namely *dilution* (incorporation) and *diffusion* methods. Each of these may be carried out by a variety of techniques and only a brief reference will be made to these methods.

Tube dilution (incorporation of drugs in media)

For quantitative estimates of antimicrobial activity, dilutions of the drug may be incorporated in broth or nutrient agar and then inoculated with a standardized suspension of the test organism. Similar tubes or agar plates should be inoculated with a standard suspension of a known sensitive organism and this set acts as a control.

After appropriate incubation, the presence or absence of growth is recorded. The lowest concentration of antibiotic showing no growth indicates the amount of antibiotic per millilitre to which the organism is susceptible. The lowest concentration is termed the minimal inhibitory concentration (MIC).

The most practical way of indicating the clinical implications of the terms 'sensitive' and 'resistant' is to state the relationship between the MICs of the antibiotic *in vitro* and the concentration obtainable in body fluids, etc., *in vivo*. This latter should be determined from material as close to the focus of infection as possible.

For most purposes, the blood level is of paramount importance. If this exceeds the MIC of the infecting microbe by a safety factor of from 2 to 4, the infection is generally amenable to treatment. The upper limit of MIC of sensitive microorganisms should therefore be one-half to one-fourth the average level of the antibiotic in the blood when ordinary dosage is given by the usual route.

Agar diffusion methods

In these tests, the surface of an agar plate is inoculated and the antibiotic (in the form of a disc, cup or hole placed or cut in the media) diffuses from this reservoir source into the medium. As the organism grows, it is exposed to a continuous gradient of antibiotic. When the organism reaches an area where the antibiotic is no longer effective and the population of the organism can overcome the effect of the antibiotic, a zone edge is formed.

Generally, these tests are used for distinguishing between susceptible and resistant strains.

Stokes method

Required

Blood agar plates, 4 mm in depth, prepared from a nutrient agar specifically designed for susceptibility testing; antibiotic discs; calipers.

Control organisms: (a) for organisms isolated from urine—*Escherichia coli* NCTC 10418; (b) other material—*Staphylococcus aureus* NCTC 6571; (c) pseudomonads—*Pseudomonas aeruginosa* NCTC 10662.

Table 27.2 Schematic guide for isolation and identification of some common organisms from specimens

Organism	Specimen	Gram stain reaction	Suggested media	Remarks on isolation and identification
Bordetella	Pernasal and pharyngeal swabs	Negative	Bordet–Gengou Lacey DPF	Serology
Brucella	Exudates, blood	Negative	Serum dextrose agar	10% CO_2 cultivation. Phage Serology—dye plates, H_2S production
Campylobacter	Faeces	Negative	Campylobacter medium	10% CO_2/N_2 at 43°C Typical spreading colonies Gram film—oxidase test
Clostridium	Wounds, pus, exudates, blood	Positive	Blood agar Cooked meat Thioglycollate	Anaerobic cultivation, sugar reactions, litmus milk Animal inoculation Nagler plate, stormy clot
Coliforms	Urine, exudates, blood, pus, CSF faeces, sputa	Negative	Blood agar MacConkey's agar	Aerobic cultivation Biochemical tests including EMVIC reactions. Serology
Corynebacterium	Nasopharynx wounds	Positive	Blood agar Tellurite agar Loeffler's	Aerobic cultivation Toxin production, serum sugar reactions, virulence tests
Gonococcus	Exudates from genitalia, eye, joints	Negative	Chocolate agar New York City medium	10% CO_2 cultivation Serum sugar reactions Oxidase test
Haemophilus	CSF, blood, sputum, exudates	Negative	Blood agar Chocolate agar	Aerobic cultivation Serology X and V factors Satellitism
Klebsiella pneumoniae	Sputum, blood, CSF exudates	Negative	Blood agar Blood broth	Aerobic cultivation Mouse inoculation Serological typing
Legionella	Tracheal aspirate Plural fluid Lung tissue	Negative	Legionella medium	Aerobic cultivation Gram and fluorescent antibody test on typical colonies Biochemical tests Gas–liquid chromatography
Meningococcus	Blood, CSF, nasopharynx	Negative	Chocolate agar	10% CO_2 cultivation Serum sugar reactions Oxidase test
Mycobacterium tuberculosis	Sputum, CSF exudates, urine, pus, faeces	Positive (not easily stained)	Lowenstein–Jensen	Aerobic cultivation Concentration by alkali methods Acid-fast stains Niacin and catalase peroxidase tests
Pasteurella	Sputum, blood, exudates, pus	Negative	Blood agar	Aerobic cultivation Growth on MacConkey, animal inoculation, sugar reactions Motility, serology
Pneumococcus	Sputum, blood, CSF, pus, exudates	Positive	Blood agar	Aerobic cultivation α-haemolysis Bile or Optochin sensitivity Typing with specific antiserum
Proteus	Urine, exudates, CSF, blood	Negative	High-concentration agar Salt-free agar	Aerobic cultivation Swarming Splitting of urea, sugar reactions
Pseudomonas	Urine, exudates, pus, CSF, blood	Negative	Blood agar	Aerobic cultivation Pigmentation Hugh and Liefson
Salmonella	Faeces, blood, urine, exudates	Negative	MacConkey's agar Desoxycholate–citrate agar Selenite F Wilson's and Blair's medium	Aerobic cultivation Sugar reactions, indole, motility, serology

Table 27.2 continued

Organism	Specimen	Gram stain reaction	Suggested media	Remarks on isolation and identification
Shigella	Faeces	Negative	MacConkey Desoxycholate–citrate media Selenite F	Aerobic cultivation Sugar reactions Indole, motility, serology
Staphylococcus	Pus, exudates, blood, CSF, faeces, sputum	Positive	Blood agar Salt medium	Aerobic cultivation Coagulase, phage typing
Streptococcus	Pus, exudates, blood, CSF, throat swabs	Positive	Blood agar	Aerobic or anaerobic cultivation Haemolysis, soluble haemolysin, Lancefield group Growth on MacConkey, heat resistance
Yeasts and fungi	Skin, nails, hair, exudates, pus, sputum, blood	—	Sabouraud's dextrose agar Penicillin and streptomycin Blood agar	Aerobic cultivation at 37°C and 22°C Needle mount Fluorescence of hair Corn meal agar ⎫ yeasts Sugar reactions ⎭ Growth on rice grains
Yersinia	Faeces	Negative	MacConkey's agar *Yersinia* medium	Cold environment, aerobic 30°C Biochemical tests Motility

Method

1. Emulsify several colonies in quarter-strength Ringer solution to give a density similar to an overnight broth culture. The inoculum should give a semi-confluent growth on the plates after overnight incubation.
2. Seed the control organism, using a sterile swab on either side of the plate, leaving a central band un-inoculated (*Figure 27.1*).

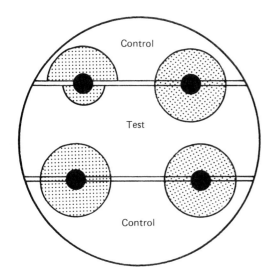

Figure 27.1. Control culture seeded on either side of the inoculated specimen

3. Seed the test organism, using a sterile swab, from the centre of the plate.
4. Apply the disc on the line between the test and control organisms.
5. Incubate overnight at 37°C or, if methicillin discs are used, inoculate at 30°C.
6. Using calipers, measure the zones of inhibition.

Results

1. Zone diameter equal to, wider than or not more than 3 mm smaller than the control—sensitive.
2. Zone diameter greater than 3 mm but smaller than the control by more than 3 mm in diameter—intermediate.
3. Zone diameter 3 mm or less—resistant.

Bauer–Kirby technique

This method is recommended by the US Food and Drug Administration as the method of antibiotic susceptibility testing in America. Provided the technique is followed carefully, the method can prove accurate and reliable. One danger of using this test is that as high potency discs are used, care must be taken that these are used only for this test, and are not used in any other method.

Method

1. Using 150 × 15 mm plates, pour 80 ml of sterile molten Mueller–Hinton agar into each dish.

Table 27.3 Zone-size interpretative chart*

Antibiotic or chemotherapeutic agent		Disc potency	Inhibition zone diameter (to nearest mm)		
			Resistant	Intermediate	Sensitive
Ampicillin	Gram-negative and enterococci	10 µg	11 or less	12–13	14 or more
	Staphylococci and highly penicillin-sensitive organisms	10 µg	20 or less	21–28	29 or more
Penicillin G	Haemophilus[a]	—	—	—	20 or more
	Staphylococci	10 units	20 or less	21–28	29 or more
	Other organisms	10 units	11 or less	12–21[e]	22 or more
Bacitracin		10 units	8 or less	9–12	13 or more
Cephaloridine		30 µg	11 or less	12–15	16 or more
Cephalothin		30 µg	14 or less	15–17	18 or more
Chloramphenicol		30 µg	12 or less	13–17	18 or more
Colistin		10 µg	8 or less	9–10	11 or more
Erythromycin		15 µg	13 or less	14–17	18 or more
Gentamicin[a]		10 µg	—	—	13 or more
Kanamycin		30 µg	13 or less	14–17	18 or more
Lincomycin		2 µg	9 or less	10–14	15 or more
Methicillin		5 µg	9 or less	10–13	14 or more
Nafcillin and oxacillin[a]		1 µg	10 or less	11–12	13 or more
Nalidixic acid[b]		30 µg	13 or less	14–18	19 or more
Neomycin		30 µg	12 or less	13–16	17 or more
Nitrofurantoin[b]		300 µg	14 or less	15–16	17 or more
Novobiocin[c]		30 µg	17 or less	18–21	22 or more
Oleandomycin		15 µg	11 or less	12–16	17 or more
Polymixin B		300 units	8 or less	9–11	12 or more
Streptomycin		10 µg	11 or less	12–14	15 or more
Sulphonamides[b,d]		300 µg	12 or less	13–16	17 or more
Tetracycline		30 µg	14 or less	15–18	19 or more
Vancomycin		30 µg	9 or less	10–11	12 or more

a = Tentative standards; b = urinary-tract infection only; c = not applicable to blood-containing media; d = any of the commercially available 300 µg or 250 µg sulphonamide discs can be used with the same standards of zone interpretation; e = this category includes some organisms, such as enterococci, which may cause systemic infections treatable by high doses of penicillin G.
*Reprinted from *University of Washington Hospital Practice*, February 1970, by courtesy of the Editor.

2. Dry at 37°C for 30 min.
3. Transfer 5 colonies of the organism under test into 4 ml of tryptose phosphate or tryptose soya broth.
4. Incubate at 37°C for 2–5 h and adjust turbidity to match an opacity tube containing 0.5 ml of 1% barium chloride in 1% sulphuric acid. Replace the standard monthly.
5. Using a sterile cotton-wool swab, streak the test culture evenly over the Mueller–Hinton plate.
6. Allow to dry and distribute the antibiotic discs* onto the plate (see *Figure 27.2*). Incubate at 37°C for 18 h.
7. Using Vernier calipers, measure the zone of inhibition for each antibiotic.
8. Determine the result by reading from *Table 27.3*.

*Automatic hand disc dispensers are available from Difco and Oxoid.

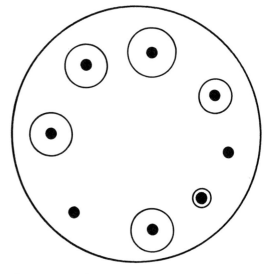

Figure 27.2. Antibiotic discs distributed on plate

Assay of antibiotics in body fluids

Another essential function of the microbiology laboratory is the assessment of antibiotic concentration in body fluids of patients being treated with antibiotics. It is often necessary to know that the treatment being given is sufficient to attain levels of antibiotics that will deal adequately with the organism causing infection, as well as keeping a check that the levels are not so high that they will harm the patient in some way.

Methods

Antibiotic assays can be performed by either tube dilution or large plate assay methods, or by more rapid methods such as EMIT (see p. 282).

For the former two methods, a number of organisms are recommended for the assay of different antibiotics (*Table 27.4*). If these organisms are not all available, satisfactory results can usually be obtained using either the Oxford staphylococcus or the standard *Escherichia coli*.

Table 27.4 Organisms used in assay of some antibiotics

Antibiotic to be used	Organism of choice
Penicillins (except carbenicillin, cloxacillin and flucloxacillin)	*Bacillus subtilis* NCTC 8236
Carbenicillin	*Pseudomonas aeruginosa* NCTC 10701
Cloxacillin Flucloxacillin }	*Staphylococcus saprophyticus*
Cephalosporins	*B. subtilis* NCTC 8236 or *S. aureus* NCTC 7447
Aminoglycosides	*Klebsiella edwardsii* NCTC 10896
Erythromycin	*Micrococcus lutea* NCTC 8340
Lincomycin Clindamycin }	*M. lutea* NCTC 8340
Fusidic acid	*Corynebacterium xerosis* NCTC 9755
Chloramphenicol	*M. lutea* NCTC 8340
Tetracyclines	*S. aureus* NCTC 8849
Rifampicin	*S. aureus* NCTC 8236 or *M. lutea* NCTC 8340

Either clotted blood or a specimen of urine are the usual body fluids monitored, and specimens are taken at intervals after the last dosage of antibiotic. Ideally, the specimens should be taken before dosage, and 1 h, 2 h, 4 h, 8 h, 12 h and 24 h thereafter. If this is not practicable two specimens, one before and the other 2 h after dosage, are often sufficient.

Only the large plate agar diffusion method will be given here.

Large plate assay

Required

Large glass or plastic assay plates; levelling tripods; puncher for cutting holes (7–8 mm diameter); Pasteur pipettes; tubes, pipettes and racks; standard antibiotic solutions; Quasi-Latin Square Design; vernier calipers; semilogarithmic graph paper.

Method

1. Place the assay plate in the levelling tripods and adjust so that the plate is level.
2. Using molten antibiotic medium, cooled to 50°C and seeded with appropriate amount of assay organisms to give confluent growth, pour plates.
3. Allow agar to solidify and keep in refrigerator (4°C) for up to 24 h.
4. Dilute the standard antibiotic solution to give 4 or 5 doubling dilutions within the range for that antibiotic. Number 1–4 (or 5).
5. Place the assay plate over the Quasi-Latin Square Design. Using the punch, cut holes corresponding to the square design.
6. Taking tube labelled 1, fill the four holes appearing over 1 of the square design.
7. Continue with tubes 2 and 3, and so on.
8. Incubate overnight at 30°C or 37°C.

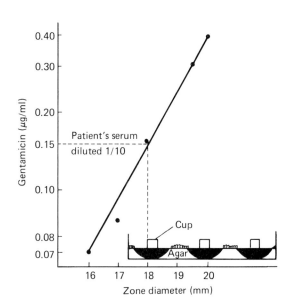

Figure 27.3. Dose–response curve for gentamicin

9. The next morning, remove plates from the incubator and place over the square design.
10. Measure the zones of inhibition and average the readings for each concentration of standard antibiotic solution and test.
11. Plot the mean inhibition zone diameters of the standard solution against the log of the antibiotic concentrations, using semilogarithmic paper.
12. Construct the best-fitting straight line connecting the points and determine the concentration of each dilution of specimen by reading from the standard line (*Figure 27.3*).

Section 5

Haematology

28

Introduction to haematology

Haematology is the study of blood, and in a routine hospital laboratory is concerned largely with abnormalities of the blood. One of the primary functions is to detect anaemia and assist in the diagnosis of the exact type of anaemia to enable the right treatment to be given. Other important aspects of haematology are the identification of disorders associated with abnormal proliferation of blood cell precursors (e.g. leukaemia), the identification of inherited blood disorders (e.g. haemophilia) and the monitoring and control of patient treatments.

Essentially, blood consists of plasma, a fluid medium in which erythrocytes (red blood cells), leucocytes (white blood cells) and thrombocytes (platelets) are suspended. Plasma is a complex solution of proteins, salts and numerous metabolic substances and acts as a transport medium carrying its constituents to specialized organs of the body. As blood passes through the intestinal circulation, nutrients are absorbed into the plasma and carried to the liver and other tissues. As the blood passes through the kidneys, waste products of metabolism are filtered off into the urine. Many of the plasma proteins such as the blood-clotting factors, antibodies (immunoglobulins) and enzymes have specialized functions.

The majority of cells suspended in the plasma are erythrocytes. They contain a high concentration of haemoglobin, the oxygen-carrying pigment which gives blood its red colour. The leucocytes are very much fewer in number, and several different forms exist, each having different but complementary roles associated with the physiological defence mechanisms. The platelets are small cells which are intimately concerned with the blood-clotting process.

Structure and function of blood cells

Erythrocytes

Unstained, these cells are seen under the microscope as non-nucleated, pale greenish-yellow biconcave discs. When stained by Romanowsky stains, they have an affinity for eosin and therefore stain a pinkish colour.

The diameter of the normal red cell in the adult is between 6.7 and 7.7 μm, with an average of 7.2 μm. The thickness of the cells is between 1.7 and 2.4 μm. Thus, in the adult the normal mean cell volume (MCV) ranges from about 80 to 95 femtolitres (fl).

There are approximately 5.00×10^{12} red cells in each litre of blood. However, the normal range is dependent upon the age and sex of the patient. In the case of an adult female, the normal red cell count is 3.95 to 5.15×10^{12} per litre, which is in contrast to 4.4 to 5.8×10^{12} per litre recorded for the adult male.

The red cell normally survives in the blood stream for 110 days, after which time it is removed by the phagocytic cells of the reticuloendothelial system, broken down and some of its constituents re-utilized for the formation of new cells.

The primary function of the red cell is to transport oxygen from the lungs, via the heart, to the tissues. The cells contain haemoglobin which has the ability to combine reversibly with oxygen. In the lungs the haemoglobin in the red cell combines with oxygen, and releases it to the tissues of the body during its circulation. Carbon dioxide, a waste product of metabolism, is then absorbed from the tissues by the red cells and transported to the lungs to be exhaled.

The red cells, because they transport carbon dioxide from the tissues to the lungs, play an important role in maintaining the acid–base balance of the blood.

If the amount of circulating haemoglobin decreases below the normal range for the individual, then a state of anaemia exists.

Leucocytes

These are nucleated cells, some of which are capable of amoeboid movement. They are present in normal blood in smaller numbers than red cells, the normal adult range being between 4.0 and 11.0×10^9 per litre of blood. As they are capable of phagocytosis (ingestion of bacteria and other particulate matter), their main function is to act as one of the body's defences. Some of the white blood cells are also connected with antibody formation.

Certain conditions, such as acute bacterial infections, are capable of producing a variation in the white cell count. Leucocytosis is the term used to describe an increase in white cells, that is above 11.0×10^9 per litre. Leucopenia is the term used to describe a decrease in white cells, that is below 4.0×10^9 per litre.

Unstained leucocytes appear almost colourless, but a thin blood film, stained by the Romanowsky method, can be seen to contain white cells of three main types; the polymorphonuclear cells (granulocytes), lymphocytes and monocytes.

Polymorphonuclear leucocytes

These cells each contain a single nucleus consisting of a number of lobes. They are also called granulocytes, as they contain small granules in their cytoplasm. There are three types of polymorphonuclear leucocytes which can be differentiated according to the staining reactions of these granules.

Polymorphonuclear neutrophil

Usually, these cells are between 10 and $12 \mu m$ in diameter and are capable of amoeboid movement.

When stained by one of the Romanowsky stains they show a lobed nucleus, which stains a purple-violet colour. Most of the cells have 2 or 3 lobes, but it is possible to see as many as 7 (see Cooke–Arneth count, p. 332). The cytoplasm stains a light pink colour and contains small, violet or pinkish staining, dust-like granules. The term 'neutrophil', a relic of earlier staining methods, is perhaps a little misleading since the granules do not stain in a neutral manner, but rather in an acidic manner.

Neutrophils are increased in acute bacterial infections such as pneumonia and are the main constituents of pus. However, an increased neutrophil count (neutrophilia) does not always indicate infection. Neutrophils, in addition to being present in the peripheral circulation, are also present in the tissues and muscles. These neutrophils are rapidly mobilized and re-enter the circulation during periods of physical stress and therefore can give rise to a neutrophil leucocytosis. This is very apparent during childbirth, where the mother's neutrophil count can increase to about 20.0×10^9 per litre.

Not all bacterial infections are associated with neutrophilia – sometimes the infection can suppress the production of these cells and give rise to a neutropenia; that is where the neutrophil count is less than 2.0×10^9 per litre.

Polymorphonuclear eosinophil

These cells are approximately the same size as a neutrophil, but usually only have 2 lobes to their nucleus, often in a 'spectacle' arrangement. The nucleus stains a little paler than the neutrophil and the cytoplasm contains many large, round or oval, deep orange-pink granules. This is due to their great affinity for the acid dye component (eosin) of Romanowsky stains.

The eosinophil is not as amoeboid as the neutrophil, but is capable of phagocytosis. The exact function of the eosinophil is still unclear, but it is known that it is involved with allergic reactions. At the site of allergic reaction, the eosinophil releases a number of chemical substances which assist the overall repair function.

The normal eosinophil count in the adult is 0.04 to 0.4×10^9 per litre. An increase in numbers (eosinophilia) is often associated with allergic reactions, and when intestinal parasites are present.

Polymorphonuclear basophil

These cells are about $8–10 \mu m$ in diameter. The nucleus is usually kidney shaped and the cytoplasm contains a mass of large, deep purple staining granules which frequently obscure the nucleus.

The function of the basophil is still obscure, although it is known that the granules contain heparin and histamine, which are both released at the site of inflammation.

Basophils are rarely increased above 0.1×10^9 per litre of blood. One condition in which these cells are increased in the peripheral blood is chronic myeloid leukaemia.

Lymphocytes

Examination of a stained blood film shows two morphological forms, the large lymphocyte and the small lymphocyte. The small lymphocyte has a diameter of $7–10 \mu m$ and has a round, deep purple staining nucleus which occupies most of the cell so that the cytoplasm, which stains a pale blue colour, can be seen only as a rim around the nucleus. The small lymphocyte is the predominant form found in normal blood.

The large lymphocyte has a diameter between 12 and 20 µm and the nucleus stains a little paler than the small lymphocyte. The cytoplasm, which may contain a few reddish granules, is more plentiful, staining a pale blue colour.

Lymphocytes play an essential role in protecting the body from 'foreign' substances, such as bacteria. Sometimes this function is directed at the body itself, and can result in auto-immune diseases. Similarly, lymphocytes play a major role in the 'rejection' of transplanted tissues which are antigenically different to the recipient.

It is now realized that there are many subfractions of the lymphocyte population, each with specific but complementary roles. From experimental work it has been possible to identify two major populations of cell, the B-lymphocyte and the T-lymphocyte.

The B-lymphocyte is derived from the bone marrow and is concerned with the production of antibodies, in response to stimulation from antigens 'foreign' to the body. The B-lymphocyte, having recognized an antigen, transforms into a plasma cell which matures and secretes a specific antibody from the lymph nodes. The antibody is carried in the plasma and lymph fluid and coats the antigen, and thus makes it more susceptible to phagocytosis.

The T-lymphocyte is derived from the thymus gland and is concerned with cell-mediated immunity, a process which involves the cells surrounding the antigenic material, causing its destruction by direct cellular involvement. Examples of this include the localized reactions to tuberculin tests and the rejection of transplanted tissues. The T-lymphocytes have a very long life span, possibly 20 years, and are thought to hold a 'memory' of previously encountered antigens such that on subsequent exposure, the body can rapidly respond.

Although it may appear that the B-lymphocytes and T-lymphocytes have different functions, it must be emphasized that they are closely related and serve to complement each other.

Identification and quantitation of T-lymphocytes and B-lymphocytes cannot be done by simple morphological examination, but is dependent upon specialized immunological tests to determine cell surface markers.

The normal lymphocyte count for an adult is between 1.5 and 4.0 $\times$ 10^9 per litre of blood. Lymphocytosis, an increase in lymphocytes, is a common feature in viral infections such as mumps and measles and very high counts are seen in whooping-cough and chronic lymphatic leukaemia. Lymphopenia, a decrease in lymphocytes, is often found in patients undergoing radiotherapy and chemotherapy.

Monocytes

Monocytes are cells capable of ingesting bacteria and particulate matter, and act as 'scavenger cells' at the site of infections. They are larger than other white cells, measuring between 16 and 22 µm in diameter. Monocytes have one large nucleus, which is usually centrally placed within the cell and often kidney shaped. This nucleus has a stranded appearance, like a loosely coiled bundle of wool, and when stained is a pale violet colour. The copious cytoplasm, staining a pale greyish-blue, contains reddish-blue dust-like granules. The cytoplasm can also contain a few clear vacuoles.

The normal monocyte count in the adult is between 0.2 and 0.8 $\times$ 10^9 per litre of blood. Monocytosis often occurs in some bacterial infections (e.g. tuberculosis) and in some protozoal infections (e.g. malaria).

Platelets (thrombocytes)

These cells appear in films stained by Romanowsky techniques as small non-nucleated oval or round cells, 2–3 µm in diameter, which stain pale blue and contain many pink granules.

On contact with collagen, exposed when blood vessels are injured, platelets rapidly adhere to the damaged vessel and with one another to form a platelet plug. During this process, the soluble blood coagulation factors are activated to produce a mesh of insoluble fibrin around the clumped platelets. This assists and strengthens the platelet plug and produces a blood clot, which prevents further blood loss.

The normal platelet count in the adult is between 150 and 400 $\times$ 10^9 per litre of blood. A decrease in platelet numbers is called thrombocytopenia and may result in either an external or internal haemorrhage. An increase in platelets is called thrombocytosis, and may follow haemorrhage, surgery and fractures of bones. An increased platelet count is clinically important not just because it predisposes to thrombosis, but also because it can be associated with haemorrhage.

Blood cell production and maturation (haemopoiesis)

In the adult, blood cells are produced in the bone marrow, spleen, liver and lymphatic tissue including the thymus; these comprise the reticuloendothelial system. Only the red-coloured bone marrow actively produces blood cells. Although the yellow bone marrow, found principally in the shafts of the long bones, is not haemopoietically active, it retains the potential for further blood production should this be required due to extra demands. This can occur in

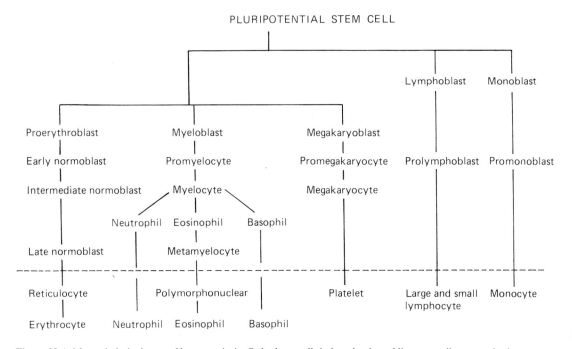

Figure 28.1. Monophyletic theory of haemopoiesis. Only those cells below the dotted line normally appear in the circulation

certain types of anaemia and myeloproliferative disorders.

The process of blood production is called haemopoiesis and the model describing the process is known as the monophyletic theory of haemopoiesis (*Figure 28.1*). This model shows that all blood cells are derived from a common precursor, the pluripotential stem cell. There are very few pluripotential stem cells in the body, but by mitosis and a feedback control mechanism they are able to supply all the blood cell requirements while maintaining their original numbers. Following the production of two daughter cells by mitosis, one of the cells retains the properties of the pluripotential cell, while the other becomes committed to produce mature blood cells. This cell, sometimes known as the committed stem cell, will, dependent upon the exact stimulus, develop into the specific precursor, or blast cell, of one of the cell lines. This phase of haemopoiesis is known as the differentiation phase.

The development of a normal red or white cell from its original blast cell progresses through three further phases. First, the blast cell divides by mitosis to produce large numbers of immature daughter cells (proliferation phase), and with each mitotic division there is a slight increase in maturity. Secondly, it is during the maturation phase that the specific properties develop which will allow the cell to fulfil its physiological function. Thirdly, the nearly mature or mature cells are released into the circulation.

The development of a normal cell from the original blast cell is accompanied by a diminution in the size of the cell because of successive divisions of the cell. The nucleus also decreases in size, the nuclear chromatin condenses and the nucleoli are lost. In the case of the red cell precursors, haemoglobin appears, and in the case of the polymorphonuclear precursors, the characteristic granules appear.

In the case of platelet production, the nucleus of the megakaryoblast increases its chromosome numbers similar to mitosis, but this is not accompanied by cell division. This therefore means that the developing megakaryocyte continues to increase in size. This process is called endoreduplication or endomitosis.

Erythropoiesis

Erythropoiesis, or red cell production, is stimulated by the hormone erythropoietin, which is produced in the kidneys. It is produced in response to a lowering of the tissue oxygen tension, and it acts by stimulating stem cells to transform into proerythroblasts. This cell is the first recognizable cell of the red cell series. It is a large cell with a large nucleus containing nucleoli, surrounded by a rim of basophilic (blue) cytoplasm. As the cell divides, haemoglobin synthesis starts in the cytoplasm, and with successive divisions the amount of haemoglobin increases. As the cell becomes smaller its cytoplasm when stained, first becomes purple and then greyish-pink. This gradual change of colour from blue to pink denotes the changes in the cytoplasmic concentrations of ribonucleic acid (RNA) and haemoglobin. These dividing cells are called normoblasts and are classified as early, intermediate or late according to (a) the amount of haemoglobin present, (b) the degree of contraction of the originally large nucleus, and (c) the size of the cell.

When the cell is fully haemoglobinized the small dense nucleus remaining is extruded, leaving a young greyish-blue cell called a polychromatic cell. These cells are also called reticulocytes because a reticular structure, representing the remnants of the ribosomes, is revealed in the cytoplasm when stained with brilliant cresyl blue. After 24–48 h in the peripheral blood, the reticulocyte matures to an adult red cell.

Leucopoiesis

In contrast to erythropoiesis, the exact nature of the factors stimulating leucopoiesis is unclear, but from *in vitro* tissue culture experiments a number of macromolecular substances have been isolated which will stimulate and produce colonies of a particular white cell line. These are called colony stimulating factors (CSFs). It is necessary to use a prefix to designate the type of colony produced, for example, granulocyte-macrophage colony stimulating factor (GM-CSF).

The granulocytes or polymorphonuclear cells arise from the myeloblast which is the first recognizable form. As development takes place through successive cell divisions the nucleus becomes smaller and loses its nucleoli, while at the same time the characteristic granules begin to appear in the cytoplasm and the cell progresses through the promyelocyte to the myelocyte stage. As the single nucleus becomes kidney-bean shaped, and then horseshoe shaped, the cell is called a metamyelocyte. When this horseshoe nucleus forms separate lobes, the cell is a true polymorphonuclear cell, which depending upon the specific granules will be either a neutrophil, eosinophil or basophil.

Although lymphoblasts are found both in the bone marrow and lymphoid tissues, the full development sequence is not completely understood. It is possible that the cells seen in the peripheral blood may undergo further transformations which have not yet been adequately demonstrated.

The monocyte develops from the monoblast, but the exact sequence of development is unclear.

Thrombopoiesis

Platelets are produced by the process of 'budding' from the cytoplasm of the megakaryocyte. It is understood that platelet production is maintained by feedback regulation mediated by a humoral substance known as thrombopoietin.

Factors required for haemopoiesis

The factors required for haemopoiesis are the same as those required for the production of any other cell. However, due to the specialized function of the red cell, and the extensive proliferation of blood cells, there are three factors which are of paramount importance to the maintenance of normal haemopoiesis. These are iron, vitamin B_{12} and folic acid.

Iron

Iron is an integral component of the haemoglobin molecule, and if excessive iron is lost from the body (e.g. due to blood loss) an iron deficiency anaemia can occur. Iron deficiency anaemia is the most common form of anaemia in the world. The chief dietary sources of iron are meats, egg yolk and green vegetables. There is considerable variation in the availability of iron for absorption in different foodstuffs. In general, iron from animal food is better absorbed than that of vegetable foods.

Vitamin B_{12} and folic acid

Both of these substances play an essential role in cell metabolism, acting as coenzymes in the chemical reactions leading to the synthesis of nucleic acids. Deficiency of one or both of these factors will lead to a megaloblastic anaemia. Vitamin B_{12} is obtained from foods, mainly those of animal protein origin, whereas folic acid is obtained from vegetable foodstuff.

Haemoglobin

Haemoglobin is a large complex protein molecule (molecular weight 64458) consisting of four polypeptide chains (globin) closely linked together. An iron-containing porphyrin called haem is attached to each polypeptide chain, and it is this part of the molecule which is principally responsible for its oxygen-carrying properties. If the ferrous iron of haem is oxidized to the ferric form, then the oxygen-carrying capacity of the haemoglobin is lost.

Haemoglobin has the property of combining reversibly with oxygen. Oxygen is rapidly taken up by the red cell in the lungs during the few microseconds the cell takes to pass through the pulmonary microcirculation. This rapid saturation of the haemoglobin molecule with oxygen, to form oxyhaemoglobin, is due to the enhancing interaction of the four haem groups in an environment with a high oxygen tension. This process is reversed when the red cell passes through tissues with a low oxygen tension. When the oxyhaemoglobin releases its oxygen, reduced haemoglobin is formed.

Haemoglobin also plays a part in the transport of carbon dioxide to the lungs. Carbon dioxide is not bound to the haemoglobin in the same way as oxygen, but is carried in the red cell in the form of bicarbonate. About 90% of the carbon dioxide is removed from the tissues in this way, the remainder being carried as bicarbonate in the plasma.

In adult women, the normal haemoglobin level is between 12.0 and 15.0 g per 100 ml of blood whereas in adult men it is between 13.0 and 17.0 g per 100 ml. The haemoglobin of a newborn infant is higher than the normal levels recorded for the adult, and may be as high as 19.0 g per 100 ml. This level falls quite rapidly in the first few weeks of life to around 15.0 g per 100 ml and then falls slowly to about 11.0 g per 100 ml during the next year or so. This then gradually increases throughout childhood, reaching adult levels at about 15 years of age.

Fate of haemoglobin

When the red cell reaches the end of its life span after approximately 110 days in the circulation, it is removed by the phagocytic macrophages of the reticuloendothelial system. Haemoglobin is released, and eventually both iron and globin are split off and bilirubin formed.

The released iron is carefully stored in the body, probably by becoming bound with a special tissue protein known as apoferritin to form the iron-containing protein, ferritin. Ferritin is a storage form of iron which circulates in very small quantities in the plasma. Normally, iron is transported in the plasma bound to a specific transport called transferrin. Although ferritin represents an important storage form of iron, haemosiderin, which is thought to be aggregates of 'ferritin-like' material, is the principal storage form. Haemosiderin can be demonstrated in the tissues of the reticuloendothelial system using Perl's stain.

Bilirubin, the iron-free residue of the haem molecule, is transported to the liver where it enters the hepatic cells and undergoes conjugation with glucuronic acid to form conjugated bilirubin. This substance passes by the bile ducts to the intestine, where by bacterial degradation, mainly in the colon, stercobilinogen and stercobilin are formed. These compounds are responsible for the brown colour of the faeces.

Haemoglobin pigments

In the circulation, haemoglobin normally takes the form of oxyhaemoglobin, or reduced haemoglobin. Certain other forms can be produced if haemoglobin is acted upon by other chemicals. These haemoglobin pigments are carboxyhaemoglobin, methaemoglobin and sulphaemoglobin.

Carboxyhaemoglobin (HbCO)

Carbon monoxide has an affinity for haemoglobin many times greater than that of oxygen. Therefore, even in low concentrations carbon monoxide will rapidly bind to haemoglobin to form carboxyhaemoglobin. It is found in high concentrations in cases of carbon monoxide poisoning, which because this compound cannot carry oxygen, can lead to death. It is also found in lower concentrations in people who smoke.

Methaemoglobin (Hi)

Methaemoglobin is formed when the ferrous iron of haemoglobin is oxidized to the ferric form. This occurs to a small extent in all red cells, but because of a series of red cell enzymes which can reverse the process, the normal levels are usually only 1–2% of the total haemoglobin. High levels of methaemoglobin can be found in individuals who are being treated with drugs (e.g. phenacetin, sulphonamides) which may cause oxidation of haemoglobin. Methaemoglobin is an inert pigment and does not carry oxygen. Methaemoglobin can also occur as a result of an inherited abnormality of the haemoglobin molecule.

Sulphaemoglobin (SHb)

Sulphaemoglobin is the name given to a group of irreversibly degraded haemoglobin pigments produced by certain drugs, such as the sulphonamides.

The molecular structure of haemoglobin

Haemoglobin, like all other proteins, is synthesized according to inherited genetic information. The genetic code for haemoglobin dictates the type and quantity of globin chains produced in the developing normoblast. In normal adults there are three molecular forms of haemoglobin, each consisting of different combinations of globin chains. Adult haemoglobin (HbA) is the predominant form (97%) and consists of two alpha globin chains and two beta chains. The alpha chains consists of 141 amino acids, whereas the beta chain has 146. The minor components, haemoglobin A_2 (HbA$_2$) and foetal haemoglobin (HbF), also have two alpha chains, but differ from HbA because they have two delta globin chains and two gamma globin chains, respectively. Like beta chains, the delta and gamma chains have 146 amino acids, but are structurally different because of their amino acid sequence.

Haemoglobin F is found in high concentrations in the foetus and represents between 70% and 90% of the haemoglobin at birth. This falls to 1–2% during the first year of life, remaining at this level throughout life. In some diseases, such as thalassaemia, HbF values may be increased.

HbF has two important characteristics. First, it has the ability to combine more readily with oxygen than HbA, a property which allows the foetus to acquire as much oxygen as possible from the placental circulation. Secondly, it resists denaturation with alkalis more than HbA. This characteristic is used to demonstrate and quantitate HbF in samples of blood.

The haemoglobinopathies

These are inherited abnormalities of haemoglobin structure and are sometimes referred to as 'haemoglobin variants'. There are many of these variants now recognized and the abnormality in all these conditions lies in the globin fraction of the haemoglobin molecule. Each type of globin chain has a specific sequence of amino acids which is genetically determined. If the amino acid sequence in any of the globin chains is altered, a variant is formed which may cause anaemia or, in the very severe forms, death. The commonest form of haemoglobin variant that is of clinical importance is haemoglobin S, so called because the red cells take on the characteristic 'sickle' shape when subjected to reduced oxygen tension.

Haemoglobin S is similar in overall structure to the HbA molecule, but differs because one of the amino acids in the beta chain has been substituted. This single amino acid alteration (i.e. the replacement of glutamic acid by valine at position 6 on the beta chain), is sufficient to account for the characteristics of this haemoglobin variant. This small change in protein structure probably is a consequence of a point mutation within the DNA gene locus for the beta chain.

The clinical abnormality caused by HbS exists in two forms, depending on whether the abnormal beta gene is inherited from one or both parents. If only one parent passes on the abnormal beta gene, the offspring is heterozygous and will produce both HbA and HbS. This is often termed sickle-cell trait, which except in unusual circumstances is a benign, asymptomatic condition, compatible with a normal life span. If both parents pass on the abnormal gene it is called homozygous and the offspring will only produce HbS; this condition is termed sickle-cell disease, and is often clinically very serious.

Haemoglobin S is found almost exclusively in Negroes, but has also been reported in communities in India, Greece, Italy and Turkey. In Africa, the incidence of the sickle abnormality varies from tribe to tribe, and in some may reach 45%.

There are many other haemoglobin variants, each having a slightly different amino acid sequence in one of the globin chains, and may also present genetically in either the heterozygous or homozygous state. Letters of the alphabet, or place names, are used to classify them (e.g. HbC, HbD, HbE and HbC Harlem). Many of these may be differentiated by haemoglobin electrophoresis.

Thalassaemia (Mediterranean anaemia)

As the name suggests, this anaemia was first discovered in people living around the Mediterranean sea, but it is now known to be far more widespread and is found in India and the Far East, and also in immigrants from these regions.

Thalassaemia is due to an inherited imbalance of globin chains caused by suppression of either the beta or alpha chains. In beta-thalassaemia there is a reduced number of beta chains produced, which if inherited as a heterozygous condition means that there is a relative decrease in the amount of HbA, associated with a relative increase in both HbA_2 and HbF. In alpha-thalassaemia the levels of HbA, HbA_2 and HbF are equally depressed since they all have alpha chains. In the absence of sufficient alpha chains, an excess of beta chains will form tetramers to produce HbH.

29

Haemostasis and blood coagulation

Maintenance of an intact vascular system, free from lesions or blockages, in which the blood can circulate in a fluid state, is controlled by the processes which comprise the haemostatic mechanism. The way in which this is achieved depends on the close interaction of numerous dynamic processes. These include the constriction of the injured vessels; the adherence and aggregation of platelets to form a platelet plug; the formation of a fibrin clot by the soluble blood coagulation factors; and the eventual dissolution of the clot by the plasma fibrinolytic enzymes. Although it is useful to consider these as separate entities, it must be emphasized that they are closely interrelated. Failure of one or more of these processes may predispose the patient to bleed, or in some cases to form blood clots in the circulation.

The role of the blood vessel

The constriction of blood vessels at the site of injury is considered to be the earliest phase in haemostasis. Direct trauma to a blood vessel will cause constriction, thereby reducing blood loss, either by the release of chemicals or by nervous stimuli. In small blood vessels, this process coupled with the formation of a platelet plug is possibly sufficient to prevent excessive blood loss. However, if large blood vessels are injured, this process alone will not be sufficient.

The role of platelets

Bleeding problems may arise because of deficiencies either in platelet numbers or in platelet function. When a blood vessel wall is injured, platelets will adhere to the exposed collagen fibres, and numerous chemicals are released into the immediate environment. These include adenosine diphosphate (ADP) and 5-hydroxytryptamine (serotonin). The precise role of some of these factors is not clearly understood, but it is known that some of them cause the platelets to aggregate. During the aggregation phase more chemicals are released which produce an irreversible aggregation of platelets (viscous metamorphosis) and the forming of an impermeable plug. This is further reinforced by the formation of a mesh of fibrin.

Blood coagulation factors

Present in the plasma of normal individuals there are a number of interacting proteins, which on activation will form insoluble fibrin. Morawitz attempted to explain this phenomenon in 1905 in his Classical Theory of Coagulation. He stated that four substances present in normal blood were responsible for blood clotting:

1. Thrombokinase, which he said was liberated from platelets when they came into contact with a water-wettable surface.
2. Prothrombin, a proteinaceous substance formed in the liver and found in plasma.
3. Fibrinogen, a plasma protein produced by the liver, and also found in plasma.
4. Free calcium ions.

Morawitz stated that when blood was shed, thrombokinase was liberated from the platelet, and reacted with the prothrombin, in the presence of calcium ions, converting the prothrombin into a substance called thrombin. The fibrinogen in the presence of thrombin was then converted into fibrin, forming a fine network of strands which trap the blood cells thus forming a typical clot:

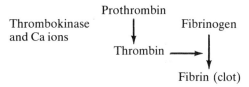

This theory is still essentially correct, but it has become apparent that the reactions leading to the conversion of prothrombin are more complicated than those suggested by Morawitz. The latter part of the classical theory, that is, the production of fibrin from fibrinogen in the presence of thrombin, is still regarded as true. However, modern workers have postulated a more complex theory termed the intrinsic and extrinsic mechanism of blood coagulation.

Intrinsic–extrinsic coagulation mechanisms

Normal blood contains certain factors which enable it to clot within 5–10 min when collected in a glass tube. Tissue contains a substance which, when added to blood, accelerates the clotting. This substance is commonly called thromboplastin.

The intrinsic–extrinsic theory of blood coagulation suggests that prothrombin can be activated to thrombin by one of two substances which are termed

(a) extrinsic thromboplastin (extrinsic prothrombin activator), and (b) intrinsic thromboplastin (intrinsic prothrombin activator).

Extrinsic thromboplastin is produced when tissue extract is acted upon by certain factors present in normal blood. The tissue extract requires to be activated by factor V, factor VII, factor X and calcium to form extrinsic thromboplastin (*Figure 29.1*).

Intrinsic thromboplastin is produced entirely from substances present in the blood. These substances are factor V, factor VIII, factor IX, factor X, factor XI, factor XII, free calcium ions, and platelet lipid factor, but no tissue extract. It is thought that factor XII, when coming into contact with a foreign surface, is activated to form activated factor XII. This then reacts with factor XI to form an activation product. The activation product then reacts with factor IX, factor VIII, factor X and factor V and the platelet lipid factor, in the presence of free calcium ions, to form intrinsic thromboplastin.

Both the intrinsic and extrinsic thromboplastins are capable of converting prothrombin to thrombin, which in turn converts fibrinogen to fibrin. The coagulation mechanism is summarized in *Figure 29.1*.

Some confusion has developed over the different terminology used by various workers in the field of blood coagulation. International agreement has been reached whereby Roman numerals are used to identify the factors. *Table 29.1* lists the coagulation factors with their synonyms.

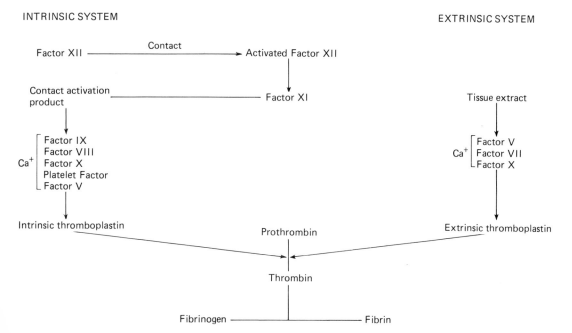

Figure 29.1. Intrinsic–extrinsic coagulation mechanism

Table 29.1 Coagulation factors and their synonyms

International nomenclature	Synonyms
Factor I	Fibrinogen
II	Prothrombin
V	Proaccelerin, labile factor
VII	Proconvertin, stable factor
VIII	Antihaemophilic globulin (AHG), antihaemophilic factor A (AHF)
IX	Christmas factor, antihaemophilic factor B, plasma thromboplastin component (PTC)
X	Stuart–Prower factor
XI	Plasma thromboplastin antecedent (PTA)
XII	Hageman factor
XIII	Fibrin-stabilizing factor

The fibrinolytic system

It has long been known that in cases of 'sudden death' blood may be incoagulable. This has been demonstrated to be due to a lack of fibrinogen caused by the action of a proteolytic enzyme present in plasma. Normally, this enzyme, plasminogen, is inactive, but it may be activated to plasmin by the action of tissue and blood activators released at the site of injury, or by products of bacterial infection. Plasmin digests fibrin(ogen) to form fibrin(ogen) degradation productions (FDPs) and this process is known as fibrinolysis. This process is completely antagonistic to the blood coagulation process, and the maintenance of haemostasis is due to the preservation of the dynamic equilibrium between these processes.

Bleeding disorders

Bleeding disorders can result from a failure of any of the previously mentioned mechanisms. In particular, thrombocytopenia, and either acquired or inherited deficiencies of the blood coagulation factors, may lead to situations where external or internal haemorrhage may occur.

The two most common inherited defects of the coagulation mechanism are haemophilia and Christmas disease. Both are inherited as sex-linked recessive conditions, and it is rare for females to be affected. Haemophilia is associated with a low activity of factor VIII, whereas Christmas disease is associated with a low activity of factor IX. Clinically, it is not possible to differentiate between these, diagnosis being entirely dependent on laboratory investigations.

Anticoagulants

Samples of blood will clot if transferred to dry containers. While this is desirable for certain laboratory investigations (such as serological examinations), the examination of blood cells requires blood which has not been allowed to clot.

As has been shown above, certain steps are involved in blood coagulation, and if one of the factors is removed or inactivated, the coagulation reaction will not take place. The substance responsible for this removal or inactivation is called an anticoagulant. Anticoagulated blood is obtained by transferring blood samples, immediately they are obtained, into bottles containing a known amount of anticoagulant. Thorough mixing of the blood in the bottle is now necessary. There are several anticoagulants in general use, some of which are described.

Oxalates

Oxalates are often used for laboratory investigations of blood, but never in transfusion work as they are poisonous. Sodium, potassium and ammonium oxalate are all used; they act by combining with the calcium in blood to form insoluble calcium oxalate. Once the calcium is so combined it cannot be utilized, and blood coagulation does not take place.

Citrate

Sodium citrate is used as an anticoagulant in blood transfusion work, coagulation studies and the Westergren ESR. It combines with calcium, thereby preventing the conversion of prothrombin to thrombin, and coagulation does not occur.

Sequestrene

This substance, which combines with calcium, is a chelating agent. It is in fact the disodium or dipotassium salt of sequestric acid, that is disodium or dipotassium ethylene diamine tetra-acetic acid (EDTA) which are normally used.

Sequestrene prevents the clumping of platelets and is therefore the anticoagulant of choice where total platelet counts are required.

Heparin

This substance is believed to inactivate thrombin, preventing conversion of fibrinogen to fibrin. Red cells are unaltered by the action of heparin, and it is a useful, although expensive, anticoagulant to use.

Leucocytes are often clumped by heparin and should not be used when these cells are to be counted. The effect of heparin may be neutralized by the addition of protamine sulphate. Heparin is also given to patients when immediate total anticoagulation is required, such as in coronary thrombosis, where oral anticoagulants will take 48 h to have any effect on the coagulation system.

Oral anticoagulants

Oral anticoagulants (e.g. warfarin) suppress the synthesis of the vitamin K dependent clotting factors (factors II, VII, IX and X) by the liver. The anticoagulant effect is therefore delayed for several days until the existing circulating clotting factors are cleared from the blood stream. It is essential that the degree of anticoagulation is controlled; usually by way of the prothrombin time.

30

Blood collection and blood film preparation

Collection of blood

For haematological investigations, capillary or venous blood may be used. It is essential that adequate mixing of the blood and anticoagulant or diluting fluid is carried out prior to any investigation. For this purpose a rotating mixer (*Figure 30.1*) is required. The type of mixer illustrated has been shown to give excellent mixing and is standard equipment in many laboratories. When not available the specimen should be mixed by slow inversion.

Capillary blood

It must be remembered that capillary blood samples, although of great value in children and in adults with 'difficult' veins, are not only subject to sampling error but tests cannot be repeated in the laboratory, as the whole sample may have been used and further tests which may be required cannot be performed.

Select a suitable site for puncture—the ball of the finger or the side of the thumb. Blood from a baby is best obtained from the base of the heel. The area

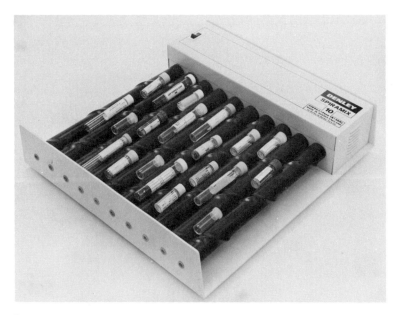

Figure 30.1. Denley Spiramix 10 rotating mixer (reproduced by courtesy of Denley Instruments Ltd)

chosen must be vigorously cleaned with 75% alcohol, and allowed to dry. This sterilizes the skin and promotes a free flow of blood. A quick stab is made, preferably with a pre-sterilized disposable blood lancet, the use of which reduces the hazard of cross-infection.

After the skin has been punctured, a little pressure is applied to ensure a free flow of blood. Undue squeezing must be avoided as this can cause lymph to dilute the blood, giving erroneous results. Undue or prolonged pressure can cause congestion and concentration of cells and haemoglobin. Wipe away the first few drops of blood, and then carefully draw blood into the appropriate pipette by means of gentle suction applied to the rubber teat attached to the pipette. Make sure that there are no air bubbles, and check that the blood level is exactly to the mark. Wipe the outside of the pipette, and slowly deliver the blood into a tube containing the appropriate diluent.

Alternatively, blood may be expressed from the puncture site into a container holding suitable anticoagulant, and stored for future processing.

Venous blood

If larger volumes are required, a venous sample of blood must be obtained. Using a dry, sterile syringe and needle, the blood is withdrawn from a suitable vein in the arm.

If serum is required, the needle of the syringe is removed and the blood slowly ejected into a clean, dry, sterile bottle.

In recent years, some laboratories have dispensed with the traditional needle and syringe as a means of blood collection. Instead, they use double-ended needles, one end of which is inserted into the patient's vein. An evacuated blood sample 'bottle', with a rubber top, is then pushed onto the other end of the needle. The blood will then flow into the bottle. The needles and evacuated sample bottles are available from several manufacturers.

Plasma

This is the fluid portion of the blood, so that when blood is maintained in a fluid state *in vitro*, by the addition of an anticoagulant, the fluid is referred to as plasma. This plasma contains all the coagulation factors except the one removed by the anticoagulant. If this substance is replaced in sufficient quantity, the plasma will clot.

Serum

This is the fluid which remains after blood has clotted. Some of the clotting factors are not present in serum, as these will have been used to produce the fibrin clot.

Blood film preparation

Gently touch a fresh drop of blood onto one end of a clean grease-free slide. Using a bevelled piece of glass a little narrower than the slide, allow the drop to spread along it. Holding the slide and 'spreader' at a suitable angle (*Figure 30.2*), push the spreader along the slide, drawing the blood behind it, until the whole of the drop has been smeared. Do not

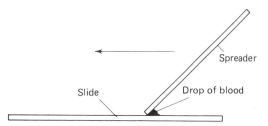

Figure 30.2. Making a blood smear

have too large a drop, or incline the spreader at too great an angle, as the film will be too thick for satisfactory microscopic examinations.

The thickness and the even distribution of the cells plays an important part in obtaining accurate results. The smear should be slightly thicker at the commencement than at the tail end. In badly prepared films, the polymorphonuclear neutrophils frequently concentrate at the edges of the preparation.

Romanowsky stains

These stains depend for their staining properties upon certain derivatives produced when alkaline methylene blue is combined with eosin. Methylene blue, when treated with alkali, forms a methylene azure. The various Romanowsky stains differ in the method of preparation of the methylene azure and in the proportion of eosin and methylene azure used to prepare the stain.

All the stains in the group are sensitive to changes in pH, the methylene blue component staining more intensely in an alkaline environment and the eosin derivative staining more intensely in an acid environment. When using these stains, buffered distilled water is used throughout the staining procedure. The alcohol used to dissolve the stain must be free from acetone, acetic acid and water.

Romanowsky stains may be purchased in powder, tablet or liquid form. For the busy laboratory, the stain already in solution is probably the most convenient, but each batch purchased or prepared should be tested for its optimum staining time.

Leishman's stain

This is a Romanowsky-type stain designed to differentiate leucocytes.

Leishman's stain

Solution 1:

Methylene blue (CI No. 52015)	1 g
Sodium carbonate, 0.5% aqueous solution	100 ml
Eosin BA (CI No. 45400) 0.1% aqueous solution	100 ml
Methyl alcohol, absolute	to 100 ml

Dissolve the methylene blue in the sodium carbonate solution. Heat at 65°C for 12 h, cool and allow the mixture to stand for 10 days. Add an equal volume of the eosin solution, mix well and allow the mixture to stand for 6–12 h. Filter and collect the precipitate. Wash the precipitate with several changes of distilled water until no more colour is extracted. Dry the precipitate in a 37°C incubator and grind to a powder in a glass mortar. Weigh out 0.15 g of the powder and triturate in a mortar with methyl alcohol, store in a tightly stoppered dark bottle and label. Allow the stain to stand for 24 h prior to use.

Buffer solution (pH 6.8)

Solution 2:

Disodium hydrogen orthophosphate Na$_2$HPO$_4$ (anhydrous), 0.067M solution (9.47 g per litre)	49.6 ml
Potassium dihydrogen orthophosphate KH$_2$PO$_4$ (anhydrous), 0.067M solution (9.08 g per litre)	50.4 ml

Dissolve the phosphates in the distilled water, check the reaction (pH 6.8) and label.

Procedure

1. Prepare thin blood films and fix in solution 1 for 1–2 min.
2. Add an equal volume of solution 2 and mix by gentle rocking. Allow the diluted stain to act for 10 min.
3. Wash and differentiate with solution 2. When correctly differentiated the smear should be a salmon-pink colour.
4. Drain and dry in the air at room temperature. Clean the back of the slide and examine microscopically.

Results

Nuclei of leucocytes, purple; eosinophilic granules, orange-red; basophilic granules, dark blue; lymphocytes, dark purple nuclei with pale blue cytoplasm; platelets, violet granules; Auer bodies, red; red blood corpuscles, salmon pink.

■ Notes

1. Leishman's stain may be purchased commercially in the form of the precipitated powder or as a ready-prepared

solution. The mode of preparation of the commercially prepared powder is similar to that described above, 0.15 g of the powder being dissolved in 100 ml of methyl alcohol. Alternatively, place the dye and alcohol together in a flask, plug with cotton wool and warm for 15 min in a water bath, shaking at intervals.
2. The use of a buffer solution for diluting the Romanowsky stains is recommended owing to the varying pH of tap water in different localities. The buffer solution should be added to the slide gently, without displacing any of the stain. After staining, the dye should be washed from the slide in such a manner that the scum is removed first.
3. When dry, the stained film can be mounted with a coverglass using a neutral medium as a mountant. Although optional, this step is preferred by some workers.

Giemsa stain

This is a Romanowsky-type stain designed to differentiate leucocytes.

Solution 1: Methyl alcohol, absolute (Analar)

Giemsa stain

Solution 2:

Azure II–eosin	3 g
Azure II	0.8 g
Glycerol, pure	200 ml
Methyl alcohol, absolute (Analar)	300 ml

Grind the two dyes together in a clean mortar and combine the alcohol with the glycerol in a 1-litre flask. Sprinkle the mixed dye carefully over the surface of the alcohol–glycerol and allow the mixture to stand for 24 h. Stir the mixture at intervals after the 24 h has elapsed to ensure that all of the dye has passed into solution. Store in a tightly stoppered dark bottle and label.

Buffer solution (pH 7.0)

Solution 3:

Disodium hydrogen orthophosphate Na$_2$HPO$_4$ (anhydrous), 0.067M solution (9.47 g per litre)	61.1 ml
Potassium dihydrogen orthophosphate KH$_2$PO$_4$ (anhydrous), 0.067M solution (9.08 g per litre)	38.9 ml

Dissolve the phosphates in the distilled water, check the reaction (pH 7.0) and label.

Procedure

1. Prepare thin blood films and fix in solution 2 for 3 min.
2. Dilute one volume of solution 2 with nine volumes of solution 3, flood the slide and allow the stain to act for 15 min.
3. Wash and differentiate with solution 3, controlling the degree of differentiation microscopically.
4. Drain and dry in the air at room temperature.

Results

Nuclei of leucocytes, reddish-purple; eosinophilic granules, red to orange; basophilic granules, blue; lymphocytes, dark purple nuclei with light blue cytoplasm; platelets, violet to purple granules.

■ Notes

Giemsa stain is available commercially either in liquid form ready for use or as a combined powder. The azure dyes frequently vary from batch to batch and for this reason most laboratories prefer to purchase the commercial product. The commercial powder is dissolved as follows: weigh out 1 g of the powder and place it in a 250 ml conical flask. Add 66 ml of pure glycerol and heat the mixture at 56°C for 90–120 min. Add 66 ml of absolute methyl alcohol, mix thoroughly and allow the solution to stand for 7 days at room temperature. Filter, store in a tightly stoppered bottle and label. The solution should be diluted for use as in the above procedure.

Staining machines

When staining large numbers of blood films it is an advantage to use a staining machine, as not only do they stain a large batch of films more quickly but they also give more uniform staining results.

The most common blood film stain used in Britain is May Grunwald–Giemsa, and it is ideally suited for use on an automatic staining machine. The May Grunwald component used in this technique is not a Romanowsky-type stain, but is a basic dye which is used to accentuate the staining reaction of the Giemsa stain.

31

The full blood count

The most often requested investigation in haematology laboratories, in the UK, is the full blood count (FBC). This is a set of complementary investigations which act together to provide information on the general pathophysiology of the blood and reticulo-endothelial system.

The number and type of investigations offered as part of the FBC varies from laboratory to laboratory and is dependent upon the technology, staff and financial resources available. In general terms, the FBC consists of (a) haemoglobin measurement, (b) white cell count, (c) packed cell volume, (d) red cell count and (e) calculation of the red cell indices, or absolute values. With the advent of sophisticated analysers, some laboratories now include a platelet count as an integral part of every FBC.

The use of semi-automated and fully-automated analysers is now accepted as standard practice in most laboratories, but it should be borne in mind that the traditional methods based on manual techniques are still important because they serve as the reference methods for most automated procedures.

The principles of visual cell counts

Most haematological requests require an assessment of the number of red cells, white cells and platelets. The earliest methods used for this involved diluting the blood specimen and loading it into a special glass counting chamber known as a haemocytometer. This consists of a heavy glass slide, with four troughs or channels extending across the slide. The centre platform thus formed is set slightly lower than the two adjacent ones (*Figure 31.1*) and is engraved to show a ruled area (*Figure 31.2*). When placed in position, the coverglass rests upon the two outer

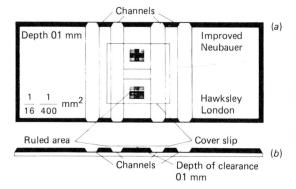

Figure 31.1. (a) Double-sided counting chamber; (b) side view of chamber

platforms, producing a clearance between itself and the rulings on the central platform. This clearance is referred to as the depth of the counting chamber. Thus the volume of diluent, between the coverglass and the engraved markings, can be calculated by multiplying the depth by the area enclosed within the markings. The number of cells in the original blood sample is achieved by counting the number of cells lying on the ruled area and performing a simple calculation using this figure, the dilution factor and the volume of diluent between the ruled area and coverglass.

Counting chambers

Although there are a number of different types of haemocytometer (e.g. Burker, Fuchs–Rosenthal), it is the Improved Neubauer counting chamber which is used for most routine cell counts.

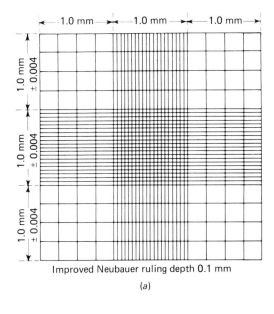

Improved Neubauer ruling depth 0.1 mm

(a)

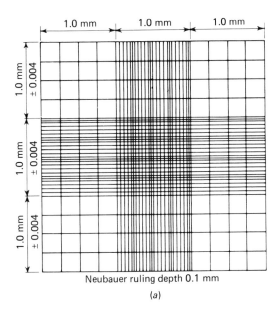

Neubauer ruling depth 0.1 mm

(a)

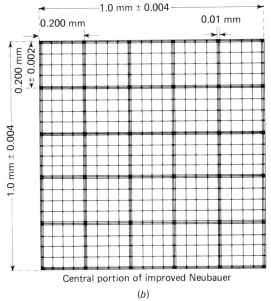

Central portion of improved Neubauer

(b)

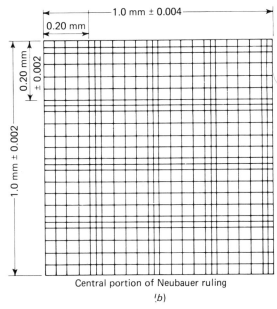

Central portion of Neubauer ruling

(b)

Figure 31.2. Ruled area of the Improved Neubauer counting chamber

Figure 31.3. Ruled area of the Ordinary Neubauer counting chamber

Ordinary Neubauer counting chamber

The central platform is set 0.1 mm below the level of the two side ones, giving the chamber a depth of 0.1 mm. The engraving covers an area of $9\,mm^2$ divided into 9 squares of $1\,mm^2$ each. The 4 corner squares are divided into 16 squares, each with an area of $\frac{1}{16}$ of a mm^2. The central ruled area of $1\,mm^2$ is divided into 16 large squares by sets of triple lines. These large squares are further subdivided into 16 small squares by single lines. It will be noticed from the diagram (*Figure 31.3*) that the width of the triple lines dividing the large squares is the same as the width of a small square. Two adjacent sides of the ruled area are bounded by triple lines, the other two by single lines. Each side is, therefore, divided into 20 equal divisions (the

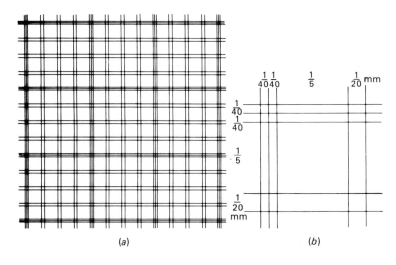

Figure 31.4. (a) Ruled area of the Burker counting chamber; (b) enlarged view showing actual measurements

width of 16 small squares and 4 sets of triple lines). Each small square is, therefore, $\frac{1}{20}$ of 1 mm squared, that is $\frac{1}{400}$ of 1 mm^2.

Burker counting chamber

Like the Neubauer counting chamber, this has a ruled area of 9 mm^2 and a depth of 0.1 mm (*Figure 31.4*).

Fuchs–Rosenthal counting chamber

This chamber was originally designed for counting cells in cerebrospinal fluid, but as such a relatively large area is covered, it is preferred by some workers for counting leucocytes. The depth is 0.2 mm and the ruled area consists of 16 mm squares divided by triple lines. These squares are subdivided to form 16 smaller squares, each with an area of $\frac{1}{16}$ of 1 mm^2 (*Figure 31.5*).

Another type of Fuchs–Rosenthal chamber is now available, which has the same depth as the one described, but is ruled over 9 mm^2 only.

Improved Neubauer counting chamber

The Improved Neubauer counting chamber (*Figures 31.1* and *31.2*) has a total ruled area of 9 mm^2 and a depth of 0.1 mm. The central area (1 mm^2) is divided into 25 squares, each with an area of 0.04 mm^2, and each of these is further marked into 16 squares. The volume of diluent contained between the central square and the coverglass is 0.1 mm^3 which is equivalent to 0.1 µl.

It is important that the correct procedure is followed when making a cell count; failure to do so may result in significant errors which will produce erroneous results. The correct procedure is as follows:

1. Thoroughly clean the counting chamber and the coverglass; place it on a flat horizontal surface and, using firm pressure, slide the coverglass into position on the counting chamber, obtaining a rainbow effect on both sides (Newton's rings).
2. Mix the dilution of blood and withdraw a quantity of fluid into a capillary tube.
3. Fill the chamber by holding the capillary tube at an angle of 45 degrees and lightly touch the tip against the edge of the coverglass. It is important that the fluid is not allowed to overflow into the channels. Should this occur, the chamber must be cleaned and refilled. Too much fluid in the chamber may raise the coverglass, causing a variation in the depth, resulting in erroneous counts.

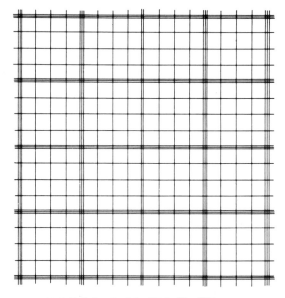

Figure 31.5. Ruled area of the Fuchs–Rosenthal counting chamber

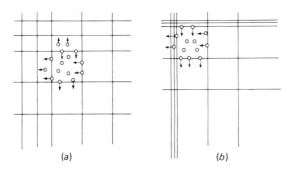

Figure 31.6. Cells to be counted within each small square: (a) ordinary Neubauer counting chamber; (b) Improved Neubauer counting chamber

4. Allow the cells to settle for 20 min, by placing the filled chamber in a petri dish, containing a piece of moist filter paper. This prevents the fluid in the chamber from evaporation, a process which would concentrate the cells and give rise to erroneous counts.
5. Place the chamber on the microscope stage and count the number of cells in a specified area using an appropriate objective. Because the cells are distributed randomly across the entire area of the counting chamber, and therefore some of them will lie on the ruled lines, it is necessary to adopt a standard counting technique. *Figure 31.6* shows the method usually adopted for including or excluding cells which lie on the ruled lines of the Improved Neubauer counting chamber.

Visual red cell counts

The most common diluent used for visual red cell counts is a solution of formol–citrate, prepared by mixing 10 ml of formalin (40% formaldehyde) with 1 litre of trisodium citrate solution (31.3 g per litre). This fluid should be filtered, and then stored in a clean glass container until required. The patient's blood sample is diluted by washing 20 µl of blood taken into a 'shellback' pipette or positive displacement pipette, into 4.0 ml of diluent to give a final dilution of 1 in 201. The diluted sample is then mixed and loaded into the counting chamber.

When the cells have settled out of suspension, the number lying on 5 of the 0.04 mm^2 areas are counted. If the number recorded is less than 500, the total central 1 mm^2 area should be counted; this will increase the confidence in the final result by decreasing the inherent statistical counting error. For the final result to be expressed as the number of cells per litre, the following calculation is necessary.

Calculation

$$\text{Red cell count} = \frac{N \times DF \times 10^6}{A \times D} \text{ per litre}$$

where N is the number of cells (e.g. 500), DF the dilution factor (e.g. 201), 10^6 converts to cells per litre, A is the area of chamber counted (e.g. 0.2 mm^2), and D the depth of chamber (e.g. 0.1 mm). Thus,

$$\text{Red cell count} = \frac{500 \times 201 \times 10^6}{0.2 \times 0.1} \text{ per litre}$$

$$= 5.03 \times 10^{12} \text{ per litre}$$

■ Notes

1. In practice, it is acceptable to regard a 1 in 201 dilution as a 1 in 200 dilution. In the above example, the final red cell count would be 5.00×10^{12} per litre.
2. Formol–citrate is not suitable as a diluent for blood samples with cold agglutinins. In these cases, a solution of 3.13% trisodium citrate should be used.

Visual white cell counts

Prior to counting the number of white cells present in a sample of blood, it is necessary to prepare a dilution which will lyse the red cells and thus make the white cells more readily visible.

A suitable diluent for this purpose, especially if light microscopy is used, is 2% acetic acid (20 ml per litre) tinged with gentian violet. This, in addition to destroying the red cells, will also stain the white cell nuclei. Alternatively, if phase contrast microscopy is used, a solution of 1% ammonium oxalate (10 g per litre) can be used to count both white cells and platelets present in the same dilution. Prior to use, the diluting fluid must be filtered to prevent dust and debris interfering with the accuracy of the count.

The patient's blood sample is diluted by washing 50 µl of blood taken into a shellback pipette, or positive displacement pipette, into 950 µl of diluent to give a final dilution of 1 in 20. The dilute sample is then mixed and loaded into the counting chamber. Using the Improved Neubauer chamber, count the white cells present in the 4 corner 1 mm^2 areas, and those in the central 1 mm^2 area. Apply the same margin rule for including or excluding cells lying on peripheral lines, as described for the red cell count.

The final white cell count for the whole blood sample is calculated using the same basic formula as described for red cell counts.

Example of white cell count calculation

The number of cells counted (N) = 200, the dilution factor (DF) = 20, the area counted (A) = 5 $\times$ 1 mm^2, and the depth of the counting chamber (D) = 0.1 mm. Therefore,

$$\text{White cell count} = \frac{200 \times 20 \times 10^6}{5 \times 0.1} \text{ per litre}$$

$$= 8.0 \times 10^9 \text{ per litre}$$

Visual platelet counts

A 1 in 20 dilution of the patient's blood is made in 1% ammonium oxalate and, after mixing for several minutes, it is loaded into an Improved Neubauer counting chamber. The chamber is then stood in a petri dish, containing a piece of moist filter paper, for 20 min to allow the cells to settle.

The cells are counted as for red cells (that is 5 of the 0.04 mm^2 areas) using either phase contrast or light microscopy. It has been recommended that phase contrast microscopy should be the preferred method for counting platelets, because they are more readily visible and more easily differentiated from dust and debris.

The whole blood platelet count is calculated using the same basic formula as described for red cell counts.

Example of platelet count calculation

The number of platelets counted (N) = 250, the dilution factor (DF) = 20, the area counted (A) = 0.2 mm^2, and the depth of the counting chamber (D) = 0.1 mm. Therefore,

$$\text{Platelet count} = \frac{250 \times 20 \times 10^6}{0.2 \times 0.1} \text{ per litre}$$

$$= 250 \times 10^9 \text{ per litre}$$

Errors associated with visual cell counts

The accuracy of any cell count is determined by two factors. First there are those technical factors where, due to bad technique and inaccurate apparatus, the final count will not be representative of the true cell concentration. These errors are avoidable and every effort must be taken to ensure that they are minimized, if not eliminated. The following list gives some of the technical errors which are likely to be encountered with visual cell counting:

1. Dirty pipettes and counting chambers.
2. Inaccurate pipettes.*
3. Inaccurate counting chambers.†
4. Inadequate mixing of blood sample.

*After cleaning, new pipettes should be checked for accuracy. The pipettes should be filled to the mark with mercury which is then expelled into a vessel and carefully weighed. 20 μl of mercury weighs 272 mg, and 50 μl of mercury weighs 680 mg. Alternatively, pipettes may be checked by performing replicate haemoglobin estimations or cell counts in comparison with pipettes where the accuracy has been previously established.
†The British Standard on Haemocytometer Counting Chambers (BS 748) specifies a tolerance of dimensions for Improved Neubauer chambers.

5. Poor dilution technique.
6. Preparation of dilution on wrong patient.
7. Inadequate mixing of dilution.
8. Over- or under-filling of counting chamber.
9. Insufficient time given for cells to settle.
10. Careless counting of cells.
11. Errors in calculation.
12. Reporting wrong result.

Secondly, there are those errors associated with the random distribution of the cells in the counting chamber. These are referred to as 'inherent errors' and can never be eliminated. However, they can be minimized by counting large numbers of cells.

Using the mathematical model known as the Poisson distribution, which describes the probability of random occurrences, it is possible to predict the inherent error associated with any cell count. From the Poisson distribution it is known that the standard deviation (S.D.) can be derived by calculating the square root of the number of cells counted ($\sqrt{N}$). Using this figure it is then possible to calculate the confidence limits for the cell count, and the percentage inherent error. Normally, the 95% confidence limits for a cell count are calculated to show the range of results which are possible. This range is calculated by taking the number of cells counted, plus or minus 2 standard deviations: ($N \pm 2\sqrt{N}$). The percentage inherent error (coefficient of variation) is calculated from

$$\text{Coefficient of variation} = \frac{\text{S.D.} \times 100}{N}$$

Table 31.1 shows that the confidence placed in any cell count (e.g. red cell count = 5.00×10^{12} per litre) increases as the number of cells counted also increases. This is due to a decrease in the coefficient of variation, or inherent error.

Table 31.1 Confidence in cell count

Number of cells (N)	Standard deviation	Coefficient of variation (%)	95% confidence limit ($\times 10^{12}$/l)
100	10	10.0	4.00–6.00
500	22	4.5	4.55–5.45
1 000	32	3.2	4.68–5.32
5 000	71	1.4	4.86–5.14
10 000	100	1.0	4.90–5.10

Haemoglobin measurement

The object of measuring haemoglobin is to estimate the oxygen-carrying capacity of blood, in addition to providing an assessment of the erythropoietic status of the reticuloendothelial system. The results assist in the detection and diagnosis of diseases which cause a deficiency or excess of haemoglobin. The former is called anaemia, whereas the latter is known as polycythaemia.

Haemoglobin concentration can be measured by several principles, all of which relate to the characteristics of the Hb molecule. The first principle is by measuring the amount of oxygen which can combine with haemoglobin. In this method, a known volume of blood is taken and the haemoglobin it contains is saturated with oxygen; the oxygen is displaced and measured in a Van Slyke apparatus. Then, applying Hufner's factor, the amount of haemoglobin in the known volume of blood can be calculated. Hufner's factor states that 1 g of haemoglobin can combine with 1.34 ml of oxygen. This method only estimates the haemoglobin capable of carrying oxygen. Inert forms such as methaemoglobin and sulphaemoglobin are not measured. It is now accepted that a more correct figure to use for Hufner's factor would be 1.36 ml oxygen per 1 g of haemoglobin. This method is of historic importance only, and is not used for routine haemoglobin measurements.

The second principle applied to the measurement of haemoglobin relates to the amount of iron contained in a known sample of blood. From chemical analysis of pure haemoglobin it has been found that there are 347 mg of iron present in 100 g of haemoglobin. Therefore, if the amount of iron is measured in a sample of haemoglobin, the actual concentration can be derived by calculation. Although this is a relatively simple principle, the actual method is too cumbersome and time-consuming for routine use.

By far the most common principle applied to haemoglobin measurement is that of colour comparison. In these methods, the colour of a dilute sample of blood is compared either by direct visual observation, or by photoelectric colorimeter, with the colour of an artificial or blood standard. The methods which employ direct visual comparison and artificial standards (e.g. Sahli method) have generally been superseded by those which use photoelectric colorimeters. (Chapter 6 gives the principle of colorimetry.)

Regardless of method, the major problem associated with the measurement of haemoglobin has been the availability of a suitable standard material. In 1966, the International Committee for Standardization in Haematology (ICSH) recommended that a suitable standard for haemoglobin measurement was a cyanmethaemoglobin solution. This standard is prepared according to strict specifications, and the concentration of haemoglobin established by spectrophotometry using the millimolar extinction coefficient of cyanmethaemoglobin. In Britain, the specifications detailing the preparation and assay of this material are contained in B.S. 3985. The cyanmethaemoglobin standard is a very stable material and is widely available from commercial sources.

The cyanmethaemoglobin method is the preferred method for measuring haemoglobin in the UK, but occasionally the oxyhaemoglobin method is used.

The cyanmethaemoglobin method

Blood is diluted in a buffered solution of potassium ferricyanide and potassium cyanide to yield cyanmethaemoglobin. The potassium ferricyanide converts the haemoglobin to methaemoglobin which is further converted to cyanmethaemoglobin by the action of the potassium cyanide. The absorbance of this solution is read in a colorimeter at a wavelength of 540 nm, or with a yellow-green filter (e.g. Ilford 625).

The original diluent used for this method was Drabkin's fluid, but because of the relatively long incubation time required to achieve complete conversion to cyanmethaemoglobin, and problems caused by precipitation of plasma proteins, the formulation has been modified several times.

Modified Drabkin's fluid (van Kampen and Zijlstra) is prepared by dissolving 200 mg potassium ferricyanide, 50 mg potassium cyanide, 140 mg potassium dihydrogen phosphate and 1 ml of non-ionic detergent (e.g. Nonidet P40; Shell Chemical Company) in distilled water and making the volume up to 1 litre. The pH of this solution should be between 7.0 and 7.4.

Modified Drabkin's fluid is photolabile and should therefore be stored in the dark. If the diluent is prepared in bulk, it should be tested at regular intervals to ensure that the pH is within the acceptable range, and also to ensure that it is free from turbidity. This can easily be ascertained by checking the absorbance of the material at 540 nm against a distilled water blank. If the absorbance is not zero, then the material should be discarded and fresh reagent prepared.

Drabkin's fluid contains cyanide, which is an extremely poisonous chemical. It is therefore imperative that proper safety precautions be observed when preparing and handling this diluent.

To measure haemoglobin concentration, an accurate dilution must be made. The exact dilution used will depend upon the sensitivity of the photoelectric colorimeter, and the range of haemoglobin levels which are to be measured. Typically, when using photoelectric colorimeters, satisfactory results are only obtained with absorbances ranging from about 0.1 to 1.0 (better still between 0.2 and 0.7), so that if possible the dilution should be adjusted to fall within this range. Different instruments may give different absorbance readings on the same dilution; this is particularly so with filter instruments and those with wide bandwidths. In routine practice, either a 1 in 201 or 1 in 251 dilution is used, but in some instances a 1 in 501 dilution may be found to be more satisfactory.

If a 1 in 251 dilution is selected, the dilution can

be prepared by washing 20 μl of blood, taken into either a shellback pipette or positive displacement pipette, into 5.0 ml of modified Drabkin's fluid. This must be allowed to stand for at least 3 min, to allow for complete conversion to cyanmethaemoglobin, before the absorbance is measured on a colorimeter. The absorbance is read against either a distilled water or reagent blank at a wavelength of 540 nm. If a calibration curve has not been prepared, then the absorbance of an aliquot of cyanmethaemoglobin standard must be measured at the same time as that of the test. The final haemoglobin result is calculated from the following:

$$Hb = \frac{T \times C \times D}{A \times 1000} \text{ g/100 ml}$$

where T is the test absorbance at 540 nm, A the standard absorbance at 540 nm, C the concentration of cyanmethaemoglobin standard (mg/100 ml), and D the dilution factor; 1000 converts from mg/100 ml to g/100 ml.

Example

If a cyanmethaemoglobin standard with an absorbance of 0.400 has a concentration of 60 mg/100 ml and the patient's sample diluted 1 in 251 has an absorbance of 0.320, then

$$Hb = \frac{0.320 \times 60 \times 251}{0.400 \times 1000} \text{ g/100 ml}$$

$$= 12.0 \text{ g/100 ml}$$

Calibration of a colorimeter for haemoglobin measurement

In routine practice it would be very time consuming, and expensive, if standard solutions were tested with every batch of haemoglobin tests, and the results calculated as previously described. It is more usual to prepare a calibration graph for each instrument. The calibration graph represents the relationship between absorbance (*y*-axis) and haemoglobin concentration (*x*-axis). Thus, the absorbance of the test dilution can be translated quickly, by reference to the graph, into haemoglobin concentration.

When preparing a calibration graph there are two factors which must be considered. First, that part of the graph which gives a linear response between absorbance and concentration must be established. This is to ensure that the Beer–Lambert law (Chapter 6) is obeyed. Secondly, on proving linearity, the graph must be calibrated with a cyanmethaemoglobin standard.

Linearity can be established very simply by taking a blood sample and removing some of the plasma to give a haemoglobin value of about 25.0 g/100 ml. From this sample a bulk dilution of cyanmethaemoglobin is prepared, and serial dilutions of

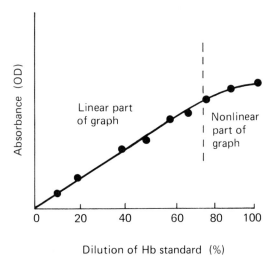

Figure 31.7. Haemoglobin calibration graph

this are made in Drabkin's fluid. The absorbance of each dilution is then established, and plotted on linear graph paper against the percentage dilution relative to the bulk dilution. *Figure 31.7* shows a typical calibration graph and shows that, at the higher concentrations of haemoglobin, there is a nonlinear response between absorbance and concentration. Thus, the calibration graph should not be extended beyond the linear region.

After establishing linearity, the colorimeter can then be calibrated against a cyanmethaemoglobin standard. This is best carried out by diluting the standard in Drabkin's fluid to give a range of dilutions (e.g. 1 in 2, 1 in 3 and 1 in 4). The equivalent whole blood haemoglobin is calculated by multiplying the cyanmethaemoglobin concentration of each dilution by the dilution factor which will be used for the routine tests. The absorbance of each dilution is then plotted on linear graph paper against its concentration, and a straight line drawn through the points. Care must be taken to avoid extending the line into the nonlinear region of the colorimeter. From this standard calibration graph it is possible to construct a chart which gives the whole blood haemoglobin level for any absorbance. The use of such a chart greatly increases the speed at which haemoglobin tests can be performed, but it should be remembered that the calibration graph and chart are unique to that instrument for the specified whole blood dilution factor.

It is also important to include control samples with every batch of tests to ensure that the test system has not changed. If the control sample results indicate a change in performance, then the fault must be found and corrected, before proceeding with further tests.

If a 1 in 501 dilution is used, it is possible to combine the linearity and calibration procedure into one experiment. This is because at a 1 in 501 dilution the cyanmethaemoglobin standard will have an equivalent whole blood haemoglobin value in the region of 30.0 g/100 ml. This is in contrast to a 1 in 201 dilution where the whole blood equivalent concentration will be about 12.0 g/100 ml, and for a 1 in 251 dilution will be 15.0 g/100 ml.

The packed cell volume (haematocrit)

The packed cell volume (PCV), or the haematocrit, is a measure of the relative mass of red cells present in a sample of whole blood.

There are several methods which can be used to determine the PCV. These are: (a) by centrifugation, (b) by calculation and (c) by radioisotope dilution technique. The latter technique is not used routinely, but may be used as a reference, or comparative procedure, in research work.

Measurement of PCV by centrifugation

The PCV can be determined by centrifuging a sample of well-mixed anticoagulated blood, contained in a parallel-sided glass tube, for a suitable period of time to ensure maximal packing of cells. The method which is most commonly used is the macrohaematocrit technique, but occasionally the microhaematocrit technique is adopted. The microhaematocrit method is preferred because of simplicity, speed and overall reproducibility. Using this method, the blood is centrifuged at approximately 12 000 g for 10 min in a special centrifuge (*Figure 31.8*) which automatically attains the correct speed. The PCV is subsequently determined by measuring the height of the red cell column and expressing this as a ratio of the height of the total blood column. A PCV reader can be obtained from commercial

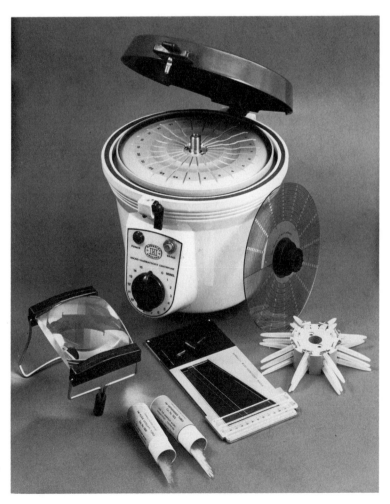

Figure 31.8. Microhaematocrit centrifuge (reproduced by courtesy of Hawksley and Sons Ltd)

sources, and can be used to determine the height of both the red cell and total blood column simultaneously, and convert these to the final result. Alternatively, the heights can be measured using linear metric graph paper.

Example

If the height of the column of red cells was 19 mm and the total blood column was 49 mm, then

$$PCV = \frac{\text{Height of red cell column}}{\text{Height of total blood column}}$$

$$= \frac{19 \text{ mm}}{49 \text{ mm}}$$

$$= 0.388 \text{ litres of red cells per litre of whole blood (l/l)}$$

Normal values

As with the normal values for haemoglobin and red cell numbers, the PCV is also dependent upon age and sex. In the adult male the 95% confidence limits are usually given as 0.390–0.530 l/l, and for females 0.350–0.490 l/l.

The appearance of the centrifuged haematocrit tube should always be examined for any abnormalities. Above the packed red cells will be a white layer of leucocytes and immediately above this a creamy layer of platelets (these layers are called the buffy coat); any increase in these cells will be easily detectable after a little experience. The plasma, which is usually straw coloured, will be bright yellow if the patient is jaundiced, colourless in iron deficiency anaemia and red if haemolysis is present.

Factors affecting the accuracy of the micro-haematocrit

Although the microhaematocrit technique is relatively simple there are a number of factors which can influence the accuracy of the final result. These are associated with (a) specimen collection, (b) the quality of capillary tubes, (c) the time and speed of centrifugation, and (d) the method used for reading the PCV result.

Specimen collection

When blood is collected into K_2EDTA it is important that the ratio of blood to anticoagulant is correct. The recommended concentration is 1.5 mg K_2 EDTA for every millilitre of blood. If there is an excess of anticoagulant, then the red cells will shrink due to the osmotic force of the K_2 EDTA, causing a water shift from the cells to the plasma. This can cause serious errors if the microhaematocrit (or macrohaematocrit) is used to determine the PCV.

Quality of capillary tubes

It is essential that the interior walls of the capillary tubes are parallel. If this is not the case, then due to the variable thickness of the column of blood, the height relationship used to determine the PCV will not be true. Similar errors may be introduced if care is not taken to ensure that the seal at the base of the tube forms a flat surface at right-angles to the side of the tube. Capillary tubes are commonly sealed with a 'putty-like' material; this has tended to replace the traditional method where the tubes were heat sealed. Although heat sealing is more difficult and requires greater skill to achieve a flat seal, it is possibly more efficient and reduces the chance of the blood being lost from the tube during centrifugation.

Capillary tubes suitable for microhaematocrit determination are described in B.S. 4316 and are available from commercial sources.

Time and speed of centrifugation

If blood is centrifuged for a short period of time, or at a low centrifugal force, plasma will be trapped between the red cells. This will give an inaccurate assessment of the height of the red cell column. This problem can be minimized if the centrifugation conditions are carefully controlled, such that the centrifugal force applied to the mid-point of the capillary tube is a minimum of 12 000 g and the centrifugation time is 10 min. Under these conditions it has been demonstrated that trapped plasma will account for approximately 1.5% of the PCV reading. If shorter centrifugation times are used, especially in those samples of blood with high PCV levels, the amount of trapped plasma will increase.

Reading PCV results

There are several reading devices available which will give reasonable results, but none is entirely satisfactory. Some of the problems can be overcome with a magnifying glass, which allows the operator to define the boundaries of the column of blood with more confidence.

Alternative PCV methods

The macrohaematocrit is an alternative centrifugation method. This method employs the use of a Wintrobe tube, which can also be used to determine the erythrocyte sedimentation rate (ESR). The Wintrobe tube is 11 cm in length, with an internal diameter of 2.5 mm. It has two graduation scales, marked in millimetres, along its length. One side is graduated from 0 to 100 mm from the bottom to the top, whereas the other side is graduated from 100 to 0 from bottom to top. The former scale is used to determine PCV, and the latter is used to measure ESR.

The Wintrobe method for determining PCV is recommended as a reference method by the ICSH, but because of technical problems and the centrifugation time required to achieve maximal packing of cells (at least 30 min), it is not used for routine measurements.

In recent years, with the introduction of automated analysers, the centrifugation procedures for measuring PCV have been superseded. Some of these instruments derive the PCV by calculation. These instruments (Chapter 33) are capable of measuring both the numbers and size of red cells present in a sample of blood. Thus, by multiplying the red cell numbers by the mean red cell volume (MCV), the relative mass of red cells can be established. This method has the advantage that it does not measure trapped plasma, and is not affected by excess anticoagulation, but has the disadvantage that there is no true standard which can be used for instrument calibration.

The red cell indices (absolute values)

These values are calculated from the red cell count, haemoglobin content and packed cell volume. The information obtained provides a valuable guide to the classification of anaemia and has made obsolete the 'colour index' which compared arbitrary normal figures with those actually calculated. The figures calculated are the average of the red cells present and may at times be within the normal range, but on examination of the stained blood film the red cells may show marked morphological changes.

As the results are dependent upon the accuracy of the various estimations, it must be remembered that the red cell count, which has the greatest potential error, must be performed with extreme care, preferably using an electronic counter.

Mean cell haemoglobin concentration (MCHC)

This refers to the amount of haemoglobin in 100 ml of packed red cells, as opposed to the amount of haemoglobin present in whole blood. It is calculated from the haemoglobin and PCV, and the results are expressed as grams per 100 ml.

Example

If the Hb value is 15.0 g/100 ml, and the PCV value is 0.450, then 0.450 dl of red cells contains 15.0 g Hb. Therefore, 1.000 dl of red cells contain

$$\frac{1.000 \times 15.0}{0.450 \times 1} \text{ g Hb}$$

or

$$MCHC = \frac{Hb}{PCV} = 33.3 \text{ g/100 ml of packed red cells}$$

The normal MCHC ranges from about 32.0 to 35.5 g/100 ml, but slightly different values may be found, dependent upon whether or not a correction has been applied to the PCV, to take account of trapped plasma.

The MCHC is usually decreased in iron deficiency anaemia. Values greater than 35.5 g/100 ml are very rare, but can be found in some cases of hereditary spherocytosis. Normally, if an increased MCHC is found it is usually associated with an inaccurate haemoglobin or PCV.

Mean cell haemoglobin (MCH)

This refers to the amount of haemoglobin (expressed as picograms) present in the average red cell. It is calculated from the haemoglobin and red cell count.

Example

A litre of blood which has a Hb value of 15.0 g/100 ml, contains 150.0 g Hb. If this sample has a red cell count of 5.00×10^{12} per litre, then 5.00×10^{12} red cells contain 150.0 g Hb. Therefore, one red cell contains

$$\frac{150.0}{5.00 \times 10^{12}} \text{ g Hb}$$

or

$$MCH = \frac{Hb \times 10}{\text{Total red cells}} = 30.0 \text{ pg}$$

(*Note*: a picogram (pg) is 10^{-12} of a gram.)

The normal MCH ranges from about 27.0 to 32.0 pg. It is decreased in microcytic hypochromic anaemias (e.g. iron deficiency, thalassaemia) and is increased in macrocytic anaemias (e.g. vitamin B_{12} and folate deficiencies).

Mean cell volume (MCV)

This is the mean volume of the red cells, expressed as femtolitres. The MCV can be derived by calculation from the PCV and red cell count, or alternatively can be established directly by electronic instruments (Chapter 33).

Example

A sample of blood with a PCV of 0.450 has a red cell count of 5.00×10^{12} per litre. Then, 5.00×10^{12} red cells occupy 0.450 litre. Therefore, one red cell occupies

$$\frac{0.450}{5.00 \times 10^{12}} \text{ litres}$$

or

$$MCV = \frac{PCV}{\text{Total red cells}} = 90 \text{ fl}$$

(*Note:* a femtolitre (fl) is 10^{-15} of a litre.)

The normal MCV ranges from about 80 to 95 fl, but published values may show variation depending upon whether or not a correction factor has been applied to take account of trapped plasma in the PCV.

The MCV is typically increased in megaloblastic anaemias and some haemolytic anaemias. It is decreased in iron deficiency anaemia and some of the haemoglobinopathies.

Erythrocyte sedimentation rate (ESR)

The ESR is a non-specific test, frequently requested along with full blood counts. If anticoagulated blood is allowed to stand undisturbed, the red cells will gradually settle to the bottom of the container, leaving a clear layer of plasma. This sedimentation occurs in three phases. First the cells tend to aggregate and form rouleaux and only fall slightly. In the second phase the speed of the fall is increased and, as the cells pack, this speed is decreased during the third phase.

Rouleaux formation is controlled by the concentration of fibrinogen and the amount of globulins present. The ESR is commonly used as a screening test at the initial clinical examination. An increased rate of fall in chronic conditions such as rheumatoid arthritis and tuberculosis is usual, and the increase or decrease in ESR is used to monitor the progress of the disease. It is also elevated in acute and chronic infections and in malignant diseases where the plasma proteins are abnormal.

Although the rate of red cell sedimentation is dependent upon the relative concentrations of plasma proteins, it is also dependent on the number of red cells, or PCV. Thus, in anaemic patients an increased ESR will be recorded because of the low PCV, and not necessarily because there is a change in the relative concentration of plasma proteins.

A decreased rate of fall is often present in polycythaemic subjects and a reading of 0 mm is not unusual. A normal ESR result does not preclude a disease process.

Certain physical conditions also affect the rate of sedimentation, and stringent precautions are therefore necessary to bring about standard conditions for the test.

There are two main methods of performing the ESR, namely Wintrobe's and Westergren's method.

Wintrobe's method

With a Pasteur pipette, a Wintrobe tube (see Alternative PCV Methods, p. 328) is filled to the top graduation with blood anticoagulated with K_2 EDTA. The tube is allowed to stand in a vertical position for 1 h, and the distance in millimetres that the red cells have fallen is recorded. The normal range for male adults is 0–9 mm in the first hour, and for females, 0–20 mm in the first hour.

Westergren's method

Apparatus and reagents

1. Westergren ESR tube. This tube looks rather like a 1 ml pipette. It is 300 mm long, with an internal diameter of 2.5 mm It is graduated from the bottom over a 200 mm scale in millimetre divisions.
2. Venous blood taken into sodium citrate. One part of 3.13% trisodium citrate to 4 parts of blood. Blood taken into K_2 EDTA may be used, but must be similarly diluted with 3.13% trisodium citrate.

Technique

The blood is well mixed and drawn into the tube to the top mark (0 mark). The tube is then stood vertically for 1 h. The level of the red cells is then read as the ESR. Normal values are: men, 3–5 mm; women, 4–7 mm.

Precautions to be taken when performing ESR tests

1. As blood is taken by venepuncture, prolonged venous congestion must be avoided.
2. The test must be set up within 3 h of blood collection or sedimentation may be retarded. Some workers have shown that blood taken into K_2 EDTA can be stored for up to 24 h at 4°C and then diluted with 3.13% trisodium citrate and a Westergren ESR performed.
3. Haemolysed blood must not be used.
4. Blood containing the slightest trace of a clot must be discarded.
5. Tests must not be performed in direct sunlight.
6. Tests should be performed between 18°C and 22°C as higher temperatures accelerate the sedimentation rate.
7. All the apparatus used must be scrupulously clean.
8. There must be no air bubbles in the sedimentation tube.
9. The tube must be placed in an absolutely vertical position.

32

Microscopical examination of blood

Although the red cell indices provide useful information about the red cells, they can in some instances appear normal even when marked red cell abnormalities exist. For example, if a patient has a population of small red cells (microcytes) and a population of large red cells (macrocytes), then it is quite possible that the MCV will be within the normal range. Thus, it must be remembered that the red cell indices only give average results and do not provide any information on the distribution of values for individual cells. To overcome this problem it is necessary to examine a well-prepared stained peripheral blood film. In addition to providing further information on the red cell series, morphological examination will also provide more information on the white blood cells and platelets.

Examination of a peripheral blood film is an important investigation which should be undertaken on the first occasion that a patient has haematological tests requested. On subsequent occasions, it may be possible to omit the blood film if no abnormalities were previously found and the results of the full blood count remain constant.

To provide valuable data, the blood film must be well prepared and stained (see Chapter 30). The procedure used to examine the blood film should be systematic and must only be carried out by individuals who have received adequate instruction.

Before any detailed examination takes place, the laboratory worker must ensure that the microscope has been adjusted to give the optimum viewing conditions of Kohler illumination (Chapter 2). The next stage involves a scan of the blood film using a low-powered objective to ensure that the distribution of cells is satisfactory, and to find an area where the cells are free from distortion. Having found a suitable area, a detailed examination of the morphology can be undertaken using a high-dry objective. This should be followed with an examination of individual cells for intracellular abnormalities using an oil-immersion objective.

Red cell morphology

Blood film assessment is subjective and it is therefore necessary to standardize the way in which the semi-quantitative data is presented. The usual procedure is to apply a grading scheme based on a one plus, two plus or three plus score, to denote the progression from a mild to marked abnormality. However, it is important to emphasize that some variation in red cell morphology is to be expected in all normal blood samples, and thus the use of a one plus score should be reserved for only those conditions showing true mild abnormalities.

There are two stages which should be followed when reporting on red cell morphology. First, the overall appearance in terms of variation in size, shape and colour of cells should be recorded. Anisocytosis and poikilocytosis are terms used to describe an abnormal variation in cell size and shape, respectively. These red cell changes are non-specific and merely indicate an abnormality of erythropoiesis. If the red cells are fully haemoglobinized, then they are termed normochromic, whereas cells which do not have a full complement of haemoglobin (denoted by an increased area of central pallor) are termed hypochromic. It is possible to find blood films which show both normochromic and hypochromic cells; this is termed anisochromasia.

The second stage involves the description of particular types of red cell which may be present. There are many types of cells, each of which have different significance. It is beyond the scope of this chapter to review all morphological types, and therefore the interested reader should refer to a standard text on this subject. However, a non-exhaustive list is given in *Table 32.1* to demonstrate the types of cells which may be observed in some conditions.

Table 32.1 Some morphological red cell types

Condition	Cell type (examples)
Vitamin B_{12}/folate deficiency	Macrocytes, ovalocytes, Howell–Jolly bodies
Iron deficiency	Microcytes, leptocytes, pencil cells
Thalassaemia	Microcytes, target cells, red cell fragments
Sickle cell anaemia	Sickle cells, target cells, red cell fagments

From the red cell morphology and the results from the FBC it is possible, in most cases, to make a statement about erythropoiesis. For example, it should be possible to state whether erythropoiesis is (a) normal; (b) abnormal—associated with inadequate haemoglobin formation (e.g. iron deficiency); (c) abnormal—associated with damage to circulating red cells (e.g. haemolytic anaemia); (d) abnormal—associated with failure of the bone marrow to produce sufficient cells (e.g. vitamin B_{12} or folate deficiency).

There are instances where the information from a blood film will be diagnostic (e.g. malaria), but in most cases further laboratory investigations are required to confirm the tentative morphological conclusions.

Differential leucocyte count

The relative numbers of each type of white blood cell is established by the differential white cell count.

Battlement method

The film is examined systematically, by being traversed 3 fields along the edge, 2 fields up, 2 fields along and 2 fields down. This sequence is continued until a minimum of 100 cells has been enumerated.

Longitudinal method

The cells are counted in one complete longitudinal strip of the film. If less than 100 cells are counted, a second strip should be similarly enumerated.

Regardless of which of the above methods is used, all leucocytes encountered must be differentiated and classified. The result of each cell type is then expressed as a percentage, and in absolute numbers of the total white cell count. *Table 32.2* shows the normal differential white cell count expected for an adult.

Differential white cell counts should preferably be reported in absolute numbers because percentage figures may be misleading. For example, from *Table 32.2* it would appear that a neutrophil count of 82% and a lymphocyte count of 18% would be abnormal. However, if this relates to a total white cell count of 9.0×10^9 per litre, then the absolute number of neutrophils would be 7.4×10^9 per litre and lymphocytes 1.6×10^9 per litre. Both these cell types would therefore be present in normal numbers.

Table 32.2 Normal range for the adult differential white cell count

Leucocyte classification	Normal range (adult)	
	Percentage	Absolute numbers ($\times 10^9$/l)
Neutrophil	40–75	2.0–7.5
Lymphocyte	20–45	1.5–4.0
Monocyte	2–10	0.2–0.8
Eosinophil	1–6	0.04–0.4
Basophil	<1	<0.1

Cooke–Arneth count

Arneth attempted to classify the polymorphonuclear neutrophils into groups according to the number of lobes in the nucleus and also according to the shape of the nucleus. The procedure was too cumbersome for routine use and was modified by Cooke, who classified the neutrophils into five classes according to the number of lobes in the nucleus:

Class I   No lobes, i.e. an early cell in which the nucleus has not started to lobulate.
Class II   Two lobes.
Class III   Three lobes.
Class IV   Four lobes.
Class V   Five or more lobes.

The lobes cannot be said to be separated if the strand of chromatin joining them is too thick. The strand must be a very fine one. Some workers suggest that the strand must be less than one-quarter of the width of the widest part of the lobe.

The count is performed by examining 100 neutrophils and placing them in their correct class. The normal proportions are:

Class I   10%.
Class II   25%.
Class III   47%.
Class IV   16%.
Class V   2%.

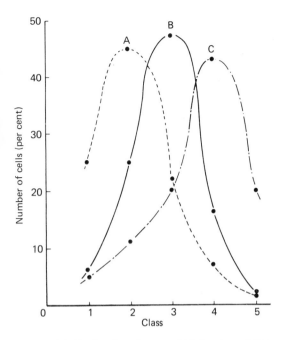

Figure 32.1. Cooke–Arneth count: (A) showing a shift to the left; (B) normal curve; (C) showing a shift to the right

When the sum of Class I and Class II exceeds 45%, a 'shift to the left' in the Arneth count can be said to exist; that is, if the figures were to be plotted on graph paper as in *Figure 32.1*, the peak of the graph would move to the left-hand side of the normal curve. The shift to the left occurs in infections, since new cells are released into the circulation from the marrow.

A 'shift to the right' can also occur; that is, the peak of the graph moves to the right-hand side of the normal graph. This occurs in certain conditions, notably in vitamin B_{12} and folate deficiencies.

Reticulocyte count

Reticulocytes (immature erythrocytes) are slightly larger than mature red cells, and by using a supravital staining technique, basic dyes, such as brilliant cresyl blue, are precipitated into a mesh-work (called reticulum) within the cell. This meshwork appears deep blue against a relatively unstained background. The reticulum is remnants of basophilic ribonucleoprotein (normally found in the cytoplasm), and the more mature the cell the less reticulum present.

Apparatus and reagent

Small glass tubes, clean slides and spreader, Miller's microscope eyepiece, 37°C incubator, and brilliant cresyl blue.

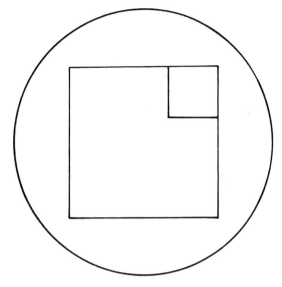

Figure 32.2. Miller ocular eyepiece used for counting reticulocytes; it consists of two squares whose areas have a ratio 1:9

Sodium citrate	0.6 g
Sodium chloride	0.7 g
Distilled water	100.0 ml
Dissolve and add:	
Brilliant cresyl blue G	1.0 g

Dissolve and filter. The solution is now ready.

Technique

1. Place 2–3 drops of the dye in the glass tube.
2. Add 2–4 drops of the patient's blood; gently mix.
3. Incubate at 37°C for 15–20 min.
4. Gently resuspend the cells.
5. Make blood films and allow them to dry quickly.
6. Using the Miller eyepiece* (*Figure 32.2*) and the 2 mm oil objective, examine the unfixed, uncounterstained film. Normal red cells appear greenish-blue, reticulocytes greenish-blue with deep blue intracellular precipitate.
7. Count at least 1000 red cells and calculate the percentage of reticulocytes present.
8. Using the reticulocyte percentage and the total red cell count, calculate the absolute number of reticulocytes.

*This graticule is used in some laboratories to reduce the tedium of counting large numbers of cells. It is inserted into the eyepiece of the microscope. All red cells (Rbc) and reticulocytes are counted in the small square (one-ninth of total area), and similarly all reticulocytes in the complete large square. Twenty fields, with an even distribution of cells, are examined and counted. The reticulocyte percentage is calculated as follows:

$$\text{Reticulocyte } (\%) = \frac{\text{Retics} \times 100}{(\text{Rbc} + \text{Retics.}) \times 9}$$

Example

If the red cell count is 5.00×10^{12} per litre and the reticulocyte percentage is 1.5%, then the absolute number will be 75×10^9 per litre.

The normal range for reticulocytes in a sample of adult blood is between 10 and 100×10^9 per litre. A decreased reticulocyte count indicates that the bone marrow is not producing sufficient cells, whereas an increased count indicates active erythropoiesis.

33

Automation in haematology

The use of manual methods to measure cell numbers, haemoglobin, PCV and the subsequent calculation of red cell indices has to a great extent been superseded by semi-automated and fully automated methods.

Electronic methods for counting cells first began to be used in laboratories during the early 1960s. Since then, these relatively simple counting instruments have developed into very sophisticated analysers capable of producing simultaneous counts on all of the three blood cell types, haemoglobin values and the red cell indices. In recent years the analytical scope of these instruments has been extended, such that they are producing data relating to the variation in cell size, as well as being able to provide data on the differential white cell count.

These instruments have been able to offer much greater precision, accuracy and speed of analysis and, because of this, the doctor who uses laboratory data is able to make clinical decisions with greater confidence. In addition, these instruments have provided for more economical use of laboratory resources.

With the introduction of automated procedures, new problems developed which were related to the rapid throughput of work. The first of these was associated with the maintenance of high-quality work in the face of rapid sample processing. It was for this reason that more attention was paid to the formal procedures of quality control, and not because the results from automated methods were less reliable than those from manual techniques. Quality control is an essential part of all laboratory procedures, regardless of how the results are produced.

The second problem which emerged with the increase in automation was related to the vast amount of data produced in short periods of time. It

was for this reason that some laboratories introduced computers. These offer a means for efficient data collection, storage and retrieval, and thus contribute to the overall effectiveness of the laboratory service.

Contrary to popular belief the use of electronic counters and computerized procedures is not just a case of 'pushing the button'. Those who use these techniques must be fully acquainted with the theoretical and operational principles, and must be able to identify situations which could produce erroneous results, and also be able to take corrective and remedial action in those situations.

The automated full blood count

There are many commercial companies who market semi-automated and fully automated instruments capable of providing data for the FBC. However, even though differences in operating principles exist from one manufacturer to another, the instruments can be considered to function on the basis of either a conductivity change, or an interruption of a beam of light, caused by the passage of a cell through the 'sensing' compartment of the instrument.

'Impedance' cell counters

In the UK this is the most common type of cell counter used in haematology laboratories. The impedance principle for counting cells was first used by Coulter Electronics Ltd, but now has been adopted with minor changes by other manufacturers.

The method of cell counting and sizing used by Coulter is based on the detection and measurement of changes in electrical resistance (impedance) produced by a particle (e.g. a red cell) suspended in

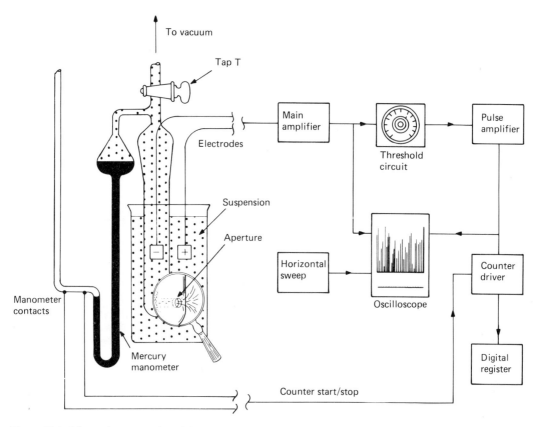

Figure 33.1. Schematic presentation of the Coulter principle for counting cells (reproduced by courtesy of Coulter Electronics Ltd)

a conductive liquid, passing through a small aperture.

Blood cells are essentially non-conductors of electricity. When they are suspended in a conductive diluent they function as discrete insulators. When a dilute suspension of cells is drawn through a small aperture, the passage of each cell momentarily increases the resistance of the electrical path between two submerged electrodes, located on either side of the aperture. *Figure 33.1* illustrates the passage of a cell through a typical aperture. The change in resistance produces a voltage pulse, whose magnitude is proportional to the volume of the particle.

The voltage pulses are fed into a threshold circuit which acts as a discriminator of cell size. Only those pulses that exceed the threshold levels are counted. Thus, very small particles which may be present in the diluent can be excluded from the cell count. Because the magnitude (height) of the voltage pulse is proportional to the cell volume, it is possible to analyse the pulse heights to provide data related to cell volume. This is the principle which is used to measure the MCV on this type of equipment.

Coulter Electronics Ltd, like many manufacturers, offer a large selection of instruments, ranging from multi-purpose, semi-automated cell counters to fully automated whole blood analysers. Using the multi-purpose, semi-automated cell counters (e.g. Coulter[TM] Model ZF; *Figure 33.2*), a separate dilution is required for each type of cell count. For the white cell count, a 1 in 500 dilution of blood is prepared in a suitable diluent (Isoton[R] II) and a few drops of stromalysing solution (e.g. Zap-oglobin[R]) are added. The stromalysing solution will remove all cell membranes and will thus destroy red blood cells completely, while maintaining the white cell nuclei intact. It is the passage of the nuclei through the aperture of the counter that produces the white cell count.

To perform a red cell count on this type of instrument it is necessary to dilute the blood sample 1 in 50 000. No further sample preparation is required, because since the white blood cells are so few in number they will not significantly alter the accuracy of the red cell count. Platelets, although present in greater numbers, will in most cases be excluded from the count because the voltage pulses

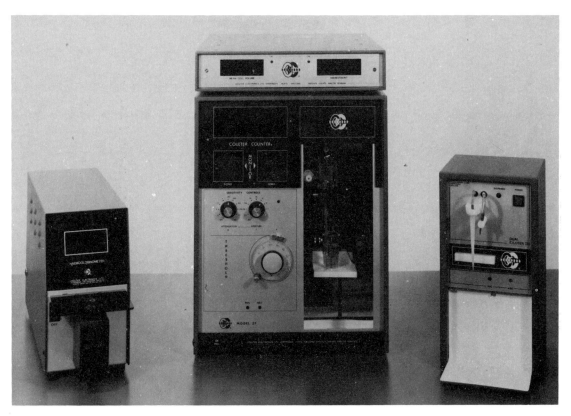

Figure 33.2. The Coulter Model ZF haemoglobinometer and sample diluter (reproduced by courtesy of Coulter Electronics Ltd)

they produce will fail to exceed the red cell threshold limit.

Platelet counts are more difficult to perform on multi-purpose semi-automated impendance counters because it is necessary to use centrifugal and double threshold procedures to discriminate between the platelets and other blood cells. In most cases the counts derived from these procedures will compare favourably with phase contrast platelet counts, but in others there may be significant errors due to the inclusion of microcytic red cells, or exclusion of large platelets from the count.

In the more sophisticated fully-automated analysers from Coulter Electronics Ltd (e.g. Coulter S-Plus™ series; *Figure 33.3*), red cells, white cells and platelets are counted in triplicate and the count automatically averaged. If one of the triplicate counts falls outside preset limits it is rejected and the result calculated on the remaining two. If two of the counts disagree, the count is rejected completely, and no result is given. This facility increases the precision and accuracy of the results.

The MCV is measured on these instruments by pulse-height analysis. This result is used in conjunction with the red cell count to give the PCV. There

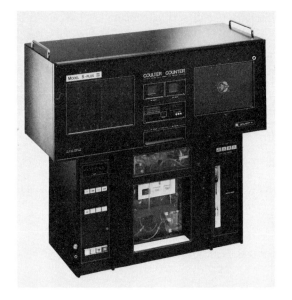

Figure 33.3. The Coulter S-Plus analyser (reproduced by courtesy of Coulter Electronics Ltd)

are therefore no problems associated with trapped plasma. Haemoglobin is measured using a 'cyan-methaemoglobin-like' method, and along with the red cell count, MCV and PCV is used to calculate the MCH and MCHC.

The new generation of Coulter instruments permit the selective counting of cells within very narrow size-distribution ranges by electronic selection of the pulses they generate. This facility has made possible accurate measurement of the size distribution of cells in the blood sample. In the case of red cells and platelets, these instruments give measurements that approximate with the visual assessment of 'anisocytosis' on the blood film. In the case of white cells, the selective counting of cells by volume analysis has developed to a stage where they can be differentially classified into three populations. These approximate with the lymphocyte, granulocyte and monocyte populations found on the blood film. Although this type of analysis cannot substitute for a visual differential white cell count in those patients with marked abnormalities, it is possible to use this data as a screen for white cell distribution abnormalities.

'Optical' cell counters

Instruments which incorporate an optical sensing system for counting and sizing blood cells are also commonly used in haematology laboratories. These work on a similar principle to reverse dark-field microscopy.

Figure 33.4 shows a schematic representation of the optical system used in instruments produced by Technicon Instruments; the illustration demonstrates that the beam of light focused on the cuvette is interrupted by the passage of cells and causes the light to be scattered. The scattered light rays radiate out beyond the periphery of the dark-field disc. These are collected by a photomultiplier tube that generates electrical pulses which are then counted. When no cells flow through the cuvette, the dark-field disc catches all light rays, and therefore no pulses are generated by the photomultiplier tube.

This principle has been applied by many manufacturers. For example, Technicon have utilized it for many years on a range of haematology analysers. Their most recent instrument, the H6000 (*Figure 33.5*) in addition to producing FBC results, also incorporates a method for differential white cell counts. This is based on the light absorption and scattering characteristics of each white cell type, stained by a number of cytochemical reactions.

Automated blood cell morphology

From the previous section it is apparent that both the impedance and optical cell counting principles are being adapted to give data that relates to blood cell morphology. An alternative method used to automate blood film assessment is that known as digital image analysis. These instruments assess morphology directly from a stained blood film, using computerized methods. The cells on the blood film are illuminated on a modified microscope, and the images produced are collected and transformed into digital data. This is analysed according to predefined classification criteria, and the cell types recorded. Thus, by scanning a large number of fields, the instrument produces a blood film assessment.

Quality control

With the advent of automation and rapid sample analysis, it became more apparent that there was a need for formal procedures to measure and maintain the performance of laboratory procedures. Thus, side-by-side with the growth of automated laboratory methods, quality control procedures have developed from relatively simple and insensitive occasional checks, into sophisticated laboratory management techniques. There is no single quality control procedure which will measure and maintain laboratory performance. Rather, many techniques are employed to monitor different functions within the laboratory. The maintenance of laboratory performance is an all-embracing task and must not

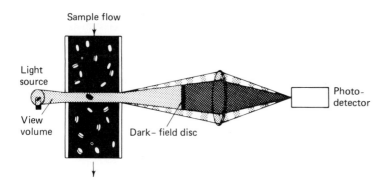

Sample flow

Light source

View volume

Dark-field disc

Photo-detector

Figure 33.4. Dark-field optics—schematic diagram of cell counting

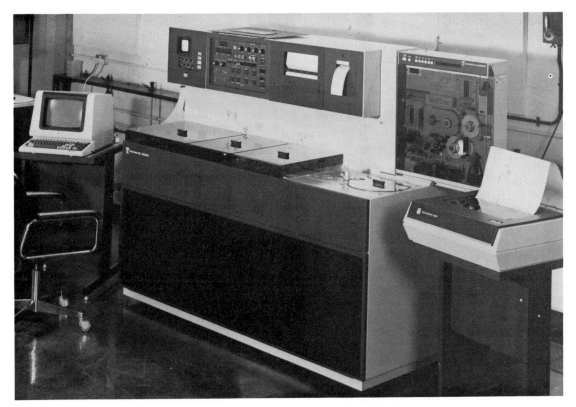

Figure 33.5. The Technicon H6000 (reproduced by courtesy of Technicon Instruments Co. Ltd)

be considered to be concerned with only the analytical stages of sample handling.

In its simplest form, laboratory performance is mainly dependent upon three phases of activity: (a) those activities which involve the input of the elements required to perform the analysis (e.g. reagents, methods, instruments, staff); (b) the actual analytical process; (c) those activities which involve the issue of the final report to the clinician.

It is the second of these (analytical process control), which will be dealt with in the remainder of this section, but the reader should be aware that the other phases of activity require monitoring if the overall laboratory standard is to be upheld.

Basic elements of quality control

Quality control is the activity which measures deviations from planned performance and initiates corrective action. The basic elements of a quality control technique are:

1. A statement, usually by way of a standard, specifying expected performance.
2. A measurement of actual performance.
3. A comparison of the actual with the expected performance.
4. A statement of significant deviation.
5. A feedback mechanism which will initiate correction of any significant deviation.

Analytical process control is exercised in laboratories by information feedback. In general, a feedback system gathers information on past performance from the output of a technique (e.g. results), and through an effector mechanism that manipulates the input elements (e.g. reagents) is able to govern future performance. To be of value, quality control procedures must generate information as near as possible to the time of analysis. If the lag time between analysis and data interpretation becomes too great, then the quality control procedure becomes less effective. In some instances this can add to laboratory problems because the corrective action indicated by the quality control procedure may be applied to a system that, for some reason, has changed from the time of performance assessment.

Quality control procedures

There are many procedures that can be used to monitor and maintain performance. Within the scope of analytical process control, most of those are procedures which involve the analysis of a control or reference material, and the subsequent interpretation of the data, usually by statistical methods. The control or reference materials can either be prepared in the laboratory or bought from commercial sources. These represent the statement of expected performance. When they are analysed along with the patient samples they generate information on the actual performance of the method. The comparison of actual with expected results can be accomplished using a number of charting or statistical methods. Two methods which are used to control semi-automated and fully automated procedures in haematology are (a) the Levey–Jennings plot and (b) the cumulative sum plot, known as 'cusum'.

Levey–Jennings plot

If a control sample is subjected to replicate analysis and a frequency distribution graph of the results is prepared, then this will approximate with a Normal (Gaussian) distribution. From theoretical considerations of the Normal distribution it is known that approximately 95% of all results will fall within ±2 S.D. of the mean (target value). Thus, it can be said

that if the control sample is subsequently analysed and the method has remained stable, then 95 out of every 100 control results should be within the ±2 S.D. limits. If the stability of the method has changed from the time that the target value was established, then the frequency of control results occurring outside these confidence limits will increase. In practice, a graph of the results (*Figure 33.6a*) is prepared and the occurrence of data points is continually monitored for signs of method bias.

Cumulative sum plot

A weakness of the Levey–Jennings plot is its insensitivity to low-level bias. To overcome this problem, some laboratory workers prefer to use the cusum technique, which highlights minor shifts in analytical accuracy.

The cusum plot is easily constructed. First, the mean or target value is measured by replicate analysis. It is important at this stage to ensure that the analytical process is correct, because the calculated target value will be used to measure changes in accuracy, relative to this point. The second stage in the cusum calculation is to subtract

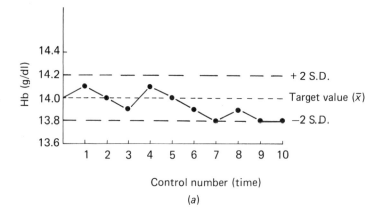

(a)

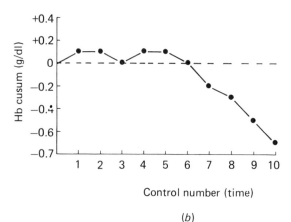

(b)

Figure 33.6. Levey–Jennings (a) and cumulative sum (b) plots for the quality control of haemoglobin measurements. Notice how the 'cusum' highlights small deviations from target values

the target value from every control result, to yield the difference. This is followed by adding together the differences, taking account of the algebraic sign, to give the cumulative sum of the differences. The final stage is to plot the cumulative sum of the differences (*y*-axis) against control sample number (*x*-axis) on linear graph paper. To achieve optimum sensitivity with the cusum plot, it has been recommended that the distance between each control result on the *x*-axis should be equal to the distance between 2 S.D. on the *y*-axis. If this rule is followed, then an angle of 45° will be produced if the analytical procedure deviates at a constant 2 S.D.

If the analytical process remains in control, then the cusum graph should oscillate between positive and negative values, and the best-line-of-fit through the points should be parallel to the *x*-axis. *Figure 33.6(b)* shows a cusum graph constructed from the same data used in *Figure 33.6(a)*. Note that the cusum plot highlights the minor shift in accuracy which has occurred, while the Levey–Jennings plot fails to demonstrate the same effect. Thus, the cusum plot will show to maximum effect any minor changes in accuracy by the fact that the plotted line will not remain parallel to the reference line.

Although the cusum plot is extremely sensitive to low-level bias, it is also this sensitivity which creates two major problems with this technique when applied to the parameters of the FBC. First, it is sometimes difficult to define the true target value with confidence because of random sampling error. If the target value is not 'true', then the plotted line for subsequent control analysis will show a deviation. Secondly, if fresh blood samples or stored blood preparations are used as controls, it is inevitable that 'prolonged' storage will cause a shift in the target value due to biological deterioration; this again will show as a deviant line. These problems can be overcome to a certain extent by periodically adjusting the target values. However, this can make interpretation difficult, and therefore decisions on analytical performance may be impaired.

Computers in haematology

The primary aim of any clinical laboratory should be the production of a laboratory report at the time and place it is required. It would be ideal for the patient if the clinician could request a laboratory investigation and immediately receive the results. Unfortunately this is not the case, since real world constraints impose many steps between the writing of the request and the return of the laboratory report.

As the laboratory workload increases, then the time lag between request and report may increase if the clerical system is unable to cope. It is in this respect that computers are finding a role in the laboratory.

Figure 33.7 illustrates the major steps between the laboratory request and the issue of the final laboratory report. The clinician writes the request, the specimen is collected and, after transport to the laboratory, it is formally received as a valid request by allocation of a unique laboratory number. The analysis is carried out, usually on a piece of

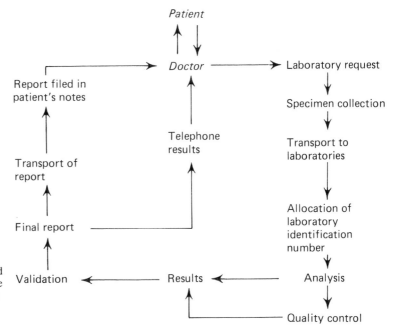

Figure 33.7. The major steps involved in specimen processing, from the time of patient–doctor encounter until the result is interpreted and acted on by the doctor

analytical equipment, and the result is coupled with the request to produce the report. This is then returned to the ward or out-patient department, and there used by the clinician for the continuing treatment of the patient.

Of the steps listed, a laboratory computer can subsequently improve as well as shorten the requesting stage, some portions of the analytical stage and almost all of the reporting function. Transport of the specimen from patient to laboratory will still have to be done by a person, or by a mechanical transport device, but the return of the report to the patient's records could be achieved with a computer, since this function is only information transfer and can be accomplished electronically.

Computers can also store large amounts of data, and are therefore ideal storage and retrieval systems for accumulated laboratory records.

It is not every laboratory that requires a computerized laboratory data management system, either because the existing clerical system is efficient or the cost is not justified in the face of a low workload. It should also be remembered that laboratory reports produced more quickly by a computer are not necessarily better reports. The value of a laboratory report is only achieved if the information it contains substantially improves the clinical decisions relating to the patient. Thus, to be effective in patient care a computer must be able to achieve this objective.

34

Beyond the full blood count

The information generated from the FBC analysis and blood film examination is unlikely to provide a complete picture of a patient's underlying pathology. In some instances the data will act as a powerful indicator of haematological disease and will thus enable the clinician to form a diagnosis. In other cases, the FBC data will merely indicate to the clinician that an abnormality may exist. In these cases further investigations will be required to confirm or refute the initial observations. A complete catalogue of confirmatory investigation is outside the scope of this book and the interested reader should refer to a standard haematology text for further information. However, some of the more common investigations will be noted, merely to show the type of work which may be undertaken in a haematology laboratory.

Measurement of iron status

The most common form of anaemia found throughout the world is iron deficiency anaemia, and is typically associated with microcytic and hypochromic red blood cells. However, because these blood cell changes are not specific for this type of anaemia, and can be associated with other haematological conditions where 'iron therapy may be contraindicated (e.g. thalassaemia), it is imperative that the patient's iron status be assessed. This can be achieved either by measurement of serum iron and iron binding capacity, or measurement of body iron stores by ferritin assay or quantitation of stainable iron present in bone marrow. This latter technique, however, is invasive and is not preferred for routine iron assessment.

Serum iron and iron binding capacity are measured by the reaction of ferric iron, split from transferrin and reduced to the ferrous form, with a chromogenic substance (e.g. bathophenanthronine or ferrozine), to form a coloured complex. The amount of coloured complex produced is directly proportional to the amount of iron present. The normal range of serum iron is 13–32 μmol/l and total iron binding capacity (TIBC) 45–70 μmol/l.

Although the serum iron and TIBC are extremely useful and extensively used to assess iron status, some laboratories measure storage iron in the form of ferritin by either radioimmunoassay or immunoradiometric assay. This measurement provides a more reliable measurement of body iron stores, and is not susceptible to the same variables which cause natural fluctuations in serum iron levels.

Measurement of vitamin B_{12} and folate

Deficiency of either vitamin B_{12} or folate will cause a megaloblastic anaemia, and typically gives a macrocytic blood picture. These vitamins can be assayed by microbiological techniques using microorganisms which do not multiply in number unless they have an external source of either vitamin. Thus, if an extract of a patient's sample is mixed with a culture media deficient in one of these vitamins, and inoculated with a suitable organism, then the amount of growth after incubation will be related to the amount of vitamin present in the test material.

Microbiological methods have been used for many years but because of technical limitations they are gradually being superseded by competitive protein binding assays which employ radioisotopic tracers. These assay procedures make use of the principle of radioisotope dilution, where a measured amount of radioisotopic tracer (e.g. vitamin B_{12} labelled with a radioisotope of cobalt) is mixed with an extract of the patient's blood sample and allowed to equilibrate. An aliquot of the equilibrated mixture is bound to a specific binding protein (e.g. intrinsic factor or transcobalamin for vitamin B_{12}) and this is separated from the unbound vitamin. The amount of radioactivity in the bound phase is inversely related to the amount of vitamin present in the test material.

The normal range for these vitamins varies slightly depending upon the assay procedures used, but in general terms the following values can be used as guidelines:

Serum vitamin B_{12}	150–1000 ng/l
Serum folate	2–10 µg/l
Red cell folate	150–800 µg/l

Identification of variant haemoglobins

The red blood cells of an individual may contain three or four different molecular forms of haemoglobin. The differences are in the protein (globin) portion of the haemoglobin molecule. Some of these haemoglobin species are of clinical significance, and it is therefore essential that techniques are available for their identification.

For purposes of clinical diagnosis, some of the variant haemoglobins may be readily identified using electrophoresis. This is because differences in amino acid composition of the globin chains may produce a variation in the electrophoretic mobility of the haemoglobins on the supporting medium. Although electrophoresis is used extensively to separate haemoglobin variants, there are some cases where the exact identification may prove difficult due to some variants having the same electrophoretic mobility. For example, HbS and HbD have the same mobility on cellulose acetate. To differentiate HbS, which is of great clinical importance, from other variants with the same mobility, many laboratories use the solubility test.

The solubility of HbS is not very different from that of HbA and other variants in the oxygenated state, but in the reduced (deoxygenated) state HbS is about one-fiftieth as soluble. Thus, it is the marked insolubility of reduced HbS which is used to confirm the presence of this haemoglobin variant.

Solubility test for HbS

Method

1. Add 100 mg of sodium dithionite to 10 ml of stock buffer solution.

Buffer solution (pH 7.1):

Potassium dihydrogen orthophosphate	33.78 g
Dipotassium hydrogen orthophosphate	59.33 g
White saponin	2.50 g
Distilled water	to 250 ml

2. Add 20 µl of well-mixed blood to 2.0 ml of buffer containing dithionite; mix and incubate at room temperature for 5 min.
3. Centrifuge at 1200 g for 5 min.
4. Examine each tube for the presence of HbS which forms a red precipitate on top of the soluble haemoglobin.

In a case of HbS disease (i.e. homozygous S), the subnatant solution will appear colourless, whereas in HbS trait (i.e. heterozygous S) the subnatant will be red. If HbS is not present, then there will be no precipitate.

■ **Notes**

1. Always include a positive and negative control with every batch of tests. The positive control should be from a person heterozygous for HbS.
2. If the patient is anaemic, it is preferable to remove some plasma from the sample to yield a normal PCV.

Identification of haemoglobin pigments

The absorption spectra which are obtained when white light is passed through haemoglobin solutions are useful in distinguishing between the haemoglobin pigments. Oxyhaemoglobin shows three absorption bands: a narrow band of light absorption at a wavelength of 578 nm, a wider band at 542 nm, and a third band at 415 nm. Reduced haemoglobin shows only one broad band with its centre at 559 nm. The chemical variants of haemoglobin (methaemoglobin, carboxyhaemoglobin and sulphaemoglobin), also have characteristic absorption spectra. Methaemoglobin shows three ill-defined bands at 630 nm, 500 nm and 406 nm. Carboxyhaemoglobin has an absorption spectrum closely resembling that of oxyhaemoglobin. The absorption peaks are at 570 nm, 535 nm and 418 nm. Sulphaemoglobin, on the other hand, has an ill-defined absorption spectrum with peaks of absorption at 618 nm, 577 nm and 541 nm.

The simplest, but possibly the least sensitive, method used for the identification of Hb pigments is direct vision spectroscopy (see Chapter 6). More commonly, either a Hartridge reversion spectroscope or a scanning spectrophotometer is used.

Examination of a dilute solution of haemoglobin will provide valuable evidence of the presence of Hb pigments, particularly if combined with chemical tests.

Red cell fragility test

Red blood cells suspended in an isotonic solution of saline remain intact. As the salt concentration is

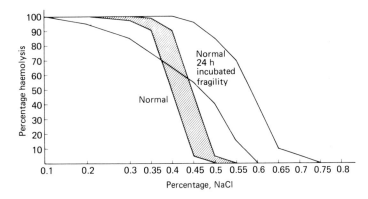

Figure 34.1. Osmotic fragility curves

decreased (making a hypotonic solution), the cells disrupt, causing haemolysis. The red cell fragility test is performed to find the salt concentration at which lysis takes place.

Normal blood shows slight haemolysis at 0.45–0.39%, complete haemolysis occurring at 0.33–0.30%. In some diseases the fragility of the cells is increased (hereditary spherocytosis) and in others the fragility is decreased (hypochromic anaemia).

As the differences in salt concentrations are extremely small, great care and accuracy must be exercised when performing this test.

Apparatus and reagents

1. *Stock sodium chloride solution* (pH 7.4), osmotically equivalent to 10% sodium chloride. Sodium chloride 18 g, disodium hydrogen orthophosphate (Na_2HPO_4) 2.731 g, sodium dihydrogen orthophosphate ($NaH_2PO_4.2H_2O$). Dissolve the salts in 200 ml of glass distilled water and store in a well-stoppered bottle.
2. *Test concentrations.* Dilute the stock sodium chloride solution 1 in 10 with distilled water to produce a solution with an osmotic equivalent of 1% sodium chloride. From this solution prepare 100 ml amounts of the following dilutions: 0.85, 0.70, 0.65, 0.60, 0.55, 0.50, 0.45, 0.40, 0.35, 0.30, 0.20, 0.10%. These solutions can be conveniently prepared by adding the stock saline solution from a burette into 100 ml volumetric flasks. The volume is then made up to the 100 ml mark with glass-distilled water.
3. Venous blood (heparinized or defibrinated).

Method

1. Set up two racks of 13 test-tubes.
2. Into tubes 1–12 measure 5 ml of the test concentrations, and into tube 13 add 5 ml of distilled water.
3. Add 50 μl of well-mixed aerated blood to each tube, using the blood under test for one rack and

a control specimen for the other. This gives a dilution of 1 in 100.

4. Mix and allow to stand at room temperature for at least 30 min. Centrifuge the tubes gently and read the supernatant fluids in a colorimeter using a tube of buffered saline as a blank and a yellow-green filter (Ilford No. 625) or at 540 nm.
5. Lysis is recorded as a percentage (using tube 13 as a 100% lysis) and plotted against percentage sodium chloride to obtain a 'fragility curve' (*Figure 34.1*). The curve obtained with the patient's blood is compared against that of the normal control. It is also useful to record the concentration of saline causing 50% lysis, which is referred to as the median corpuscular fragility (MCF).

■ Note

The use of oxalated or citrated blood is not recommended for this test owing to the additional salts added to the blood.

Before adding the blood to the tubes (step 3 above) it must be well aerated. This may be achieved by blowing air, using a Pasteur pipette fitted to the positive pressure side of a vacuum pump, through the blood.

A direct visual examination of the tubes can be made and the findings reported as commencement of haemolysis and completion of haemolysis for both test and normal blood.

Incubated osmotic fragility

Red cells from patients with hereditary spherocytosis have a greater increase in osmotic fragility when their blood is incubated at 37°C for 24 h. An incubated fragility is performed exactly as the technique described above, but the patient's blood and the control blood are incubated at 37°C for 24 h prior to performing the test.

35

Investigations for haemostatic abnormalities

In order to study patients thought to be suffering from blood clotting defects, various tests may be carried out. The simplest are the platelet count, bleeding time, whole blood clotting time, one-stage prothrombin time and kaolin cephalin time. It must be emphasized that normal results in these five tests do not exclude a haemorrhagic disorder. Further tests are necessary before the patient can be said to have a normal haemostatic mechanism.

Bleeding time

Duke's method

1. With the patient in a sitting position place a towel on the shoulder to prevent blood accidentally dropping onto the patient's clothing.
2. Sterilize the patient's ear lobe with 75% alcohol and puncture to a depth of about 2 mm with a sterile needle or lancet. Start a stopwatch at the same time as the ear is punctured.
3. Touch the formed drops of blood with the edge of a filter paper every 30 s. Avoid touching the skin or the result may be affected.
4. Take the time when bleeding stops. If the bleeding time exceeds 15 min, apply pressure to the puncture to stop the bleeding and report as greater than 15 min.

Normal range 2–5 min.

Ivy's method

1. Place a sphygmomanometer cuff around the patient's upper arm and raise the pressure in the cuff to 40 mmHg.
2. After sterilizing the skin, make five punctures in the pronator surface of the forearm (the front of

the forearm), avoiding any blood vessels or scar tissue. The punctures should preferably be made with a sterile Frank's automatic lancet to a depth of 3 mm.

Normal range 1.5–4 min.

Whole blood clotting time

Lee and White

1. Take four test-tubes with an internal diameter of 8 mm and place them in a 37°C water bath.
2. Take venous blood with a clean dry syringe, taking care that no tissue juices enter the syringe. Start a stopwatch immediately blood enters the syringe.
3. Deliver 1 ml amounts of the blood into each of the four warmed test-tubes. Examine them at 30 s intervals and observe for clotting by gently tilting the tube.
4. The clotting time is reported as the average of the times given by the four tubes.

Normal range 5–11 min (usually 6–9 min at 37°C).

One-stage prothrombin time

This technique is so-called because it was designed to measure prothrombin on the basis of Morawitz's Classical Theory of Coagulation.

The test employs a tissue extract which is added to plasma in the presence of excess calcium. The time taken for the mixture to clot is recorded.

It is apparent from the extrinsic clotting system that deficiency of factor V, factor VII and factor X will give an abnormal result, as well as a deficiency of prothrombin and hypofibrinogenaemia.

Reagents

(A) Dried brain extract (brain thromboplastin). This can be purchased commercially or prepared as follows:

1. Use a fresh human brain removed at post-mortem. It should be removed as soon as possible after death and certainly within 24 h.
2. Remove the superficial blood vessels and membrane. Cut the brain into small pieces with scissors and place in a large mortar.
3. Add a volume of acetone equal in volume to the brain and macerate the brain in the acetone.
4. Allow to settle and pour off the acetone. Repeat the process at least four times.
5. The material can be dried on a suction filter, or it can be placed between sheets of blotting paper and placed in the incubator, but it must not be left at 37°C for more than 15 min.
6. Material can then be stored in a vacuum desiccator over phosphorus pentoxide at 4°C. Alternatively, it can be placed into ampoules in convenient amounts and sealed in an atmosphere of dried nitrogen.
7. For use, take 0.3 g of the powder and add 5 ml of phenol saline (0.5% phenol in physiological saline). Place in the water bath at 37°C for 30 min, inverting periodically to mix.
8. Centrifuge lightly. Remove the cloudy suspension for use, discarding the large coarse particles in the bottom of the tube.

(B) 0.025M calcium chloride. Dissolve 2.775 g of anhydrous calcium chloride in some distilled water and make up to 1000 ml.

(C) Control and test plasma. The blood is taken by venepuncture and 9 parts of blood are added to 1 part of 3.13% sodium citrate solution.

Centrifuge as soon as possible after the blood has been taken and remove the plasma.

Test

1. Place 100 µl of test plasma into each of three small test-tubes and place in a 37°C water bath.
2. Add 100 µl of the brain suspension to each tube and allow the contents to reach 37°C.
3. Add 100 µl of calcium chloride solution to the first tube, simultaneously starting a stopwatch.
4. Mix and leave the tube in the bath for 9–10 s, then remove and examine for clot formation, stopping the watch at the first sign of a clot.
5. Note time taken to clot, and repeat procedure with the other two tubes.
6. Repeat the whole procedure using the control normal plasma. In practice, it is advisable to perform this test first, so that any possible errors in the test procedure will be recognized immediately. This normal plasma should clot between 11 and 14 s after the addition of the calcium chloride.

Recording of results

1. Results can be reported as the time taken in seconds for the test to clot, quoting also the clotting time of the control plasma, or
2. Results can be expressed as a prothrombin index, which is calculated as follows:

$$\text{Prothrombin time} = \frac{\text{Normal plasma clotting time} \times 100\%}{\text{Test plasma clotting time}}$$

■ **Note**

The percentage arrived at by this method has no relation to the percentage read off a dilution curve (see below).

3. A dilution curve can be prepared from normal plasma. The normal plasma is diluted to give 10, 20, 30% etc., to 90 and 100% dilution in normal saline, and the prothrombin time of each dilution is obtained. The clotting times are plotted on graph paper against the concentrations of prothrombin, assuming the normal plasma to contain 100% prothrombin activity. The prothrombin times of the tests can then be read off this graph and given as percentage prothrombin activity.

■ **Note**

Unfortunately, dilution of the plasma with normal saline also dilutes other clotting factors. Some workers, therefore, prefer to use prothrombin-free normal plasma as a diluent instead of saline. This can be obtained by treating the plasma with aluminium hydroxide. The shape of the graph obtained will vary from one laboratory to another and also with the strength of the brain suspension used. It is therefore necessary to prepare a new dilution curve for every batch of thromboplastin used.

4. Results can be expressed as a ratio:

$$\text{Prothrombin ratio} = \frac{\text{Test plasma clotting time}}{\text{Normal plasma clotting time}}$$

■ **Note**

This method is preferred, since it is not ambiguous.

Kaolin cephalin time (KCT)

This test simulates and therefore tests for deficiencies in the intrinsic clotting system. Citrated plasma is preincubated at 37°C with an agent (i.e. kaolin) which activates the contact factors so that the time-consuming reactions associated with contact activation are completed prior to the addition of calcium. Phospholipid is supplied to the test system to substitute for the platelet factor 3 activity.

Reagents

1. Kaolin

Kaolin BP is suspended in barbitone buffer (pH 7.4) at a concentration of 5 g/l. The suspension is stable at room temperature.

2. Phospholipid (Bell and Alton's platelet substitute)

Take 1 g of acetone-dried brain (see One-stage prothrombin time, p. 346) and extract this with 20 ml acetone. Incubate at room temperature for 2 h and centrifuge. Discard the supernatant and dry the residue in an evacuated desiccator. The dried powder is further extracted at room temperature with 20 ml of chloroform. This is filtered, and the filtrate is evaporated at 37°C in an evacuated desiccator. Suspend the residue in 10 ml of physiological saline (9.0 g/l). The resulting suspension is diluted 1 in 100 with saline for use in the test system.

3. Calcium chloride

0.025M calcium chloride (see One-stage prothrombin time reagents, p. 347).

4. Control and test plasma

The blood is taken by venepuncture and 9 parts of blood are added to 1 part of 3.13% sodium citrate solution. Centrifuge as soon as possible after the blood has been taken and remove the plasma.

Test

1. Mix equal volumes of kaolin suspension and phospholipid and incubate at 37°C.
2. Add 200 µl of well-mixed kaolin/phospholipid suspension to a 75 × 12 mm test-tube. Follow this with the addition of 100 µl of either patient's plasma or the normal control plasma. Start a stopwatch and leave the plasma–kaolin–phospholipid mixture at 37°C for 10 min (mix occasionally to resuspend the kaolin).
3. After exactly 10 min incubation, add 100 µl of 0.025M calcium chloride and start a second stopwatch. Record the time taken to clot.

Normal range

A normal control plasma should give a clotting time in the range 35–43 s. A result which is 7 s or more greater than the normal control should be considered abnormal.

Significance of results

The bleeding time is a combined measurement of capillary function, platelet numbers and platelet function, and therefore an increased result will indicate an abnormality of one or more of these. The whole blood clotting time is a relatively insensitive test because even in patients with severe haemostatic defects, sufficient thrombin may be generated to give a normal result. However, a prolongation of the whole blood clotting time in a patient who is not being treated with anticoagulants may indicate a deficiency of factor VIII (haemophilia) or a deficiency of factor IX (Christmas disease).

The prothrombin time is a non-specific measurement of the extrinsic blood coagulation mechanism, and therefore an abnormal result will indicate a deficiency in one or more of factors V, VII and X. Marked deficiencies of factors I and II may give a prolongation of the prothrombin time.

The prothrombin time is commonly used to monitor the degree of anticoagulation in patients treated with oral anticoagulants (e.g. warfarin). This is because these anticoagulants interfere with the *in vivo* synthesis of factors II, VII, IX and X.

The KCT is a non-specific test for deficiencies in the intrinsic clotting system. An abnormal result is to be expected in deficiencies of factors II, V, VIII, IX, X, XI or XII. The test is a useful screening test for haemophilia and Christmas disease, but it will not, however, distinguish between the two.

Normal results for any of these investigations do not preclude an abnormality in a patient with a suspect haemostatic defect. Further investigations will be required to confirm or refute the possibility.

Section 6

Blood transfusion technique

36

Introduction to blood transfusion

Blood transfusions are now commonplace throughout the hospitals of the world, and although apparently undertaken as a routine procedure, it should be remembered that blood is a tissue (albeit in a fluid state) and that every unit of blood transfused is in effect a tissue transplantation.

Although the administration of blood to a patient is a potentially life-saving procedure, if insufficient care is taken with the grouping and crossmatching of donor and recipient the results may be fatal. This fact cannot be too strongly emphasized.

The transfer of blood from a healthy individual to a sick one is an ancient idea. Drinking of animal blood was practised during medieval times, but this did not produce the desired results. Little progress was made until 1916, when William Harvey advanced his theory of circulation. Christopher Wren, better known as an architect, then suggested the injection of substances into veins, and with the aid of a quill as a sort of intravenous needle, blood was transfused from one dog to another.

In 1667, a French physician performed a transfusion of lamb's blood to a human patient, but after the death of the second patient no further transfusions were attempted.

James Blundell of Guy's Hospital, London, showed that blood from one species could not successfully be transfused to another. He subsequently became the first recorded doctor to perform a successful transfusion between members of the same species. His patients were several women who had suffered severe blood loss during childbirth.

Two major problems still remained: first, the blood which was being transfused frequently clotted during the procedure, since anticoagulants were not in use. Secondly, many patients suffered severe,

often fatal, reactions to the donated blood.

The breakthrough came in 1900, when Karl Landsteiner demonstrated the ABO blood grouping system. Following the discovery of the ABO groups and the recognition of their importance in the safe transfusion of blood, it was suggested that these blood groups were inherited characters. This was subsequently shown to be true. In 1927, Landsteiner and Levine described two further blood group systems—the MN system and the P system.

The discovery of the Rhesus system, in 1939, also led to the recognition of the cause of haemolytic disease of the newborn.

With the advent of new techniques in the field of blood grouping (especially those techniques detecting antibodies which, although attached to the red cell, were unable to produce any visible reaction) came the discovery of a number of new blood group systems including the Lutheran, Kell, Lewis, Duffy and Kidd systems.

Since then, vast amounts of data have been accumulated about previously described blood group systems. New information about these systems has shown that the original theories were, in fact, an oversimplification. Many of the systems have been shown to be very complex with large numbers of polymorphisms of red cell antigens. There have also been major advances in obtaining information about the structure and biochemistry of blood group antigens which has greatly increased our knowledge about blood group systems.

With the introduction of new blood grouping techniques, further blood group systems have been identified, and it is expected that more new techniques will result in the discovery of yet more new systems.

The routine hospital blood transfusion laboratory is mainly concerned with the blood grouping of patients, provision of suitable blood for transfusion and detection of atypical antibodies which may complicate blood transfusions and/or pregnancy.

Blood transfusion centres are concerned with the bleeding and testing of blood donors and provision of suitable blood, blood products and reagents to hospital laboratories. In addition, they act as a reference centre to confirm hospital laboratory findings and to perform tests and solve problems beyond the scope of a hospital laboratory.

37

Blood group immunoglobulins

Man lives in an environment in which he is surrounded by potentially dangerous bacteria and viruses. It is necessary that the body has a suitable defence in order to remove foreign organisms which have entered it. This is carried out in several ways, one of which is the production of an antibody which reacts with the foreign organism or antigen.

An antigen may be defined as a substance which stimulates the production of antibodies, and when mixed with the antibody reacts in some observable way.

An antibody is a protein formed in the spleen or lymph nodes in response to the presence of an antigen, and reacts specifically with that particular antigen in some observable way.

Antibodies are immunoglobulins and may be divided into five subclasses, all of which have a similar basic structure.

Each immunoglobulin molecule (*Figure 37.1*) is made up of four polypeptide chains: two long heavy chains which are distinct for each class of immunoglobulin, and two short light chains which exist in two forms, either kappa or lambda. Most antibodies are a mixture of both kappa and lambda forms,

although both light chains will be the same for each immunoglobulin molecule.

The heavy chains are joined to each other by disulphide bonds, and the light chains are joined to the heavy chains by similar bonding. The disulphide bonds give the molecule strength, although allowing flexibility.

The variable region occurs at the end of both light and heavy chains. It is the sequence of amino acids making up the protein in this area that defines the specificity of the antibody. The large number of possible amino acid combinations in this region enables great diversity of antibody specificity.

There are, however, marked differences in the structure of the heavy chains, and immunoglobulins may be divided into subclasses on the basis of these. The classes are known as IgG, IgA, IgM, IgE and IgD. Blood group antibodies are almost exclusively IgG, IgM and IgA (*Figure 37.2*).

The differences in molecular weight and size between IgG and IgM are marked and have *in vivo* significance. The IgG molecule has a molecular weight of 155000, whereas the IgM molecule is larger, having a molecular weight of 900000.

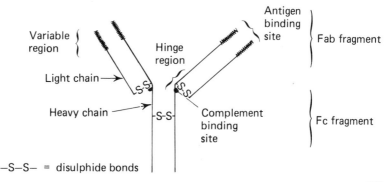

Figure 37.1. Structure of an immunoglobulin molecule   −S−S− = disulphide bonds

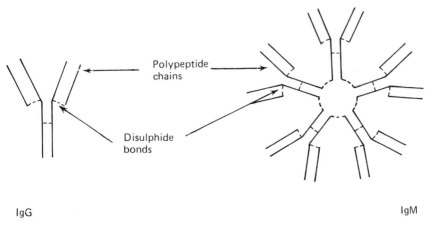

Polypeptide
chains

Disulphide
bonds

IgG   IgM

Figure 37.2. Structure of IgG and IgM immunoglobulins

IgG antibodies are able to cross the placental barrier and enter the foetal circulation, whereas IgM antibodies are too large to do so. Therefore, when considering the possible effects of maternal antibodies on the foetus, it is the IgG antibodies which are of importance.

The immune response

When an antigen is introduced into an individual, antibodies are produced in response to the stimulation. The production and increase in antibody is known as the immune response (*Figure 37.3*). The peak of this reaction usually occurs at an interval of 10–20 days after the initial stimulation. The response to the antigen depends on whether the individual has previously been exposed to that particular antigen. The response after the first dose, known as the primary or sensitizing dose, is usually slow and weak, but subsequent exposure to the same antigen produces a strong response with large amounts of antibody being produced quickly. These may remain in the circulation for many years. The antibodies initiated by the primary response are predominantly IgM, while subsequent exposure to the antigen results in the production of IgG antibodies.

Antigen–antibody reactions

The forces holding an antigen–antibody complex together are: ionic bonds, hydrogen bonds, Van der Waals forces and hydrophobic bonds. In blood grouping, the two most commonly observed results of antigen–antibody reactions are agglutination or clumping of red cells, caused by crosslinking by a multivalent antibody, and haemolysis, where the antigen–antibody reaction results in breakdown or lysis of the red cell.

Red cells suspended in saline, although appearing to touch each other when viewed under the microscope, in fact do not as they are surrounded by what is referred to as an ionic cloud. Red cells have a net negative electrostatic charge on their surface due to the ionization of the carboxyl groups of sialic acid present at the cell membrane which attracts positive ions from the surrounding medium; this positive layer subsequently attracts negatively charged ions to its surface. This process continues in layers until there is insufficient force to attract more ions, and the outer edge is called the surface of shear. The electrostatic charge is referred to as the zeta potential.

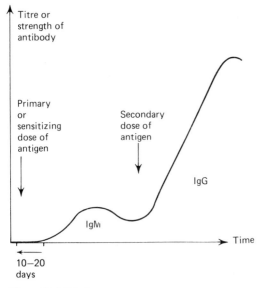

Figure 37.3. The immune response

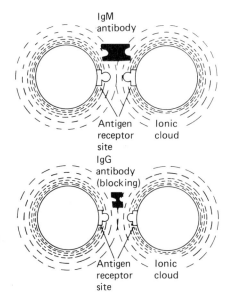

Figure 37.4. Effect of the ionic cloud on IgM and IgG antibodies

The relative size of the immunoglobulins and the techniques for demonstrating specific red cell antigens and antibodies takes into account the surrounding ionic cloud. The IgM or complete antibodies are large enough to bridge the ionic cloud and therefore agglutination can occur in a saline medium. The IgG or complete antibodies are much smaller and because of this the majority are unable to straddle the ionic cloud, producing blocking of the receptor site, but no agglutination in saline (*Figure 37.4*). These red cells can be said to be sensitized.

Each molecule of IgG and IgA has two antigen binding sites, whereas IgM has ten. This may facilitate agglutination in saline by IgM antibodies.

In order for an IgG antibody to agglutinate two red cells, it would have to bind each of its two antigen binding sites onto separate cells. An IgM antibody, having many more antigen binding sites, would be able to bind more than one antigen binding site to each red cell.

Complement

Complement is a complex group of serum globulins which are present in fresh normal serum, and are able to lyse red cells and destroy certain bacteria. Eleven components of complement are recognized, C1–9, C1 having three sub-units C1q, C1r and C1s. Complement, in a similar way to the blood coagulation and fibrinolytic systems, is a triggered enzyme cascade system where activation of one component leads to activation of others.

Complement activation can occur in at least two ways, (a) the classical pathway, where antibody binding leads to haemolysis of the cell by the later stages of the sequence, and (b) the alternate pathway where antibody is not essential for activation to take place.

When antigen–antibody reactions occur on the cell surface, some are capable of binding complement to the red cell. During binding, the antibody is thought to undergo configurational change, exposing a complement activation site on the antibody molecule. The final stages of the sequence lead to lysis of the red cell as a result of enzymic digestion of small areas of the red cell membrane.

IgM antibodies are better at activating complement than IgG. The complement activation site is positioned on the Fc portion of the antibody molecule (see *Figure 37.1*) and it is necessary for two Fc portions to interact in order to activate the complement pathway. This interaction is achieved when two adjacent antigen sites are bound by antibody. Because of the larger number of combining sites possessed by the IgM molecules, there is a much greater chance of adjacent sites being bound by antibody, and it has been shown that a single IgM molecule is capable of initiating complement binding. Although it is possible for IgG to activate complement, the chance of two molecules binding adjacent sites during random association between antigen and antibody is low.

Another contributing factor is the distribution of antigen sites on the cell surface. Some antigen sites are thought to be clustered together, thus facilitating complement activation, while others are so far apart that even binding of two adjacent sites will not lead to activation.

The activation of the classical complement pathway can be divided into three main steps:

1. The recognition stage where the first component of complement C1 is activated by the exposed complement binding site on the Fc portion of the immunoglobulin molecule.
2. The activation stage which leads to the formation of a C2–C4 complex which acts on C3. Part of C3 and its activating enzyme form another enzyme which, in turn, bring about the formation of C5.
3. The final stage or membrane attack sequence involves components C6–9 which interact to produce cell lysis by means of circular holes punched in the red cell membrane.

In some instances, although complement binding occurs, the sequence does not proceed to lysis of the cell. However, it is possible to detect the complement bound onto the red cell in these cases using anti-complement antibodies.

Because complement deteriorates on storage, it is essential that fresh samples are used in blood banking wherever possible, since complement binding, resulting in lysis, is indicative of an antigen–antibody reaction on the cell surface.

Factors affecting antigen–antibody reactions

The speed at which antigen–antibody reactions take place and the strength of the reaction are affected by many factors. The sensitivity of blood grouping tests is dependent on the use of optimum antigen and antibody concentrations. An increase in the number of antibodies that are bound to each red cell results in an increase in the strength of the reaction.

Conditions of the test, such as pH and temperature, are important. Most blood group antibodies show optimum activity between pH 6.5 and 7.5, and the majority show maximum rate of formation of antigen–antibody complexes at 37°C, with a reduction in this rate at lower temperatures.

An increase in the rate of association between antigen and antibody can be observed if the ionic strength of the medium is decreased. This results in an increase in zeta potential, causing an increased attraction between the negatively charged cells and antibody molecules, most of which are positively charged.

Since the titre of most antibodies can be increased by diluting the serum in low ionic strength saline, and because of the increased rate of antigen–antibody association, it is possible to reduce incubation time of blood grouping and crossmatching tests without any loss of sensitivity. This fact has led to the widespread routine use of low ionic strength saline in hospital laboratories.

A marked reduction in ionic strength has been associated with non-specific antibody uptake onto red cells. A low ionic strength of saline with glycine, with a molarity of 0.03, has been found to combine maximum increase in sensitivity without large numbers of false positive results (physiological saline has a molarity of 0.17).

38

Techniques used in blood transfusion

Although IgG antibodies are mostly unable to cause agglutination of red cells in a saline medium (see page 354) they are of significance when grouping and crossmatching. Several techniques may be used to demonstrate these antibodies.

Use of bovine albumin

The use of a medium which is able to dissipate electric charge (and therefore disperse the ionic cloud surrounding the red cell) allows the cells to become more closely associated. Agglutination of the cells by IgG or incomplete antibodies is then possible.

Use of proteolytic enzymes

The net negative charge which the red cell carries is due to the ionization of the carboxyl groups of sialic acid present at the cell surface. As a result of proteolytic action, some enzymes are able to liberate sialic acid residues from the cell membrane. This has the effect of decreasing the negative charge at the red cell surface, thus allowing cells to approach one another more closely. IgG antibodies are then able to bring about agglutination of the cells. A further effect of the action of these enzymes is to increase the accessibility of some antigen sites by removal of the sialic acid residues.

There are four enzymes available:

1. Papain, extracted from paw-paw fruits.
2. Bromelin, extracted from pineapples.
3. Ficin, extracted from figs.
4. Trypsin, extracted from pancreas.

Enzyme techniques can be performed using either of two different methods. The first of these is the two-stage technique where cells are pretreated with enzyme before setting up the test. This is the more sensitive of the two methods and is ideal for tests where the same cells are tested against a number of sera (e.g. antibody screening, antibody identification). The second method is the one-stage technique where the serum, enzyme and cells are layered in the tube and the cells become enzyme treated as they fall through the enzyme layer into the serum. This method is used more frequently in situations where many different cells are used (e.g. crossmatching) since pretreatment of cells required for the two-stage technique is time consuming.

When using enzyme techniques it should be remembered that proteolytic enzymes will destroy some antigens when they remove sialic acid from the red cells. These are the M, N and Fy^a antigens.

Because of this it is important that enzyme techniques are not used on their own, but together with other techniques where these antigens are not destroyed.

The anti-human globulin test

This test was introduced in 1945 by Dr R. Coombs and is also known as the Coombs test or antiglobulin test. It is considered to be one of the most sensitive techniques in the detection of complement binding and IgG antibodies. It is one of the essential tests used in the crossmatching of blood in order to check that the donor blood is compatible with the recipient's blood.

If human serum is injected into an animal such as a goat, sheep or rabbit, it will, as a result of this, produce a broad spectrum antibody directed against all components of human serum. In the same way, it is possible to stimulate the production of a more specific antibody by injection of single components

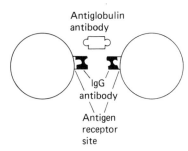

Antiglobulin
antibody

IgG
antibody

Antigen
receptor
site

Figure 38.1. Diagrammatic representation of the principles of the antiglobulin test

of the serum, such as IgG or complement fractions. The animal will also produce an anti-species antibody (in this case, anti-man), since the serum which was introduced was from another species. This anti-man antibody can be removed by absorption with human red cells, and if the remaining anti-human globulin is mixed with human serum the globulins will be precipitated (*Figure 38.1*).

After an initial screening test to determine that the produced antiglobulin serum is potentially suitable for routine use, a full series of standardization tests is undertaken. The serum is inactivated to destroy complement and mixed with group A and group B cells to remove unwanted agglutinins. Doubling dilutions (1 in 2, 1 in 4, 1 in 8, etc.) of the antiglobulin serum are prepared and each dilution is tested against red cells which have been sensitized with varying amounts of IgG antibody and complement binding antibody. The complexity of this standardization is to ensure that the antiglobulin serum will detect even small amounts of IgG and complement binding antibodies.

The detection of cells sensitized with IgG antibodies or complement binding antibodies using anti-human globulin serum may be performed in two ways:

1. *The direct antiglobulin test*, also referred to as the direct Coombs test or DCT. This test is performed directly on the patient's washed red cells to establish if they have been coated with antibody *in vivo*, i.e. antibody attaching itself to the patient's own red cells while still circulating in the vascular system. This test is often positive in haemolytic disease of the newborn, incompatible transfusion reactions and in some cases of auto-immune haemolytic anaemia.

2. *The indirect antiglobulin test* or indirect Coombs test. This test detects *in vitro* sensitization, i.e. sensitization following the incubation of cells and sera in a tube. One example of how this technique may be used is to detect antibodies in a patient's serum by incubating fully genotyped red cells with the patient's serum at 37°C to establish if any antibody present will sensitize the red cells *in vitro*. After incubation, the red cells are washed, antiglobulin serum is added and the presence or absence of agglutination is noted. By using a 'panel' of fully genotyped red cells and incubating the patient's serum with each, it is possible to determine the specificity of any antibody or mixture of antibodies present. Any red cells which do not agglutinate after the addition of antiglobulin serum will not contain the antigen to the specific antibody. The cells which do agglutinate will have been sensitized by the antibody and will contain the specific antigen to this antibody. By a series of eliminations the specificity of the antibody may be determined. The indirect antiglobulin test may also be used to detect unknown red cell antigens using antibodies of known specificity (genotyping) and to detect unknown red cell antigens using unknown antibodies (crossmatching).

As all human serum contains globulins, it is essential that any globulin not attached to the red cells is removed by washing in copious volumes of saline before the addition of antiglobulin serum. If these are not removed the antiglobulin serum will be neutralized by the 'free' contaminating globulins and false negative reactions obtained. The cells should be washed at least three times, and in laboratories which perform large numbers of antiglobulin tests this procedure is tedious and use is made of a cell-washing centrifuge which automatically washes the cells, and in some models automatically adds the antiglobulin serum.

39

The ABO blood group system

Landsteiner observed that the red cells of some individuals were agglutinated by the serum of other individuals. He demonstrated that these people could be classified into four groups according to which of two antigens were detectable, A, B, AB and, if neither of these antigens were present, group O. He also showed that an individual possesses antibodies against the antigen or antigens that he lacks on his red cells. This can be summarized as follows:

Antigen on red cell	Antibody in serum
A	Anti-B
B	Anti-A
AB	None
O	Anti-A + B

Because of the presence of these antibodies the ABO system is of major importance when transfusing blood in an individual, and wherever possible blood should not be transfused if it carries an ABO antigen which the recipient lacks.

The presence of these anti-A and anti-B agglutinins means that ABO grouping can be performed on both cells and serum. This acts as a double check to ensure that the correct ABO group has been determined.

Biochemistry of red cell antigens

The specificity of the ABO antigens is determined by a precursor substance which is acted upon by the H gene and converted to H substance (*Figure 39.1*). This is then acted on by the various A, B and O genes, and the terminal end sugar, which in H substance is fucose, adds further sugars depending on which specific gene is present. The A gene adds *N*-acetylgalactosamine and the B gene D-galactose. If the O gene is present, the H substance remains unaltered and therefore the terminal sugar is fucose.

If the H gene is not present, then the precursor substance is not able to be converted to H substance. This in turn means that the A, B or O genes cannot work to produce the appropriate antigens. This unusual situation results in the rare Bombay group, probably less than one per 1 000 000

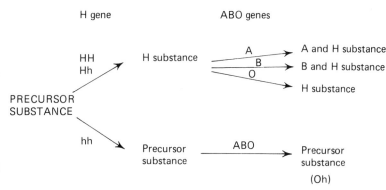

Figure 39.1. Interaction of ABO and H genes

but thought to have a much higher incidence in areas around Bombay.

Conversion to A or B chains is never complete and all red cells, except Bombay blood, have the H antigen, with group O having the largest amount.

ABO antigens

The A and B antigens can be detected at an early stage in the foetus, but are still not fully developed at birth. There is no problem in grouping cord blood cells with potent antisera, but weaker subgroups may be difficult to detect.

There are many antigen sites on a single red cell which express the presence or absence of the various blood groups, and each of these has to be represented many times over. It has been calculated that the A antigen alone in a single adult red cell is represented approximately 1 000 000 times and the B antigen approximately 700 000 times. In a group AB adult, the number of sites is reduced, there being approximately 500 000 A sites. The ABO antigens are also present on the white cells, platelets and tissue cells.

Group specific substances

Blood group factors A and B are not only present in red cells, but are also widely distributed in tissue cells and body fluids in hapten form (carbohydrate) and are non-antigenic, hence the name given them.

One of the richest and most readily available sources of group specific substances is saliva. When testing to detect the presence of these substances in an individual, it is usual to test the saliva. Individuals whose saliva contains the appropriate ABO substances are called secretors. Absence of the substance in saliva indicates absence throughout all tissue and body fluids. Secretion is controlled by a pair of allelomorphic genes, Se and se, giving rise to three genotypes:

$$\left.\begin{array}{ll} Se & Se \\ Se & se \end{array}\right\} 80\%$$

se   se   20%

There are two distinct forms of substance:

1. A water-soluble form present in body fluids and tissues.
2. An alcohol-soluble form present in red cells and some other tissues but absent from body fluids.

The presence of the water-soluble form is controlled by the secretor gene, the alcohol-soluble form is not. Thus, red cells and tissue of all persons contain an alcohol-soluble form whether secretor or not, but the secretor in addition possesses the water-soluble form in the body fluids. Only the substances present in the red cells can also be present in the tissues and body fluids. Group O substance is not secreted and secretors' saliva contains H substance.

Group A secretor	A and H
Group B	B and H
Group AB	A, B and H
Group O	H

To detect substances in solution, advantage is taken of the fact that soluble substance is capable of specifically neutralizing its corresponding agglutinin. The neutralization is reflected in the complete or partial inhibition of the agglutinin titre.

Subgroups of A

In 1911, Van Dungern and Hirszfeld described two different types of the A antigen now known as A_1 and A_2. Nearly all anti-A produced by group B individuals contains two anti-A antibodies, namely anti-A and anti-A_1. Anti-A agglutinates cells of the groups A_1, A_2, A_1B and A_2B, but anti-A_1 agglutinates only the cells of groups A_1 and A_1B.

The A_2 antigen reacts more weakly than the A_1 antigen when mixed with anti-A. This is because there are fewer antigen sites to which the anti-A can become attached.

The anti-A component of group O serum (anti-A + B) reacts more strongly with A_2 cells than with the anti-A produced by B individuals, even if the antibodies are of the same titre. This is because anti-A + B possesses a different serological activity from mixtures of anti-A and anti-B produced by group B and group A individuals, respectively.

The antibody A_1 occurs naturally as a cold agglutinin in about 2% of A_2 individuals and in about 25% of A_2B individuals. In some individuals the antibody becomes active at 37°C and will rapidly destroy any transfused A_1 cells. These individuals should be transfused with group A_2 blood. The A_2 antigen is not in any way attacked by the anti-A; therefore, no damage to the red cells occurs in these individuals.

No specific antibody to the antigen A_2 has been described, but the use of anti-H specific for the H antigen may be used. The H antigen is present in a higher amount in A_2 cells than A_1 cells, suggesting that the A_2 gene is able to convert less H substance than the A_1 gene (see *Figure 39.1*).

Further weak subgroups of A have been described.

Incidence of the ABO groups

The incidence of the ABO groups varies strikingly in different parts of the world and certain races have a predominance of different groups to others; for example, Negroes have a higher percentage of group B within their ethnic group. The approximate incidence of the ABO groups in Britain is given below, but even in this small part of the world there is a difference between the north and south of the country:

Group O = 47%
Group A = 42%
Group B = 8%
Group AB = 3%.

ABO antibodies

These antibodies are frequently referred to as 'naturally occurring', but it seems unlikely that they should appear without any stimulation from an antigen. It is suggested that these antibodies, which are not present at birth, are stimulated by the inhalation or ingestion of bacteria, seeds and foodstuffs which have similar chemical structures to the ABO antigens. To support this theory, experiments performed on animals showed that if they are kept from birth in a sterile environment they do not produce any antibody. The production of ABO antibodies in infants does not begin until about 4 months of age, which means that it may only be possible to determine an infant's ABO type from a cell group. However, antibody may be detected in the cord blood which has been transferred via the placenta from the mother.

These 'natural' antibodies are also referred to as 'allo' antibodies, and as they react maximally at 4°C are also called 'cold' antibodies. They have the following properties:

1. React maximally at 4°C, but the thermal range of activity includes 37°C.
2. Agglutinate cells suspended in saline.
3. Are absorbable.
4. The agglutinated cells adhere very strongly and agglutinates are difficult to break up.

Anti-A and anti-B levels are highest between the ages of 5 and 10 years, after which they decrease and are sometimes difficult to detect in elderly patients.

ABO antibodies, like other antibodies, are found in the globulin fraction of plasma. They can be demonstrated in other body fluids which contain plasma globulins, such as lymph, exudates and milk. They are not usually found in tears, saliva, urine, CSF or amniotic fluid.

Anti-A and anti-A_1

Serum from a group B individual contains two specific antibodies: anti-A which reacts with A_1 cells, A_2 cells and A_3 cells; anti-A_1 which reacts only with A_1 cells.

If the serum is absorbed using A_2 cells, this removes the anti-A and leaves a specific anti-A_1 which will only react with A_1 cells. If the antibody that has been absorbed by the A_2 cells is removed

(eluted) from the cells it can be shown to react with A_1 cells, A_2 cells and A_3 cells.

Anti-A_1 is found in 2% of group A_2 individuals and in 25% of A_2B individuals.

The following are weak subgroups of A.

A_3

The subgroup A_3 may be identified by the typical appearance of the agglutination it produces with anti-A and anti-A + B, notably a number of clumps of agglutinated cells in a sea of unagglutinated cells. This type of agglutination is known as mixed field agglutination. Anti-A_1 has been described in the serum of some A_3 individuals, but it is not commonly found. The frequency of the subgroup is about 1 in 1000 group A persons. Saliva of A_3 secretors contains both A and H substances.

A_x

The cells of the subgroup A_x may not be agglutinated by anti-A from group B individuals, although the antibody has been found to be absorbed onto the cell surface. The cells are, however, agglutinated by anti-A + B, thus showing the importance of using anti-A + B when ABO grouping. A_x individuals usually produce anti-A_1 and the frequency of the subgroup has been suggested to be 1 in 40000. The saliva of A_x secretors contains H but no A substance.

A_{int}

A_{int} has acquired its name because of the weak reaction the cells give with anti-A_1. It is more commonly found in Negroes than in whites. It has more H than A_2 individuals, despite the fact that it has been thought to be intermediate between A_1 and A_2 because of the reactions given with anti-A_1. Saliva of secretors contains both A and H substances.

A_m

The cells of this subgroup are agglutinated weakly, if at all, by anti-A and anti-A + B, but are capable of absorbing anti-A onto the red cell surface. It is then possible to remove or elute the antibody from the cell. A_m individuals do not usually produce anti-A_1, and saliva of secretors contains both A and H substances.

A_{end}

The A_{end} subgroup gives very weak reactions with both anti-A and anti-A + B. Secretors have H but no A substance in their saliva, and serum from A_{end} individuals does not contain anti-A_1.

A_{el}

No visible reactions are given with anti-A or anti-A + B by cells of this group, but antibody is absorbed onto the cell. An eluate prepared from these cells shows anti-A specificity. Saliva of secretors contains H but no A substance, and anti-A$_1$ may be present in the serum of these individuals.

A_{bantu}

A$_{bantu}$ accounts for approximately 4% of Bantu group A bloods. The serum of these individuals contains anti-A$_1$ and the saliva of secretors H, but no A substance. The cells give weak reactions with both anti-A and anti-A + B.

A_{finn}

This subgroup is more commonly found in Finland and can be distinguished from the subgroup A$_{end}$ by its enhanced reaction when using enzyme or antiglobulin techniques. The resulting agglutination is mixed field agglutination. The saliva of secretors contains H but no A substance and anti-A$_1$ has been described in all sera tested.

The presence of antigens on the red cells is determined by genes. The genes are carried on chromosomes which are present in the nucleus of all cells of the body. There are 46 chromosomes arranged in 23 pairs in each nucleus, with the exception of the sex cells which contain only 23 chromosomes, so that only one chromosome from each pair is present in the ovum and sperm. The fusion of the ovum and sperm brings the total number back again to 23 pairs. The two genes (one from each parent) which control the ABO group can be the same or different. If the two genes are the same the person is called homozygous for that character and, if different, heterozygous. The genes which can occupy the same site or locus on a chromosome are called allelomorphic or alleles.

Ignoring the question of subgroups, the inheritance of the ABO groups depends upon three genes A, B and O, which can be broadly described as co-dominant, although in practice the A and B genes express themselves dominantly to O. The O gene is called an amorph which is a recessive gene showing no observable change when present in the homozygous form. An individual inherits the A, B and O gene from one parent and the A, B or O gene from the other, thereby making a pair of genes called the genotype. Therefore, six genotypes can occur: AA, AB, BB, AO, BO and OO. It is not possible to differentiate red cells of genotype AA or AO, BB or BO and the term phenotype is used to describe the observed reactions. AB cells and OO cells are both a phenotype and the genotype.

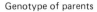

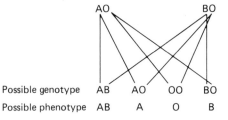

Figure 39.2. Diagrammatic representation of the possible genes being passed from parent to offspring

Laws of heredity

Two laws of inheritance have been proved in accordance with Bernstein's theory (*Figure 39.2*):

1. The offspring cannot possess the antigen A or B, alone or in combination, except that it be inherited from one or both parents.
2. The parent of group AB cannot produce an offspring of group O, nor can a parent of group O give rise to a child of group AB. This is because the group AB is heterozygous, so that the A gene must come from one parent and the B gene from the other.

The only possible results from the matings of various blood groups are shown in *Table 39.1*.

Table 39.1 Results from matings of various blood groups

Phenotypes of parents	Possible phenotypes of offspring
O × O	O
O × A	O or A
O × B	O or B
O × AB	A or B
A × A	A or O
A × B	A, B, AB or O
A × AB	A, B or AB
B × B	B or O
B × AB	A, B or AB
AB × AB	A, B or AB

Inheritance of the subgroups

The antigens A$_1$ and A$_2$ genetically are co-dominant, but in practice the genes A$_1$ and A$_2$ are expressed dominantly over the O gene; the A$_1$ gene is also expressed dominant to the A$_2$ gene. The genotypes in *Table 39.2* may therefore be present from each of the phenotypes shown.

Table 39.2 Phenotypes and their possible genotypes

Phenotype	Possible genotypes
O	OO
A_1	A_1A_1, A_1A_2 or A_1O
A_2	A_2A_2 or A_2O
B	BB or BO
A_1B	A_1B
A_2B	A_2B

Laws of heredity

The following laws of inheritance have been proved:

1. The antigen A_1 cannot occur in an offspring unless obtained from one or both parents, but since the phenotype A_1 can have the genotype A_1A_2, two parents of this genotype can produce an A_2 offspring.
2. The matings $A_1 \times B$ and $A_1B \times A_1B$ cannot produce A_2B offspring because there is no genotype of A_1B that contains the A_2 gene.
3. In matings $A_1 \times O$, $A_1 \times A_1$, $A_1 \times B$ and $A_1 \times A_1B$, the subgroups A_2 and A_2B are impossible in an offspring if it can be proved that a sibling (brother or sister) from the same parents is either B or O. The reason for this is that the genotypes of the B and O siblings must be BO or OO so that an O gene must have been obtained from an A_1 parent, thus revealing the genotype of this parent

Table 39.3 Combinations of phenotypes

Phenotype of parents	Possible phenotype of offspring
$A_1 \times O$	A_1, A_2 or O
$A_1 \times A_1$	A_1, A_2 or O
$A_1 \times A_2$	A_1, A_2 or O
$A_1 \times B$	A_1, A_2, B, A_1B, A_2B or O
$A_1 \times A_2B$	A_1, A_2, B, A_1B or A_2B
$A_1B \times O$	A_1 or B
$A_1B \times A_1$	A_1, B, A_1B or A_2B
$A_1B \times A_2$	A_1, B or A_2B
$A_1B \times A_2B$	A_1, B, A_1B or A_2B
$A_1B \times B$	A_1, B or A_1B
$A_1B \times A_1B$	A_1, B or A_1B
$A_2 \times O$	A_2 or O
$A_2 \times A_2$	A_2 or O
$A_2 \times B$	A_2, B, A_2B or O
$A_2B \times O$	A_2 or B
$A_2B \times A_2$	A_2, B or A_2B
$A_2B \times B$	A_2, B or A_2B
$A_2B \times A_2B$	A_2, B or A_2B

to be A_1O, which cannot give the offspring an A_2 gene.

The inclusion of the subgroups of parents greatly increases the possible phenotypes of an offspring, and the complete combinations are as shown in *Table 39.3*.

ABO grouping serum

This is usually obtained from selected donors whose antibody levels are suitable for use as a laboratory reagent. Standard anti-A serum should have a titre of 1 in 512 and anti-B a titre of 1 in 256 when titred against A and B cells, respectively. Serial dilutions of the serum are made in saline, and cells of the appropriate group added. The titre is the reciprocal of the highest dilution at which agglutination occurs. Although some sera may conform to these requirements, the avidity of the antibody may not be suitable. Avidity is the power of the antibody to agglutinate quickly and strongly. In order to detect weak subgroups of A, it is necessary for the anti-A to show a higher titre and avidity than the anti-B. Group O serum (anti-A + B) must conform to the same standards used for anti-A and anti-B, and should be capable of detecting weak A subgroups such as A_x. No other antibodies should be present other than those specifically required, and thorough testing of the serum is necessary against as many red cell antigens as possible. The serum must not cause cells to form rouleaux and should be free from fat.

Lectins

Extracts from certain plants, particularly their seeds, contain substances capable of causing agglutination of red cells. In most cases the agglutination occurs regardless of the antigens present, but some show blood group specificity. It should be noted that these substances are not antibodies but have a similar effect. The two most commonly used extracts from seeds used in blood grouping are:

1. *Dolichos bifloris* (Indian cattle bean, commonly known as horse gram or grain) can be diluted so as to react specifically with the A_1 antigen and therefore differentiate A_1 and A_1B cells from A_2 and AB cells.
2. *Ulex europaeus* (common gorse) has an anti-H specificity and agglutinates A_2, A_2B and O cells far more strongly than A_1B or B cells.

40

The Rhesus system

In 1940, Landsteiner and Wiener injected the red cells of the Rhesus monkey into rabbits, thereby producing an antibody which not only agglutinates Rhesus monkey red cells but also the red cells of approximately 85% of Caucasians (a term used by anthropologists to describe the white races). As these people apparently possessed an antigen similar to the Rhesus monkey, these individuals were called Rhesus positive, and the remainder whose cells did not agglutinate were called Rhesus negative. The antigen was called D and the antibody anti-D. It is now known that the antigen present on the red cells of the monkey, and its corresponding antibody produced in rabbits, is not identical to the human form, but for all clinical purposes time has sanctioned the continuance of the term Rhesus (Rh). Subsequent investigations proved the existence of further Rhesus antigens and antibodies and the basis of the Rhesus system was explained.

The Rhesus system is a very complex one, in which more than 40 antibodies have been described. However, at the level of general use there are six common Rhesus genes—C, D and E and their allelomorphs c, d and e (i.e. a chromosome can carry C or c but not both). Each chromosome can carry the genes in only eight possible combinations, which are CDe, cDE, cDe, CDE, Cde, cdE, CdE or cde. As these combinations are difficult to say without causing some confusion, a shorthand system for easy identification is essential (*Table 40.1*).

The three genes C or c, D or d and E or e are carried on the same chromosome and are positioned close together. We know this because an individual receiving, for example, cde from one parent and CDe from another passes on to his offspring either cde or CDe. If the genes were positioned at some distance apart on the chromosome and 'crossing-over', or the chromosomes occurred freely, the

Table 40.1 Shorthand system for Rhesus antigens

Rhesus antigens	Shorthand
CDe	R_1
cDE	R_2
cDe	R_0
CDE	R_z
Cde	r'
cdE	r''
CdE	r_y
cde	r

genetic frequencies would differ widely from those observed. The linkage can therefore be said to be close.

Since there will be two Rh chromosomes found in the red cell, the eight combinations can be paired in 36 different ways, resulting in 36 possible Rhesus genotypes. With the exception of the antigen d, the other five Rhesus antigens are capable of stimulating the formation of a specific antibody. Extensive studies have failed to find an antibody anti-d, and indicate that there is no antigen d.

Table 40.2 shows the reactions of red cells with the five Rhesus antisera available, the Rhesus phenotype, commonest and therefore probable genotype, shorthand symbol and approximate percentage frequency in the UK.

After the A and B antigens of the ABO system, the D antigen is the most antigenic. This means that the introduction of the D antigen into an individual lacking that antigen is more likely to stimulate antibody production than other Rhesus antigens. Because of this, it is usual to determine only the presence or absence of the D antigen in the routine hospital laboratory. As the vast majority of patients in hospital are grouped as the potential recipients of

Table 40.2 Reactions of red cells with Rhesus antisera

Rhesus antisera					Rh phenotype	Commonest genotype	Symbol	Approximate % frequency in UK
Anti-C	Anti-c	Anti-D	Anti-E	Anti-e				
+	+	+	−	+	CcDee	CDe/cde	R_1r	31
+	−	+	−	+	CCDee	CDe/CDe	R_1R_1	16
−	+	−	−	+	ccddee	cde/cde	rr	15
+	+	+	+	+	CcDEe	CDe/cDE	R_1R_2	13
−	+	+	+	+	ccDEe	cDE/cde	R_2r	13
−	+	+	+	−	ccDEE	cDE/cDE	R_2R_2	3
−	+	+	−	+	ccDee	cDe/cde	R_0r	1

a blood transfusion, the determination of the D antigen only is not hazardous. The reason for this is because a donor grouped as D negative by the National Blood Transfusion Service will have been fully genotyped and determined as a true Rhesus negative individual, having the genotype cde/cde (rr).

A patient being grouped as D positive and, for example, lacking the E antigen, as in the genotype CDe/CDe (R_1R_1), may well be transfused with blood containing the E antigen. The possibility of an anti-E antibody developing cannot be discounted. Similarly, any antigen transfused which is lacking in the recipient may well give rise to the production of the specific antibody, but in clinical practice the problem is not common, with the exception, as previously stated, of the D antigen.

It must be emphasized that determination of the presence or absence of the D antigen alone in a potential blood donor is not sufficient and the full Rhesus genotype should be determined where possible.

The D^u antigen

A number of rare genes exist in the Rhesus system, but the most important of these for the routine laboratory worker is the D^u antigen. The D^u antigen appears to be a weaker form of the D antigen.

It has been postulated that the D antigen is in fact made up of a mosaic of four parts, Rh^A, Rh^B, Rh^C and Rh^D. An individual who is RhD positive possesses all four parts of the mosaic, whereas none of these parts is present in the RhD negative individual. In some people, however, one or more of the parts of the mosaic may be missing and their red cells are agglutinated by some, but not all, anti-D sera. The anti-D serum should react with all four parts of the mosaic, but some may fail to react with one part, hence variable reactions may occur. The D^u antigen does not usually react with complete anti-D, but will react with varying numbers of different incomplete anti-D sera depending on whether it is a high grade or a low grade D^u antigen.

When the D^u antigen is present, any anti-D serum which does not agglutinate the cells will have sensitized the cells, that is to say the red cells will have been coated with the antibody and this may be demonstrated using the antiglobulin test.

A D^u person if given RhD positive blood may, although rarely, form an anti-D, and similarly D^u blood given to a RhD negative person may well stimulate the formation of an anti-D. It is therefore accepted that a D^u individual is considered as Rhesus positive as a donor and Rhesus negative as a recipient.

Although the incidence of the D^u antigen is highest among the Negro races, it also occurs in about 1% of the population in the UK.

Apparent D^u

An apparent D^u can occur in some people with the genotype R_1r' (CDe/Cde). The C on the other chromosome (in the *trans*-position) suppresses the D antigen so that cells will give similar reactions to D^u cells. However, when the R_1 gene is passed on to the next generation the D antigen will appear normal.

Haemolytic disease of the newborn

In 1939, it was demonstrated by Levine and Stetson that maternal antibodies crossing the placenta could damage foetal red cells possessing the antigen specific for the maternal antibody. This results in a condition known as Haemolytic Disease of the Newborn (HDN). Since only IgG antibodies are able to cross the placenta (IgM antibodies are too large), it is these antibodies when active at 37°C which can cause HDN, and almost all specificities of these antibodies have been implicated. However, in the majority of cases the causative antibody is anti-D, the mother being RhD negative and the foetus having inherited the D antigen from the father.

The first child is seldom affected by HDN since the stimulation of the antibody is frequently due to a transplacental haemorrhage from the foetus to the mother during delivery. If a pregnancy with a second Rhesus positive foetus occurs, then small bleeds from foetus to mother may further stimulate antibody production. The antibody produced as a result of the primary dose of the antigen will be mainly IgM, but on subsequent exposure to the antigen IgG production replaces IgM. It is these IgG antibodies which are able to cross the placenta, enter the foetal circulation and destroy red cells.

The affected infant usually presents with anaemia and jaundice. The anaemia is usually accompanied by an increase in reticulocytes and a high nucleated red cell count. Bilirubin levels performed on cord blood give an indication of the degree of jaundice. It should be remembered that not all jaundice is a result of HDN but may be 'physiological' jaundice; however, this usually arises about 24 h after birth whereas jaundice due to HDN is present at birth. The measurement of serum bilirubin in affected infants is of great importance, since high levels which in an infant are predominantly in the form of unconjugated bilirubin may cause irreversible brain damage. Tests on the blood of the infant should also include grouping and a direct anti-human globulin test (DCT). When infant's cells have been sensitized by maternal antibody, a positive DCT is usually seen. In HDN caused by an ABO incompatibility, the DCT may be weak or negative. The specificity of the sensitizing antibody may be determined by performing tests against an antibody identification panel using an eluate prepared from the infant's cells.

When the infant is severely affected by the disease it may be necessary to perform an exchange transfusion. This serves to lower dangerous bilirubin levels, treat anaemia and remove the sensitized cells from the circulation. The blood given should be negative for the antigen against which the maternal antibody is directed. Thus if the causative antibody is anti-D, then ABO compatible Rhesus negative blood is given to the infant.

A number of tests are performed on the mother during pregnancy in order to determine if the infant may be affected by the disease. On their first attendance at the clinic, all pregnant women should have blood taken for grouping and an antibody screening test. If an antibody is found it should be tested in order to determine the specificity and strength. The strength of the antibody is measured by a titre, usually performed using the anti-human globulin technique. A rising titre during pregnancy may indicate that the infant is positive for the antigen against which maternal antibody is directed, and gives an indication of the severity of the disease. Amniocentesis is suggested if the titre reaches 1 in 32 or more. A sample of amniotic fluid is tested for bilirubin pigments which will be present if the infant is affected. If the foetus is severely affected, an intra-uterine transfusion may be necessary, but after 36 weeks of pregnancy delivery is usually performed by caesarean section. Exchange transfusion can then be performed if necessary.

Since the most common causative antibody of HDN is anti-D, a large number of cases can be prevented by giving an injection of a potent anti-D immunoglobulin to Rhesus negative women bearing Rhesus D positive children. If given within 72 h of delivery, the anti-D is able to destroy any RhD positive foetal cells before they reach the sites of antibody production.

Other blood group systems

Over 100 blood group antigens may be demonstrated using the specific antisera, and these have been classified into blood group systems. Many of these antigens fortunately have no clinical significance, but as the blood group systems are inherited quite independently from each other, they are of immense value as genetic markers. Some of the other blood group systems apart from the ABO and Rhesus are called as follows: MNSs, P Kell, Lewis, Lutheran, Duffy, Kidd and I. For further information about these groups more specialized textbooks (such as Race and Sanger's *Blood Groups in Man*) should be referred to.

Medico-legal aspects of blood groups

In paternity disputes, the blood grouping of all the parties concerned can do no more than exclude one of the parents. Usually it is the father who is in dispute and he is excluded if antigens which he genetically must pass on are not present in the child; also, if the child possesses an antigen which both he and the mother lack, the disputed father must be excluded. This type of work is not usually carried out in the hospital laboratory because of the legal implications.

Forensic aspects

The determination of the blood group antigens of an individual are nearly as exclusive as the fingerprints. This fact is used frequently by police departments throughout the world during the investigation of criminal cases. The techniques are often those used in the clinical laboratory, but highly sophisticated methods are available in detecting blood group antigens in dried stains and also the determination of blood group substances in saliva and other body fluids.

41

Collection and storage of blood

National Blood Transfusion Service

In England, blood is predominantly collected by the National Blood Transfusion Service (NBTS). The country is divided into regions, with each region having its own Transfusion Centre responsible for supplying blood, blood products and grouping sera to the hospital laboratories in its catchment area. Donors are bled twice a year and are notified when to attend a donor session, which is operating in the locality where they live. The mobile collecting teams, which consist of a medical officer, driver, clerks and donor attendants, also visit factories and offices as well as local halls and establish a temporary but efficient blood collection service. The collected blood is then transported to the appropriate Transfusion Centre where it is fully tested for its suitability as donor blood, labelled and stored before its final journey to the hospital blood bank.

Blood donors

A blood donor must be within the ages of 18 and 65 of either sex and conform to the National Standard of Fitness as laid down by Act of Parliament. Male donors should have a haemoglobin level of at least 13.5 g/dl and females a level of at least 12.5 g/100 ml. The haemoglobin level of the donor is checked prior to donation. A drop of blood from a finger prick is carefully delivered into a copper sulphate solution of specific gravity where it immediately forms copper proteinate. Male donors are accepted if their blood sinks in a copper sulphate solution having a specific gravity of 1.055 and female donors if it sinks in a solution having a specific gravity of 1.053. If blood contains less than the required concentration of haemoglobin it will rise to the surface before finally sinking. Should this happen the individual is unacceptable as a blood donor.

It is perhaps unnecessary to state that all donors must be fit and well before donating their blood, but certain diseases may remain hidden and must be excluded so as to prevent transmission to the recipient. Every donation is tested to exclude syphilis and any donation giving a positive result is discarded. Red cells of donors who have recently visited or who have lived in a country where malaria is present are also discarded, although their plasma may be used for the preparation of 'blood products'. Malarial parasites resist storage at 4°C and may easily be transmitted to the recipient of any such red cells.

Potential donors who give a previous history of jaundice, allergy or who have had a recent illness are not bled.

The donor is bled into a plastic blood pack, which may be a single bag with or without one or two 'satellite' bags, depending upon what the donation will be used to provide. The bag contains 75 ml of anticoagulant, to which is added about 420 ml of blood. This should be well mixed to prevent clotting of the collected blood. The anticoagulant should not cause deterioration of the red cells, nor must it be toxic to the recipient of the transfusion.

Although they are no longer used in the UK, glass bottles are still in use in some Third World countries where plastic blood bags are unavailable.

One of the original anticoagulants used for the transfer of blood from one individual to another was sodium citrate. Later it was found that the volume of anticoagulant required could be reduced and that better preservation of the blood was obtained if the solution was acidified and glucose added. These observations led to the widespread use of acid–

367

citrate dextrose (ACD) which has the following composition:

Trisodium citrate	2.2 g
Citric acid	0.8 g
Dextrose	2.5 g
Distilled water (pyrogen-free)	to 100 ml

However, citrate–phosphate dextrose adenine (CPD–adenine) has widely replaced ACD as the anticoagulant used for storage of blood for transfusion. This is because better preservation of an important red cell enzyme, and hence better oxygen carrying capacity, has been demonstrated with this anticoagulant.

Each 100 ml of CPD–adenine solution contains:

Sodium citrate	2.63 g
Dextrose	2.90 g
Citric acid	327 mg
Sodium acid phosphate	251 mg
Adenine	27.5 mg

Blood stored at 4°C is well preserved in CPD–adenine and may be used up to 35 days after the date of collection. Beyond this time there is considerable loss of viability of the blood.

Although red cells may be satisfactorily stored, platelets survive storage poorly and are not viable after 24 h. White cells remain viable for longer, and some lymphocytes may survive for up to 21 days. As platelet and leucocyte antibodies can be demonstrated in recipients of multiple transfusions, it must be assumed that although these cells may not survive storage, their antigenic structure remains intact. Coagulation factors diminish rapidly on storage, especially factors V and VIII which disappear within 24 h of collection.

Hepatitis B

One of the most serious risks involved in the transfusion of blood is the danger of transmitting hepatitis. This is a condition ascribed to a viral infection which causes inflammation of the liver and may prove fatal.

The fact that hepatitis could be transmitted by transfusion of blood and certain blood products has been known for many years, but it was not until 1967 that the antigen responsible for the infection—Australia antigen—was discovered. This antigen is also known as hepatitis B surface antigen (HB$_s$Ag) and is a marker of the infective agent of hepatitis B.

Donations can be screened for hepatitis by the means of a test for HB$_s$Ag, and the incidence of hepatitis post-transfusion has decreased since this has been performed routinely on all donations. The most commonly used method for detecting HB$_s$Ag is radioimmunoassay.

■ Note

Any blood sample entering the laboratory may contain the hepatitis B surface antigen. These samples should be treated with extreme care in the laboratory and the recommendations laid down in the Department of Health publication 'Safety in Laboratories' strictly adhered to.

Storage of blood

Blood deteriorates rapidly if not kept under ideal conditions, and blood which has haemolysed or become infected may well be lethal to the recipient.

Blood must be stored in specially constructed refrigerators which have high insulation properties and a very sensitive thermostat. The refrigerator must maintain a temperature of 4°C, with a maximum range of 2–6°C. It is essential that the temperature does not exceed 6°C or fall below 2°C or damage to the red cells may occur. To prevent this, the blood bank must have a temperature recorder so that it is possible to tell the temperature at a glance, and also be able to keep a record of the stability of temperature. The blood bank must also be connected to an alarm system, preferably a loud bell or buzzer, which will give an audible signal if the temperature rises or falls outside the prescribed limits. The alarm must also sound in a place where the staff are always on duty, thereby ensuring that a responsible person will take the predetermined action even when the laboratory is closed. The alarm should also sound if the electricity supply fails; it therefore follows that the alarm system must be battery operated.

On no account must blood be stored in a domestic refrigerator such as is found in most hospital wards. These refrigerators exhibit marked fluctuations in temperature and it is not unusual for this type of cabinet to fall below 0°C.

If there is any doubt regarding the storage of blood once it has left the laboratory blood bank, it must be discarded and not returned to the stock to be re-crossmatched for another patient. It is the laboratories' responsibility to continually educate all persons who handle blood (this includes medical, nursing and portering staff) as to the importance of the correct storage procedures in the individual hospital.

Transportation of blood

The National Blood Transfusion Service delivers the majority of its blood by road, using specially designed refrigerated vans or insulated vans with large ice containers, the bags of blood being held safely in metal crates. If the blood is to be sent by rail, a purpose-built insulated box is used. The insulated box is strong and designed to take an ice insert in the centre. Using this type of insulated box, blood will keep at a temperature of 4–6°C for at least 6 h.

Frozen blood

Blood for transfusion may be kept for a much longer period than 28 days if it is kept frozen solid at −80°C. In order to prevent damage to the red cells by ice crystals, the addition of glycerol is essential. When the blood is required for transfusion, all traces of glycerol must be removed immediately the blood has thawed. This is achieved by washing the cells serially in lowering concentrations of isotonic glycerol solutions. The recovery rate of red cells stored by this method is good and they may be kept at −80°C for up to two years.

Another low-temperature storage method is to freeze red cells at −196°C in liquid nitrogen. The red cells are preserved in aluminium canisters, since the standard plastic packs disintegrate in liquid nitrogen. The freezing, thawing and recovery of cells ready for transfusion requires special techniques and apparatus, but blood may be stored for 10 years in this way.

The latter method has been adopted by most centres with established banks of frozen cells.

Frozen blood, although very expensive to maintain, does have many advantages over blood stored in the usual way at 4°C. Red cells having rare antigen combinations or lacking common antigens may be stored for extremely long periods, and will be available for patients who have developed antibodies to the majority of red cells. Alternatively, patients who have very rare blood groups may be bled at intervals so that they may receive their own blood during surgery; this is called auto-transfusion.

Since blood stored at low temperatures has a greatly prolonged shelf life, it is possible to store large quantities as a reserve to offset any deficiency in donor blood or meet increased demands which may occur.

It is of value to store small quantities of red cells in glycerol and liquid nitrogen as reference cells in the laboratory. The recovery of small volumes of red cells frozen in glycerol is much easier to achieve, as they may be dialysed against isotonic saline and are ready for use in 2 h. Likewise with red cells stored in liquid nitrogen; these may be thawed quickly in a warmed sucrose solution. Red cells frozen in liquid nitrogen are in the form of small peas or pellets, and the appropriate number are removed as they are required.

42

Blood products and substitutes

Blood products

With the advent of more intensive and sophisticated methods of clinical management, the demands for blood have greatly increased. In order to keep up with these demands it has been necessary to split blood into its various components so that a patient receives only the component or components which he requires. In this way the same amount of blood may be used to treat many more patients.

To meet increasing demands for many of the blood products now available, it is necessary to remove plasma before the red cells are issued. This has led to a decrease in the number of available units of whole blood. These have been replaced by red cell concentrates. Whole blood transfusions are used predominantly to replace blood loss from acute haemorrhage or surgical operations, although many hospitals use a proportion of red cell concentrates in these cases. Red cell concentrates are given to anaemic patients who need the additional haemoglobin, but not the plasma fraction which may precipitate cardiac failure.

These red cell concentrates may be prepared by removal of about 200 ml of plasma from a unit containing 450 ml of blood in 75 ml anticoagulant. The plasma removed can be used in the production of other blood products.

Fresh frozen plasma

The plasma used for the production of fresh frozen plasma must be separated from red cells within a few hours of collection and stored at −20°C. The plasma is stored in individual units, and since ABO agglutinins are present, should be transfused to ABO compatible recipients.

Fresh frozen plasma contains clotting factors and can be used for treatment of multiple clotting factor deficiencies.

Dried human plasma

This is prepared from pooled plasma and dried by freeze drying; it is a light to deep cream-coloured powder. To ensure cross-neutralization of the ABO antibodies by the soluble blood group substances, plasma from donors of A, O and either B or AB groups are mixed in the approximate ratio 9:9:2. No more than 10 separate donations are pooled. The dried plasma must be stored at a room temperature below 25°C, preferably protected from the light. Provided the Viscap remains intact, preventing the entry of moisture, the storage life of the dried plasma is 8 years. Dried plasma is reconstituted by adding 400 ml of sterile, pyrogen-free distilled water and should completely dissolve within 10 min at 15–20°C. Any signs of lumpiness indicate the presence of denatured protein, and the bottle contents must be discarded. In the UK, dried human plasma is no longer used and has been replaced by plasma protein fraction.

Plasma protein fraction (PPF)

This is a solution of the proteins of human plasma and is a clear, amber fluid. It is prepared from pooled plasma which has been precipitated with suitable organic solvents, and redissolved in water. The final solution is made isotonic by adding sodium chloride, and further substances added to stabilize it to heat. It is sterilized by filtration and heated at 60°C for 10 h to prevent transmission of the hepatitis B virus. PPF contains not less than 4.3% w/v of total protein, contains no fibrinogen, little if any immunoglobulin, and has a storage life of 3 years at 2–25°C. It is used mainly to replace depleted plasma volume and may be used in place of blood in an emergency while awaiting issues of blood. More recently, the name of this solution has been changed to Human Albumin Solution 4.5%.

Albumin

Albumin is produced by further processing of the PPF-containing fraction. This reduces the salt concentration, hence the product is often known as salt-poor albumin. Before freeze drying, the albumin is heat treated for 10 h at 60°C which inactivates the hepatitis B virus.

Salt-poor albumin is frequently used for treating hypoalbuminaemia resulting from liver or renal disease.

Dried human fibrinogen

This is prepared from plasma by precipitating with organic solvents, the precipitate being redissolved in a solution of sodium chloride and sodium citrate and then freeze dried. It is a white powder or friable solid and is reconstituted for use by the addition of sterile, pyrogen-free distilled water. Fibrinogen therapy is only indicated for the specific replacement of fibrinogen when bleeding is due to lowered levels, or lack of this coagulation factor. This is no longer available in the UK and fresh frozen plasma (FFP) is used (see p. 370).

Cryoprecipitate

This is prepared from fresh plasma which is frozen solid in a mixture of solid CO_2 (dry ice) and ethanol, and allowed to thaw slowly at 4°C for 24 h. Thawing leaves a cold-insoluble precipitate rich in antihaemophilic factor (factor VIII), which is kept after the plasma has been centrifuged and the supernatant removed. The precipitate is stored at −20°C, and for use thawed at 37°C, re-suspended and usually injected intravenously using a syringe and needle. Cryoprecipitate contains about 56% of the original factor VIII in less than 3% of the original plasma volume, together with a small amount of fibrinogen, but no significant amounts of other coagulation factors are present. It is used predominantly in the treatment of classical haemophilia and sometimes in diseases where the factor VIII level is reduced to the extent that bleeding occurs.

Factor VIII concentrates

Factor VIII concentrates have widely replaced cryoprecipitate for the treatment of haemophilia. The level of factor VIII in cryoprecipitate varies from donation to donation which makes it difficult to calculate how many packs are required for the treatment of a disorder. Concentrated fractions of factor VIII, which are prepared from multiple donations of fresh plasma, contain freeze-dried material of known potency which is stated in international units on each concentrate. Thus, it is possible to calculate accurately the number of concentrates required for the treatment of factor VIII deficiencies.

Platelets

Platelets may be used for the treatment of thrombocytopenia, a condition which has become more common with the use of cytotoxic drugs for the treatment of leukaemia and malignant tumours. Platelets may be harvested from platelet-rich plasma, obtained by spinning blood collected into double or triple plastic blood bags at low speeds. The platelet-rich plasma is transferred to a satellite bag and a concentrate obtained by spinning the bag hard to throw down platelets into a button. The supernatant plasma can be returned to the red cells, leaving a platelet concentrate. This method can be reversed, starting with a hard spin to throw down platelets and white cells on top of the red cells. This layer of white cells and platelets, known as the *buffy coat*, can be transferred to a satellite pack and a slower spin yields a platelet concentrate.

In order to produce a significant rise in platelet count in the recipient, platelets from four donations of blood are pooled. Because the platelets cannot be pooled in a closed system, this reduces the shelf life due to the risk of infection.

There has been a great deal of discussion concerning ideal storage temperatures for platelets. Concentrates stored at 22°C yield platelets which have a longer life span in the recipient than those stored at 4°C. However, haemolytic activity is better immediately after transfusion of platelets stored at 4°C than those stored at 22°C. The latter may take up to 24 h to recover full haemostatic activity. Thus, storage temperature may depend on the clinical reason for platelet transfusion.

White cells

The transfusion of white cells—in particular granulocytes—has been successfully used in patients with leucopenia in order to combat life-threatening infection. The main problem is the large number of granulocytes needed to treat a patient, since the life span of the transfused cells is only 6–7 h.

The white cells may be obtained in the form of buffy coat preparations pooled from a number of donations. A more successful method of collecting large numbers of white cells involves a special cell separator that enables the donor's blood to be passed through a centrifuge where white cells can be removed and the remaining components of the blood returned to the patient. Platelets may also be harvested in this way.

It should be noted that platelet and white cell transfusions may result in the production of antibodies directed against antigens present on the surface of these cells. Platelets and white cells for transfusion should therefore be used only when essential, and if repeated transfusions are indicated it may be necessary to find donors with antigens matching those possessed by the recipient of the transfusion.

Blood substitutes

A number of solutions are available which, although they are not blood products, enable blood volume to be replaced. It must be emphasized that none of these substances will increase the oxygen-carrying capacity of the blood; only the transfusion of red cells will achieve this.

Dextran

Dextran is the collective name given to the polysaccharide formed when a solution of sucrose is broken down by the action of *Bacterium leuconostoc mesenteroides*. Dextrans of various molecular weights can be made, but the ideal molecular weight is approximately 70000. If the molecules are too small they are rapidly excreted in the urine, and if too large may cause undesirable physiological effects. The solution is usually 6% dextran in isotonic saline, and is used to replace the blood volume, particularly after acute haemorrhage, allowing time for whole blood to be crossmatched. All dextrans have the property of greatly increasing rouleaux formation, which can cause crossmatching errors unless the antiglobulin technique is used. It is advisable that blood for crossmatching is taken before dextran is given.

Gelatin solutions

These are soluble derivatives of collagen, and are used in a 3–5% solution which is stable when stored at room temperature for 7 years. Of the three main types of gelatin solutions available, the urea-linked gelatin (Haemaccel) is the most commonly used.

Gelatin solutions may be used as an alternative to dextran.

Other crystalloid solutions

These include 4% glucose–saline, Hartmann's lactate solution and isotonic saline. These solutions are used predominantly to maintain the blood volume and prevent dehydration after major surgery.

Artificial blood

Much effort has been concentrated on finding a suitable substitute for blood, it being essential that this substitute should be able to transport oxygen. Fluorocarbons are effective synthetic oxygen carriers, but are unable to transport oxygen as efficiently as haemoglobin.

Another substance being studied is stroma-free haemoglobin which has been found to be much safer than some of the earlier solutions studied.

43

Compatibility testing (crossmatching)

In most blood transfusion cases, even though the blood donor's and the recipient's ABO and Rhesus groups are the same, it is essential that crossmatch techniques are performed. This is to ensure that the donor blood will not give rise to any reaction from antibodies the recipient may have formed to any other blood group systems. As it is probably true to say that no blood given will exactly match the antigenic structure of the recipient's red cells, it is vital that every precaution is taken to prevent harm to the patient. The crossmatch is performed by testing the donor red cells against the recipient's serum using several different techniques, although different laboratories use different combinations of these techniques.

Usually included is the saline technique at room temperature which detects most cold antibodies, and checks for ABO errors; saline 30°C or 37°C to detect any cold antibodies with wide thermal range and of clinical significance; albumin addition and/or an enzyme technique to detect incomplete warm antibodies. The enzyme technique is particularly sensitive for Rhesus antibodies, and the indirect antiglobulin technique is the most sensitive and for that reason should always be included in cross-matching tests. All these techniques are usually incubated for 1 h. As mentioned previously, if low ionic strength saline is used these incubation times may be reduced.

Blood should ideally never be given to a patient without crossmatching. An emergency crossmatch can be performed using reduced incubation times; the majority of clinically significant antibodies will be detected by these methods.

If blood is required in an emergency, and it is necessary to issue uncrossmatched blood, the requesting clinician then assumes responsibility.

In most hospital blood banks, two units of group O Rhesus negative blood are available in case of emergencies. This 'Flying Squad' blood can be issued in cases where there is insufficient time to perform a rapid group on the patient. It should be remembered that it is always better to issue uncrossmatched blood of the patient's own group rather than O Rhesus negative blood. In all cases the units of blood should be fully crossmatched as soon as possible, even if this means crossmatching units of blood once the used blood bags have been returned to the laboratory.

Transfusion reactions

If a patient receives blood against which he has antibodies, rapid destruction of the transfused cells may result. This destruction of red cells may be accompanied by fever, shivering, nausea and low back pain, together with an increase in pulse rate and fall in blood pressure. Subsequently, jaundice, haemoglobinuria and a reduced urine output may be observed.

There are two ways in which cells may be eliminated from the circulation. First, cells may be haemolysed as a result of the action of complement activated by antigen–antibody reactions. This results in *intravascular haemolysis*, and produces severe transfusion reactions. The second way in which cells may be eliminated is by the removal of antibody-coated cells from the circulation by tissue macrophages in the spleen and liver. This removal results in a slower rate of destruction than is seen in intravascular haemolysis and is known as *extravascular haemolysis*.

A laboratory investigation of any reported transfusion reaction should be performed. A number of specimens are required:

1. The unit responsible for the reaction must be returned to the laboratory. The transfusion of contaminated blood may cause very severe, even fatal transfusion reactions. A sample of blood from the blood bag must be cultured to eliminate this. Cells from the unit should be grouped.
2. *Pre-transfusion sample.* This sample should be regrouped and recrossmatched with cells from the returned unit. A full antibody screen should be performed.
3. *Post-transfusion sample.* This should be grouped, crossmatched with cells from the returned unit and a full antibody screen performed. A direct anti-human globulin test should be performed on the cells to test for *in vivo* sensitization of cells. Post-transfusion samples should also be examined for haemoglobin, bilirubin levels and haptoglobin levels. The first sample of urine to be passed after the transfusion reaction should be tested for haemoglobin and its derivatives.

If an antibody is only detected in the post-transfusion samples this may be because pre-transfusion samples have been stored for too long or at the wrong temperature, resulting in loss of antibody strength. It may also be because the antibody causing the reaction was produced as a result of the transfusion. However, this usually causes a milder, delayed transfusion reaction.

It is possible that an antibody may be detected in the pre-transfusion sample but not in the post-transfusion sample, due to absorption of the antibody by the transfused blood.

It should be remembered that high titre antibodies present in the plasma of the donor blood may cause destruction of the recipient's red cells and may result in a transfusion reaction.

A transfusion reaction accompanied by chills and fever without any of the other more serious symptoms is known as a febrile reaction. These are mostly due to the presence of antibodies directed against transfused white cells. In order to prevent these reactions, patients known to have white cell antibodies should be issued with white cell depleted blood. This is produced by spinning and removing the buffy coat, and/or passing the blood through a micro-aggregate filter. If the patient still suffers febrile reactions to blood tested in this way, it may be necessary to provide washed blood.

Blood grouping technique

The performance of any blood grouping technique demands a high degree of concentration and technical competence. Under ideal conditions the scientific officer should work in a quiet atmosphere and not be disturbed by the telephone or by the talking of colleagues. In practice this is difficult to achieve, but every effort should be made to attain the quietest conditions possible.

Specimens

All blood for grouping and crossmatching must be correctly labelled, and as a minimum requirement must have the patient's name and hospital registration number clearly legible. If there is any doubt as to the identification of the sample it must be discarded and a fresh sample obtained. Blood grouping tests should be performed daily, so that samples are fresh and risk of bacterial contamination and haemolysis minimized. After grouping, serum specimens should be kept frozen at $-30°C$ for one week; this will allow for rechecking should this be found to be necessary.

Apparatus

This is essentially very simple, but at all times must be kept scrupulously clean so as to ensure that no contamination will occur due to bacteria, chemicals or foreign proteins. Tubes used for grouping and crossmatching should be clear polystyrene and disposable, or glass, which can be washed using a suitable washing machine. Basically only two sizes of tube are required; one approximately $75 \times 12\,mm$ for cell suspensions, the antiglobulin test and various other procedures, sometimes called a 'postal-tube', the other is the *precipitin tube*, $50 \times 6\,mm$, which is used in all grouping procedures where the 'standard tube technique' is used. Since the precipitin tube is so small it has the advantage that only small quantities of reagents are required, and since the column of serum–cell mixtures is relatively high in the narrow-bore tube, the cells will therefore take longer to fall, allowing more contact for antigen–antibody reaction.

Isotonic saline (0.9% sodium chloride) should be prepared freshly each day. Large aspirators of isotonic saline should not be kept, as algae will grow and the pH will gradually fall due to absorption of CO_2 from the atmosphere. Similarly, in laboratories using low ionic strength saline (LISS), this should be made up frequently. Care should be taken not to confuse physiological saline and LISS; therefore, all containers should be clearly labelled.

Since LISS is more expensive than physiological saline, most workers use the latter for rinsing pipettes and washing antiglobulin tests. This can be done without detrimental effect. Wash-out pots must be thoroughly cleaned at least once daily and preferably after each batch of tests.

Clerical errors

These are without doubt the commonest mistakes encountered in the blood group laboratory. They can only be avoided by careful checking and concentration; a quiet atmosphere is of considerable help in excluding clerical errors. All results must be recorded onto sheets which have a laboratory protocol printed on them. Results must be entered directly on the protocol and not transferred from a rough working sheet, which may increase the possibility of clerical error.

Storage of grouping serum

The antibody content of untreated human serum deteriorates if kept at room temperature and therefore grouping antisera, unless stated, must be kept frozen preferably at $-30°C$, where its strength will be maintained almost indefinitely. Serum kept between $2°C$ and $4°C$ is preserved for a variable period. Serum should not be kept in large amounts as continued thawing and freezing, a daily occurrence, will also accelerate deterioration and increase the risk of bacterial contamination, another cause of deterioration.

Commercial antisera must be stored according to the manufacturer's instruction, and usually this is at $4°C$ and not frozen. These sera do not resemble human serum in their composition and often contain bovine albumin. Although very expensive, commercial antisera from reputable sources have the advantage of being very potent and show consistency of reaction from batch to batch.

Bovine albumin

This is available in two concentrations, 20% and 30%. It is usually the 20% concentration which is used in the clinical laboratory, and this may be stored at $4°C$.

Techniques

Although there is some variation in the techniques used in the field of blood group serology, most laboratories employ the same basic methods.

It is essential that adequate controls are included with each batch of tests performed. It must be emphasized that proficiency in blood grouping and the detection of antibodies can only be achieved with considerable practice, and although the techniques described appear simple, experience is essential to obtain consistently reliable results.

Recording of results

As previously mentioned, all results must be recorded into a protocol, but the strength of

Table 43.1 A method of recording agglutination

Macroscopic agglutination	Microscopic agglutination
C = complete—no free cells in surrounding fluid	+++ = very large agglutinates with free cells
V = visual—agglutinates easily visible with free cells	++ = large agglutinates with many free cells
	+ = agglutinates of 8–16 cells
	+ or W = agglutinates of 3–8 cells
	− = no agglutination
	R = rouleaux formation
	L or H = haemolysis

reaction is important and therefore each laboratory must agree on a method of recording the various reactions which all staff must abide by. A suggested method of scoring agglutination is given in *Table 43.1*.

ABO grouping—rapid or tile method

Most laboratories use this method only for emergency grouping and results are usually confirmed using the tube technique or automated grouping technique. It is essential that the antisera should give clear-cut results extremely quickly.

One volume of 20% patient's cells is mixed with one volume of anti-A, anti-B and anti-A + B, respectively, on an opal glass tile. One volume of patient's serum is mixed with one volume of A_1 cells and B cells, respectively.

The cells and sera in each square are mixed and the tile rocked gently. The tile should be examined under a good light within 2–5 min and the presence or absence of agglutination noted. Care should be taken to read groups within this time, otherwise reagents and cells may dry giving rise to false positive results.

Controls must be set up with any group performed. The anti-A, anti-B and anti-A + B must be controlled with A_1 cells, B cells and O cells.

Before use, the opal glass tile must be scrubbed with soap and water, thoroughly rinsed, and dried using a clean cloth. The Pasteur pipettes used for antisera and cell suspensions must be thoroughly rinsed with clean saline between each sample.

ABO grouping—standard tube technique

Using this method, both the patient's cells and serum are tested and the results compared.

Into a grouping rack are placed the requisite number of precipitin tubes; these are used for the

Table 43.2 Results of typical reactions encountered are shown in the following protocol (see also Table 43.1)

Cell group	1	2	3	4	5	6	7	8	9	10	A_2	A_2	B	O
Anti-A	C	–	C	–	+++	+++	++	++	–	–	C	+++	–	–
Anti-B	–	C	C	–	–	–	V	V	–	–	–	–	C	–
Anti-A + B	C	C	C	–	C	C	C	C	–	–	C	C	C	–
Patient's serum	–	–	–	–	–	–	–	–	–	–		*Controls*		
Serum group														
A_1 cells	–	C	–	C	–	+	–	+	–	H				
A_2 cells	–	V	–	C	–	–	–	–	–	H				
B cells	C	–	–	C	C	C	–	–	–	H				
O cells	–	–	–	–	–	–	–	–	–	–				

Interpretation: 1. Group A
2. Group B
3. Group AB
4. Group O
5. Group A—confirm using lectin A_1 or specific anti-A_1
6. Group A_2 with anti-A_1 serum—confirm using lectin A_1 or specific anti-A_1. Test serum with A_2 cells—no reaction if anti-A_1
7. Group A_2B—confirm using lectin A_1 or specific anti-A_1
8. Group A_2B with anti-A_1 in serum—confirm using lectin A_1 or specific anti-A_1. Test serum with A_2 cells—no reaction if anti-A_1
9. Group O. Cord blood. Note absence of 'naturally occurring' anti-A and anti-B
10. Group O. Note presence of haemolysis rather than agglutination

cell–serum mixtures. A postal tube for the patient's cell suspension is also required.

One volume (usually one drop from a Pasteur pipette is satisfactory) of both the unknown cells or serum is added to each tube, and an equal volume of the known cells or serum added to the appropriate tubes.

A 2–5% suspension of patient's cells is tested against

Anti-A
Anti-B
Anti-A + B

Patient's serum is tested against

A_1 cells ⎫
A_2 cells ⎪
B cells   ⎬ 2–5% cell suspension
O cells   ⎪
Patient's own cells ⎪
(auto-control) ⎭

The tubes are gently mixed and allowed to stand undisturbed at room temperature for 2 h.

Controls are essential and are set up in the same way as the test, using the following combinations:

Anti-A, anti-B and anti-A + B against 3% A_1 cells, A_2 cells, B cells and O cells

The tests are read by gently tapping the tube and looking for the presence of agglutination and recording the strength on the protocol. All negative reactions must be examined microscopically; this is easily done by removing a little of the cell–serum mixture from the tube and gently spreading it out onto a glass slide. The slide is examined using the low-power objective.

The auto-agglutination control (patient's serum against patient's cells) must be negative; any agglutination of the A_1, A_2, B or O cells in the presence of a positive auto-agglutination control is discussed under causes of false positive results (see below).

Differentiation of group A_1 and group A_2

Using the tile method, one volume of 20% patient's red cells are mixed with one volume of *Dolichos bifloris* lectin. Agglutination is rapid and very strong if the cells are A_1. A negative reaction with *Dolichos bifloris* extract in conjunction with a positive reaction with standard anti-A indicates that the cells are group A_2 (*Table 43.2*).

Causes of false positive results in ABO grouping

Rouleaux formation

Sometimes called 'pseudo-agglutination', this rarely gives trouble to an experienced worker. If the rouleaux formation is marked, the auto-agglutination control will be positive and any cells added to the patient's serum will give a similar reaction. If the serum is diluted 1 in 2 or 1 in 3 with physiological saline, the rouleaux formation should disappear, while true agglutination will persist. Rouleaux formation is not true agglutination, as it is not due to an absorbable agglutinin. The commonest mistake due to formation of rouleaux is delay in reading the result when using a tile method; a 'graininess' appears which may be read as a weak positive, but will usually disappear when a drop of saline or albumin is added to the mixture. Occasionally, rouleaux may be present in the cell grouping tubes, in which case repeat the test using washed red cells.

Infected red cells (the Thomsen phenomenon)

Several types of bacteria are capable of causing red cells to agglutinate by any normal serum, animal or human, except young infants, and the cells are called polyagglutinable. The bacteria are able to expose the T antigen and most sera contain the T antibody, thereby causing agglutination. The reaction may become apparent within 18 h at 4°C or within shorter periods at room temperature. It is important to use only fresh cells or cells which have been stored for the shortest time in the refrigerator. In blood stored in the form of a clot, the phenomenon is rarely found.

Infected serum

Occasionally this gives a false positive reaction, but invariably it gives a false negative reaction.

Cold agglutinins

The higher the titre of cold agglutinins, the higher the temperature at which they will react (this will seldom be above 25°C), and therefore if active at room temperature the auto-agglutination control will be positive as will the A_1, B and O cells, this type of reaction being termed pan-agglutination. High titre cold antibodies are sometimes formed during viral or atypical pneumonia (the causative organism often being *Mycoplasma pneumoniae*), lymphoma and rarely with infectious mononucleosis. They usually have blood group specificity with the I/i system (for further information of this system it is suggested that reference is made to a standard blood group serology textbook). When this type of reaction is encountered, the patient's red cells should be washed in warm saline at 37°C to remove the cold antibody, and the test repeated. The serum grouping must be repeated at 37°C and the auto-agglutination control should be negative, although at this temperature any anti-A or anti-B present will still react.

Causes of false negative results in ABO grouping

These are usually due to impotent sera which have

deteriorated by being stored incorrectly or repeatedly frozen and thawed.

Failure to recognize the time factor in the tube method may cause false negative results to be reported.

Failure to recognize that haemolysis must be reported as such and not recorded as negative because no agglutination can be seen, may cause false negative results to be reported.

Rhesus grouping

Standard tube technique

A number of techniques are available for the detection of the Rhesus antigens, but the most widely used are enzyme and albumin addition techniques to detect the D antigen. Two sera of different batches are used. As the Rhesus group cannot be 'back-checked' by using the patient's serum, as in the ABO system, the use of two sera adds confidence to the results.

Albumin addition technique

To one volume of 2–5% patient's red cells add one volume albumin operating antiserum, mix and incubate undisturbed at 37°C for 1 h. Add, without disturbing the settled button cells, one volume of 20% bovine albumin; reincubate for a further 15–30 min at 37°C. Examine for agglutination macroscopically by gently tapping the tube. Results are usually clear-cut, but all apparent negative reactions must be examined microscopically.

Positive and negative cells must be included as controls using an identical technique to that of the test.

As a further control, 1 volume of the 2–5% suspension of patient's cells should be mixed with 1 volume of AB serum and treated in the same way as the tests, i.e. incubated at 37°C with the addition of albumin after 1 h.

This control should be negative. A positive result indicates that the patient's cells have been coated with antibody *in vivo* and it is the addition of albumin to the sensitized cells rather than the anti-D which may be causing positive reactions in the tests. These samples can be regrouped with an IgM or saline-reacting anti-D.

The detection of the Rhesus antigens, C, D, E, c and e is technically the same for each, provided care is taken to ensure that the relevant technique is used, according to the manufacturer's instructions.

Emergency Rhesus grouping

This is commonly performed using a tile technique in the same way as the ABO grouping. If a commercial reagent is used, the manufacturer's instructions should be followed. Rhesus D positive and D negative cells should be tested against the anti-D as a control.

Antibody screening

It is important that antibody screening tests will detect both IgG and IgM antibodies; therefore, it is usual to perform screening tests by a combination of methods. The test cells should possess all the common blood group antigens, and must be group O so that there will be no interference from any anti-A or anti-B which may be present in the serum.

If the screening test is positive, further tests will be necessary to determine the specificity of the antibody. A panel of red cells possessing various blood group antigens is used so that by a process of elimination the specificity of the antibody can be determined. The technique used will include a combination of the red cells being suspended in saline, enzyme-treated cells, and the use of the indirect anti-human globulin test.

Saline technique

Add one volume of a 2–5% cell suspension to one volume of patient's serum. Incubate either at room temperature (22°C) or 37°C for 1–1.5 h. Negatives must be checked microscopically for weak agglutination.

Enzyme-treated red cells

Treatment of red cells with enzymes will enable both IgM and IgG antibodies to be detected. The method of treating red cells with papain (Low's method) is described. This is the most commonly used enzyme.

Papain 2 g
Sorensen's buffer,* pH 5.4, 100 ml
Grind in a mortar and centrifuge for 10 min
Add 10 ml cysteine hydrochloride 0.5 ml
Make solution up to 200 ml with Sorensen's buffer and incubate at 37°C for 1 h

One-stage technique

Add one volume of activated papain to one volume of patient's serum followed by one volume of the appropriate 2–5% red cells. Incubate at 37°C for 1 h and read macroscopically.

*Sorensen's buffer—stock solution: (A) 0.067M potassium dihydrogen KH_2PO_4 (9.08 g/l). (B) 0.067M disodium hydrogen orthophosphate $Na_2HPO_4.2H_2O$ (11.88 g/l). For pH 5.4 add 9.6 parts of solution A to 0.4 parts solution B. For pH 7.0 add 3.9 parts of solution A to 6.1 parts solution B.

Two-stage technique

The pretreatment of red cells with papain gives greater sensitivity and this is usually the method of choice:

1 volume activated papain solution
9 volumes Sorensen's buffer, pH 7.0

Add equal volumes of papain and washed packed red cells and incubate in a water bath at 37°C for 20 min. Wash the red cells twice in saline and dilute to 2–5%. To one volume patient's serum add one volume 2–5% pretreated red cells and incubate at 37°C for 1 h. Read macroscopically.

The anti-human globulin tests (Coombs tests)

The direct anti-human globulin test (DAHGT)

This test is performed on the patient's red cells without any prior incubation, and demonstrates the sensitization of the red cells *in vivo* with antibody.

Patient's red cells are washed four times in physiological saline using 75 × 12 mm disposable plastic tubes.

The anti-human globulin serum is added to the washed cells and the cells and serum mixed thoroughly and centrifuged according to the manufacturer's instructions. The contents of the tube should be carefully transferred to a glass slide and examined microscopically.

The agglutination of the red cells with anti-human globulin serum indicates that antibody has attached itself to the red cells in the patient's circulation.

Controls

The anti-human globulin is tested against red cells which have previously been sensitized with a weak IgG antibody, usually an incomplete anti-D, and washed as in the test. The use of this control indicates that the anti-human globulin serum being used is capable of detecting cells weakly sensitized with IgG, but in no way indicates that the anti-human globulin serum is operating in the tube containing the actual test. There are a number of reasons for this, but the commonest cause is that the patient's red cells have been inadequately washed leaving free globulin present which has neutralized the anti-human globulin serum. To ensure that the anti-human globulin serum is operating in the tube containing the test, it is essential that to each negative test is added a volume of sensitized red cells, and that agglutination is noted after a further short spin. If the test remains negative, the test should be repeated.

A positive direct anti-human globulin test may be found in cases of auto-immune haemolytic anaemia. This is a condition in which an individual will produce antibodies to antigens which he possesses and may result in the increased rate of destruction of the individual's red cells. In some instances the cause of the condition is unknown, but it has also been associated with some malignant diseases and has been seen in patients treated with certain drugs.

The indirect anti-human globulin test (IAHGT)

This test is used for

1. Detection of unknown antibody using known red cell antigens.
2. Detection of unknown red cell antigens using known antibodies (antisera).
3. Detection of unknown red cell antigens using unknown antibodies.

Six volumes of serum are incubated with 2 volumes of a 2–5% cell suspension. The tubes are incubated for 1 h at 37°C. After incubation, the test is performed exactly as for the direct anti-human globulin test described above.

Positive and negative controls should be included with each batch of tests. As a positive control, use Rhesus D positive cells sensitized with an incomplete anti-D serum and well washed. As a negative control, non-sensitized washed red cells should be used.

Causes of false negative results

1. Inadequate washing of cells.
2. Contamination of pipettes, tubes, saline or AHG reagent with human serum.
3. Failure to add AHG reagent.
4. Loss of reactivity of AHG reagent due to incorrect storage.

Causes of false positive results

1. Bacterial contamination of reagents.
2. Test performed on red cells from clotted blood stored in a refrigerator. Normal cold agglutinins will cause complement uptake.

Crossmatching technique

Although each laboratory uses its own combination of methods to perform a crossmatch, the most widely used techniques are described here.

A sample of donor red cells are obtained by removing a section of the tube attached to the plastic blood bag. Care should be taken that the tube is adequately sealed above any cut made in the tube, so that the contents of the bag remain sterile.

The donor cells are washed three times in saline and resuspended to give a 2–5% cell suspension.

Saline room temperature technique

Using precipitation tubes, one volume of donor cells is added to one volume of patient's serum, mixed and incubated at room temperature (22°C) for 1–1½ h. The contents of the tube should be examined microscopically for agglutination.

Saline 37°C

This is set up in the same way as the saline room temperature technique, except that incubation is at 37°C. A water bath or incubator heated to 37°C is suitable.

Enzyme technique—papain

The one-stage enzyme technique is usually performed for crossmatching. One volume of patient's serum is added to a precipitin tube. A volume of papain (see p. 378) is added and on top of this is layered one volume of donor cells.

The tubes are incubated at 37°C for 1 h, after which the contents are examined macroscopically on a glass tile.

Anti-human globulin technique

Six volumes of patient's serum are mixed with two volumes of donor cells and incubated at 37°C for 1 h. After this time, the cells are washed four times, the anti-human globulin reagent added and the tubes spun at a low speed for 30 s.

The contents of the tube are examined microscopically.

Controls should be performed with each batch of tests (see p. 378).

44

Automation and computerization

Automated blood grouping

Much of the tedium of grouping large numbers of blood samples has been eliminated with the development of automated blood grouping systems. This has also led to increased reliability and sensitivity.

There are predominantly two types of automated systems available. The first is the Technicon Auto Analyzer continuous flow system, which was originally used for clinical chemistry procedures but has been successfully adapted for ABO and rhesus blood typing. A double probe samples centrifuged, anticoagulated samples, simultaneously aspirating red cells and plasma. Reagents are drawn through the system by means of rollers compressing the pump tubes, the diameter of these tubes governing the flow rate of the reagents. The cells and sera are mixed with the appropriate reagents and pass into the manifold or reaction coil. Each sample is separated from the next by means of air bubbles which also clean the walls of the tubing, thus avoiding contamination. Rouleaux-inducing agents bring cells into close contact with each other and with the aid of enzymes speed up any reaction taking place. The rouleaux are later dispersed by saline, leaving true agglutination. The agglutinates are decanted, free cells are lysed and the degree of lysis read using a colorimeter. This method of obtaining results has enabled antibody quantitation to be automated in the same way, since the absorbance is dependent on the number of free cells lysed.

The earlier machines were only partially automated, since the system was dependent on visual interpretation of a series of agglutination reactions decanted onto filter paper. The addition of an electrical readout system and positive sample identification by means of a laser scanner has led to a fully automated system. This updated machine is known as the Technicon Autogrouper 16C (*Figure 44.1*).

The second type of machine available is the Groupamatic (Roche Bioelectrics). This system is based on the photometric reading of tile reactions, and in 1971–72 was first introduced into blood transfusion centres. Samples of patient's serum and cells are incubated with reagents in a cuvette and then centrifuged. Agitation of the mixtures at different speeds then occurs in order to resuspend all unagglutinated red blood cells, while any agglutinates collect in the central area of the cuvette.

Two photometric readings are made for each reaction cuvette—a central measurement and a peripheral measurement—and the results of these measurements compared. The absence of any variation between the two readings characterizes a negative result, while a significant variation indicates a positive result. The machine is able to compare, interpret and print out the results. Samples are identified by means of a laser scanner capable of reading bar code labels attached to the specimen tubes.

Semi-automated blood grouping

Automated blood grouping has been used for many years in blood transfusion centres and larger hospital laboratories, but until recently, smaller hospital blood banks have had no alternative to the use of manual tube grouping.

During the past few years a semi-automated system using microtitre plates has been successfully introduced into both hospitals and blood transfusion

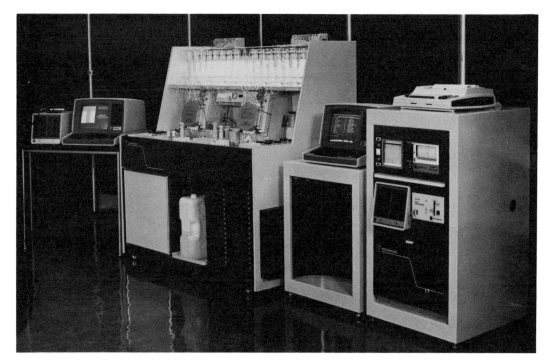

Figure 44.1. The Technicon Autogrouper 16C (reproduced by courtesy of Technicon Instruments Co. Ltd)

centre laboratories. The cells and serum are mixed in the 'U'-bottomed wells of a microtitre plate and, after suitable incubation, may be read. This is done either manually by tipping the plate and looking for agglutinates or automatically by placing the plate on a reader where light is passed through the wells. The amount of light passing through each well is measured, interpreted and may be stored in a microprocessor or transferred onto a computer.

Computerization

The introduction of computers in blood transfusion laboratories has been successfully used to meet the demand for maximum efficiency and safety. Many of the time-consuming, tedious aspects of blood transfusion work can be undertaken by computer and, since boredom has been shown to lead to an increase in clerical errors, has provided greater accuracy. The relative inflexibility of a computer system has been advantageous, since it is not possible to take short cuts in checking procedures, which may be a temptation with manual procedures.

With increasing pressures upon Blood Transfusion Centres to provide blood and components, the use of computers has helped with blood collection programmes, donor administration and stock control, and has led to a more efficient service.

Quality control

Reagents, equipment and laboratory workers must conform to standards of clinical effectiveness and safety. Every laboratory should have a procedure which is carefully followed to ensure that all reagents and equipment are working satisfactorily. A valuable contribution to quality control are the national and regional proficiency testing schemes which are available in the UK. Samples are provided for grouping, antibody identification and cross-matching and should be treated in exactly the same way as patient's samples entering the laboratory. A comparison of the results obtained by all participants is made available, thus enabling individual laboratories to check the accuracy and safety of the methods which are employed.

Bibliography

The following works are recommended for further reading:

General

FARR, A.D. (1982). *Learn, That You May Improve*, 1st edn. Billingshurst, Sussex; Denley Instruments Ltd

HMSO (1978). 'The Code of Practice for the Prevention of Infection in Clinical Laboratories and Postmortem Rooms (Howie Code)'. London; HMSO

HMSO (1984). 'Categorisation of Pathogens according to Hazard and Categories of Containment'. London; HMSO

WHO (1977). 'The SI for the Health Professions'. Geneva; WHO

Clinical chemistry

BELL-EMSLIE SMITH, G.H. and PATERSON, C.R. (1980). *Textbook of Physiology and Biochemistry*, 10th edn. Edinburgh; Churchill-Livingstone

VARLEY, H., GOWERLOCK, A.H. and BELL, M. (1976, 1980). *Practical Clinical Biochemistry*, 5th edn, Volumes 1 and 2. London; Heinemann

ZILVA, J.F. and PANNALL, P.R. (1984). *Clinical Chemistry in Diagnosis and Treatment*, 4th edn. London; Lloyd-Luke

Cellular pathology

CORN, H. and LILLIE, R.D. (1977). *Biological Stains*, 9th edn. Baltimore; Williams and Wilkins

CULLING, C.F.A., ALLISON, R.T. and BARR, W.T. (1985). *Cellular Pathology Technique*, 4th edn. London; Butterworths

SDC/ASTC&C (1971). *Colour Index*, 3rd edn, Volumes 1–5. Bradford; Society of Dyers and Colourists/American Society of Textile Chemists and Colorists

SDC/ASTC&C (1982). *Colour Index*, 3rd edn (revised), Volumes 5–7. Bradford; Society of Dyers and Colourists/American Society of Textile Chemists and Colorists

Microbiology

BAKER, F.J. and BREACH, M.R. (1980). *Medical Microbiological Techniques*. London; Butterworths

COWAN, S.T. (1974). *Cowan and Steel's Manual for the Identification of Medical Bacteria*. London; Cambridge University Press

DIFCO LABORATORIES INC. (1984). *Difco Manual*, 10th edn. Detroit; Difco

DUGUID, J.P., MARMION, D.P. and SWAIN, P.H.A. (1978). *Mackie and McCartney's Medical Microbiology*, 13th edn, Volumes 1 and 2. Edinburgh; Churchill-Livingstone

OXOID LTD (1982). *The Oxoid Manual*, 5th edn. Basingstoke, Hants; Oxoid

ROITT, I. (1975). *Essential Immunology*, 2nd edn. Oxford; Blackwell

STOKES, E.J. and RIDGWAY, G.L. (1980). *Clinical Bacteriology*, 5th edn. London; Edward Arnold

Haematology, and blood transfusion technique

BOORMAN, K.E., DODD, B.E. and LINCOLN, P.J. (1977). *Blood Group Serology*, 5th edn. Edinburgh; Churchill-Livingstone

DACIE, J.V. and LEWIS, S.M. (1984). *Practical Haematology*, 6th edn. Edinburgh; Churchill-Livingstone

HALL, R. and MALIA, R.G. (1984). *Medical Laboratory Haematology*. London; Butterworths

INGRAM, G.I.C., BROZOVIC, M. and SLATER, N.G.P. (1982). *Bleeding Disorders: Investigation and Management*, 2nd edn. Oxford; Blackwell

ISSIT, P.D. and ISSIT, C.H. (1976). *Applied Blood Group Serology*, 2nd edn. Biological Corporation of America Publications

RICHARDS, J.D.M., LINCH, D.C. and GOLDSTONE, A.H. (1983). *A Synopsis of Haematology*. Bristol; Wright

SPIRAK, J.L. (1983). *Fundamentals of Clinical Haematology*. London; Harper and Row

STRIKE, P.W. (1981). *Medical Laboratory Statistics*. Bristol; Wright

THOMASON, J. (1980). *Blood Coagulation and Haemostasis*, 2nd edn. Edinburgh; Churchill-Livingstone

Appendix I: Manufacturers' names and addresses

Alpha Laboratories, 40 Parham Drive, Eastleigh, Hants SO5 4NU.

American Optical, Instrument Division, Box 123, Buffalo, NY 14240-0123, USA.

Ames Co. Division of Miles Laboratories Ltd, PO Box 37, Stoke Court, Stoke Poges, Slough SL2 LLY.

Amicon Ltd, Upper Mill, Stonehouse, Gloucester GL10 2BJ.

Astec Environmental Systems Ltd, 31 Lynx Crescent, Weston Industrial Estate, Weston-super-Mare, Avon BS24 9DJ.

BCL (see under Boehringer Corporation)

BDH plc, Poole, Dorset BH12 4NN.

Beckman-RIIC Ltd, Progress Road, Sands Industrial Estate, High Wycombe, Bucks HP12 4JL.

Becton Dickinson (UK) Ltd, York House, Empire Way, Wembley, Middlesex HA9 0PS.

Beecham Research Laboratories, Brentford, Middlesex TW8 9BD.

Bethlehem Instruments Ltd, PO Box 101, Hemel Hempstead, Herts.

Boehringer Corporation (London) Ltd (BCL), Mannheim House, Bell Lane, Lewes, East Sussex BN7 1LG.

Chemical Concentrates (RBS) Ltd, 8 Lebanon Road, London SW18 1RE.

Chemlab Instruments Ltd, Hornminster House, 129 Upminster Road, Hornchurch, Essex RM11 3XJ.

Clandon Scientific, Lysons Avenue, Ash Vale, Aldershot, Hants GU12 5QR.

Corning Medical & Scientific, Halstead, Essex CO9 2DX.

Coulter Electronics Ltd, Northwell Drive, Luton, Beds LU3 3RH.

Decon Laboratories Ltd, Conway Street, Hove, East Sussex BN3 3LY.

Denley Instruments Ltd, Natts Lane, Billingshurst, Sussex RH14 9EY.

Difco Laboratories, PO Box 14b, Central Avenue, East Molesey, Surrey KT8 0SE.

Eaton Laboratories, Reagent House, The Broadway, Woking, Surrey GU21 5AP.

The Elga Group, Lane End, Bucks.

Gallenkamp, PO Box 290, Technico House, Christopher Street, London EC2P 2ER.

Harleco, c/o American Hospital Supplies (UK), Station Road, Didcot, Berks.

Hawksley and Sons Ltd, 12 Peter Road, Lancing, West Sussex BN15 8TH.

Hilger Analytical, Westwood, Margate, Kent CT9 4JL.

Hughes and Hughes Ltd, Elms Industrial Estate, Church Road, Harold Wood, Romford.

Raymond A. Lamb, 6 Sunbeam Road, North Acton, London NW10 6JL.

E. Leitz (Instruments) Ltd, 48 Park Street, Luton LU1 3HP.

LKB Instruments Ltd, 232 Addington Road, South Croydon, Surrey CR2 8YD.

London Analytical and Bacteriological Media Ltd, Ford Lane, Salford M6 6PB.

Miles Scientific (see under Ames Co.)

Millipore (UK) Ltd, 11 Peterborough Rd, Harrow, Middx.

Nuclear Enterprises Ltd, Sighthill, Edinburgh, Scotland EH11 4BY.

Oxoid Ltd, Wade Road, Basingstoke, Hants RG24 0PW.

Wm Pearson Ltd, Clough Road, Hull HU6 7QA.

The Projectina Co. Ltd, Skelmorlie, Ayrshire, Scotland.

Reichert-Jung Ltd, 820 Yeovil Road, Slough SL1 4JB.

Roche Products Ltd, Welwyn Garden City, Herts AL7 3AY.

Shandon Southern Products Ltd, Chadwick Road, Astmoor, Runcorn, Cheshire WA7 1PR.

Shell Chemical UK Ltd, 1 Northumberland Avenue, Trafalgar Square, London WC2N 5LA.

Sigma Chemical Co. Ltd, Fancy Road, Poole, Dorset BH17 7NH.

Slee Medical Equipment Ltd, Lanier Works, Hither Green Lane, London SE13 6QD.

TCS (see under Tissue Culture Services Ltd).

Technicon Instruments Co. Ltd, Evans House, Hamilton Close, Basingstoke, Hants RG21 2YE.

Tintometer Ltd, The Colour Laboratory, Waterloo Road, Salisbury SP1 2JY.

Tissue Culture Services Ltd, 10 Henry Road, Slough SL1 2QL.

Warner Lambert Technologies Inc., Box 123, Buffalo, NY 14240, USA.

Carl Zeiss, D-7082 Oberkochen, West Germany.

Appendix II: Useful information

British Standard colours for medical gas cylinders*

Nature of gas	Colour of cylinder
Air	Grey bottom with black and white top
Carbon dioxide	Grey
Cyclopropane	Orange
Ethylene	Mauve
Helium	Brown
Hydrogen	Red
Nitrogen	Grey with black top (white spot = oxygen-free)
Nitrous oxide	Blue
Oxygen	Black with white top
Oxygen and carbon dioxide mixture	Black bottom with grey and white top
Oxygen and helium mixture	Black bottom with brown and white top

Conversion factors

Fahrenheit (F) and Celsius (Centigrade) (C) temperatures

To convert °F into °C:

Subtract 32 and multiply by $\frac{5}{9}$

To convert °C into °F:

Multiply by $\frac{9}{5}$ and add 32

*For safety's sake, the contents of all cylinders should be checked by name and colour. Reliance should not be placed on the colour alone.

Dilution of solutions

The following equation is useful when the dilution of solutions of known strengths is required:

$$\frac{R \times V}{O} = \begin{array}{l} \text{Volume of original solution to be} \\ \text{diluted with distilled water to the final} \\ \text{volume required} \end{array}$$

where R is the required concentration, V the total volume of solution required, and O the original concentration.

Example

The original solution is 70%: 45 ml of 30% solution is required. Using the equation

$$\frac{30 \times 45}{70} = 19.3$$

Therefore, 19.3 ml of 70% solution must be diluted with 25.7 ml of distilled water to obtain 45 ml of a 30% solution.

Measurement conversion

Temperature	
Centigrade	Fahrenheit
− 30	− 22
− 20	− 4
− 10	+ 14
− 5	+ 23
0	+ 32
+ 5	+ 41
+ 10	+ 50
+ 20	+ 68

Temperature (cont.)

Centigrade	Fahrenheit
+ 30	+ 86
+ 36.9*	+ 98.4*
+ 40	+104
+ 50	+122
+ 60	+140
+ 70	+157
+ 80	+176
+ 90	+194
+100	+212

*Normal body temperature.

Metres–Feet

m	ft or m	ft
0.305	1	3.281
0.610	2	6.562
0.914	3	9.842
1.219	4	13.123
1.524	5	16.404
1.829	6	19.685
2.134	7	22.966
2.438	8	26.247
2.743	9	29.528
3.048	10	32.808
7.620	25	82.022

Litres–Gallons

l	gal or l	gal
4.45	1	0.22
9.09	2	0.44
13.64	3	0.66
18.18	4	0.88
22.73	5	1.10
27.28	6	1.32
31.82	7	1.54
36.37	8	1.76
40.91	9	1.98
45.46	10	2.20
90.92	20	4.40
136.38	30	6.60
181.84	40	8.80
227.30	50	11.00

Kilograms–Pounds

kg	lb or kg	lb
0.453	1	2.205
0.907	2	4.409
1.360	3	6.614
1.814	4	8.818
2.268	5	11.023
2.721	6	13.228
3.175	7	15.432
3.628	8	17.637
4.082	9	19.841
4.535	10	22.046
11.339	25	55.116

Boiling points

The following boiling points are correct to the nearest degree Celsius.

Substance	°C
Acetic acid	118
Acetone	56
Amyl alcohol	130
Benzene	80
Butyl alcohol	118
Caprylic alcohol	180
Carbon disulphide	46
Chloroform	62
Ether	34
Ethyl alcohol (ethanol)	78
Methyl alcohol (methanol)	65
Toluene	111
Water	100
Xylenes	138–144

Solutions of acids and alkalis

Dilution of concentrated acids and alkalis to make approximately molar solutions.

	Millilitre diluted to 1000 ml with distilled water
Acids	
Acetic (glacial)	60
Hydrochloric	100
Nitric	63
Sulphuric	56
Alkalis	
Ammonium hydroxide	50
Potassium hydroxide (solid)	58 g
Sodium hydroxide (solid)	42 g

Buffer solutions

(After Clark and Lubs)

pH	Amount of 0.2M HCl in ml	pH	Amount of 0.2M NaOH in ml
	To 50 ml 0.2M KH phthalate (40.844 g/l), add the following amounts of 0.2M HCl and dilute to 200 ml		To 50 ml 0.2M KH phthalate add the following amounts of 0.2M NaOH (CO_2 free), and dilute to 200 ml
2.2	46.60	4.0	0.40
2.4	39.60	4.2	3.65
2.6	33.00	4.4	7.35
2.8	26.50	4.6	12.00
3.0	20.40	4.8	17.50
3.2	14.80	5.0	23.65
3.4	9.95	5.2	29.75
3.6	6.00	5.4	35.25
3.8	2.65	5.6	39.70
		5.8	43.10
		6.0	45.40
		6.2	47.00

pH	Amount of 0.2M NaOH in ml	pH	Amount of 0.2M NaOH in ml
	To 50 ml 0.2M KH_2PO_4 (27.219 g/l) add the following amounts of 0.2M NaOH and dilute to 200 ml		To 50 ml 0.2M KCl.H_3BO_3 (14.912 g KCl + 12.369 g H_3BO_3/l), add the following amounts of 0.2M NaOH and dilute to 200 ml
6.0	5.70	7.8	2.61
6.2	8.60	8.0	3.97
6.4	12.60	8.2	5.90
6.6	17.80	8.4	8.50
6.8	23.65	8.6	12.00
7.0	29.65	8.8	16.30
7.2	35.00	9.0	21.30
7.4	39.50	9.2	26.70
7.6	42.80	9.4	32.00
7.8	45.20	9.6	36.85
8.0	46.80	9.8	40.80
		10.0	43.90

■ Notes

1. Provided the salts are in correct ratio to one another, the exact degree of the final dilution is not important.
2. Use the purest chemicals available when preparing buffer solutions.
3. Use freshly distilled or de-ionized water with pH 6.7–7.3.
4. Store the buffer solutions in polythene bottles or Pyrex glass with closely fitting stoppers.

5. Provided the reagents are in correct ratio to one another, the exact degree of the final dilution is not important.
6. A series of differing buffers and their composition can be found in the *Scientific Tables of Documenta Geigy* (published by Geigy).

Walpole's sodium acetate–hydrochloric acid buffer (pH range 0.65–5.20)

pH	Vol. in ml of 1.0M $NaC_2H_3O_2$	Vol. in ml of 1.0M HCl	Vol. in ml of distilled water to make 250 ml
0.65	50	100.0	100
0.75	50	90.0	110
0.91	50	80.0	120
1.09	50	70.0	130
1.24	50	65.0	135
1.42	50	60.0	140
1.71	50	55.0	145
1.85	50	53.50	146.5
1.99	50	52.50	147.5
2.32	50	51.0	149
2.64	50	50.0	150
2.72	50	49.75	150.25
3.09	50	48.50	151.5
3.29	50	47.50	152.5
3.49	50	46.25	153.75
3.61	50	45.0	155.0
3.79	50	42.50	157.5
3.95	50	40.0	160
4.19	50	35.0	165
4.39	50	30.0	170
4.58	50	25.0	175
4.76	50	20.0	180
4.92	50	15.0	185
5.20	50	10.0	190

Walpole's sodium acetate–acetic acid buffer (pH range 2.7–6.52)

pH	Vol. in ml of 0.2M $NaC_2H_3O_2$	Vol. in ml of 0.2M $CH_3.CO.OH$
2.70	—	20.0
2.80	0.1	19.9
2.91	0.2	19.8
2.99	0.3	19.7
3.08	0.4	19.6
3.15	0.5	19.5
3.20	0.6	19.4
3.32	0.8	19.2
3.42	1.0	19.0
3.56	1.5	18.5
3.72	2.0	18.0
3.90	3.0	17.0
4.05	4.0	16.0
4.16	5.0	15.0
4.27	6.0	14.0
4.36	7.0	13.0
4.45	8.0	12.0
4.53	9.0	11.0
4.62	10.0	10.0
4.71	11.0	9.0
4.80	12.0	8.0
4.90	13.0	7.0
4.99	14.0	6.0
5.11	15.0	5.0
5.23	16.0	4.0
5.38	17.0	3.0
5.58	18.0	2.0
5.90	19.0	1.0
6.21	19.5	0.5
6.52	20.0	—

Saturated solutions

(After Bayley)

Substance	Solubility in g per 100 ml of distilled water		
	0°C	Various temperatures	100°C
Ammonium chloride	29.7		75.8
Ammonium oxalate	2.54		34.8
Ammonium sulphate	70.6		103.8
Aniline		3.4 at 20 °C	
Barium chloride	31.0		59.0
Barium sulphate		0.00023 at 18 °C	
Barium sulphide		Decomposes in water	
Benzidine		Only slightly soluble	
Benzoic acid		0.27 at 18 °C	
Bromine		3.58 at 20 °C	
Calcium carbonate		0.0014 at 25 °C	
Calcium chloride (anhyd.)	59.5		
Calcium chloride (cryst.)	279.0		
Calcium hydroxide	0.185		0.077
Calcium oxalate		0.0014 at 95 °C	
Cholesterol		Only slightly soluble	
Citric acid	130.0	116 °C at 25 °C	
Copper hydroxide		Insoluble in water	
Copper oxide		Insoluble in water	
Cupric sulphate	31.6		203.3
Cuprous sulphate		Decomposes in water	
Ferric ammonium sulphate		124 at 25 °C	
Ferric chloride	74.4		535.7
Ferric oxide		Insoluble in water	
Lithium carbonate		1.33 at 20 °C	0.72
Magnesium carbonate		Only slightly soluble	
Magnesium sulphate		71.0 at 20 °C	
Mercuric chloride		6.9 at 20 °C	61.3
Naphthalene		Insoluble in water	
Osmium tetroxide		6.23 at 25 °C	
Oxalic acid		9.5 at 15 °C	
Phenol		6.7 at 16 °C	
Phloroglucinol		Only slightly soluble	
Phosphorus pentoxide		Decomposes in water	
Picric acid		1.4 at 20 °C	
Potassium acetate		253 at 20 °C	
Potassium carbonate		112 at 20 °C	156
Potassium chloride		34.7 at 20 °C	56.7
Potassium chromate		62.9 at 20 °C	79.2
Potassium dichromate	4.9		102
Potassium hydroxide		107 at 15 °C	178
Potassium iodide	127.5		208
Potassium metabisulphite		Only slightly soluble	
Potassium nitrate		31.6 at 20 °C	247
Potassium nitrite		313 at 25 °C	413
Potassium oxalate		33 at 16 °C	
Potassium permanganate		6.33 at 20 °C	
		25.0 at 65 °C	
Silver nitrate	122.0		
Sodium acetate	76.2		
Sodium carbonate	7.1		45.5
Sodium chloride	35.7		39.12
Sodium citrate		92.6 at 25 °C	250.0
Sodium hydroxide	42.0		347.0
Sodium nitrate	73.0		180.0
Sodium nitrite		83.3 at 15 °C	
Sodium oxalate		3.7 at 20 °C	6.33
Sodium thiosulphate	79.4	291.1 at 45 °C	
Zinc hydroxide		Insoluble in water	
Zinc sulphate		86.5 at 80 °C	

Some elements and their symbols

Element	Symbol	Atomic no.	Molecular weight
Aluminium*	Al	13	26.9815
Arsenic	As	33	74.9216
Barium*	Ba	56	137.34
Bromine	Br	35	79.909
Calcium*	Ca	20	40.08
Carbon	C	6	12.01115
Chlorine	Cl	17	35.453
Chromium*	Cr	24	51.996
Copper (Cuprum)*	Cu	29	63.54
Gold (Aurium)*	Au	79	196.967
Hydrogen	H	1	1.00797
Iodine	I	53	126.9044
Iron (Ferrum)*	Fe	26	55.847
Lead (Plumbarr)*	Pb	82	207.19
Lithium*	Li	3	6.939
Magnesium*	Mg	12	24.312
Manganese*	Mn	25	54.9380
Mercury (Hydrargyrum)*	Hg	80	200.59
Nitrogen	N	7	14.0067
Oxygen	O	8	15.9994
Phosphorus	P	15	30.9738
Potassium (Kallium)*	K	19	39.102
Silicon	Si	14	28.086
Silver (Argentum)*	Ag	47	107.870
Sodium (Natrium)*	Na	11	22.9898
Sulphur	S	16	32.064
Tin (Stannum)*	Sn	50	118.69
Tungsten (Wolfram)*	W	74	183.85
Uranium*	U	92	283.03
Zinc*	Zn	30	65.37

Note: The atomic weights are taken from *International Atomic Weights*, 1961. The metallic elements are marked with an asterisk.

Index